Heat packs, neck
Standard terry cover
Neck terry cover
Fluorimethane
Cold spray
Ice bags
Ice bags, Cramer
Kwik-heat pack
Cramer Atomic Rub Down
Flexi-wrap (small, large)
Flexi-wrap handles
Lotion, 1 gal

First Aid
Cotton rolls (nose plugs)
Tongue depressors
Pocket masks
Cotton tip applicators
Cotton tip applicators (sterile)
Sani Cloths
Latex gloves (medium, large)
Cotton balls
Skin-preps
Save-A-Tooth
Penlights
Biohazard bags
Safety goggles

Taping Accessories
Heel and lace pads
Tape adherent spray
Tape remover

Sharps
Stainless steel prep blades
Scalpel blades, #10, #11 (sterile)
Scissors bandage
Scissors, small

Tweezers
Tweezers (sterile)
Suture sets
Nail clippers (large, small)
Tape cutters
Stethoscopes
Shark refill blades

Inhalants
Afrin

Antiseptics
Triadine
Peroxide
Rubbing alcohol
Betasept, small bottles
Betasept, 1-gal jug
Antimicrobial skin cleaner
Super Quin 9
Zorbicide Spray

Skin Treatments
Polysporin
Bacitracin
1% tolnaftate powder
Lamisil
1% hydrocortisone
Second skin
Collodion
2% miconazole
10% hydrocortisone
Baby powder
Tincture of benzoin

Eye Treatment
Dacriose Irrigation
Saline
Eye wash

ReNu contact cleaning agent
Penlights

Teeth Treatment
Blue mouth guards, 25/box
Clear mouth guards, 25/box

Oral Medications
Acetaminophen bottle
Acetaminophen, 2 pk
Cepastat
Chlorpheniramine, 4 mg
Diphenhydramine, 25 mg
Ibuprofen bottle
Ibuprofen, 2 pk
Imodium AD
Pepto-Bismol tabs
Q-fed pkg
Sudodrin, 2 pk
Titralac
Robitussin DM

Crutches
Large
Medium
Small
Large aluminum

Water
Bottle carriers
Water bottles
Coolers (3-, 7-, 10-gal)
Chest

Other
Stools
Spray bottles
Bucket
Cloth towels

Principles of

ATHLETIC TRAINING

A Competency-Based Approach

FIFTEENTH EDITION

William E. Prentice, PhD, ATC, PT, FNATA

Professor, Coordinator of Sports Medicine Program
Department of Exercise and Sport Science
The University of North Carolina at Chapel Hill
Chapel Hill, North Carolina

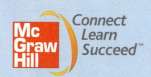

McGraw Hill

Connect
Learn
Succeed™

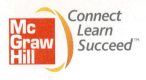

PRINCIPLES OF ATHLETIC TRAINING: A COMPETENCY-BASED APPROACH, FIFTEENTH EDITION

Published by McGraw-Hill, a business unit of The McGraw-Hill Companies, Inc., 1221 Avenue of the Americas, New York, NY 10020. Copyright © 2014 by The McGraw-Hill Companies, Inc. All rights reserved. Printed in the United States of America. Previous editions © 2011, 2009 and 2006. No part of this publication may be reproduced or distributed in any form or by any means, or stored in a database or retrieval system, without the prior written consent of The McGraw-Hill Companies, Inc., including, but not limited to, in any network or other electronic storage or transmission, or broadcast for distance learning.

Some ancillaries, including electronic and print components, may not be available to customers outside the United States.

This book is printed on acid-free paper.

6 7 8 9 DOW 21 20 19 18 17 16

ISBN 978-0-07-802264-7
MHID 0-07-802264-9

Senior Vice President, Products & Markets: *Kurt L. Strand*
Vice President, General Manager, Products & Markets: *Michael Ryan*
Vice President, Content Production & Technology Services: *Kimberly Meriwether David*
Managing Director: *Gina Boedeker*
Senior Brand Manager: *Bill Minick*
Executive Director of Development: *Lisa Pinto*
Managing Development Editor: *Sara Jaeger*
Developmental Editor: *Gary O'Brien*
Marketing Specialist: *Alexandra Schultz*
Editorial Coordinator: *Adina Lonn*
Director, Content Production: *Terri Schiesel*
Project Manager: *Erin Melloy*
Cover Designer: *Studio Montage, St. Louis, MO*
Cover Image: *© Adam Gault/Getty Images/RF*
Buyer: *Laura Fuller*
Media Project Manager: *Sridevi Palani*
Compositor: *MPS Limited*
Typeface: *10/12 Meridian Roman*
Printer: *R.R. Donnelley*

All credits appearing on page or at the end of the book are considered to be an extension of the copyright page.

Library of Congress Cataloging-in-Publication Data

Prentice, William E.
    Principles of athletic training : a competency-based
approach / William E. Prentice, PhD, ATC, PT, FNATA, professor, coordinator of Sports Medicine
Program, Department of Exercise and Sport Science, the University of North
Carolina Chapel Hill, North Carolina. — Fifteenth edition.
        pages cm
    Includes bibliographical references and index.
    ISBN 978-0-07-802264-7 (alk. paper)—ISBN 0-07-802264-9 (alk. paper)
        1. Athletic trainers.   2. Physical education and training.   I. Title.

RC1210.A75 2013
617.1'027—dc23   2012036184

Brief Contents

Contents

PART VI

General Medical Conditions   805

Appendixes

Preface

PHILOSOPHY

The publication of this fifteenth edition marks the 50-year anniversary for this text! Since the first edition was published in 1963, the profession of athletic training has experienced amazing growth, not only in numbers but also in the associated body of knowledge. During those years, the authors of this text have taken it as a personal responsibility to provide the reader with the most current evidence-based and clinically based information available in athletic training and sports medicine. This text has always been considered by many as the leading text in this field.

Dr. Daniel Arnheim, the original and long term author of this text established it's initial philosophy which continues with this edition. The text is designed to lead the student from general foundations to specific concepts relative to injury prevention, evaluation, management, and rehabilitation. As the student progresses from beginning to end, he or she will gradually begin to understand the complexities of the profession of athletic training. As in past editions, a major premise is that the student should be able to apply the appropriate techniques and concepts in the day-to-day performance of his or her job. The changes and additions in this fifteenth edition are a reflection of my commitment and passion toward continuing Dr. Arnheim's tradition.

THE ATHLETIC TRAINER AS A HEALTH CARE PROVIDER

Over the years since the origins of the athletic training profession in the 1930s, the majority of athletic trainers have been employed at colleges and universities, and in secondary schools, providing services almost exclusively to an athletic population. Historically, this work environment has been referred to as the "traditional setting" for employment for athletic trainers.

During the past decade, the role of the athletic trainer has gradually evolved into one that is unquestionably more aligned with that of a health care provider. Today, more than 40% of certified athletic trainers are employed in clinics and hospitals or in industrial and occupational settings, working under the direction of a physician as physician extenders. Although many athletic trainers continue to work in colleges, universities, and secondary schools, others can be found working as health care providers in all kinds of professional sports, including rodeo and NASCAR; in performing arts and the entertainment industry; in medical equipment sales and support; in the military; with law enforcement departments; and with government agencies, including NASA, the U.S. Senate, and the Pentagon.

This expansion of potential employment settings has forced the profession not only to change the methods by which health care is delivered to a variety of patient populations but also to change athletic training education programs to teach and/or establish professional competencies and proficiencies that are universal to all settings.

Depending on the employment settings in which they work, athletic trainers no longer provide health care only to athletes, nor do they only provide health care to individuals who are injured as a result of physical activity. Thus, the athletic trainer is more closely aligned with other allied health professionals, and athletic training has gained recognition as a clinical health care profession.

ADDRESSING THE ATHLETIC TRAINING EDUCATIONAL COMPETENCIES

The Professional Education Council (PEC) established by the National Athletic Trainers' Association, is responsible for identifying the knowledge and skills that must be included in educational programs preparing students to enter the athletic training profession. The PEC developed a list of educational competencies according to eight domains that comprise the role of the athletic trainer. The athletic training educational programs that are accredited by the Committee for Accreditation of Athletic Training Education (CAATE), as well as those seeking accreditation, must integrate the extensive list of educational competencies into their curriculums. This move toward competency-based athletic training education programs enhanced the need for a comprehensive text for athletic training students. My goal in this fifteenth edition is to make certain that each and every one of the educational competencies identified by the Professional Education Council is specifically covered at some point in this text.

WHO IS IT WRITTEN FOR?

Principles of Athletic Training: A Competency-Based Approach should be used by athletic trainers in courses concerned with the scientific, evidence-based, and clinical foundations of athletic training and sports medicine. Practicing athletic trainers, physical therapists, and other health care professionals involved with physically active individuals will also find this text valuable.

CONTENT ORGANIZATION

The 29 chapters in the fifteenth edition are organized into six sections: Professional Development and Responsibilities, Risk Management, Pathology of Sports Injury, Management Skills, Musculoskeletal Conditions, and General Medical Conditions.

As in previous editions, developing the fifteenth edition included serious consideration and incorporation of suggestions made by students, as well as detailed feedback from reviewers and other respected authorities in the field. Consequently, this fifteenth edition reflects the major dynamic trends in the field of athletic training and sports medicine. Furthermore, it is my hope that this newest edition will help prepare students to become competent health care professionals who will continue to enhance the ongoing advancement of the athletic training profession.

In addition to the inclusion of material that addresses specific competencies, this newest edition continues to undergo changes in content. The changes and additions are reflective of the ever-increasing body of knowledge that is expanding the scope of practice for the athletic trainer.

Throughout the text, information relevant to athletic trainers working in a variety of employment settings is included. As is the case for those working in secondary schools and colleges or universities, athletic trainers working in clinical, hospital, corporate, or industrial settings must be competent in preventing and recognizing injuries, and supervising injury rehabilitation programs. However, staff athletic trainers working in these settings treat and rehabilitate a wider range of patients both in terms of age and physical condition. The athletic trainer may provide care to pediatric, adolescent, young adult, adult, and geriatric patients. Patients may have physical ailments that may or may not be related to physical activity.

WHAT IS NEW IN THIS EDITION?

This latest edition of *Principles of Athletic Training: A Competency-Based Approach* continues to evolve in concert with the profession. Historically, the authors have tried diligently to stay on the cutting edge of the athletic training profession with regard not only to presenting a comprehensive and ever expanding body of knowledge but also with the latest techniques of delivering educational content to students. Most evident in this edition is the addition of photos showing pertinent surface anatomy landmarks and specific joint motions, as well as 3D photos showing primarily mechanisms of injury for a variety of conditions. In addition to the hard copy of this text, the author has created an online library of approximately 1300 instructional videos that clearly demonstrate specific clinical techniques, injury evaluation skills, rehabilitative exercises, and manual therapy skills that are used by experienced athletic trainers. There is also an online eBook version of this text that will facilitate direct access to the instructional videos from within the body of the text.

Principles Connect was developed by Amanda Benson, PhD., ATC from Troy University, and Linda Bobo, PhD., ATC from Stephen F. Austin Slate University. *Connect* is a Web-based assignment and assessment platform that gives students the means to better connect with their coursework, their instructors, and the important concepts that they need to know for success now and in the future. Students can practice important skills at their own pace and on their own schedule, receive instant feedback on their work, and track performance on key activities. With *Connect*, students get 24/7 online access to an eBook—an online edition of the text—to aid them in successfully completing their work, wherever and whenever they choose. With *Connect,* instructors can deliver assignments, graphing questions, quizzes, and tests easily online.

CHAPTER-BY-CHAPTER ADDITIONS

Chapter 1

- Material on the responsibilities of the athletic trainer according to the five domains identified in the latest Role Delineation Study has been reorganized
- New extensive discussion of the new competency that deals with evidence-based medicine and how the clinician should incorporate that into clinical practice
- Updated discussion on professional education of the athletic training student and addressed the reorganization of the 12 competency areas to eight
- Updated discussion of future directions for the athletic training profession

Chapter 2

- New discussion and new Focus Box on what items should be included in a medical record

- New information on the transition from paper to electronic records
- New information on health maintenence and personal hygiene screening
- New discussion on sickle cell trait screening
- Additional information of the National High School Sports-Related Injury Surveillance Study

Chapter 3

- Updated the discussion of efforts to obtain third-party reimbursement of athletic trainers

Chapter 4

- Changed the title to "Fitness and Conditioning Techniques" to better reflect the material that is covered in this chapter

Chapter 5

- Additional information on Food Labels
- New discussion of ChooseMyPlate
- New information on the glycemic index and selecting foods with a high GI
- New information on caffeine energy drinks

Chapter 6

- New information and guidelines for measuring rectal temperature

Chapter 7

- New photos showing the newest types of equipment
- Updated information on mouthquards
- Updated information on using cleated shoes

Chapter 8

- Changed the terms *bandage* and *bandaging* to *wrap* and *wrapping*
- Repositioned figures and line drawings to be more closely aligned with text
-

Chapter 9

- Clarified distinction between tendinopathy and tendinitis
- Reorganized information on fractures

Chapter 10

- New information on prolotherapy
- New information on platelet-rich plasma (PRP) injections

Chapter 11

- New discussion of the cognitive appraisal model that better describes the athlete's psychological reaction to injury

Chapter 12

- Updated information on the latest American Red Cross techniques of CPR/AED
- New section on using airway adjunct devices, including manual suction, oropharyngeal airways, nasopharyngeal airways, and supraglottic airways
- Updated information on the recommended technique for placing an injured athlete on a spine board
- New section on using a cane

Chapter 13

- New information on the positron emission tomography imaging technique
- New information on pulse oximetry
- New information on using a glucometer
- New information on using a peak flow meter

Chapter 15

- Reorganized the way in which the therapeutic modalities are organized according to the types of energy they produce
- Clarified information on the Hunting Response
- Updated figure on types of waveforms

Chapter 17

- Updated list of agencies and regulations that govern pharmaceutical care
- Updated list of information that must be included on prescription labels
- Updated procedure for using a metered dose inhaler
- Updated information on currently used and recommended medications throughout
- New information on abuse of crystal methamphetamine, ecstasy, ADHD medication, and oxycontin
- Updated list of drugs banned by the NCAA and USADA

Chapters 18–25

- New photos in each of these chapters, showing (1) surface anatomy landmarks, (2) specific joint movements, and (3) 3-D photos to show mechanisms of injury for the most common injuries

Chapter 26

- Information on concussions extensively updated and reorganized to include the latest findings
- New information on the widely used Sport Concussion Assessment Toll
- New guidelines for graduated return to play following concussion

Chapter 27

- New photos showing surface anatomy landmarks and specific joint movements
- New information on traveler's diarrhea

Chapter 28

- New photos showing different types of wounds
- New photos that better show the skin appearance

Chapter 29

- Updated information on complex regional pain syndrome
- "Sexually transmitted infections (STIs)" changed to "sexually transmitted diseases (STDs)"

INSTRUCTOR'S RESOURCE MATERIALS

Connect Principles of Athletic Training

Connect Principles of Athletic Training developed by Dr. Amanda Andrews and Dr. Linda Stark-Bobo, is a new online learning system composed of interactive exercises and assessments, like those that appear on the new Board of Certification exam. Videos, animations, and other multimedia features enable students to visualize complicated concepts and practice skills. All of the activities are automatically graded and can be submitted to the instructor's grade book. For more information, visit www.mcgrawhillconnect.com.

Instructor's Resources

Formerly the Instructor's Manual, this guide includes all the useful features of an Instructor's Manual, including learning objectives, brief chapter overviews, key terminology, discussion questions, class activities, worksheets, and the accompanying answer keys, media resources, and Web links. It also integrates the text with image clips and all the health and human performance resources McGraw-Hill offers including the Online Learning Center, The guide also includes references to relevant print and broadcast media.

Test Bank

The test bank includes approximately 2,000 examination questions. Each chapter contains true-false, multiple choice, and completion test questions. The worksheets in each chapter also include a separate test bank of matching, short-answer, listing, essay, and personal or injury assessment questions that can be used as self-testing tools for students or as additional sources for examination questions.

Computerized Test Bank CD-ROM

McGraw-Hill's EZ Test is a flexible and easy-to-use electronic testing program. The program allows instructors to create tests from book specific items. It accommodates a wide range of question types and instructors may add their own questions. Multiple versions of the test can be created, and any test can be exported for use with course management systems such as WebCT, BlackBoard, or PageOut. The program is available for Windows and Macintosh environments.

PowerPoint Presentation

Developed for the fifteenth edition by Jason Scibek, PhD, ATC, of Duquense University, a comprehensive and extensively illustrated PowerPoint presentation accompanies this text for use in classroom discussion. The PowerPoint presentation may also be converted to outlines and given to students as a handout. You can easily download the PowerPoint presentation from the Online Learning Center at www.mhhe.com/prenticel5e. Adopters of the text can obtain the login and password to access this presentation by contacting your local McGraw-Hill sales representative.

Instructional Videos

Instructional videos are available on *Connect Principles of Athletic Training*. These visual aids are designed to illustrate key concepts, promote critical thinking, and engage students on the most relevant topics in athletic training.

ACKNOWLEDGMENTS

I would like to express my sincere appreciation to my Developmental Editor, Gary O'Brien who, as always, has provided invaluable guidance throughout the development of this edition. In truth, Gary should share authorship with me on this project. Through his efforts he has demonstrated ownership and a personal investment in making this text the best it can be. His input, patience with me, and dedication to this project has been indispensable and I truly respect his opinions and direction on all of our projects. I would be hard pressed to complete any of our projects without his help.

During the revision process for the fifteenth edition, we relied heavily on input solicited from our reviewers. My personal thanks are extended to:

Emily Webster
Central Michigan University

Katie Grove
Indiana University-Bloomington

Kristi White
Angelo State University

Gen Ludwig
Pacific Lutheran University

Marilyn Oliver
University of La Verne-La Verne

Mike Pribyl
Iowa Western Community College-Council Bluffs

I also wish to extend my sincere appreciation to our technical reviewers for their critique of selected chapters. Their input was most valuable to the completion of this edition.

Amy Sauls, PharmD
Director of the Pharmacy
Campus Health Services
The University of North Carolina at Chapel Hill

Jason Mihalik, PhD, ATC
Assistant Professor, Department of Exercise
  and Sport Science,
The University of North Carolina at Chapel Hill

Finally, I want to thank my wife Tena, and our sons, Brian and Zach, for their enduring support and encouragement. They constantly help me to keep my perspective on both my professional and personal life.

William E. Prentice

Applications at a Glance

PART I

Professional Development and Responsibilities

1

The Athletic Trainer as a Health Care Provider

■ Objectives

When you finish this chapter you should be able to

- Recognize the historical foundations of athletic training.
- Identify the various professional organizations dedicated to athletic training and sports medicine.
- Identify various employment settings for the athletic trainer.
- Differentiate the roles and responsibilities of the athletic trainer, the team physician, and the coach.

- Define evidence-based practice as it relates to the clinical practice of athletic training.
- Explain the function of support personnel in sports medicine.
- Discuss certification and licensure for the athletic trainer.

■ Outline

■ Key Terms

patient
athletic training clinic
evidence-based practice

PICO
ATC

Athletic trainers are health care professionals who specialize in preventing, recognizing, managing, and rehabilitating injuries. In cooperation with physicians, other allied health personnel, administrators, coaches, and parents, the athletic trainer functions as an integral member of the health care team in clinics, secondary schools, colleges and universities, professional sports programs, and other athletic health care settings. As you will see throughout the course of this text, athletic trainers provide a critical link between the medical community and individuals who participate in all types of physical activity (Figure 1–1).

> The certified athletic trainer is a highly educated and skilled professional specializing in health care for the physically active.

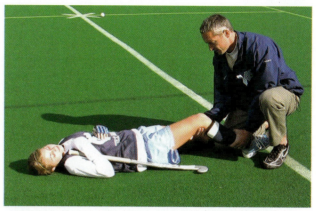

FIGURE I–I   The field of athletic training provides a critical link between the medical community and the physically active individual.

HISTORICAL PERSPECTIVES

Early History

The drive to compete was important in many early societies. Sports developed over a period of time as a means of competing in a relatively peaceful and nonharmful way. Early civilizations show little evidence of highly organized sports. Evidence indicates that in Greek and Roman civilizations there were coaches, trainers (people who helped the athlete reach top physical condition), and physicians (such as Hippocrates and Galen) who assisted the athlete in reaching optimum performance. Many of the roles that emerged during this early period are the same in modern sports.

> The history of athletic training draws on the disciplines of exercise, medicine, physical therapy, physical education, and sports.

For many centuries after the fall of the Roman Empire, there was a complete lack of interest in sports activities. Not until the beginning of the Renaissance did these activities slowly gain popularity. Athletic training as we know it came into existence during the late nineteenth century with the firm establishment of intercollegiate and interscholastic

athletes in the United States. Because the first athletic trainers of this era possessed no technical knowledge, their athletic training techniques usually consisted of a rub, the application of some type of counterirritant, and occasionally the prescription of various home remedies and poultices. It has taken many years for the athletic trainer to attain the status of a well-qualified allied health care professional.[64]

Evolution of the Contemporary Athletic Trainer

The terms *training* and *athletic training, trainer,* and *athletic trainer* are often used interchangeably and are frequently confused with one another. Historically, *training* implies the act of coaching or teaching. In comparison, athletic training has traditionally been known as the field that is concerned with the athlete's health and safety. A trainer is someone who trains dogs or horses or functions in coaching or teaching areas. The *certified athletic trainer* is one who is a specialist in athletic training. Athletic training has evolved over the years to play a major role in the health care of a variety of patient populations in general and the athlete in particular. This evolution

> A certified athletic trainer provides health care to physically active individuals.

occurred rapidly after World War I with the appearance of the athletic trainer in intercollegiate athletics. During this period, the major influence in developing the athletic trainer as a specialist in preventing and managing athletic injuries came from the work of S. E. Bilik, a physician who wrote the first major text on athletic training and the care of athletic injuries, called *The Trainer's Bible,* in 1917.[8]

In the early 1920s, the Cramer family in Gardner, Kansas, started a chemical company and began producing a liniment to treat ankle sprains. Over the years, the Cramers realized that there was a market for products to treat injured athletes. In an effort to enhance communication and facilitate an exchange of ideas among coaches, athletic trainers, and athletes, Cramer began publication of *First Aider* in 1932. The members of this family were instrumental in the early development of the athletic training profession and have always played a prominent role in the education of student athletic trainers.[65]

During the late 1930s, an effort was made, primarily by several college and university athletic trainers, to establish a national organization named the National Athletic Trainers' Association (NATA). After struggling for existence from 1938 to 1944, the association essentially disappeared during the difficult years of World War II.

Between 1947 and 1950, university athletic trainers once again began to organize themselves into separate regional conferences, which would later become district organizations within NATA. In 1950, some 101 athletic trainers from the various conferences met in Kansas City, Missouri, and officially formed the National Athletic Trainers' Association. The primary purpose for its formation was to establish professional standards for the athletic trainer.[65] Since NATA was formed in 1950, many individuals have made contributions to the development of the profession.

After 1950, the growth of the athletic training profession has been remarkable. In 1974, when NATA membership numbers were first tracked, there were 4,500 members. Today those numbers have grown to more than 34,000 members. Certified athletic trainers can be found internationally with more than 400 working in twenty-five countries outside the United States. The majority of these are in Japan and Canada.[19] As the athletic training profession has grown and evolved over the last 50 years, many positive milestones have occurred that have collectively shaped the future direction of the profession, including the establishment of a certification exam; recognition of athletic trainers as health care providers; increased diversity of practice settings; the passage of practice acts that regulate athletic trainers in most states; third-party reimbursement for athletic training services; and ongoing reevaluation, revision, and reform of athletic training educational programs.

The Changing Face of the Athletic Training Profession

Over the years since the origins of the athletic training profession in the 1930s, the majority of athletic trainers have been employed at colleges and universities and in secondary schools, providing services almost exclusively to an athletic population. Historically, this work environment has been referred to as the "traditional setting" for employment for athletic trainers.

During the past decade, the role of the athletic trainer has gradually evolved into one that is unquestionably more aligned with that of a health care provider. Today more than 40 percent of certified athletic trainers are employed in clinics and hospitals, or in industrial and occupational settings working under the direction of a physician as physician extenders. Although many athletic trainers continue to work in colleges, universities, and secondary schools, others can be found working as health care providers in all kinds of professional sports, including rodeo and NASCAR; in industrial settings; in performing arts and the entertainment industry; in medical equipment sales and support; in the military; with law enforcement departments; and with government agencies, including NASA, the U.S. Senate, and the Pentagon.

This expansion of potential employment settings has forced the profession not only to change the methods by which health care is delivered to a variety of patient populations but also to change athletic training education programs to teach and/or establish professional competencies and proficiencies that are universal to all settings.

Depending on the employment settings in which they work, athletic trainers no longer provide health care only to athletes, nor do they provide health care only to individuals who are injured as a result of physical activity. Additionally, the desire to align the athletic trainer more closely with other allied health professionals and to establish athletic training as a clinical health care profession has necessitated changes in terminology that has been "traditionally" accepted as appropriate.

Certainly, athletic trainers continue to work with athletes. It has been suggested that a more appropriate term to use when treating an athlete who sustains an injury is **patient** or *client.* Thus, throughout this text the term *athlete* is used to refer to a physically active individual who participates in recreational or organized sport activities who is not currently injured. Any

patient Ill or injured athlete.

individual who is ill or injured who is being treated by an athletic trainer is referred to as a *patient.*

It has also been recommended that instead of referring to treating athletes in the athletic training room, it is more appropriate to refer to treating patients in the athletic training clinic or facility. Thus, the term **athletic training clinic** is used to refer to a health care facility for treating individuals who have an illness or injury.

> **athletic training clinic** Health care facility.

SPORTS MEDICINE AND ATHLETIC TRAINING

The Field of Sports Medicine

The term *sports medicine* refers generically to a broad field of health care related to physical activity and sport. The field of sports medicine encompasses a number of more specialized aspects of dealing with the physically active or athletic populations that may be classified as relating either to performance enhancement or to injury care and management (Figure 1–2). Those areas of specialization that are primarily concerned with performance enhancement include exercise physiology, biomechanics, sport psychology, sports nutrition, strength and conditioning coaches, and personal fitness training. Areas of specialization that focus more on injury care and management specific to the athlete are the practice of medicine, athletic training, sports physical therapy, sports massage therapy, sports dentistry, osteopathic medicine, orthotics/prosthetics,

> Athletic training must be considered a specialization under the broad field of sports medicine.

chiropractic, podiatry, and emergency medical technology. The American College of Sports Medicine (ACSM) has defined sports medicine as multidisciplinary, including the physiological, biomechanical, psychological, and pathological phenomena associated with exercise and sports.[3] The clinical application of the work of these disciplines is performed to improve and maintain an individual's functional capacities for physical labor, exercise, and sports. Sports medicine also includes the prevention and treatment of diseases and injuries related to exercise and sports.

Growth of Professional Sports Medicine Organizations

The twentieth century brought with it the development of a number of professional organizations dedicated to athletic training and sports medicine. Professional organizations have many goals: (1) to upgrade the field by devising and maintaining a set of professional standards, including a code of ethics; (2) to bring together professionally competent individuals to exchange ideas, stimulate research, and promote critical thinking; and (3) to give individuals an opportunity to work as a group with a singleness of purpose, thereby making it possible for them to achieve objectives that, separately, they could not accomplish. The organizations identified below are presented in chronological order according to their year of establishment. Addresses, phone numbers, and/or Web sites for these and other related sports medicine organizations can be found in Appendix A in the back of this text or at www.mhhe.com/prentice15e.

> Many professional organizations that are dedicated to achieving health and safety in sports developed in the twentieth century.

Several of these professional organizations also disseminate information to the general public about safe participation in sport activities in the form of guidelines or position statements. Appendix B provides a complete listing of all position, consensus, official, and support statements developed by or with support from the National Athletic Trainers Association. Also listed in this appendix are specific Web sites where these statements may be found. Links to these statements can also be located at www.mhhe.com/prentice15e.

International Federation of Sports Medicine Among the first major organizations was the Federation Internationale de Medecine Sportive (FIMS). In English it is called the International Federation of Sports Medicine. It was created in 1928 at the Olympic Winter Games in St. Moritz, Switzerland, by Olympic medical doctors with the principal purpose of promoting the study and

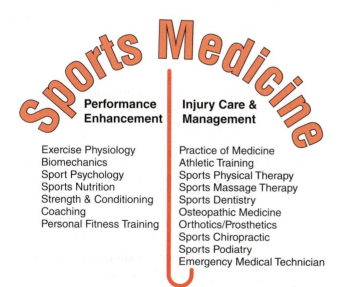

Sports Medicine

Performance Enhancement	Injury Care & Management
Exercise Physiology	Practice of Medicine
Biomechanics	Athletic Training
Sport Psychology	Sports Physical Therapy
Sports Nutrition	Sports Massage Therapy
Strength & Conditioning	Sports Dentistry
Coaching	Osteopathic Medicine
Personal Fitness Training	Orthotics/Prosthetics
	Sports Chiropractic
	Sports Podiatry
	Emergency Medical Technician

FIGURE I–2   Areas of specialization under the sports medicine "umbrella."

development of sports medicine throughout the world. FIMS is made up of the national sports medicine associations of more than 100 countries. This organization includes many disciplines that are concerned with the physically active individual. To some degree, the ACSM has patterned itself after this organization.

American Academy of Family Physicians The American Academy of Family Physicians (AAFP) was founded in 1947 to promote and maintain high-quality standards for family doctors who are providing continuing comprehensive health care to the public. AAFP is a medical association of more than 100,000 members. Many team physicians are members of this organization. It publishes *American Family Physician*.

National Athletic Trainers' Association Before the formation of the National Athletic Trainers' Association in 1950, athletic trainers occupied a somewhat insecure place in the athletic program. Since that time, as a result of the raising of professional standards and the establishment of a code of ethics, there has been considerable professional advancement. The stated mission of NATA is

> To enhance the quality of health care provided by certified athletic trainers and to advance the athletic training profession.

The association accepts as members only those athletic trainers who are properly qualified and who are prepared to subscribe to a code of ethics and to uphold the standards of the association. NATA currently has more than 34,000 members. It publishes a quarterly journal, *The Journal of Athletic Training*, and *Athletic Training Journal* on-line, and holds an annual convention at which members have an opportunity to keep abreast of new developments and to exchange ideas through clinical programs. The organization is constantly working to improve both the quality and the status of athletic training.

American College of Sports Medicine As discussed previously, the ACSM is interested in the study of all aspects of sports. Established in 1954, ACSM has a membership of more than 45,000, composed of medical doctors, doctors of philosophy, physical educators, athletic trainers, coaches, exercise physiologists, biomechanists, and others interested in sports. The organization holds national and regional conferences and meetings devoted to exploring the many aspects of sports medicine, and it publishes a quarterly magazine, *Medicine and Science in Sports and Exercise*. This journal includes articles in French, Italian, German, and English, and provides complete translations in English of all articles. It reports recent developments in the field of sports medicine on a worldwide basis.

American Orthopaedic Society for Sports Medicine The American Orthopaedic Society for Sports Medicine (AOSSM) was created in 1972 to encourage and support scientific research in orthopedic sports medicine; the organization works to develop methods for safer, more productive, and more enjoyable fitness programs and sports participation. Through programs developed by the AOSSM, members receive specialized training in sports medicine, surgical procedures, injury prevention, and rehabilitation. AOSSM's 3,000 members are orthopedic surgeons and allied health professionals committed to excellence in sports medicine. Its official bimonthly publication is the *American Journal of Sports Medicine*.

National Strength and Conditioning Association The National Strength and Conditioning Association (NSCA) was formed in 1978 to facilitate a professional exchange of ideas in strength development as it relates to the improvement of athletic performance and fitness and to enhance, enlighten, and advance the field of strength and conditioning.

NSCA has a membership of more than 30,000 professionals in 52 countries, including strength and conditioning coaches, personal trainers, exercise physiologists, athletic trainers, researchers, educators, sport coaches, physical therapists, business owners, exercise instructors, fitness directors, and students training to enter the field. In addition, the NSCA Certification Commission offers two of the finest and the only nationally accredited certification programs: the Certified Strength and Conditioning Specialist (CSCS) and the NSCA Certified Personal Trainer (NSCA-CPT). NSCA publishes both the *Journal of Strength and Conditioning Research* and *Strength and Conditioning*.

American Academy of Pediatrics, Sports Committee The American Academy of Pediatrics, Sports Committee was organized in 1979. Its primary goal is to educate all physicians, especially pediatricians, about the special needs of children who participate in sports. Between 1979 and 1983, this committee developed guidelines that were incorporated into a report, *Sports Medicine: Health Care for Young Athletes*, edited by Nathan J. Smith, M.D.

American Physical Therapy Association, Sports Physical Therapy Section In 1981, the Sports Physical Therapy Section of the American Physical Therapy Association (APTA) was officially established. The mission of the Sports Physical Therapy Section is "to provide a forum to establish collegial relations between physical therapists, physical therapist assistants, and physical therapy students interested in sports physical therapy." The Section and its 6,000 members promote the prevention, recognition, treatment, and rehabilitation of injuries in an athletic and physically active population; provide educational opportunities through sponsorship of continuing education programs and publications; promote the role of the sports physical therapist to other health professionals; and support research to further establish the scientific basis for sports physical therapy. The Section's official journal is the *Journal of Orthopaedic and Sports Physical Therapy*.

NCAA Committee on Competitive Safeguards and Medical Aspects of Sports The National Collegiate Athletic Association (NCAA) Committee on Competitive Safeguards and Medical Aspects of Sports collects and develops pertinent information about desirable training methods, prevention and treatment of sports injuries, utilization of sound safety measures at the college level, drug education, and drug testing; disseminates information and adopts recommended policies and guidelines designed to further the objectives just listed; and supervises drug-education and drug-testing programs. This committee publishes the *Sports Medicine Handbook* that contains a wealth of information related to sports medicine, that can be very useful to the athletic trainer.

National Academy of Sports Medicine The National Academy of Sports Medicine (NASM) was founded in 1987 by physicians, physical therapists, and fitness professionals; it focuses on the development, refinement, and implementation of educational programs for fitness, performance, and sports medicine professionals. According to its mission statement, "NASM is dedicated to transforming lives and revolutionizing the health and fitness industry through its unwavering commitment to deliver innovative education, solutions and tools that produce remarkable results." In addition to offering a fitness certification (Certified Personal Trainer) and performance certification (Performance Enhancement Specialist), NASM offers advanced credentials and more than 20 continuing education courses in a variety of disciplines. NASM serves more than 100,000 members and partners in 80 countries.

Other Health-Related Organizations Many other health-related professions, such as dentistry, podiatristry, and chiropractic, have, over the years, become interested in the health and safety aspects of sports. Besides national organizations that are interested in athletic health and safety, there are state and local associations that are extensions of the larger bodies. National, state, and local sports organizations have all provided extensive support to the reduction of illness and injury risk to the athlete.

Other Sports Medicine Journals Other journals that provide an excellent service to the field of athletic

training and sports medicine are *The International Journal of Sports Medicine*, which is published in English by Thieme-Stratton, Inc., New York; *The Journal of Sports Medicine and Physical Fitness*, published by Edizioni Minerva Medica SPA, ADIS Press Ltd., Auckland 10, New Zealand; the *Journal of Sport Rehabilitation* and *Athletic Therapy and Training*, both published by Human Kinetics Publishers, Inc., Champaign, Illinois; the *Physician and Sportsmedicine*, published by McGraw-Hill, Inc., New York; *Physical Therapy* and *Clinical Management*, both published by the American Physical Therapy Association, Fairfax, Virginia; *Physical Medicine and Rehabilitation Clinics* and *Clinics in Sports Medicine*, both published by W. B. Saunders, Philadelphia; *Training and Conditioning*, published by MAG, Inc., Ithaca, New York; *Sports Health*: *A Multidisciplinary Approach*, published by Sage in Thousand Oaks, California; and *Athletic Training and Sports Health Care*: *The Journal for the Practicing Clinician*, published by Slack Inc., in Thorofare, New Jersey.

There is a significant number of other journals that relate in some way to sports medicine. They are listed in Appendix C located at the end of this text.

EMPLOYMENT SETTINGS FOR THE ATHLETIC TRAINER

Opportunities for employment as an athletic trainer have changed dramatically in recent years. Athletic trainers no longer work only in athletic training clinics at the college, university, or secondary-school level. The employment opportunities for athletic trainers are more diverse than ever.[42] A discussion of the various employment settings follows (Table 1–1).

Clinics and Hospitals

Today, more than 40 percent of certified athletic trainers are employed in clinics and hospitals— more than in any other employment setting. The role of the athletic trainer varies from one clinic to the next. Athletic trainers may be employed in an outpatient ambulatory rehabilitation clinic working in general patient care; as health, wellness, or performance enhancement specialists; or as clinic administrators. Their job may also involve ergonomic assessment, work hardening, CPR training, or occasionally overseeing drug-testing programs. They may also be employed by a hospital but work in a clinic. Other clinical athletic trainers see patients during the morning hours in the clinic. In the afternoons, athletic trainers' services are contracted out to local high schools or small colleges for practice, game, or single event

> The largest percentage of certified athletic trainers are employed in clinics and hospitals.

TABLE 1–1 **Employment Settings for Athletic Trainers***

Clinic

- Hospital-based (employed by hospital; work in a clinic)
  - General patient care
  - Health/wellness/performance enhancement
  - Occupational/industrial (100%/split)
  - Administration
- Outpatient/ambulatory/rehabilitation clinic
  - General patient care
  - Health/wellness/performance enhancement
  - Occupational/industrial (100%/split)
  - Administration
- Physician-owned clinic (patient care or administration)
  - Orthopedic
  - Pediatric
  - Primary care
  - Physiatry
  - Family practice
  - Other
- Secondary school/clinic (employed by clinic; work in school)
  - Secondary school (100%)
  - Secondary school (split)
- Clinic, other

Hospital (work in a hospital but not in a hospital-based clinic)

- Administration
- Orthopedics
- Emergency department
- Other

Industrial/occupational (work on-site at an industrial or occupational facility)

- Clinic
- Ergonomics
- Health/wellness/fitness
- Other

Corporate (work for company that sells to the profession or in patient care for that company)

- Business/sales/marketing
- Ergonomics
- Health/wellness/fitness
- Patient care

College/university

- Professional staff/athletics/clinic
- Faculty/academic/research
- Split appointment
  - Division 1
  - Division 1AA
  - Division 2
  - Division 3
- Administration

Two-year institution

- Professional staff/athletics/clinic
- Faculty/academic/research
- Split appointment
- Administration

Secondary school (employed by school or district)

- High school (teacher/clinical/split)
  - Public
  - Private
- Middle school (teacher/clinical/split)
  - Public
  - Private

Professional sports

- Baseball, M
- Basketball, M/W
- Football, M
- Hockey, M
- Soccer, M/W
- Lacrosse, M
- Softball, W
- Golf, M/W
- Tennis, M/W
- Wrestling
- Boxing
- Rodeo
- Auto racing (NASCAR, Indy Car)

Amateur/recreational/youth sports

- Amateur (work for NGB, USOC, or amateur athletics)
- Recreational (work for municipal or recreational league or facility)
- Youth sports (AAU)

Performing arts

- Dance
- Theater
- Entertainment industry (Disney, casinos, tour bands)

Military/law enforcement/government

- Military (Air Force, Army, Navy, Marines, Coast Guard, Merchant Marines, National Guard)
  - Active duty/civilian
- Academy
- Hospital/clinic
- Administration
- Other
- Law enforcement
  - Local department or agency (police/fire/rescue)
  - State department or agency (police/investigation)
  - Federal department or agency (FBI, CIA, ATF)
- Government
  - Local
  - State
  - Federal (Senate, House, judicial)
  - Agencies (NASA, FDA)

Health/fitness/sports/performance enhancement clinics/clubs (work for franchise, chain, or independent club)

Independent contractor (work for themselves and are not employees)

*Modified from National Athletic Trainers' Association.

coverage. For the most part, private clinics have well-equipped facilities in which to work. In many sports medicine clinics, the athletic trainer may be responsible for formulating a plan to market or promote athletic training services offered by that clinic throughout the local community[27] (Figure 1–3A).

Physician Extenders Some athletic trainers work in clinics that are owned by physicians. Although virtually all athletic trainers work under the direction of a physician, those employed as a physician extender actually work in the physician's office, where patients of all ages and backgrounds are being treated.[61] The educational preparation for athletic trainers allows them to function in a variety of domains, including injury prevention, evaluation, management and rehabilitation, health education, nutrition, training and conditioning, preparticipation physicals, and maintenance of essential documentation.[98] Although the contact with only the physically active population may not be as great as in other employment settings, the physician extender can expect regular hours, few weekend or evening responsibilities, opportunity for growth, and, in general, better pay.[23] All these factors collectively make physician extender positions attractive for the athletic trainer. Potentially, many new jobs can be created as physicians become more and more aware of the value that an athletic trainer, functioning as a physician extender, can provide to their medical practice[21] (Figure 1–3B).

Industrial/Occupational Settings

It is becoming relatively common for industries to employ athletic trainers to oversee fitness and injury rehabilitation programs for their employees.[1] The athletic trainer working in an industrial or occupational setting must have a sound understanding of the principles and concepts of workplace ergonomics, including inspecting, measuring, and observing dimensions of the work space, as well as specific tasks that are performed at the workstation.[20] Once a problem has been identified, the athletic trainer must be able to implement proper adjustments to workplace ergonomics to reduce or minimize possible risks for injury. In addition to these responsibilities, athletic trainers may be assigned to conduct wellness programs and provide education and individual counseling. It is likely that many job opportunities will exist for the athletic trainer in industrial/occupational settings in the next few years (Figure 1–3C&D).

Corporate Settings

Opportunities are expanding for athletic trainers to use their educational background as preparation for working in business, sales, or marketing of products that other athletic trainers may use. Athletic trainers might also be employed by a company to administer health, wellness, and fitness programs or to provide some patient care to their employees.

Colleges or Universities

At the college or university level, clinical positions for athletic trainers vary considerably from institution to institution. In smaller institutions, the athletic trainer may be a half-time teacher in physical education and half-time athletic trainer. In some cases, if the athletic trainer is a physical therapist rather than a teacher, he or she may spend part of the time in the school health center and part of the time in athletic training. Increasingly at the college level, athletic training services are being offered to members of the general student body who participate in intramural and club sports. In most colleges and universities, the athletic trainer is full-time, does not teach, works in the department of athletics, and is paid by the institution.

In February 1998, the NATA created the Task Force to Establish Appropriate Medical Coverage for Intercollegiate Athletics (AMCIA) to establish recommendations for the extent of appropriate medical coverage to provide the best possible health care for all intercollegiate student-athletes. Essentially, the AMCIA task force made recommendations for the number of athletic trainers who should be employed at a college or university based on a mathematical model created by a number of variables existing at each institution. These guidelines were revised and updated in 2003. (For directions to determine the recommended number of athletic trainers, consult "*NCAA Recommendations and Guidelines for Appropriate Medical Coverage for Intercollegiate Athletics*.")[63] (http://www.nata.org/sites/default/files/AMCIA-Revised-2010.pdf) or find a link at www.mhhe.com/prentice15e. In August 2003, the NCAA Committee on Competitive Safeguards and Medical Aspects of Sports (CSMAS) recommended that NCAA institutions "examine the adequacy of their sports medicine coverage"[50]—in particular, whether the increased time demands placed on certified athletic trainers reduces their ability to provide high-quality care to all student-athletes. After reviewing the *Recommendations and Guidelines*, the CSMAS "encouraged NCAA institutions to reference the NATA AMCIA in their assessment of the adequateness of their sports medicine coverage . . . and share the responsibility to protect student athlete health and safety through appropriate medical coverage of its sports and supporting activities." (See http://www.nata.org/sites/default/files/NCAASupportofATCs.pdf or find a link at www.mhhe.com/prentice15e).

A number of athletic trainers working at colleges and universities are employed as faculty

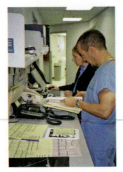

A: Clinics and Hospitals

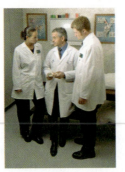

B: Physician Extenders

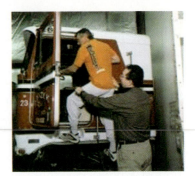

C: Industrial-Rehabilitation

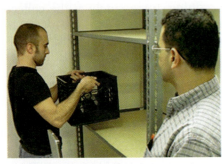

D: Work Hardening/Occupational

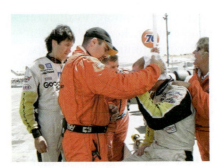

E: Professional Sports—NASCAR

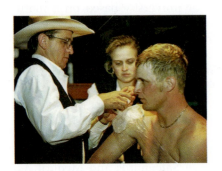

F: Professional/Sports—Rodeo

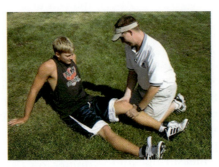

G: Youth Sports

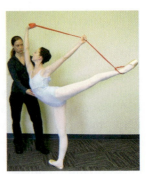

H: Performing Arts

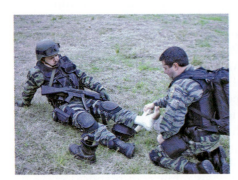

I: Military

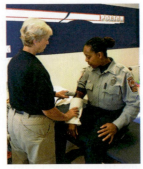

J: Law Enforcement

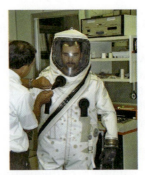

K: NASA

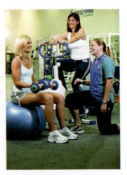

L: Health Clubs

FIGURE 1–3   Athletic trainers work in a variety of employment settings.

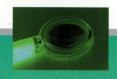

Full-time, on-site athletic trainer coverage for secondary-school athletic programs

"The National Athletic Trainers' Association, as a leader in health care for the physically active, believes that the prevention and treatment of injuries to student-athletes are a priority. The recognition and treatment of injuries to student-athletes must be immediate. The medical delivery system for injured student-athletes needs a coordinator within the local school community who will facilitate the prevention, recognition, treatment and reconditioning of sports related injuries. Therefore, it is the position of the National Athletic Trainers' Association that all secondary schools should provide the services of a full-time, on-site, certified athletic trainer (ATC) to student-athletes."

From NATA official statement *Full time, on-site athletic trainer coverage for secondary-school athletic programs* (2004) (http://www.nata.org/sites/default/files/SecondarySchool.pdf).

---

members.[36] These individuals may or may not be assigned clinical responsibilities. In addition to faculty responsibilities, it is most likely that these faculty members serve as program directors and/or as researchers.

Secondary Schools

There are more than 44,000 public and private secondary schools in the United States. It would be ideal to have certified athletic trainers serve every secondary school and middle school in the United States.[45] Many of the physical problems that occur later from improperly managed sports injuries could be avoided initially if proper care from an athletic trainer had been provided.[7] If a secondary school or middle school hires an athletic trainer, it is very often in a faculty–athletic trainer capacity.[68] This individual is usually employed as a teacher who carries a reduced teaching load and performs athletic training duties. In this instance, compensation usually is on the basis of both teaching, a stipend as an athletic trainer, or both.[37] Salaries for the secondary-school athletic trainer are continuing to improve.[5] Another means of obtaining secondary-school athletic training coverage is using a certified graduate student from a nearby college or university. The graduate student receives a graduate assistantship with a stipend paid by the secondary school or community college. In this situation, both the graduate student and the school benefit.[86] However, this practice may prevent a school from employing a certified athletic trainer on a full-time basis.

In 1995, the NATA adopted an official statement on hiring athletic trainers in secondary schools that appears in *Focus Box 1–1:* "Full-time, on-site athletic trainer coverage for secondary-school athletic programs." Based on a proposal from the American Academy of Pediatrics, in 1998 the American Medical Association adopted a policy calling for certified athletic trainers to be employed in all high-school athletic programs (see Appendix B). Although this policy was simply a recommendation and not a requirement, it was a very positive statement supporting the efficacy of athletic trainers in the secondary schools (http://www.nata.org/sites/default/files/AMA_Support.pdf).

Following the adoption of this policy, the NATA provided a second official statement on certified athletic trainers in high schools, which appears in *Focus Box 1–2:* "The use of qualified athletic trainers in secondary schools."

In 2008, the NATA published a consensus statement "Appropriate medical care for the secondary-school-age athlete" (http://www.nata.org/sites/default/files/AppropriateMedicalCare4SecondarySchoolAge Athletes.pdf) in which recommendations were provided for handling specific medical situations that can arise in the secondary-school setting.[2]

School Districts Some school districts have found it effective to employ a centrally placed certified athletic trainer. In this case, the athletic trainer, who may be full- or part-time, is a nonteacher who serves a number of schools. The advantage is savings; the disadvantage is that one individual cannot provide the level of service usually required by a typical school.

Professional Sports

Although the availability of positions for athletic trainers working at the professional level is limited, opportunities to work in this setting continue to expand. Virtually every professional team, regardless of the sport, employs at least one and occasionally as many as four certified athletic trainers.

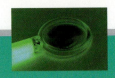
The use of qualified athletic trainers in secondary schools

"The National Athletic Trainers' Association (NATA) is confident the best way to protect the public is to allow only Board of Certification–certified athletic trainers and state licensed athletic trainers to practice as athletic trainers. NATA is not alone in these beliefs. The American Medical Association has stated that certified athletic trainers should be used as part of a high school's medical team. The American Academy of Family Physicians agrees and states on its Web site, 'The AAFP encourages high schools to have, whenever possible, a BOC-certified or registered/licensed athletic trainer as an integral part of the high-school athletic program.

"In states with athletic training regulation, allowing other individuals to continue practicing as athletic trainers without a valid state license or BOC certification places the public at risk. Athletic trainers have unique education and skills that allow them to properly assess and treat acute and traumatic injuries in high-school athletics. In coordination with the team physician, they routinely make decisions regarding the return-to-play status of student-athletes. Other allied health professionals are not qualified to perform these tasks. Finally, most situations encountered by athletic trainers should not be left to a coach or layperson who does not have the necessary education and medical and emergency care training."

From NATA Official statement *Use of qualified athletic trainers in secondary schools* (2004) (http://www.nata.org/sites/default/files/ATsInHSs.pdf)

Athletic trainers work with both male and female professional teams, including football, basketball, baseball, hockey, soccer, lacrosse, softball, golf, and tennis. They are also employed in professional rodeo, auto racing (NASCAR), and wrestling. The athletic trainer for professional sports teams usually performs specific team athletic training duties for 6 to 8 months out of the year; the other 4 to 6 months are spent in off-season conditioning and individual rehabilitation. The athletic trainer working with a professional team is involved with only one sport and is paid according to contract, much as a player is. Playoff and championship money may be added to the yearly income (Figure 1–3E&F).

Amateur/Recreational/Youth Sport

Athletic trainers are working at all levels of amateur sport. The United States Olympic Committee employs athletic trainers and interns at three training centers. Every national governing body (NGB) for each of the Olympic sports employs either a single athletic trainer or a group of athletic trainers to work with the national teams and developmental programs for younger athletes. Some municipal or community-based recreational programs employ athletic trainers either full-time or as independent contractors to cover their programs. The Amateur Athletic Union (AAU) also employs athletic trainers to cover its tournaments (Figure 1–3G).

Performing Arts

A relatively new and expanding employment opportunity exists in the performing arts and entertainment industry. Athletic trainers can be found working with dance companies and theater performance groups. They are employed by Disney and the large casinos. Some touring bands even employ athletic trainers to work with their performers and road crew who sustain injuries while traveling (Figure 1–3H).

The Military/Law Enforcement/Government

The United States military, particularly the Navy, the Marines, and the Army, have demonstrated increased emphasis on injury prevention and health care for the troops.[59] Treatment centers are being developed that closely resemble and, to a great extent, function as athletic training clinics. The centers are staffed by sports medicine physicians, orthopedists, athletic trainers, physical therapists, and support staff. Injured personnel are seen as soon as possible by an athletic trainer, who evaluates an injury, makes decisions on appropriate referral, and begins an immediate rehabilitation program. Currently, over 100 athletic trainers are in the military as either active duty or reserve personnel.[59] Occasionally, some contract positions are available. It is likely that the role of the athletic trainer in the military will increase substantially over the next several years (Figure 1–3I).

Opportunities are increasing for athletic trainers to become involved with local, state, and federal law enforcement groups and agencies. Athletic trainers are working with police and firefighters as well as with agencies such as the FBI and the American Federation of Teachers (AFT) (Figure 1–3J). Other athletic trainers are employed by government agencies such as the United States Senate, NASA, and the Pentagon (Figure 1–3K).[41]

Health and Fitness Clubs

It is likely that a significant number of job opportunities for athletic trainers exist in health and fitness clubs. Some clubs may offer patient care, but it is more likely that the athletic trainer is a performance-enhancement specialist or an instructor. These clubs may be a chain, a franchise, or an independent club (Figure 1–3L).

Treating Physically Active Populations

In the various employment settings, athletic trainers no longer treat only athletes, but instead a physically active population. *Physically active* individuals engage in athletic, recreational, or occupational activities that require physical skills and utilize strength, power, endurance, speed, flexibility, range of motion, and agility. *Physical activity* consists of athletic, recreational, or occupational activities that require physical skills and utilize strength, power, endurance, speed, flexibility, range of motion, and agility.

The Adolescent Athlete Children have always been physically active. But in today's society, playtime or physical activity for many adolescents is focused on organized competition. Certainly, many relevant sociological issues arise in answer to questions such as how old children should be when they begin to compete and when a child should begin training and conditioning. Skeletally immature adolescents present a particular challenge to the athletic trainer involved in some aspect of their health care. Adolescents cannot be approached either physically or emotionally in the same manner as adults. Thus, the athletic trainer must be aware of patterns of growth and development and all the special considerations that this process brings with it.

The Aging Athlete Aging involves a lifelong series of changes in physiological and performance capabilities. These capabilities increase as a function of the growth process throughout adolescence, peak sometime between the ages of 18 and 40 years, then steadily decline with increasing age. However, this decline may be due as much to the sociological constraints of aging as to biological effects. In most cases, after age 35, qualities such as muscular endurance, coordination, and strength tend to decrease. Recovery from vigorous exercise requires a longer amount of time. Regular physical activity, however, tends to delay and in some cases prevent the appearance of certain degenerative processes.

It is possible for individuals to maintain a relatively high level of physiological functioning if they maintain an active lifestyle. Consistent participation in vigorous physical activity can result in improvement of many physiological parameters regardless of age. The effects of exercise on the aging process and the long-term health benefits of exercise have been convincingly documented.

Generally, exercise is considered a safe activity for most individuals. ACSM has recommended that individuals under age 40 who are apparently healthy with no significant risks can generally begin an exercise program without further medical evaluation, as long as the exercise program progresses gradually and moderately, and no unusual signs or symptoms develop.[3] Individuals who are over age 40 or who are at high risk should have a complete medical examination and undergo an exercise test before beginning an exercise program.

The Occupational Athlete The occupational, industrial, or worker "athlete" often engages in strenuous, demanding, or repetitive physical activities while performing his or her job. Like other athletes, these activities can lead to accidents and injuries. Although an objective of any athletic trainer remains the immediate, accurate, and appropriate medical care of those injured in physical activity, the significant reduction of workers' compensation costs and improved employee productivity becomes critically important in the corporate or industrial world. Training a worker to use appropriate ergonomic techniques while engaging in the physical demands of the job is essential for preventing or at least minimizing the incidence of injury. Should injury occur, intervention strategies that correct faulty body mechanics, strength deficits, or lack of flexibility can help the worker return to performing his or her normal job.

ROLES AND RESPONSIBILITIES OF THE ATHLETIC TRAINER

Of all the professionals charged with injury prevention and health care provision for an injured patient, perhaps none is more intimately involved than the athletic trainer. The athletic trainer is the one individual who deals with the patient throughout the period of rehabilitation, from the time of the initial injury until the patient's complete, unrestricted return to activity. Certainly, providing effective health care for an injured athlete requires input from a cadre of individuals who compose the sports medicine team, including the physicians, coaches, and many other support personnel.[11] The athletic trainer is most directly responsible for all phases of health care, including preventing injuries from occurring, providing initial first aid and injury management, evaluating injuries, and designing and supervising a timely and effective program of rehabilitation that can facilitate the safe and expeditious return to activity.

The athletic trainer must be knowledgeable and competent in a variety of specialties encompassed under the umbrella of "sports medicine" if he or she is to be effective in preventing and treating injuries. The specific roles and responsibilities of the athletic trainer differ and to a certain extent are defined by the situation in which he or she works.[10]

Board of Certification Domains of Athletic Training

In 2010 the Board of Certification (BOC)* completed the latest Role Delineation Study,** which defined the profession of athletic training.[10] This study was designed to examine the primary tasks performed by the entry-level athletic trainer and the knowledge and skills required to perform each task.

> **Five Domains of Athletic Training**
> - Injury/illness prevention and wellness protection
> - Clinical evaluation and diagnosis
> - Immediate and emergency care
> - Treatment and rehabilitation
> - Organizational and professional health and well-being

The panel determined that the roles of the practicing athletic trainer could be divided into five major domains: (1) injury/illness prevention and wellness protection; (2) clinical evaluation and diagnosis; (3) immediate and emergency care; (4) treatment and rehabilitation; and (5) organizational and professional health and well-being.

Prevention A primary responsibility of the athletic trainer is to make the competitive environment as safe as possible to minimize the risk of injury. If injury can be prevented initially, there will be no need for first aid and subsequent rehabilitation. The athletic trainer should educate all of those individuals who are in some way either directly or indirectly responsible for the health care of the athlete.

The athletic trainer can minimize the risk of injury by (1) conducting preparticipation exams; (2) ensuring appropriate training and conditioning of the athlete; (3) monitoring environmental conditions to ensure safe participation; (4) selecting, properly fitting, and maintaining protective equipment; (5) making certain that the athlete is eating properly; and (6) making sure the athlete is using medications appropriately, while discouraging substance abuse.

Conducting Preparticipation Physical Examinations The athletic trainer, in cooperation with the team physician, should obtain a medical history and conduct physical examinations of the athletes before participation as a means of screening for existing or potential problems (see Chapter 2). The medical history should be reviewed closely, and clarification should be sought for any point of concern.

The preparticipation examination should include the measurement of height, weight, blood pressure, and body composition. The physician examination should concentrate on cardiovascular, respiratory, abdominal, genital, dermatological, and ear, nose, and throat systems, and may include blood work and urinalysis. A brief orthopedic evaluation would include range of motion, muscle strength, and functional tests to assess joint stability. When the athletic trainer knows at the beginning of a season that an athlete has a physical problem that may predispose that athlete to an injury during the course of the season, he or she may immediately implement corrective measures that may significantly reduce the possibility of additional injury.

Developing Training and Conditioning Programs Perhaps the most important aspect of injury prevention is making certain that the athlete is fit and thus able to handle the physiological and psychological demands of competition. The athletic trainer works with the coaches to develop and implement an effective training and conditioning program for the athlete (see Chapter 4). It is essential that the athlete maintain a consistently high level of fitness during the preseason, the competitive season, and

*The Board of Certification (BOC) has been responsible for the certification of athletic trainers since 1969. Upon its inception, the BOC was The Certification Committee for NATA, the profession's membership association. However, in 1989, the BOC became an independent nonprofit corporation. Formerly known as the NATABOC, the BOC officially changed its name in 2004.

**The 2010 Role Delineation Study went into effect in 2011 and continues through 2016.

the off-season. This consistent level of fitness is critical not only for enhancing performance parameters but also for preventing injury and reinjury. An athletic trainer must be knowledgeable in the area of applied physiology of exercise, particularly with regard to strength training, flexibility, improvement of cardiorespiratory fitness, maintenance of body composition, weight control, and nutrition. Many colleges and most professional teams employ full-time strength coaches to oversee this aspect of the total program. The athletic trainer, however, must be acutely aware of any aspect of the program that may have a negative impact on an athlete or a group of athletes and must offer constructive suggestions for alternatives when appropriate. At the high-school level, the athletic trainer may be totally responsible for designing, implementing, and overseeing the fitness and conditioning program for the athletes.

Ensuring a Safe Playing Environment by Minimizing Safety Hazards
To the best of his or her ability, the athletic trainer must ensure a safe environment for competition. This task may include duties not typically thought to belong to the athletic trainer, such as collecting trash, picking up rocks, or removing objects (e.g., hurdles, gymnastics equipment) from the perimeter of the practice area, all of which might pose potential danger to the athlete. Athletic trainers must also identify safety hazards involving issues such as workplace ergonomics, equipment considerations, maintenance, and sanitation. The athletic trainer should call these potential safety hazards to the attention of an administrator. The interaction between the athletic trainer and a concerned and cooperative administrator can greatly enhance the effectiveness of the sports medicine team.

The athletic trainer should also be familiar with the potential dangers associated with practicing or competing under inclement weather conditions, such as high heat and humidity, extreme cold, or electrical storms. Practice should be restricted, altered, or canceled if weather conditions threaten the health and safety of the athlete. If the team physician is not present, the athletic trainer must have the authority to curtail practice if the environmental conditions become severe (see Chapter 6).

Selecting, Fitting, and Maintaining Protective Equipment
The athletic trainer works with coaches and equipment personnel to select protective equipment and is responsible for maintaining its condition and safety (see Chapter 7). Because liability lawsuits have become the rule rather than the exception, the athletic trainer must make certain that high-quality equipment is purchased and that it is constantly being worn, maintained, and reconditioned according to specific guidelines recommended by the manufacturers.

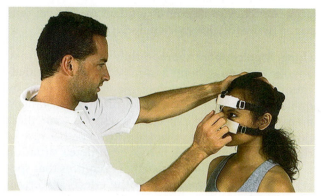

FIGURE 1–4 The athletic trainer should be responsible for taping and for the fitting of protective devices.

Protective equipment and devices can consume a significant portion of the athletic budget. The person responsible for purchasing protective equipment is usually inundated with marketing literature on a variety of braces, supports, pads, and other types of protective equipment. Decisions on purchasing specific pieces or brands should be based on research data that clearly document effectiveness in reducing or preventing injury (Figure 1–4).

Equipment is expensive, and schools are certainly subject to budgeting restrictions. However, purchasing decisions about protective equipment should always be made in the best interest of the athlete. Most colleges and professional teams hire full-time equipment managers to oversee this area of responsibility, but the athletic trainer must be knowledgeable about and aware of the equipment being worn by each athlete.

The design, building, and fitting of specific protective orthopedic devices are also responsibilities of the athletic trainer. Once the physician has indicated the problem and how it may be corrected, the athletic trainer should be able to construct an orthopedic device to correct it.

Explaining the Importance of Diet and Lifestyle Choices
Good nutrition can have a substantial impact on health and well-being. Poor nutritional habits can certainly have a negative effect on ability to perform at the highest level possible. However, for all the attention that athletes, coaches, and athletic trainers direct at practicing sound nutritional habits, good nutritional decisions are still subject to a tremendous amount of misunderstanding, misinformation, and occasionally quackery. An athletic trainer is often asked for advice about matters related to diet, weight loss, and weight gain and is occasionally asked about disordered eating. The athletic trainer does not need to be an expert on nutrition but must possess some understanding of the basic principles of nutrition[95] (see Chapter 5). The athletic trainer should also be able to discuss non-health lifestyle habits, such as alcohol, tobacco, and

drug use. They must educate and encourage patients to make healthy lifestyle choices.

Using Medications Appropriately The athlete, like anyone else, may benefit greatly from using medications prescribed for various medical conditions by qualified physicians. Under normal circumstances, an athlete would be expected to respond to medication just as anyone else would. However, because of the nature of physical activity, the athlete's situation is unique; intense physical activity requires that special consideration be given to the effects of certain types of medication.

For the athletic trainer who is overseeing the health care of the athlete, some knowledge of the potential effects of certain types of drugs on performance is essential. Occasionally, the athletic trainer must make decisions regarding the appropriate use of medications based on knowledge of the indications for use and of the possible side effects in athletes who are involved in training and conditioning as well as in injury rehabilitation programs. The athletic trainer must be cognizant of the potential effects and side effects of over-the-counter and prescription medications on the athlete during rehabilitation as well as during competition (see Chapter 17).

In addition, the athletic trainer should also be aware of the problems of substance abuse, both in ergogenic aids that may be used in an effort to enhance performance and in the abuse of so-called recreational or street drugs. The athletic trainer may be involved in drug testing of the athlete and should thus be responsible for educating the athlete in drug use and substance abuse.

Clinical Evaluation and Diagnosis Frequently, the athletic trainer is the first person to see a patient who has sustained an injury. The athletic trainer must be skilled in recognizing the nature and extent of an injury through competency in injury evaluation. Once the injury has been diagnosed, the athletic trainer must be able to provide the appropriate first aid and then refer the patient to appropriate medical personnel.

The athletic trainer must be able to efficiently and accurately diagnose an injury and illnesses. Information obtained in an initial evaluation may be critical later on when swelling, pain, and guarding mask some of the functional signs of the injury.

It is essential that the athletic trainer be alert and observe, as much as possible, everything that goes on in practice. Invaluable information regarding the nature of an injury can be obtained by seeing the mechanism of the injury.

The subsequent off-the-field examination should include (1) a brief medical history of exactly what happened, according to the athlete; (2) observation; (3) palpation; and (4) special tests, which might include tests for range of motion, muscle strength, or joint stability or a brief neurological examination. Information obtained in this initial examination should be documented by the athletic trainer and given to the physician once the athlete is referred. The team physician is ultimately responsible for providing medical diagnosis of an injury. The initial clinical diagnosis often provides the basis for this medical diagnosis (see Chapter 13).

Understanding the Pathology of Injury and Illness The athletic trainer must be able to recognize both general medical conditions and the various types of musculoskeletal and nervous system injuries that can occur in the physically active population. Based on this knowledge of different injuries, the athletic trainer must possess some understanding of both the sequence and time frames for the various phases of healing, realizing that certain physiological events must occur during each of the phases (see Chapter 10). Anything done during training and conditioning or during a rehabilitation program that interferes with this healing process will likely delay a return to full activity. The healing process must have an opportunity to accomplish what it is supposed to. At best, the athletic trainer can only try to create an environment that is conducive to the healing process. Little can be done to speed up the process physiologically, but many things may be done to impede healing both during training and conditioning and during rehabilitation.

Referring to Medical Care After the initial management of an injury, the athletic trainer should routinely refer the patient to a physician for further evaluation and to confirm the diagnosis. If an athlete requires treatment from medical personnel other than the team physician, such as a dentist or an ophthalmologist, the athletic trainer should arrange appointments as necessary. Referrals should be made after consultation with the team physician.

Referring to Support Services If needed, the athletic trainer must be familiar with and should have access to a variety of personal, school, and community health service agencies, including community-based psychological and social support services available to the patient. With assistance and direction from these agencies, the athletic trainer, together with the athlete, should be able to formulate a plan for appropriate intervention following injury.

Immediate and Emergency Care The athletic trainer is often responsible for the initial on-the-field injury assessment and diagnosis following acute injury. Once this initial diagnosis is done, the athletic trainer then must assume responsibility for administering appropriate first aid and for making correct

1–3 Clinical Application Exercise

A high-school basketball player suffers a grade 2 ankle sprain during midseason of the competitive schedule. After a 3-week course of rehabilitation, most of the pain and swelling have been eliminated. The athlete is anxious to get back into practice and competitive games as soon as possible, and subsequent injuries to other players have put pressure on the coach to force the athlete's return. Unfortunately, the athlete is still unable to perform the functional tasks (cutting and jumping) essential in basketball.

? Who is responsible for making the decision regarding when the athlete can fully return to practice and game situations?

decisions in the management of acute injury (see Chapter 12). Although the team physician is frequently present at games or competitions, in most cases he or she cannot be at every practice session, where injuries are more likely to occur. Thus, the athletic trainer must possess sound skills not only in the initial recognition and evaluation of potentially serious or life-threatening injuries and/or illnesses but also in emergency care.

The athletic trainer must be certified in cardiopulmonary resuscitation and the use of automated external defibrillators (AEDs) by the American Red Cross, the American Heart Association, or the National Safety Council. Athletic trainers must also be certified in first aid by the American Red Cross or the National Safety Council. Many athletic trainers have gone beyond these essential basic certifications and have completed emergency medical technician (EMT) requirements.

The athletic trainer should establish well-defined emergency action plans in cooperation with local rescue squads and the community hospitals that can provide emergency treatment.[70] Emergency care is expedited, and the injured athlete's frustration and concern are lessened if arrangements regarding transportation, logistics, billing procedures, and appropriate contacts are made before an injury occurs.

Treatment and Reconditioning An athletic trainer must work closely with and under the direction of the team physician with respect to designing rehabilitation and reconditioning protocols that make use of appropriate therapeutic exercise, rehabilitative equipment, manual therapy techniques, or therapeutic modalities. The athletic trainer should then assume the responsibility of overseeing the rehabilitative process, ultimately returning the patient to full activity (see Chapter 16).

Designing Rehabilitation Programs Once an injury or illness has been evaluated and diagnosed, the rehabilitation process begins immediately. In most cases, the athletic trainer designs and supervises an injury rehabilitation program, modifying that program based on the healing process. It is critical for an athletic trainer to have a sound background in anatomy. Without this background, an athletic trainer cannot evaluate an injury. And if the athletic trainer cannot evaluate an injury, there is no point in the athletic trainer knowing anything about rehabilitation because he or she will not know at what phase the injury is in the healing process. The athletic trainer must also understand how to incorporate therapeutic modalities and appropriate therapeutic exercise techniques into the rehabilitation program if it is to be successful.

Supervising Rehabilitation Programs The athletic trainer is responsible for designing, implementing, and supervising the rehabilitation program from the time of initial injury until return to full activity. It is essential that the athletic trainer has a solid foundation in the various techniques of therapeutic exercise and an understanding of how those techniques can be incorporated most effectively into the rehabilitation program. The athletic trainer must establish both short-term and long-terms goals for the rehabilitation process and then be able to modify the program to meet those goals. The athletic trainer should constantly reassess the status of an existing injury so that correct decisions can be made about altering and/or progressing the rehabilitation program. All those individuals who are in some way involved with the rehabilitative process, such as coaches, parents, administrators, and other health care professionals, should be consistently informed of the patient's progress toward full return to activity, while maintaining the necessary confidentiality regarding the patient's injury.

Incorporating Therapeutic Modalities Athletic trainers use a wide variety of therapeutic modalities in the treatment and rehabilitation of injuries. Modality use may involve a relatively simple technique, such as using an ice pack as a first-aid treatment for an acute injury, or may involve more complex techniques, such as the stimulation of nerve and muscle tissue by electrical currents. Certainly, therapeutic modalities are useful tools in injury rehabilitation, and when used appropriately these modalities can greatly enhance the patient's chances for a safe and rapid return to athletic competition. It is essential for the athletic trainer to possess knowledge about the scientific basis and the physiological effects of the various modalities on a specific injury (see Chapter 15). Modalities, though important, are by no means the single most critical factor in injury treatment. Therapeutic exercise that forces the injured anatomical structure to perform its normal function is the key to successful rehabilitation. However, therapeutic modalities play an important role in reducing pain and are extremely useful as an adjunct to therapeutic exercise.

Offering Psychosocial Intervention The psychological aspect of dealing with an injury is a critical yet often neglected aspect of the rehabilitation process. Injury and illness produce a wide range of emotional reactions. Therefore, the athletic trainer needs to develop an understanding of the psyche of each patient (see Chapter 11). Patients vary in terms of pain threshold, cooperation and compliance, competitiveness, denial of disability, depression, intrinsic and extrinsic motivation, anger, fear, guilt, and ability to adjust to injury. Principles of sport psychology may be used to improve total performance through visualization, self-hypnosis, and relaxation techniques. The athletic trainer plays a critical role in social support for the injured patient.[6] Athletic trainers should recognize that patients may exhibit abnormal social, emotional, and mental behaviors. Athletic trainers should also be able to recognize the role of mental health in injury and recovery, and use intervention strategies to maximize the connection between mental health and restoration of participation. If the athletic trainer recognizes that a problem exists, he or she should refer the patient to the appropriate medical personnel for intervention.

Organizational and Professional Health and Well-Being The athletic trainer is responsible for the organization and administration of the training clinic, including the maintenance of health and injury records for each patient, the requisition and inventory of necessary supplies and equipment, the supervision of assistant or athletic training students, and the establishment of policies and procedures for day-to-day operation of the athletic training program (see Chapter 2).[5]

Record Keeping Accurate and detailed record keeping—including medical histories, preparticipation examinations, injury reports, treatment records, and rehabilitation programs—are critical for the athletic trainer, particularly in light of the number of lawsuits directed toward malpractice and negligence in health care. Many athletic trainers are responsible for filing insurance claims for reimbursement. Although record keeping may be difficult and time consuming for the athletic trainer who treats and deals with a large number of patients each day, it is an area that simply cannot be neglected.

Ordering Equipment and Supplies Although tremendous variations in operating budgets exist, depending on the level and the institution, decisions regarding how the available money may best be spent are always critical. The athletic trainer must keep on hand a wide range of supplies to enable him or her to handle whatever situation may arise. At institutions with severe budgetary restrictions, prioritization based on experience and past needs must become the mode of operation. A creative athletic trainer can make do with very little equipment, which should include at least a taping and treatment table, an ice machine, and a few free weights. As in other health care professions, the more tools available for use, the more effective the practitioner can be, as long as he or she understands how to use those tools most effectively.

Supervising Personnel In an athletic training environment, the quality and efficiency of the assistants and athletic training students in carrying out their specific responsibilities are absolutely essential.[14] The person who supervises these assistants has a responsibility to design a reasonable work schedule that is consistent with their other commitments and responsibilities outside the clinic. It is the responsibility of the head athletic trainer to provide an environment in which assistants and athletic training students can continually learn and develop professionally.[17] The supervision of athletic training students necessitates constant visual and auditory interaction and the ability to intervene physically on behalf of the patient or student.

Establishing Policies for the Operation of an Athletic Training Program Although the athletic trainer must be able to easily adjust and adapt to a given situation, it is essential that specific policies, procedures, rules, and regulations be established to ensure the smooth and consistent day-to-day operation of the athletic training program. A plan should be established for emergency management of injury. Appropriate channels for referral after injury and emergency treatment should be used consistently.

Policies and procedures must be established and implemented that reduce the likelihood of exposure to infectious agents by following universal precautions, which can prevent the transmission of infectious diseases (see Chapter 2).

Professional Responsibilities of the Athletic Trainer
The Athletic Trainer and Continuing Education The athletic trainer should assume personal responsibility for continuously expanding his or her own knowledge base and expertise within the field. This professional development may be accomplished by attending continuing education programs offered at state, district, and national meetings. Athletic trainers must also routinely review professional journals and consult current textbooks to stay abreast of the most up-to-date techniques. The athletic trainer should also make an effort to be involved professionally with

1–4 Clinical Application Exercise

A young athletic trainer has taken his first job at All-American High School. The school administrators are extremely concerned about the number of athletes who get hurt playing various sports. They have charged the athletic trainer with the task of developing an athletic training program that can effectively help prevent the occurrence of injury to athletes in all sports at that school.

? What actions can the athletic trainer take to reduce the number of injuries and to minimize the risk of injury in the competitive athletes at that high school?

national, regional, or state organizations that are committed to enhancing the continued growth and development of the profession.

The Athletic Trainer as an Educator The athletic trainer must take time to help educate athletic training students. The continued success of any profession lies in its ability to educate its students. Education should not simply be a responsibility; it should be a priority.

To be an effective educator, the athletic trainer needs an understanding of the basic principles of learning and methods of classroom instruction. The athletic trainer should seek and develop competence in presenting information to students through the use of a variety of instructional techniques.[44] The athletic training educator should also make an effort to stay informed about the availability of relevant audiovisual aids, multimedia, newsletters, journals, workshops, and seminars that can enhance the breadth of the students' educational experience.[97] The athletic trainer must also be able to evaluate student knowledge and competencies through the development and construction of appropriate tests.[17] The athletic training educator should also assume some responsibility for helping the students secure a professional position following graduation. Guiding the athletic training student in constructing an appropriate resume will help in this effort (see Appendix D at the end of this text or go to the link at www.mhhe.com/prentice15e).

Students of athletic training must be given a sound academic background in a curriculum that stresses the competencies that are outlined in this chapter and presented in detail throughout this text. They must be able to translate the theoretical base presented in the classroom into practical application in a clinical setting if they are to be effective in treating patients.[14] The athletic training educator accomplishes this application by organizing appropriate laboratory and/or clinical experiences to evaluate the students' clinical competencies.[75] Certainly, the clinical instructor can have a significant impact on the development of the athletic training student.[44]

The athletic trainer must also educate the general public, in addition to a large segment of the various allied medical health care professions, as to exactly what athletic trainers are and the scope of their roles and responsibilities. This education is perhaps best accomplished by organizing workshops and clinics in the community and with corporate and industrial groups, holding professional seminars, meeting with local and community organizations, publishing research in both scholarly and popular journals, and, most important, doing a professional job of providing health care to an injured patient.

The Athletic Trainer as a Counselor The athletic trainer should take responsibility for informing parents and coaches about the nature of a specific injury and how it may affect the ability of the patient to compete. The athletic trainer should be concerned primarily with counseling and advising the patient not only with regard to the prevention, rehabilitation, and treatment of specific injuries but also on any matter that might be of help to the patient.[56,57] Perhaps one of the most rewarding aspects of working as an athletic trainer can be found in the relationships that the athletic trainer develops with individual patients.

During the period of time that athletes are competing, the athletic trainer has the opportunity to get to know them very well on a personal basis because he or she spends a considerable amount of time with them. Athletes often develop a degree of respect for and trust in the athletic trainer's judgment, which carry over from their athletic life into their personal life. It is not uncommon for an athletic trainer to be asked questions about a number of personal matters, at which point he or she crosses a bridge from athletic trainer to friend and confidant. This considerable responsibility is perhaps best handled by first listening to the problems, presenting several options, and then letting the athlete make his or her own decision. Certainly, the role of counselor and advisor cannot be taken lightly.[76,79]

The Athletic Trainer as a Researcher As the athletic training profession continues to gain credibility as an allied health care profession, it is essential that athletic trainers work to enhance their visibility and credibility by engaging in research and scholarly publication.[91] Certainly, not everyone who works as an athletic trainer, in every employment setting, would be expected to engage in research as part of his or her job responsibilities. Although it is true that many clinical athletic trainers publish case studies, assist in large research studies, and even conduct their own research, most often the research that is published in professional journals is conducted by individuals who are program directors, faculty members, or doctoral students employed in colleges and universities.[84] These individuals, along with graduate students seeking masters degrees at most

CAATE-accredited Post-Professional Athletic Training Education Programs are required to conduct research either as part of their job description or as a requirement for attaining their degree. It is likely that, as the numbers of educators, academicians, and graduate students continue to increase, more and more scholarly papers will be submitted for publication in professional journals.[90] Regardless of whether an individual possesses the inclination or the ability to conduct research, each certified athletic trainer must at the very least take responsibility for developing some comprehension of basic research design and statistical analysis and thus be able to interpret and evaluate new research. The athletic training profession cannot continue to move forward unless its members generate their own specific body of knowledge.[67]

Although the transition to evidence-based practice will be difficult for some, it is absolutely essential that the entire athletic training profession must become familiar and comfortable with that process as it becomes a standard in our clinical practice.[46]

The Importance of Engaging in Evidence-Based Practice for the Athletic Trainer

Athletic trainers, like other health care professionals, must routinely integrate evidence-based practice into patient care. Most simply, **evidence-based practice** is making decisions about the clinical care of individual patients based on the current best available evidence in the professional literature.[33,85] Practicing evidence-based medicine means integrating external clinical evidence from systematic research with clinical expertise while focusing on patient values and preferences (Figure 1–5). Individual clinical expertise is the proficiency and judgment that individual clinicians acquire through clinical experience and clinical practice.[72] External clinical evidence is clinically relevant research either from the basic sciences or medicine, or from patient-centered clinical research into the accuracy and precision of preventive, therapeutic, and rehabilitative techniques.[52] For athletic trainers, the evidence-based

> **evidence-based practice** Making clinical care decisions based on supporting evidence available in the literature.

1–5 Clinical Application Exercise

A secondary school athletic trainer is concerned about the number of anterior cruciate ligament injuries that are occurring in the female athletes in all sports. She wants to find out whether incorporating a jump-landing training program will have any effect on reducing the number ACL injuries.

? How should she go about answering this clinical question?

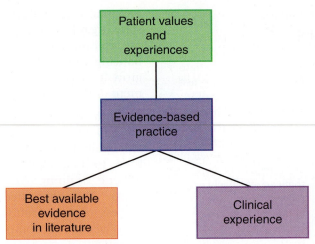

FIGURE 1–5   The Evidence-Based Practice Model

approach raises questions about specific evaluative tests, certain rehabilitation techniques, or the effectiveness of using therapeutic modalities.[13] External clinical evidence often invalidates previously accepted clinical techniques and treatments and replaces them with new ones that are more appropriate and efficient.[94] Without making use of the current best available evidence, clinical practice is in danger of becoming rapidly out of date, and this will undoubtedly have a negative impact on patient care.[31]

In evidence-based practice, there are five steps that athletic training clinicians should take when attempting to determine the efficacy of using a specific clinical technique: (1) develop a clinical question; (2) search the literature to find the best evidence; (3) evaluate the strength of that evidence; (4) apply the evidence in the literature to clinical experience and specific patient needs; and (5) assess the outcome or effectiveness of the treatment.[85]

> **Five Steps in Evidence-Based Practice**
>
> (1) Develop a clinical question.
> (2) Search the literature.
> (3) Appraise the evidence.
> (4) Apply the evidence.
> (5) Assess the outcomes.

Developing a Clinical Question When developing a clinical question, a **PICO** format which is based on three or four specific components should be used. PICO is an acronym for (1) **P**atient problems or condition; (2) **I**nterventions that are possible treatment options; (3) a **C**omparison of the alternatives that might be used in the intervention (a clinical question does not always need a specific

> **PICO =**
>
> • **P**atient condition
> • **I**nterventions
> • **C**omparison
> • **O**utcome

comparison, in which case the acronym would simply be **PIO**); and (4) the **O**utcome that you want the patient to achieve.[85]

Searching the Literature When conducting a literature search, several different bibliographic databases will likely be used most often by athletic trainers, including Articles Plus, Google Scholar, PubMed/MEDLINE, CINAL, SPORTDiscus, and EBSCO host. These databases are called "pre-appraised," or EBP, databases. Enter key words from the clinical question you are interested in answering into a search within the database. For example, if your clinical question is *"Is ultrasound effective in treating ankle sprains?"* enter the key term "ultrasound," which would be what is referred to as a *medical subject heading term* (MeSH). If you enter "ultrasound AND/OR ankle sprains" you would be using a *Boolean Operator* that searches for articles that include both terms.[77]

Evaluating the Strength of the Evidence When evaluating the strength of the evidence found in the literature, it is important to understand that many different types of research studies exist that have different purposes and individual strengths and weaknesses.[43] Among the different types of research studies are case studies, case-control studies, cohort studies, randomized controlled trials, clinical practice guidelines, narrative reviews, systematic reviews and meta-analyses. Case studies provide the least scientific rigor while a meta-analysis is more rigorous and allows for less bias or systematic error.[52] The type of study can certainly have an effect on the quality of the information that study provides relative to the original clinical question.

Critical assessment of results When critically assessing the results of a study, the evidence-based medicine approach requires you to answer three primary questions:

1. Are the results valid, and did the study measure what it was supposed to measure?
2. Are the results reliable and can they be reproduced?

3. Are the results clinically applicable to the original research question?

Critical appraisal papers (CAPs) or critical appraisal topics (CATs) are scholarly papers that analyze the level or quality of the evidence of a specific research study or topic, that is developed and written based on these three questions.[51] Scholarly journals are beginning to include the publication of CAPs and CATs as stand-alone papers.

Rating the level of evidence There are two commonly used scales that assess the level or quality of the evidence in a specific research study.[54] The two scales are the *Oxford Centre for Evidence-Based Medicine (CEBM)* and the *Strength of Recommendation Taxonomy (SORT)*. Both scales look at the *level of evidence*, which is based on the validity of the study. The CEBM scale assigns a number from 1–5 (1 is highest) to rate its quality based on the type of research study (see Table 1–2). Levels 1, 2, and 3 of evidence are further subdivided into subcategories a, b, and c, again based on the type of study. The SORT scale uses 1–3 levels of evidence, but there are no subcategories. Both of these scales also provide a *grade of recommendation*, which indicates the degree of confidence for the evidence to be used in clinical practice. In the CEBM this is a letter A–D or I (insufficient), and in the SORT scale it is A–C (A is the highest).[54] (Table 1–3).

TABLE 1–2	Levels of Evidence
1.	Randomized controlled trial
	a. Meta-analysis/systematic reviews of randomized controlled trials
	b. Randomized controlled studies with small standard deviation
	c. All or none studies
2.	Cohort studies
	a. Systematic reviews of cohort studies
	b. Outcomes research
	c. Cohort studies with little standard deviation
	d. Outcomes studies
3.	Case-control studies
	a. Systematic reviews of case controlled studies
	b. Individual case-control studies
4.	Case reports/studies
5.	Anecdotal evidence

Types of Research Studies

Meta-analyses	Most Rigorous
Systematic reviews	↑
Narrative reviews	
Cohort studies	
Randomized controlled trials	
Clinical practice guidelines	
Case-control studies	
Case studies	Least Rigorous

TABLE I-3 Grades of Recommendation

Grade	CEBM	SORT
A	Strong—Level 1 evidence	Strong
B	Fair—Level 2 or 3 evidence	Moderate
C	Conflicting—Level 4 evidence	Weak
D	Insufficient evidence to make a recommendation	
I	Insufficient	

Using Systematic Reviews Several additional databases publish systematic reviews and meta-analyses of the existing research. These systematic reviews provide clinicians with pre-filtered evidence, save time, and minimize the need for appraisal expertise. They provide the "state-of-the-art" information relative to a given research question.[77] The *Cochrane Database of Systematic Reviews* currently contains the largest database, and it is recommended that athletic trainers begin their search of systematic reviews here. *Scientific American Medicine* and the *ACP Journal Club* are databases that provide systematic overviews of the literature relative to a specific clinical question. These databases identify, review, synthesize, and appraise all of the high-level research evidence, to provide the clinician with recommendations as to which techniques should be incorporated into clinical practice. But simply locating these systematic reviews is only part of the process. The clinician must be able to further distinguish those systemic reviews that are high quality and those that are not. The type of research study design, the analysis of data, and the way the data are reported determine the overall quality of the study.

> The Cochrane Database is the most comprehensive collection of systematic reviews.

There are a number of scales and systems that rate the quality of these systematic reviews and meta-analyses.[92] Among the more commonly used scales to rate study quality are the Physiotherapy Evidence Database (PEDro), the Jadad Scale, and the New Castle—Ottawa Scale (NOS). These scales cannot be universally applied to all types of research designs. For example, the PEDro scale is designed to be used with systematic reviews and randomized controlled trials, whereas the NOS is designed to review nonrandomized studies with meta-analyses. The scales have totally different scoring systems, and scores from one scale cannot be compared to scores from a different scale.[85]

Standardized reporting guidelines assist authors with organizing critical pieces of information to include in doing a systematic review, and include Quality of Reports of Meta-Analyses of Randomized Controlled Trials (QUORUM), Standards for the Reporting of Diagnostic Accuracy Studies (STARD), Quality Assessment of Studies of Diagnostic Accuracy included in Systematic Reviews (QUADAS), Consolidated Standards of Reporting Trials (CONSORT), and Strengthening the Reporting of Observational Studies in Epidemiology (STROBE).

Applying the Evidence Once the research that appears in the literature has been evaluated to determine the level of evidence and a level of recommendation for incorporating a specific technique into clinical practice, it becomes the responsibility of the clinician to understand those recommendations if they are to be correctly applied.[80] Additionally, the clinician must then define the circumstances unique to each patient, and ask the patient whether he or she has any other existing problems that might influence the effectiveness or the safety of the treatment. The patient's preferences, values, and rights should also be taken into consideration. The best available research evidence should be integrated with the patient's specific clinical circumstances and wishes in order to come up with a correct and meaningful decision about management.[53]

It is critical to bridge the barriers between research evidence and clinical decision making to ensure that patients receive optimal treatment. It is recommended that the current best available evidence be expeditiously incorporated into clinical decision making to minimize the delay between the generation of evidence and its clinical application.[28] This should serve to increase the number of patients who can potentially benefit from the current best clinical treatments available.

Assessing the Outcomes of a Treatment After the clinician has implemented a treatment technique that is supported by the best available evidence in the research literature, there needs to be some assessment of the effectiveness of that intervention on the ability of a patient to function normally. Outcomes research is done in an attempt to understand the end results of specific health care practices and interventions. In athletic training, examples of interventions could involve the use of a particular special test in evaluating an injury, a specific treatment technique, or the effectiveness of using a therapeutic modality.

Outcomes assessment measures change in a patient's functional status. These assessments may be based on either disease or condition-oriented evidence or patient-oriented evidence. Traditionally, disease or condition-oriented evidence has focused on mechanisms of the condition or injury, pathophysiology (ligament injury), impairments (strength, ROM, swelling), prevalence, functional limitations, and prognosis, and are based primarily on clinician-centered measures. The most recent trend in outcomes research has become to focus more on patient-oriented evidence that looks at the effects of the disease on the patient's over-all health status (physical and mental health) and quality of life (social, emotional and physical well-being). Patient-oriented evidence takes into consideration the patient's perceptions and experiences from a patient-reported outcomes scale on variables that are important to the patient. If clinicians can systematically identify clearly defined patient-centered goals, they will be more likely to provide treatment and care that is patient-centered. As a result, the approach may be more effective in determining whether a treatment or intervention meets the established goals.[92]

The Disablement Model Outcomes assessment is based on a *disablement model*, which is an evaluation and treatment model that looks at functional loss due to a specific impairment and the associated impact on quality of life instead of focusing solely on a medical diagnosis.[83] A number of disablement models have been proposed, including the Nagi Model, the National Center for Medical Rehabilitation Research Disablement Model (NCMRR), and, the World Health Organization International Classification of Functioning Model (IFC). Although differences exist among their terminology, all models consistently stress the whole individual beginning with the *origin* of the existing pathology (what type of tissue is injured); the *organ* level, which describes specific impairments associated with that body system; the *person* level, which looks at specific functional limitations; and the *social* implications created by the patient's disability and its effect on quality of life (Figure 1–6). Disablement models should help the athletic training clinician to a more comprehensive view of overall health-related quality of life (HRQOL), rather than a concentration on specific functional impairments.[83]

Patient–Reported Outcome Scales (PROs) Although the disablement model serves the foundation for outcomes research, clinical outcome assessments are the measuring tools that determine a patient's health-related quality of life.[92] Patient-reported outcome scales (PROs) gather information directly from the patient using structured questionnaires that have been demonstrated to provide meaningful, quantitative assessments of how the patient feels and how they are able to function with their disorders as a result of a treatment or intervention. Several different types of PROs are available to look at health status and quality of life:

- *Generic* instruments look at a broad range of aspects of health status and the consequences of illness or conditions that may be found in a wide range of primarily healthy populations (e.g., SF-36—Medical Outcomes Study 36-Item Short-Form Health Survey, Musculoskeletal Function Assessment).
- *Dimension-specific instruments* focus on one specific aspect of health status concentrating primarily on psychological well-being (e.g., McGill Pain Questionnaire).
- *Disease-specific* instruments are specific to a particular patient group that share a common disease (e.g., The Asthma Quality of Life Scale).
- *Site or region specific* instruments assess health problems in a specific part of the body (e.g., The Oxford Hip Score).
- *Summary-item* instruments include single items and may be specific to either a region or disease.[92]

Global Rating of Change Scales Athletic trainers commonly ask their patients whether their injury has gotten better or worse with treatment, and then they use this information to determine the efficacy of a particular treatment or to guide future injury management decisions. *Global rating of change (GRC)* scales are commonly used in clinical research particularly with musculoskeletal injuries.[39] With GRC

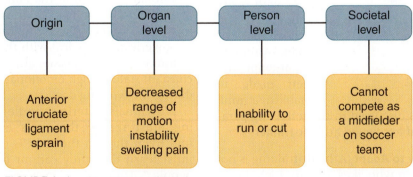

FIGURE 1–6   Disablement Model

scales the patient must assess a particular aspect of their current health status (e.g., pain), then also be able to recall that status at a previous point in time, and finally to calculate the difference between the two. The magnitude of this difference is then scored on a balanced 7–11 point numerical or visual scale with written descriptors on the ends and at the midpoint. The *minimum detectable change* of a measure gives an indication of the degree to which scores change. However, what the clinician is really interested in is the *minimally clinically important change*, which is the change that is likely to be clinically relevant to a patient. The simplicity, ease of administration, and ease of interpretation of GRC scales makes them an attractive alternative to the more complex and time-consuming PROs (e.g., SF-36) for use in clinical practice.[39]

Patient-centered clinical outcomes assessments are a critical component in evidence-based practice. Athletic training clinicians and researchers must make concerted efforts to focus on patient-based outcomes that ultimately guide and direct the practice of athletic training.[78,83,92,94]

Professional Behaviors of the Athletic Trainer

Personal Qualities There is probably no field of endeavor that can provide more work excitement, variety of tasks, and personal satisfaction than athletic training.[38] A person contemplating going into this field must love sports and must enjoy the world of competition, in which there is a level of intensity seldom matched in any other area.

An athletic trainer's personal qualities, not the facilities and equipment, determine his or her success.[4] Personal qualities are the many characteristics that identify individuals in regard to their actions and reactions as members of society. Personality is a complex mix of the many characteristics that together give an image of the individual to those with whom he or she associates.[71] The personal qualities of athletic trainers are important, because they in turn work with many complicated and diverse personalities. Although no attempt has been made to establish a rank order, the qualities discussed in the following paragraphs are essential for a good athletic trainer.

Personal qualities of the athletic trainer:
• Stamina and ability to adapt
• Empathy
• Sense of humor
• Ability to communicate
• Intellectual curiosity
• Ethics

Stamina and Ability to Adapt Athletic training is not the field for a person who likes an 9-to-5 job. Long, arduous hours of often strenuous work will sap the strength of anyone not in the best of physical and emotional health. Athletic training requires abundant energy, vitality, and physical and emotional stability.[81] Every day brings new challenges and problems that must be solved. The athletic trainer must be able to adapt to new situations with ease.[16]

As a member of a helping profession, the athletic trainer is subject to burnout.

A problem that can happen in any helping profession and does on occasion occur among athletic trainers and athletic training students is burnout.[96] This problem can be avoided if addressed early. The term *burnout* is commonly used to describe feelings of exhaustion and disinterest toward work.[40] Clinically, burnout is most often associated with the helping professions; however, it is seen in athletes and other types of individuals engaged in physically or emotionally demanding endeavors.[40] Most persons who have been associated with sports have known athletes, coaches, or athletic trainers who just drop out.[15] Such workers have become dissatisfied with and disinterested in the profession to which they have dedicated a major part of their lives.[89] Signs of burnout include excessive anger, blaming others, guilt, being tired and exhausted all day, sleep problems, high absenteeism, family problems, and self-preoccupation.[40] Athletic trainers who have high levels of perceived stress tend to experience higher emotional exhaustion and depersonalization and lower levels of personal accomplishment.[29] Persons experiencing burnout may cope by consuming drugs or alcohol.

The very nature of athletic training is one of caring about and serving the patient. When the emotional demands of work overcome the professional's resources to cope, burnout may occur.[22] Too many athletes to care for, coaches' expectations to return an injured athlete to action, difficulties in caring for chronic conditions, and personality conflicts involving athletes, coaches, physicians, or administrators can leave the athletic trainer physically and emotionally drained at the end of the day. Sources of emotional drain include little reward for one's efforts, role conflicts, lack of autonomy, and a feeling of powerlessness to deal with the problems at hand. Commonly, the professional athletic trainer is in a constant state of high emotional arousal and anxiety during the working day.

Individuals entering the field of athletic training must realize that it is extremely demanding. Even though the field is often difficult, they must learn that they cannot be "all things to all people." They must learn to say no when their health is at stake, and they must make leisure time for themselves beyond their work.[38] Perhaps most important, athletic trainers must make time to spend with their family, friends, and loved ones.[49]

Empathy Empathy is the capacity to enter into the feeling or spirit of another person. Athletic training is a field that requires both the ability to sense when an athlete is in distress and the desire to alleviate that stress.

Sense of Humor Many patients rate having a sense of humor as the most important attribute that an athletic trainer can have. Humor and wit help release tension and provide a relaxed atmosphere. The athletic trainer who is too serious or too clinical will have problems adapting to the often lighthearted setting of the sports world.[82]

Ability to Communicate Athletic training requires a constant flow of both oral and written communication. As an educator, a psychologist, a counselor, a therapist, and an administrator, the athletic trainer must be a good communicator. The athletic trainer must communicate on a daily basis with athletes, coaches, physicians, administrators, school boards, and members of the patient's family.

Intellectual Curiosity The athletic trainer must always be a student. The field of athletic training is so diverse and ever changing that it requires constant study. The athletic trainer must have an active intellectual curiosity. Through reading professional journals and books, communicating with the team physician, and attending professional meetings, the athletic trainer stays abreast of the field.

Ethics The athletic trainer must act at all times with the highest standards of conduct and integrity.[25,34,74,87,93] To ensure this behavior, the NATA has developed a code of ethics, which was approved in 1993[60] and was most recently revised in 2005. The complete code of ethics appears in Appendix E at the end of this text or go to www.mhhe.com/prentice15e. The four basic ethics principles are as follows:

1. Members shall respect the rights, welfare, and dignity of all.
2. Members shall comply with the laws and regulations governing the practice of athletic training.
3. Members shall maintain and promote high standards in their provision of services.
4. Members shall not engage in conduct that could be construed as a conflict of interest or that reflects negatively on the profession.

Members who act in a manner that is unethical or unbecoming to the profession can ultimately lose their certification.

Professional Memberships It is essential that an athletic trainer become a member of and be active in professional organizations. Such organizations are continuously upgrading and refining the profession. They provide an ongoing source

> As a health care professional, the athletic trainer must be a member of and be active in professional organizations.

of information about changes occurring in the profession and include the NATA, district associations within the NATA, various state athletic training organizations, and ACSM. Some athletic trainers are also physical therapists. Increasingly, physical therapists are becoming interested in working with physically active individuals. Physical therapists and athletic trainers often have a good working relationship. Other athletic trainers may also be occupational therapists (OTs), physician assistants (PAs), certified strength and conditioning specialists (CSCS), nurses, or performance enhancement specialists (PESs).

The Athletic Trainer and the Athlete

The major concern of the athletic trainer should always be the injured patient. It is essential to realize that decisions made by the physician, coach, and athletic trainer ultimately affect the athlete. Athletes are often caught in the middle between coaches telling them to do one thing and medical staff telling them to do something else. Thus, the injured athlete must always be informed and made aware of the why, how, and when that collectively dictate the course of an injury rehabilitation program.

The athletic trainer should make it a priority to educate the student-athlete about injury prevention and management. Athletes should learn about techniques of training and conditioning that may reduce the likelihood of injury. They should be well informed about their injuries and taught how to listen to what their bodies are telling them to prevent reinjury.

The Athletic Trainer and the Athlete's Parents In the secondary-school setting, the athletic trainer must take the time to explain to and inform the parents about injury management and prevention.[24] With a patient of secondary-school age, the parents' decisions regarding health must be a primary consideration.

In certain situations, particularly at the high-school and junior-high levels, many parents will insist that their child be seen by their family physician rather than by the individual designated as the team physician. It is also likely that the choice of a physician that the athlete can see will be dictated by the parents' insurance plan (that is, their

HMO or PPO). This creates a situation in which the athletic trainer must work and communicate with many different "team physicians." The opinion of the family physician must be respected even if the individual has little or no experience with injuries related to sports.

The coach, athletic trainer, and team physician should make certain that the athlete and his or her family are familiar with the Health Insurance Portability and Accountability Act (HIPAA), which regulates how individuals who have health information about an athlete can share that information with others and not be in violation of the privacy rule.[32,35] HIPAA was created to protect a patient's privacy and limit the number of people who can gain access to medical records. HIPAA regulations are discussed in more detail in Chapter 2.

The Athletic Trainer and the Team Physician

In most situations, the athletic trainer works primarily under the direction of the team physician, who is ultimately responsible for directing the total health care of the athlete (Figure 1–7). In cooperation with the team physician, the athletic trainer must make decisions that ultimately have a direct effect on the patient.

From the viewpoint of the athletic trainer, the team physician should assume a number of roles and responsibilities with regard to injury prevention and the health care of the athlete.[47] (See *Focus Box 1–3:* "Duties of the team physician.")

The physician should be an advisor to the athletic trainer. However, the athletic trainer must be given the flexibility to function independently in the decision-making process and must often act without the advice or direction of the physician. Therefore, it is critical that the team physician and the athletic trainer share philosophical opinions regarding injury management and rehabilitation programs; this cohesion will help minimize any discrepancies or inconsistencies that may exist.[55] Most athletic trainers would prefer to work with, rather than for, a team physician.

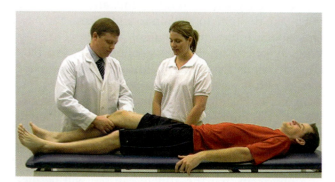

FIGURE 1–7   The athletic trainer carries out the directions of the physician.

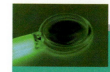

Compiling Medical Histories The team physician should be responsible for compiling medical histories and conducting physical examinations for each athlete, both of which can provide critical information that may reduce the possibility of injury. Preparticipation screening done by both the athletic trainer and the physician are important in establishing baseline information to be used for comparison, should injury occur during the season.

Diagnosing Injury The team physician should assume responsibility for making a medical diagnosis of an injury and should be keenly aware of the program of rehabilitation as designed by the athletic trainer after the diagnosis. Athletic trainers should be capable of doing an accurate initial evaluation after acute injury and determining a clinical diagnosis. Input from that evaluation may be essential to the physician, who may not see the patient for several hours or perhaps days after the injury. However, the physician has been trained specifically to diagnose injuries and to make recommendations to the athletic trainer for treatment based on that medical diagnosis. The athletic trainer, with a sound background in injury rehabilitation, designs and supervises an effective rehabilitation scheme. The closely related yet distinct roles of the physician and the athletic trainer require both cooperation and close communication if they are to be optimized.

Deciding on Disqualification and Return to Play The physician determines when a recommendation should be made that an athlete be disqualified from competition on medical grounds and must have

> Team physicians must have absolute authority in determining the health status of an athlete who wishes to participate in the sports program.

the final say as to when an injured athlete may return to activity.[30] Any decision to allow an athlete to resume activity should be based on recommendations from the athletic trainer.[48] An athletic trainer often has an advantage in that he or she knows the injured athlete well, including how the athlete responds to injury, how the athlete moves, and how hard to push to return the athlete safely to activity. The physician's judgment must be based not only on medical knowledge but also on knowledge of the psychophysiological demands of a particular sport.[88]

Attending Practices and Games A team physician should make an effort to attend as many practices, scrimmages, and competitions as possible. This attendance obviously is difficult at an institution that has twenty or more athletic teams. Thus, the physician must be readily available, should the athletic trainer (who generally is at most practices and games) require consultation or advice.

If the team physician cannot attend all practice sessions and competitive events or games, it is sometimes possible to establish a plan of rotation involving a number of physicians. In this plan, any one physician needs to be present at only one or two activities a year. The rotation plan has proved practical in situations in which the school district is unable to afford a full-time physician or has so limited a budget that it must ask for volunteer medical coverage. In some instances, the attending physician is paid a per-game stipend.

Commitment to Sports and the Athlete Most important, the team physician must have a strong love of sports and must be generally interested in and concerned about the young people who compete. Colleges and universities typically employ someone to act as a full-time team physician. High schools most often rely on a local physician who volunteers his or her time. To serve as a team physician for the purpose of enhancing social standing in the community can be a frustrating and potentially dangerous situation for everyone involved in the athletic program.

When a physician is asked to serve as a team physician, arrangements must be made with the employing educational institution about specific required responsibilities. Policies must be established regarding emergency care, legal liability, facilities, personnel relationships, and duties.[18] It is essential that the team physician at all times promotes and maintains consistently high-quality care for the athlete in all phases of the sports medicine program.

Academic Program Medical Director Accredited athletic training education programs must have a physician medical director who is responsible for the coordination and guidance of the medical aspects of the program. The medical director—who may or may not be the team physician—should provide input to the program's educational content and provide classroom, laboratory, and/or clinical instruction.

The Athletic Trainer and the Coach

It is critical for the coach to understand the specific roles and responsibilities of each individual who could be involved in treating an injured patient. This is even more critical if there is no athletic trainer to oversee the health care and the coach is forced to assume this responsibility. Individual states differ significantly in the laws that govern what nonmedical personnel can and cannot do when providing health care. **It is the responsibility of coaches to clearly understand the limits of their ability to function as a health care provider in the state where they are employed.**

The coach is directly responsible for preventing injuries by seeing that athletes have undergone a preventive injury conditioning program. The coach must ensure that sports equipment, especially protective equipment, is of the highest quality and is properly fitted. The coach must also make sure that protective equipment is

> All head and assistant coaches should be certified in CPR, AED, and first aid.

properly maintained. A coach must be keenly aware of what produces injuries in his or her sport and what measures must be taken to avoid them (Figure 1–8). When necessary, a coach should be able to apply proper first aid. This knowledge is especially important in serious head and spinal injuries. **All coaches (both head and assistant) should be certified in cardiopulmonary resuscitation (CPR) and AED** by the American Red Cross, the American Heart Association, or the National Safety Council. **Coaches should also be certified in first aid** by the American Red Cross or the National Safety Council.[73] For the coach, obtaining

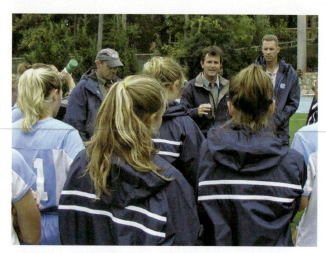

FIGURE 1–8   The coach, in conjunction with other members of the sports medicine team, is responsible for preventing injuries in his or her sport.

these certifications is important so that he or she is able to provide correct and appropriate health care for the injured athlete. But it is also true that not having these certifications can have some negative legal implications for the coach and his or her employer.

It is essential that a coach have a thorough understanding of the skill techniques and environmental factors that may adversely affect the athlete. Poor biomechanics in skill areas such as throwing and running can lead to overuse injuries of the arms and legs, whereas overexposure to heat and humidity may cause death. Just because a coach is experienced in coaching does not mean that he or she knows proper skill techniques. Coaches must engage in a continual process of education to further their knowledge in their sport. When a sports program or specific sport is without an athletic trainer, the coach very often takes over this role.

Coaches work closely with athletic trainers; therefore, both must develop an insight into each other's problems, so that they can function effectively. The athletic trainer must develop patience and must earn the respect of the coaches, so that his or her judgment in all medical matters is fully accepted. In turn, the athletic trainer must avoid questioning the abilities of the coaches in their fields and must restrict opinions to athletic training matters. To avoid frustration and hard feelings, the coach must coach, and the athletic trainer must conduct athletic training matters. In terms of the health and well-being of the athlete, the physician and the athletic trainer have the last word. This position must be backed at all times by the athletic director.

This is not to say, however, that the coach should not be involved with the decision-making process. For example, during the time the athlete is rehabilitating an injury, there may be drills or technical instruction sessions that the athlete can participate in that will not exacerbate the existing problem. Thus, the coach, the athletic trainer, and the team physician should be able to negotiate what the athlete can and cannot do safely in the course of a practice.

Any personal relationship takes some time to grow and develop. The relationship between the coach and the athletic trainer is no different. The athletic trainer must demonstrate to the coach his or her capability to correctly manage an injury and guide the course of a rehabilitation program. It will take some time for the coach to develop trust and confidence in the athletic trainer. The coach must understand that what the athletic trainer wants for the athlete is exactly the same as what the coach wants—to get an athlete healthy and back to practice as quickly and safely as possible.

REFERRING THE PATIENT TO OTHER MEDICAL AND NONMEDICAL SUPPORT SERVICES AND PERSONNEL

In certain situations, an individual may require treatment from or consultation with a variety of both medical and nonmedical services or personnel other than the athletic trainer or team physician. After the athletic trainer consults with the team physician about a particular matter, either the athletic trainer or the team physician can arrange for appointments as necessary. When referring an athlete for evaluation or consultation, the athletic trainer must be aware of the community-based services available and the insurance or managed care plan coverage available for that athlete.

A number of support health services and personnel may be used. These services and personnel include school health services; nurses; physicians, including orthopedists, neurologists, internists, family medicine specialists, ophthalmologists, pediatricians, psychiatrists, dermatologists, gynecologists, and osteopaths; dentists; podiatrists; physician's assistants; physical therapists; strength and conditioning specialists; biomechanists; exercise physiologists; nutritionists; sport psychologists; massage therapists; occupational therapists; social workers; emergency medical technicians; sports chiropractors; orthotists/prosthetists; equipment personnel; and referees.

School Health Services

Colleges and universities maintain school health services that range from a department operating with one or two nurses and a physician available on a part-time basis to an elaborate setup comprised of a full complement of nursing services with a staff of full-time medical specialists and complete laboratory and hospital facilities. At the secondary-school level, health services are usually organized so that one or two nurses conduct the program under the direction of the school physician, who may serve a number of schools in a given area or district. This organization poses a problem, because it is often difficult to have qualified medical help at hand when it is needed. Local policy determines the procedure for referral for medical care. If such policies are lacking, the athletic trainer should see to it that an effective method is established for handling all athletes requiring medical care or opinion. The ultimate source of health care is the physician. The effectiveness of athletic health care service can be evaluated only to the extent to which it meets the following criteria:

1. Availability at every scheduled practice or contest of a person qualified and delegated to render emergency care to an injured or ill participant
2. Planned access to a physician by phone or nearby presence for prompt medical evaluation of the health care problems that warrant this attention
3. Planned access to a medical facility, including plans for communication and transportation

Nurse (RN, LPN, NP)

As a rule, the nurse is not usually responsible for the recognition and management of sports injuries. However, in certain institutions that lack an athletic trainer, the nurse may assume the majority of the responsibility in providing health care for the athlete. The nurse works under the direction of the physician and in liaison with the athletic trainer and the school health services. A nurse practitioner (NP) is a registered nurse with advanced education and clinical training. NPs diagnose and treat common acute and chronic problems, and prescribe and manage medications.

Physician (MD)

A number of physicians with a variety of specializations can aid in treating the patient (see *Focus Box 1–4:* "Specializations for physicians").

Osteopath (DO)

An osteopath is a trained medical doctor who emphasizes the role of the musculoskeletal system in health and disease using a holistic approach to the patient. An osteopath incorporates a variety of manual and physical treatment interventions in the prevention and treatment of disease.

Dentist (DDS, DMD)

The role of team dentist is somewhat analogous to that of team physician. He or she serves as a dental consultant for the team and should be available for first aid and emergency care. Good communication between the dentist and the athletic trainer should ensure a good dental program. There are three areas of responsibility for the team dentist:

1. Organizing and performing the preseason dental examination
2. Being available to provide emergency care when needed
3. Conducting the fitting of mouth protectors

Podiatrist (DPM)

Podiatry, the specialized field dealing with the study and care of the foot, has become an integral part of sports health care. Many podiatrists are trained in surgical procedures, foot biomechanics, and the fitting and construction of orthotic devices for the shoe. Like the team dentist, a podiatrist should be available on a consulting basis.

Physician Assistant (PA)

Physician Assistants (PAs) are trained to assume many of the responsibilities for patient care traditionally done by a physician. A Physician Assistant is licensed to triage, conduct patient evaluations, diagnose and treat patients, arrange for various hospital-based diagnostic tests, and prescibe appropriate medications without conferring with or being seen by a physician. PAs have a physician supervisor but there are several levels of supervision to include the physician being available by phone. A number of athletic trainers have also become PAs in recent years.

Physical Therapist (PT)

Some athletic trainers use physical therapists to supervise the rehabilitation programs for injured athletes, whereas the athletic trainer concentrates primarily on getting a player ready to practice or compete. In many sports medicine clinics, athletic

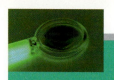

Specializations for physicians

Dermatologist A dermatologist should be consulted for problems and lesions occurring on the skin.

Family medicine physician A physician who specializes in family medicine supervises or provides medical care to all members of a family. Many team physicians in colleges and universities, and particularly at the high-school level, are engaged in family practice.

Gynecologist A gynecologist is consulted when health issues in the female reproductive system are of primary concern.

Internist An internist is a physician who specializes in the practice of internal medicine. An internist treats diseases of the internal organs by using methods other than surgery.

Neurologist A neurologist specializes in treating disorders of and injuries to the nervous system. There are common situations in athletics in which consultation with a neurologist is warranted, such as for head injury or peripheral nerve injury.

Ophthalmologist Physicians who manage and treat injuries to the eye are ophthalmologists. An optometrist evaluates and fits patients with glasses or contact lenses.

Orthopedist The orthopedist is responsible for treating injuries and disorders of the musculoskeletal system. Many colleges and universities have a team orthopedist on their staff.

Osteopath (DO) An osteopath emphasizes the role of the musculoskeletal system in health and disease, using a holistic approach to the patient. An osteopath incorporates a variety of manual and physical treatment interventions in the prevention and treatment of disease.

Pediatrician A pediatrician cares for and treats injuries and illnesses that occur in young children and adolescents.

Psychiatrist Psychiatry is a medical practice that deals with the diagnosis, treatment, and prevention of mental illness.

---

trainers and physical therapists work in teams, jointly contributing to the supervision of a rehabilitation program. A number of athletic trainers are also physical therapists. A physical therapist can be certified as a sports certified specialist (SCS). The physical therapist is prepared to treat a variety of patient populations with different types of injuries, whereas the athletic trainer is focused primarily on treating and working with the physically active population.

Strength and Conditioning Specialist (CSCS)

Many colleges and universities and some high schools employ full-time strength coaches to advise athletes on training and conditioning programs. Athletic trainers should routinely consult with these individuals and advise them about injuries to a particular athlete and exercises that should be avoided or modified relative to a specific injury. A strength coach can be certified by the National Strength and Conditioning Association as a CSCS.

Biomechanist

An individual who possesses some expertise in the analysis of human motion can also be a great aid to the athletic trainer. The biomechanist uses sophisticated video and computer-enhanced digital analysis equipment to study movement. By advising the athlete, coach, and athletic trainer on matters such

as faulty gait patterns or improper throwing mechanics, the biomechanist can reduce the likelihood of injury to the athlete.

Exercise Physiologist

The exercise physiologist can significantly influence the athletic training program by giving input to the athletic trainer regarding training and conditioning techniques, body composition analysis, and nutritional considerations. Exercise physiologists monitor and assess cardiovascular and metabolic effects and mechanisms of exercise, replenishment of fluids during exercise, and exercise for cardiac and musculoskeletal rehabilitation.

Nutritionist (RD)

Increasingly, individuals in the field of nutrition are becoming interested in athletics. Some large athletic training programs engage a nutritionist as a consultant who plans eating programs that are geared to the needs of a particular sport. He or she also assists individual athletes who need special nutritional counseling.

Sport Psychologist

The sport psychologist can advise the athletic trainer on matters related to the psychological aspects of the rehabilitation process. The way the athlete feels about the injury and how it affects his or her social, emotional, intellectual, and physical dimensions can have a substantial effect on the course of a treatment program and how quickly the athlete may return to competition. The sport psychologist uses different intervention strategies to help the athlete cope with injury. Sport psychologists can seek certification through the Association for the Advancement of Sport Psychology.

Massage Therapist (NCBTMB)

The mission of the American Massage Therapy Association (AMTA) is "to serve its members while advancing the art, science, and practice of massage therapy." Many massage therapists choose to become nationally certified in massage therapy, whereas others are required by their states to pass a national certification exam administered by the National Certification Board for Therapeutic Massage and Bodywork (NCBTMB). National certification indicates that these massage therapists possess core skills, abilities, knowledge, and attributes to practice safely and competently, as determined by the NCBTMB. The massage therapy profession is regulated in most states in the form of either a license, registration, or certification making it illegal for anyone to work as a massage therapist unless he or she has a license.

Occupational Therapist (OT)

Occupational therapists work with patients who have conditions that are mentally, physically, developmentally, or emotionally disabling to improve their ability to perform tasks in their daily living and working environments. Some occupational therapists treat individuals whose ability to function in a work environment has been impaired. These practitioners arrange employment, evaluate the work environment, plan work activities, and assess the client's progress.

Emergency Medical Technician (EMT) and Paramedic

There are four levels of emergency medical service (EMS) providers: First Responder, EMT-Basic, EMT-Intermediate, and EMT-Paramedic. First Responders are the first to arrive at the scene of an incident and are trained to provide basic emergency medical care. The EMT-Basic, also known as EMT-1, is trained to care for patients at the scene of an accident and while transporting patients by ambulance to the hospital under medical direction. An EMT-Intermediate (EMT-2 and EMT-3) has more advanced training that allows the administration of intravenous fluids, the use of manual defibrillators, and the application of advanced airway techniques. Paramedics (EMT-4) provide the most extensive prehospital care by administering drugs orally and intravenously, interpreting electrocardiograms (ECGs), performing endotracheal intubations, and using monitors and other complex equipment.

Sports Chiropractor (DC)

Chiropractors emphasize diagnosis and treatment of mechanical disorders of the musculoskeletal system, believing that these disorders affect general health by way of the nervous system. Chiropractors make use of spinal and extremity manipulations in their treatments.

Orthotist/Prosthetist (ROT)

These individuals custom fit, design, and construct braces, orthotics, and support devices based on physician prescriptions.

Equipment Personnel

Sports equipment personnel are becoming specialists in the purchase and proper fitting of protective equipment. They work closely with the coach and the athletic trainer.

Referee

Referees must be highly knowledgeable regarding rules and regulations, especially those that relate to the health and welfare of the athlete. They work cooperatively with the coach and the athletic trainer. They must be capable of checking the playing facility for dangerous situations and equipment that may predispose the athlete to injury. They must routinely check athletes to ensure that they are wearing adequate protective pads.

Social Worker

Occasionally, athletes or their families need a referral for social support services within the community. Social workers can offer counseling and support for a variety of personal or family difficulties, such as substance abuse or family planning.

RECOGNITION AND ACCREDITATION OF THE ATHLETIC TRAINER AS AN ALLIED HEALTH CARE PROFESSIONAL

In June 1990, the American Medical Association (AMA) officially recognized athletic training as an allied health care profession. The primary purpose of this recognition was to have the profession of athletic training recognized in the same context as other allied health care professions and to be held to similar professional and educational expectations, as well as to allow for the accreditation of educational programs.[26] Overseen by NATA's Professional Education

Committee (PEC), since 1969 athletic training education programs became the responsibility of the AMA. The AMA's Committee on Allied Health Education and Accreditation (CAHEA) was charged with developing the requirements (*Essentials and Guidelines*) for the structure and function of academic programs to prepare entry-level athletic trainers. The Joint Review Committee on Athletic Training (JRC-AT) was originally charged with evaluating athletic training education programs seeking accreditation and making recommendations to CAHEA as to whether those educational programs met the necessary criteria to become an accredited program in athletic training education. The JRC-AT was made up of representatives from the NATA, the American Academy of Pediatrics, the American Orthopedic Society for Sports Medicine, and the American Academy of Family Physicians. As of 1993, all entry-level athletic training education programs became subject to the CAHEA accreditation process.

In June 1994, CAHEA was dissolved and was replaced immediately by the Commission on Accreditation of Allied Health Education Programs (CAAHEP). The CAAHEP is recognized as an accreditation agency for allied health education programs by the Council for Higher Education Accreditation (CHEA). CHEA is a private, nonprofit national organization that coordinates accreditation activity in the United States. Formed in 1996, its mission is to promote academic quality through formal recognition of higher education accreditation bodies and to work to advance self-regulation through accreditation. Recognition by CHEA affirms that standards and processes of accrediting organizations are consistent with the quality, improvement, and accountability expectations that CHEA has established. Entry-level bachelors and masters athletic training education programs that were at one time approved by NATA, and subsequently accredited by CAHEA, were accredited by CAAHEP through 2005.

> **Evolution of athletic training education accreditation bodies:**
> - PEC, 1969
> - Recognition of ATC as an allied health professional, 1990
> - CAHEA, 1993
> - CAAHEP, 1994
> - JRC-AT, 2003
> - CAATE, 2006

1-6 Clinical Application Exercise

A second-semester college sophomore has decided that she is interested in becoming a certified athletic trainer. She happens to be in an institution that offers an advanced masters degree in athletic training yet does not offer an entry-level CAATE-approved curriculum.

? How can this student most effectively achieve her goal of becoming a certified athletic trainer?

In 2003, the JRC-AT leadership decided that the profession of athletic training had matured and outgrown the structure and constraints of CAAHEP and that the profession would be better served if the JRC-AT became an independent accrediting agency like those in the other allied health professions. This change meant that, instead of the JRC-AT making accreditation recommendations to CAAHEP, the JRC-AT would accredit athletic training education programs. In 2006, the JRC-AT had officially become the Committee for Accreditation of Athletic Training Education (CAATE). As of 2007, CAATE was officially recognized by the Council for Higher Education Accreditation (CHEA). Through recognition by CHEA, CAATE is in the same context/level as CAAHEP and other national accreditors.

The effects of CAATE accreditation are not limited to just educational aspects. In the future, this recognition may affect regulatory legislation, the practice of athletic training in nontraditional settings, and insurance considerations. This recognition will continue to be a positive step in the development of the athletic training profession.

Other Health Care Organization Accrediting Agencies

Although CAATE is the accrediting organization for athletic training, other organizations accredit various health care agencies and organizations.

Joint Commission on Accreditation of Healthcare Organizations The Joint Commission on Accreditation of Healthcare Organizations (JCAHO) is the nation's largest standards-setting and accrediting body in health care. JCAHO accredits more than 18,000 health care organizations and programs in the United States. Its mission is to improve the quality of care provided to the public through the provision of health care accreditation and related services that support performance improvement in health care organizations.

Commission on Accreditation of Rehabilitation Facilities (CARF) The Commission on Accreditation of Rehabilitation Facilities (CARF) is an accrediting organization that promotes quality rehabilitation services by establishing standards of quality for organizations to use as guidelines in developing and offering their programs or services to consumers. CARF uses the standards to determine how well an organization is serving its consumers and how it can improve. CARF standards are developed with input from consumers, rehabilitation professionals, state and national organizations, and funders. Every year the standards are reviewed and new ones are developed to keep pace with changing conditions and current consumer needs.

CAATE Accredited Entry-Level Athletic Training Education Programs

As of June 2012, 357 institutions across the United States offered entry-level athletic training education programs (333 entry-level bachelors and 19 entry-level masters), all of which are accredited by the Committee for Accreditation of Athletic Training Education (CAATE). In addition, more than 50 institutions are in the process of seeking CAATE accreditation. Using a medical-based model, athletic training students are educated to serve in the role of allied health care professional, with an emphasis on clinical reasoning skills.

Education Council Competencies and Clinical Proficiencies In 1997, the leadership of the NATA established the Education Council to dictate the course of educational preparation for the athletic training student.

The Board of Certification (BOC) defined the minimum competencies required to practice as an athletic trainer and thus reflects the contemporary standards of practice. The Education Council determines the competencies that should be taught in CAATE-accredited education programs. Entry-level athletic training education programs use a competency-based approach both in the classroom and in clinical settings.[17]

Educational content is based on cognitive (knowledge), psychomotor (manipulative and motor skills), and clinical proficiencies (decision making and skill application). In the document "Athletic Training Education Competencies" (5th edition), the Professional Education Council has assigned the competencies to eight areas.[58] These competencies are required for both curriculum development and the education of students enrolled in entry-level athletic training education programs. They define the educational content that students enrolled in these programs must master. The eight areas currently established by the Professional Education Council are (1) evidence-based practice, (2) prevention and health promotion, (3) clinical examination and diagnosis, (4) acute care of injury and illness, (5) therapeutic interventions, (6) psychosocial strategies and referral, (7) health care administration, and (8) professional development and responsibility.

Foundational Behaviors of Professional Practice These affective competencies can be found in every aspect of the educational program, including lecture, laboratory, and clinical instruction. They represent the "people" components of professional practice.[58] Some are easily defined; others must be modeled by instructors. Foundational behaviors include the following:

1. Recognizing that the primary focus of practice should be the patient

2. Understanding that competent health care requires a team approach
3. Being aware of the legal components of patient care
4. Practicing in an ethical manner[66]
5. Advancing the knowledge base in athletic training
6. Appreciating the cultural diversity of individual patients
7. Being an advocate and model for the athletic training profession

Post-Professional Athletic Training Education Programs

There are currently fifteen Post-Professional Athletic Training Education Programs that are now accredited by CAATE. The CAATE-accredited Post-Professional Athletic Training Education Programs are designed to enhance the academic and clinical preparation of individuals who are already certified athletic trainers and those who have completed the requirements for certification.

Specialty Certifications

The NATA is in the process of developing specialty certifications to further enhance the professional development of certified athletic trainers by expanding their scope of practice. Entry-level athletic training education programs provide a general educational foundation, whereas specialty certifications build on this foundation. Specialty certifications in athletic training will be voluntary areas of postgraduate study, and certification in areas more advanced than entry level. According to the NATA Postprofessional Athletic Training Education Committee, the purpose is to "provide the athletic trainer with an advanced clinical practice credential that demonstrates the attainment of knowledge and skills that will enhance the quality of patient care, optimize clinical outcomes, and improve patients' health-related quality of life, in specialized areas of athletic training practice." Specialization in any field of health care requires significant clinical experience in a specific content area and a continuous training effort, which ultimately results in a credential that signifies clinical expertise.

REQUIREMENTS FOR CERTIFICATION AS AN ATHLETIC TRAINER

An athletic trainer who is certified by the BOC is a highly qualified health care professional educated and experienced in dealing with the injuries that occur with physical activity. Candidates for

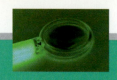
Board of Certification requirements for certification as an athletic trainer

Purpose of certification

The Board of Certification (BOC) was incorporated in 1989 to provide a certification program for entry-level athletic trainers and recertification standards for certified athletic trainers. The purpose of this entry-level certification program is to establish standards for entry into the profession of athletic training. Additionally, the BOC has established the continuing education requirements that a certified athletic trainer must satisfy to maintain current status as a BOC-certified athletic trainer.

The process

Annually, the Board of Certification reviews the requirements for certification eligibility and standards for continuing education. Additionally, the board reviews and revises the certification examination in accordance with the test specifications of the BOC role delineation study, which is reviewed and revised every 5 years. The Board of Certification uses a criterion-referenced passing point for the examination.

Requirements for candidacy for the 3 BOC certification examination

1. Successful completion of an entry-level athletic training program accredited by CAATE

   Students who have begun their last semester or quarter of college are permitted to apply to take the certification examination prior to graduation, provided all academic and clinical requirements of the section used for candidacy have been satisfied. A candidate is permitted to take the examination on the date closest to his or her date of graduation.
2. Endorsement of the examination application by the CAATE Accredited Program Director
3. Proof of current certification in CPR/AED (Note: CPR/AED certification must be current at the time of initial application and at any subsequent exam retake registration.)

certification are required to have an extensive background of both formal academic preparation and supervised practical experience in a clinical setting, according to CAATE guidelines.[26] The guidelines listed in *Focus Box 1–5:* "Board of Certification requirements for certification as an athletic trainer" have been established by the BOC.[10] As of 2004, the only way that a candidate can become certified is by completing an entry-level athletic training education program that has been accredited by CAATE.

The Certification Examination

Once the requirements have been fulfilled, applicants are eligible to sit for the certification examination. The certification examination was developed by the BOC in conjunction with an independent examination development and administration company and is currently administered at various locations throughout the United States.[62] The examination consists of 175 items. In 2007, the certification examination became a computer-based exam (CBE). The CBE tests for knowledge and skill in five major domains: (1) injury/illness prevention and wellness protection; (2) clinical evaluation and diagnosis; (3) immediate and emergency care; (4) treatment and rehabilitation; and (5) organizational and professional health and well-being. Successful performance on the certification examination leads to BOC certification as an athletic trainer with the credential of **ATC**. (For the latest information on certification requirements, visit the BOC Web site at www.bocact.org.) BOC certification is a prerequisite for licensure in most states.

ATC Certified athletic trainer.

Continuing Education Requirements

To ensure the ongoing professional growth and involvement by the certified athletic trainer, BOC has established requirements for continuing education.[9,67] The purposes of the requirements are to encourage certified athletic trainers to continue to obtain current professional development information, to explore new knowledge in specific content areas, to master new athletic training–related skills and techniques, to expand approaches to effective athletic training, to further develop professional judgment, and to conduct professional practice in an ethical and appropriate manner.

To maintain certification, all certified athletic trainers must document a minimum of 75 continuing education units (CEUs) attained during each 3-year recertification term. CEUs may be awarded for attending symposiums, seminars, workshops, or conferences; completing webinars or home study courses; serving as a speaker, panelist, or certification exam writer; authoring a research article in a professional journal; authoring

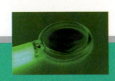

FOCUS 1–6 Focus on Organizational and Professional Health and Well-Being

State regulation of the athletic trainer*

Alabama (L)
Arizona (L)
Arkansas (L)
Colorado (E)
Connecticut (L)
Delaware (L)
Florida (L)
Georgia (L)
Hawaii (E)
Idaho (L)
Illinois (L)
Indiana (L)
Iowa (L)
Kansas (L)
Kentucky (C)
Louisiana (C)
Maine (L)
Maryland (L)
Massachusetts (L)

Michigan (L)
Minnesota (R)
Mississippi (L)
Missouri (L)
Montana (L)
Nebraska (L)
Nevada (L)
New Hampshire (L)
New Jersey (L)
New Mexico (L)
New York (C)
North Carolina (L)
North Dakota (L)
Ohio (L)
Oklahoma (L)
Oregon (R)
Pennsylvania (C)
Rhode Island (L)
South Carolina (C)

South Dakota (L)
Tennessee (L)
Texas (L)
Utah (L)
Vermont (L)
Virginia (L)
Washington (L)
West Virginia (R)
Wisconsin (L)
Wyoming (E)

States with no regulation: Alaska, California

*As of 2012.
E = exempt from existing licensure standards; C = certification; R = registration; L = licensure. For additional information about individual state regulating boards, visit www.nata.org.

---

or editing a textbook; and completing postgraduate course work. All certified athletic trainers must also demonstrate proof of current CPR/AED certification.

STATE REGULATION OF THE ATHLETIC TRAINER

During the early 1970s, the leadership of the NATA realized the necessity of obtaining some type of official recognition by other medical allied health organizations of the athletic trainer as a health care professional. Laws and statutes specifically governing the practice of athletic training were nonexistent in most states.

Based on this perceived need, the athletic trainers in many states organized their efforts to secure recognition by seeking some type of regulation by state licensing agencies. To date, this ongoing effort has resulted in 48 of the 50 states enacting some type of regulatory statutes governing the practice of athletic training.[64]

Forms of state regulation:
- Licensure
- Certification
- Registration
- Exemption

Rules and regulations governing the practice of athletic training vary tremendously from state to state. Regulation may be in the form of licensure, certification, registration, or exemption (see *Focus Box 1–6:* "State regulation of the athletic trainer").

For the most part, legislation regulating the practice of athletic training has been positive and to some extent protects the athletic trainer from litigation. However, in some instances, regulation has restricted the limits of practice for the athletic trainer. The leadership of the NATA has strongly encouraged athletic trainers in all states to seek licensure.

1–7 Clinical Application Exercise

A certified athletic trainer moves to a different state to take a new job. She discovers that in that state the ATC must be licensed to practice athletic training.

? Because she was registered as an athletic trainer in the other state, must she go through the process of licensure in her new state?

Licensure

Licensure limits the practice of athletic training to those who have met minimal requirements established by a state licensing board. Through this licensing board, the state limits the number of individuals who can perform functions related to athletic training as dictated by the practice act. Requirements for licensure vary from state to state, but most require a specific educational and training background, evidence of good moral character, letters of recommendation from current practitioners, and minimal acceptable performance on a licensing examination. Licensure is the most restrictive of all the forms of regulation. Individuals who are providing health care services to an athlete cannot call themselves athletic trainers in a particular state unless they have met its requirements for licensure.[12]

Certification

State certification as an athletic trainer differs from certification as an athletic trainer by the BOC. An individual who has passed the BOC exam does not automatically obtain a state certification. Although certification does not restrict the use of the title of athletic trainer to those certified by the state, it can restrict the performance of athletic training functions to only those individuals who are state certified. State certification indicates that a person possesses the basic knowledge and skills required in the profession and has passed a certification examination. Many states that offer certification use the BOC exam as a criterion for granting state certification.[12]

Registration

Registration means that, before an individual can practice athletic training, he or she must register in that state. The individual has paid a fee for being placed on an existing list of practitioners. The state may or may not have a mechanism for assessing competency. However, registration does prevent individuals who are not registered with the state from calling themselves athletic trainers.[12]

Exemption

Exemption means that a state recognizes that athletic trainers perform functions similar to those of other licensed professions (e.g., physical therapy) yet allows them to practice athletic training despite the fact that they do not comply with the practice acts of other regulated professions. Exemption is most often used in those states in which there are not enough practitioners to warrant the formation of a state regulatory board.[12]

FUTURE DIRECTIONS FOR THE ATHLETIC TRAINER

Certified athletic trainers possess a strong, highly structured academic background in addition to a substantial amount of closely supervised clinical experience in their chosen area of expertise. The athletic trainer continues to gain credibility and recognition as a health care professional. Certainly, recognition as an allied health profession by the American Medical Association in 1990 was a major milestone for the profession. In the future, this recognition may affect regulatory legislation, the practice of athletic training in nontraditional settings, and third-party reimbursement. Without question, this recognition will continue to be a positive factor in the development of the athletic training profession.

Future directions for athletic training will be determined by the efforts of the NATA and its membership and will likely include the following:

- Athletic trainers, like other health care professionals, routinely integrate evidence-based practice into patient care.
- Ongoing reevaluation, revision, and reform of athletic training education programs will continue to be a priority.
- Recognition of CAATE by the Council for Higher Education Accreditation will further enhance the credibility of athletic training as an allied health profession.
- Athletic trainers must continue to actively seek third-party reimbursement for athletic training services provided.
- Eventually, every state will regulate the practice of athletic training, and there will be a move to standardize the state practice acts to make them more consistent from state to state.
- Athletic trainers will seek and achieve specialty certifications to better assist in expanding their scope of practice.
- It is very likely that the greatest number of job opportunities during the next decade will be in public and private secondary and middle schools.
- Although the largest percentage of athletic trainers currently work in clinical settings, the number of clinics owned and staffed by athletic trainers will increase.
- Recognition of the athletic trainer as a physician extender who can be incorporated into the daily operations of a physician's office will increase.
- The potential for expansion of athletic trainers in the military is great.
- The potential exists for increasing job opportunities for certified athletic trainers in industrial and corporate settings.
- There will be opportunities for athletic trainers to work with children and teenagers as sport performance specialists.
- Opportunities for athletic trainers working in fitness and wellness settings will increase.
- As the general population continues to age, opportunities for athletic trainers to work with the elderly physically active population will increase.

- Athletic trainers must continue to enhance their visibility through research efforts and scholarly publication. Certified athletic trainers must strive to develop some comprehension of basic research design and statistical analysis to be able to interpret new research.
- Athletic trainers should continue to make themselves available for local and community meetings to discuss the health care of the athlete.

- The certified athletic trainer will become recognized internationally as a health care provider and will be found in Canada, South America, Europe, Asia, and Australia.
- Most important, athletic trainers must continue to focus on injury prevention and to provide appropriate, high-quality health care to physically active individuals regardless of the setting in which injury occurs.

SUMMARY

- Athletic trainers are health care professionals who specialize in preventing, recognizing, managing, and rehabilitating injuries.
- A number of organizations dedicated to athletic training and sports medicine have developed over the years. They devise and maintain professional standards of practice, exchange ideas, stimulate research, and collectively work toward a common goal. Among these organizations are the National Athletic Trainers' Association and the American College of Sports Medicine.
- Athletic trainers are employed in a variety of settings, including clinics, hospitals, industries, corporations, colleges and universities, secondary schools, professional sports, amateur and youth sports, the performing arts, the military, law enforcement, the government, and health or fitness clubs.
- The primary roles of an athletic trainer include injury prevention, clinical evaluation and diagnosis, immediate care, treatment, rehabilitation and reconditioning, organization and administration, and professional responsibilities.

- Practicing evidence-based health care means integrating external clinical evidence from systematic research with clinical expertise while focusing on patient values and preferences.
- Athletic trainers should exhibit professional behavior characteristics that will allow them to communicate and work in cooperation with patients, clients, athletes, administrators, physicians, parents, and coaches.
- They may refer to or consult with variety of both medical and nonmedical services and/or personnel to obtain help and advice in overseeing the health care needs of the physically active population.
- Educational programs for athletic trainers are accredited by the Committee for Accreditation of Athletic Training Education (CAATE). Once an individual completes an accredited program, she or he is eligible to become certified as an athletic trainer (ATC). In most states, a state licensing board regulates certified athletic trainers' practices.

WEB SITES

National Athletic Trainers' Association: www.nata.org
This site describes the athletic training profession, how to become involved in athletic training, and the role of an athletic trainer.

American Sports Medicine Institute: www.asmi.org
The American Sports Medicine Institute's mission is to improve through research and education the understanding, prevention, and treatment of sports-related injuries. In addition to stating this mission, the site provides access to current research and journal articles.

American Academy of Orthopaedic Surgeons: www.aaos.org
This site provides some information for the general public as well as information to its members. The public information is in the form of patient education brochures; the site also includes a description of the organization and a definition of orthopedics.

American Orthopaedic Society for Sports Medicine: www.sportsmed.org
This site is dedicated to educating health care professionals and the general public about sports medicine. The site

provides access to the American Journal of Sports Medicine and a wide variety of links to related sites.

Athletic Trainer.com: http://athletictrainer.com
This Web site is specifically designed to give information to athletic trainers, including students, and those interested in athletic training. It provides access to interesting journal articles and links to several informative Web sites.

National Collegiate Athletic Association: www.ncaa.org
This site gives general information about the NCAA and the publications that the NCAA circulates. This site may be useful for those working in the collegiate setting.

NATA Education Council: www.nataec.org
This site contains information pertaining to the academic preparation of the athletic trainer.

Board of Certification: www.bocatc.org
This site provides up-to-date information on requirements for certification as well as a listing of certification test dates and sites.

SOLUTIONS TO CLINICAL APPLICATION EXERCISES

1–1 To some extent, the role of the clinical athletic trainer is dictated by that state's regulation of the practice of athletic training. Certainly, the clinical and academic preparation of athletic trainers should enable them to effectively evaluate an injured patient and guide that patient through a rehabilitative program. The athletic trainer should treat only those individuals who have sustained injury related to physical activity and not patients with neurological or orthopedic conditions. The athletic trainer may work part-time in the clinic and then cover one or several high schools around the area. The athletic trainer and physical therapist should work as a team to maximize the effectiveness of patient care.

1–2 Although emergency medical technicians are qualified to handle emergency situations, an athletic trainer is able to provide comprehensive health care to the All-American High School athletes. An athletic trainer is responsible for the prevention of athletic injuries; the recognition, evaluation, and assessment of injuries; and the treatment and rehabilitation of athletic injuries.

1–3 Ultimately, the team physician is responsible for making that decision. However, that decision must be made based on collective input from the athletic trainer, the coach, and the athlete. Remember that everyone on the sports medicine team has the same ultimate goal—to return the athlete to full competitive levels as quickly and safely as possible.

1–4 To help prevent injury, the athletic trainer should (1) arrange for physical examinations and preparticipation screenings to identify conditions that predispose an athlete to injury; (2) ensure appropriate training and conditioning of the athletes; (3) monitor environmental conditions to ensure safe participation; (4) select and maintain properly fitting protective equipment; and (5) educate parents, coaches, and athletes about the risks inherent in sport participation.

1–5 The athletic trainer should make use of an evidence-based practice approach to find an answer to her clinical question "Can incorporating a jump-landing training program reduce the number of ACL injuries in female athletes?" The next step is to search the literature to find the best evidence and then evaluate the strength of that evidence. She needs to apply the evidence that she finds in the literature and use her clinical experience to address the specific goal of reducing the incidence of ACL tears. Finally she needs to assess the outcome or effectiveness of having integrated this jump-landing training program in reducing ACL injuries in her female athletes.

1–6 As of 2004, everyone must graduate from a CAATE-accredited program to take the BOC exam and become a certified athletic trainer. Therefore, she must transfer to an institution that offers an entry-level CAATE-approved program, in which she must complete course work and directly supervised clinical experience.

1–7 The laws regarding regulation of the certified athletic trainer vary from state to state. It is likely that she will have to apply for a license through the athletic training licensing board in her new state to get a license to practice in that state. It is not likely that there is reciprocity between the two states.

REVIEW QUESTIONS AND CLASS ACTIVITIES

1. How do modern athletic training and sports medicine compare with early Greek and Roman approaches to the care of the athlete?
2. What professional organizations are important to the field of athletic training?
3. Why is athletic training considered a team endeavor? Contrast the coach's, athletic trainer's, and team physician's roles in athletic training.
4. Define evidence-based practice as it relates to athletic training clinical practice.
5. What qualifications should the athletic trainer have in terms of education, certification, and personality?
6. What are the various employment opportunities available to the athletic trainer?
7. Explain the criteria for becoming certified as an athletic trainer.
8. Discuss the methods by which different states regulate the practice of athletic training.

REFERENCES

1. Albensi RJ: The impact of health problems affecting worker productivity in a manufacturing setting. *Athletic Therapy Today* 8(3):13, 2003.
2. Almquist J, McLeod T, Cavanna A: Summary statement: Appropriate medical care for the secondary school–aged athlete, *J Athl Train* 43(4):417, 2008.
3. American College of Sports Medicine: ACSM's resource manual: For guidelines for exercise testing and prescription, Baltimore, 2009, Lippincott, Williams & Wilkins.
4. Arnold B, Gansneder B, VanLunen B: Importance of selected athletic trainer employment characteristics in collegiate, sports medicine clinic, and high school settings, *J Athl Train* 33(3):254, 1998.
5. Arnold B, VanLunen B, Gansneder B: 1994 athletic trainer employment and salary characteristics, *J Athl Train* 31(3):215, 1996.
6. Barefield S, McCallister S: Social supports in the athletic training room: Athletes' expectations of staff and student athletic trainers, *J Athl Train* 32(4):333, 1997.
7. Berry J: High school athletic therapy, Part 2, *Athletic Therapy Today* 3(1):47, 1998.
8. Bilik SE: *The trainer's bible*, New York, 1956, Reed (originally published 1917).
9. Board of Certification (BOC), Continuing Education Office: *Continuing education file 2012–2015*, Dallas, 2007, BOC.
10. Board of Certification: *Role delineation study*, ed 6, Raleigh, NC, 2010, Castle Worldwide.
11. Brukner P, Khan K: Sports medicine: The team approach. In Brukner P, editor: *Clinical sports medicine*, ed 3, Sydney, 2010, McGraw-Hill.
12. Campbell D, Konin J: Regulation of athletic training. In Konin J: *Clinical athletic training*, Thorofare, NJ, 1997, Slack.
13. Casa D: Question everything: The value of integrating research into an athletic training education (editorial), *J Athl Train* 40(3):138, 2005.
14. Coker CA: Consistency of learning styles of undergraduate athletic training students in the traditional classroom versus the clinical setting, *J Athl Train* 35(4):441, 2000.
15. Craig, D: Educating students on athletic training political involvement, *Athletic Therapy and Training* 14(2):3, 2009.
16. Cuppett M, Latin R: A survey of physical activity levels of certified athletic trainers, *J Athl Train* 37(3):281, 2002.
17. Curtis N, Helion J, Domsohn M: Student athletic trainer perceptions of clinical supervisor behaviors: A critical incident study, *J Athl Train* 33(3):249, 1998.
18. Editorial: The ethics of selecting a team physician. "Show me the money" shouldn't be part of the process, *Sports Med Digest* 23(4):37, 2001.
19. Ferrara M: Globalization of the athletic training profession, *J Athl Train* 41(2):135, 2006.
20. Fícca M: Injury prevention in the occupational setting, *Athletic Therapy Today* 8(3):6, 2003.
21. Finkam S: The athletic trainer or athletic therapist as physician extender, *Athletic Therapy Today* 7(3):50, 2002.

22. Giacobbi P: Low burnout and high engagement levels in athletic trainers: Results of a nationwide random sample, *J Athl Train*, 44(4):370–77, 2009.

23. Green J, Finkam S: Athletic trainers in an orthopedic practice, *Athletic Therapy Today* 9(5):62, 2004.

24. Gould TE: Secondary-school administrators' knowledge and perceptions of athletic training, *Athletic Therapy Today* 8(1):57, 2003.

25. Graber G: Ethics 101, *Athletic Therapy Today* 8(2):6, 2003.

26. Grace P: Milestones in athletic trainer certification, *J Athl Train* 34(3):285, 1999.

27. Gray R: The role of the clinical athletic-trainer. In Konin J: *Clinical athletic training,* Thorofare, NJ, 1997, Slack.

28. Haynes B, Haines A: Barriers and bridges to evidence based clinical practices, *British Medical Journal* 317(7135):273–76, 1998.

29. Hendrix AE, Acevedo EO, Hebert E: An examination of stress and burnout in certified athletic trainers at division 1-A universities, *J Athl Train* 35(2):139, 2000.

30. Herring SA, Bergfeld J, Boyd J, et al.: Sideline preparedness for the team physician: A consensus statement, *Med Sci Sports Exerc* 33(5):846, 2001.

31. Hertel J: Research training for clinicians: The crucial link between evidence-based practice and third-party reimbursement (editorial), *J Athl Train* 40(2):69, 2005.

32. Hunt V: Meeting clarifies HIPAA regulation, *NATA News*, February 10, 2003.

33. Ingersoll C: It's time for evidence, *J Athl Train* 41(1):7, 2006.

34. Jonas J: Ethics in injury management, *Athletic Therapy Today* 11(1):28, 2006.

35. Jones D: HIPAA: Friend or foe to athletic trainers? *Athletic Therapy Today* 8(2):17, 2003.

36. Judd M, Perkins S: Athletic training education program directors' perceptions on job selection, satisfaction, and attrition, *J Athl Train* 39(2):185, 2004.

37. Kahanov L, Andrews L: A survey of athletic training employers' hiring criteria, *J Athl Train* 36(4):408, 2001.

38. Kaiser D: Finding satisfaction as an athletic trainer, *Athletic Therapy Today* 10(6):18, 2005.

39. Kamper S, Maher C, Mackay G: Global rating of change scales: A review of strengths and weaknesses and considerations for design, *Journal of Manual and Manipulative Therapy* 17(3):163–70, 2009.

40. Kania M, Meyer B, Ebersole K: Personal and environmental characteristics predicting burnout among certified athletic trainers at National Collegiate Athletic Association institutions, *J Athl Train* 44(1): 58–66, 2009.

41. Kirkland MK: A case study of athletic training at the Kennedy Space Center, *Athletic Therapy Today* 8(3):9, 2003.

42. Kirkland M: Increasing diversity of practice settings for athletic trainers, *Athletic Therapy Today* 10(5):1, 2005.

43. Knight K: Study/experimental/research design: Much more than statistics, *J Athl Train* 45(1):98–100, 2010.

44. Laurent T, Weidner T: Clinical instructors and student athletic trainers' perceptions of helpful clinical instructor characteristics, *J Athl Train* 36(1):58, 2001.

45. Lyznicki JM, Riggs JA, Champion HC: Certified athletic trainers in secondary school: Report of the Council on Scientific Affairs, American Medical Association, *J Athl Train* 34(3):272, 1999.

46. Manspeaker S, Van Lunen B: Overcoming barriers to implementation of evidence-based practice concepts in athletic training education: Perceptions of select educators, *J Athl Train* 46(5):514–22, 2011.

47. Matheson G: Advocating injury prevention: The team physician's role, *Physician Sportsmed* 33(8):1, 2005.

48. Matheson G: Return-to-play decisions: Are they the team physician's responsibility? *Clinical Journal of Sport Medicine* 21(1):25, 2011.

49. Mazerolle S, Pitney W, Casa D: Assessing strategies to manage work and life balance of athletic trainers working in the National Collegiate Athletic Association Division I setting, *J Athl Train* 46(2):194–205, 2011.

50. Mitten M: Support for certified athletic trainers in intercollegiate athletics, Memorandum from National Collegiate Athletic Association, August 14, 2003.

51. McKeon P: Assessment of the quality of clinically relevant research, *Athletic Therapy and Training* 14(3):4–9, 2009.

52. McKeon P, Medina J, Hertel J: Hierarchy of research design in evidence-based sports medicine, *Athletic Therapy Today* 11(4):42, 2006.

53. McKeon P, Medina McKeon J, Mattacola C, Latterman C: Finding context: A new model for interpreting clinical evidence, *Athletic Therapy and Training* 16(5):10–13, 2011.

54. Medina J, McKeon P, Hertel J: Rating the levels of evidence in sports medicine research, *Athletic Therapy Today*, 11(1):38–41, 2006.

55. Mellion MB, Walsh WM: The team physician. In Mellion MB, editor: *Sports medicine secrets*, Philadelphia, 2002, Hanley-Balfus.

56. Misasi S, Davis C, Morin G: Academic preparation of athletic trainers as counselors, *J Athl Train* 31(1):39, 1996.

57. Moulton M, Molstad S, Turner A: The role of counseling collegiate athletes, *J Athl Train* 32(2):148, 1997.

58. National Athletic Trainers' Association: *Athletic training competencies*, ed 5, Dallas, 2010, National Athletic Trainers' Association.

59. National Athletic Trainers' Association: A closer look at the military setting, *NATA News* 12:30, 2003.

60. National Athletic Trainers' Association: *NATA code of ethics*, NATA, Dallas, 1995.

61. National Athletic Trainers' Association: What is the physician extender? *NATA News* 1:12, 2004.

62. National Athletic Trainers' Association Board of Certification: *Study guide for the NATABOC entry level athletic trainer certification examination,* Philadelphia, 1995, Davis.

63. National Athletic Trainers' Association Education Council: *NCAA Recommendations and Guidelines for Appropriate Medical Coverage for Intercollegiate Athletics*, 2003, National Athletic Trainers' Association.

64. National Athletic Trainers' Association Government Affairs & Advocacy: http://www.nata.org/government-affairs-advocacy.

65. O'Shea M: *A history of the National Athletic Trainers' Association,* Greenville, NC, 1980, National Athletic Trainers' Association.

66. Peer K, Schlabach G: Ethics education: The cornerstone of foundational behaviors of professional practice, *Athletic Therapy Today* 12(1):2, 2007.

67. Pittney W: Continuing education in athletic training: An alternative approach based on adult learning theory. *J Athl Train* 33(1):72, 1998.

68. Pittney W: A qualitative examination of professional role commitment among athletic trainers working in the secondary school setting, *J Athl Train* 45(2):198–204, 2010.

69. Pitney W, Parker J: Qualitative inquiry in athletic training: Principles, possibilities, and promises. *J Athl Train* 36(2):185–89, 2001.

70. Potter B: Developing professional relationships with emergency medical services providers, *Athletic Therapy Today* 11(3):18, 2006.

71. Raab S, Wolfe B, Gould D: Characterizations of a quality certified athletic trainer, *J Athl Train* 46(5):672–79, 2011.

72. Raina P, Massfeller H, Macarthur C: Athletic therapy and injury prevention: Evidence-based practice, *Athletic Therapy Today* 9(6):10, 2004.

73. Ransone J, Dunn-Bennett L: Assessment of first-aid knowledge and decision making of high school athletic coaches, *J Athl Train* 34(3):267, 1999.

74. Ray R.; Ethical practice in athletic training: A thing of the past? *Athletic Therapy Today* 8(2):1, 2003.

75. Rich V: Clinical instructors' and athletic training students' perceptions of teachable moments in an athletic training clinical education setting, *J Athl Train* 44(3):294–303, 2009.

76. Rock J, Jones M: A preliminary investigation into the use of counseling skills in support of rehabilitation from sport injury, *J Sport Rehabil* 11(4):284, 2002.

77. Rosenberg W, Donald A: Evidence-based medicine: An approach to clinical problem-solving, *BMJ* 310:1122, 1995.

78. Sauers E: A team approach: Demonstrating sport rehabilitation's effectiveness and enhancing patient care through clinical outcomes assessment. *Journal of Sport Rehabilitation* 20(1):3, 2011.

79. Scriber K, Alderman M: The challenge of balancing our professional and personal lives, *Athletic Therapy Today* 10(6):14, 2005.

80. Sexton, P: Clinical decision making: Assumptions made in the absence of evidence, *Athletic Therapy and Training* 16(2):1–3, 2011.

81. Shelley GA: Practical counseling skills for athletic therapists, *Athletic Therapy Today* 8(2):57, 2003.

82. Shibinski K, Martin M: *The role of humor in enhancing the classroom climate, Athletic Therapy and Training* 15(5): 27–29, 2010.

83. Snyder A, Parsons J, Valovich-McLeod T: Using disablement models and clinical outcomes assessment to enable evidence-based athletic training practice, Part I: Disablement models, *J Athl Train* 43(4):428–36, 2008.

84. Starkey C, Ingersoll C: Scholarly productivity of athletic training faculty members, *J Athl Train* 36(2):156, 2001.

85. Steves R, Hootman J; Evidence-based medicine: What is it and how does it apply to athletic training? *J Athl Train* 39(1):83, 2004.

86. Stiller-Ostrowski J, Ostrowski J: Recently certified athletic trainers' undergraduate educational preparation in psychosocial intervention and referral, *J Athl Train* 44(1):67–75, 2009.

87. Swisher J, Nyland J, Klossner D: Professionalism & ethics—ethical issues in athletic training: A foundational descriptive investigation, *Athletic Therapy and Training* 14(2), 2009.

88. Team physician consensus statement, *Med-Sci Sports Exerc* 32(4):877, 2002.

89. Terranova A, Henning, J: National Collegiate Athletic Association division and primary job title of athletic trainers and their job satisfaction or intention to leave athletic training, *J Athl Train* 46(3):312–18, 2011.

90. Turocy P: Overview of athletic training education research publications, *J Athl Train* 37(4S):s162, 2002.

91. Turocy P: Survey research in athletic training: The scientific method of development and implementation, *J Athl Train* 37(4S):s174, 2002.

92. Valovich-McLeod T, Snyder A, Parsons J: Using disablement models and clinical outcomes assessment to enable evidence-based athletic training practice, Part II: Clinical outcomes assessment, *J Athl Train* 43(4):437–45, 2008.

93. Velasquez BJ: Sexual harassment in the athletic training room: Implications for athletic trainers, *Athletic Therapy Today* 8(2):20, 2003.

94. Vesci B: Current evidence guiding clinical practice in athletic training, *Athletic Training & Sports Health Care: The Journal for the Practicing Clinician* 2(2):57, 2010.

95. Vinci DM: Nutrition communication and counseling skills, *Athletic Therapy Today* 6(4):34, 2001.

96. Walter J, Van Lunen B, Walker S: An assessment of burnout in undergraduate athletic training education program directors, *J Athl Train* 44(2):190–96, 2009.

97. Wiksten D, Spanjer J, LaMaster K: Effective use of multimedia technology in athletic training education, *J Athl Train* 37(4S):213, 2002.

98. Xerogeanes J: The athletic trainer as orthopedic physician extender, *Athletic Therapy Today* 12(1):1, 2007.

ANNOTATED BIBLIOGRAPHY

Amato H, Cole S, Hawking C: *Clinical skills documentation guide for athletic training*, Thorofare, NJ, 2006, Slack.

Reflects the standards and specific outcomes of the NATA Clinical Proficiencies by presenting clinical skills set following a checklist design format.

Bilik SE: *The trainer's bible*, ed 9, New York, 1956, Reed.

A classic book, first published in 1917, by a major pioneer in athletic training and sports medicine.

Board of Certification: *Role delineation study*, ed 5, Philadelphia, 2010, F.A. Davis.

Contains a complete discussion of the 2004 role delineation study that redefined the responsibilities of the athletic trainer.

Cartwright L, Pittney W: *Athletic training for student assistants*, Champaign, IL, 2001, Human Kinetics.

A practical guide for student athletic training assistants, including their roles and responsibilities within the sports medicine team.

Hannum S: *Professional behaviors in athletic training*, Thorofare, NJ, 2000, Slack.

Focuses on essentials of effective career development. Addresses many of the skills students will require to build their image as health care professionals, such as communication, critical thinking, networking, interpersonal skills, and recognition of cultural differences.

Laurent T: *Athletic training clinical education guide 2009*, Delmar Learning.

Provides a structured format for goal setting, reflection, skills verification, and journaling.

Long B, Hale C: *Athletic Training Exam review*. Baltimore, 2009, Lippincott, Williams & Wilkins.

Provides a framework for athletic students to begin their certification examination preparation.

Mueller F, Ryan A: *Prevention of athletic injuries: the role of the sports medicine team*, Philadelphia, 1991, F.A. Davis.

Provides an in-depth discussion of the various members of the sports medicine team.

National Athletic Trainers' Association: *Code of ethics 1993*, Dallas, 1993, National Athletic Trainers' Association.

Contains a revision of the previous code of ethics; includes ethical principles, membership standards, and certification standards.

National Athletic Trainers' Association: *Far beyond a shoe box: fifty years of the National Athletic Trainers' Association*, Dallas, 1999, National Athletic Trainers' Association.

An interesting text about the history of NATA that should be read by any student interested in athletic training as a career.

Van Ost L, Manfre K: *Athletic training exam review: a student guide to success*, Thorofare, NJ, 2009, Slack.

Emphasizes the roles and responsibilities of student athletic trainers necessary to make them successful as health care professionals.

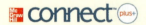

Health Care Organization and Administration in Athletic Training

■ Objectives

When you finish this chapter you should be able to

- Establish a strategic plan for conducting an athletic training program in secondary-school, collegiate, professional clinic, corporate, and industrial settings.
- Plan a functional, well-designed athletic training clinic for a secondary-school, collegiate, or professional setting.
- Discuss issues relative to operating an athletic training program in secondary-school, collegiate, and professional settings.

- Identify policies and procedures that should be enforced in the athletic training clinic.
- Discuss issues relative to operating an athletic training program in clinic, hospital, corporate, and industrial settings.
- Explain the importance of the preparticipation physical examination.
- Construct the necessary records that must be maintained by the athletic trainer.
- Describe current systems for gathering injury surveillance data.

■ Outline

■ Key Terms

accident   injury   epidemiology

■ Connect Highlights Mc Graw Hill connect™ plus+

Visit connect.mcgraw-hill.com for further exercises to apply your knowledge:

- Clinical application scenarios covering athletic training clinic design, risk management, policies, and procedures
- Click-and-drag questions covering budgeting, athletic training clinic design, and preparticipation physical examination
- Multiple-choice questions covering preparticipation physical examination, maintaining records, and developing a strategic plan for an athletic training clinic
- Selection questions covering preparticipation physical examination and classification of sport

Operating an effective athletic health care program requires careful organization and administration regardless of whether the setting is a secondary school, college, university, or professional team or a clinical, hospital, or industrial facility. Besides being a clinical practitioner, the athletic trainer must be an administrator who performs both managerial and supervisory duties.[11] This chapter looks at the administrative tasks required of the athletic trainer for successful operation of the program, including facility design, policies and procedures, budget considerations, personnel management, administration of physical examinations, record keeping, and injury data collection.

ESTABLISHING A SYSTEM FOR ATHLETIC TRAINING HEALTH CARE

Developing a Strategic Plan

Perhaps the first step in establishing a health care program in athletic training is to determine why such a program is needed and what the goals of this program should be.[16] The basic questions in the strategic planning process must be answered by clinic, hospital, or school administrators; athletic directors; or school boards who, in most cases, will ultimately be responsible for funding and supporting the health care program in athletic training.[35] The depth of the commitment from these decision makers toward providing quality health care will, to a large extent, determine the size of the staff, the size of the facility, and the scope of operation of the health care program. A clearly written mission statement will help focus the direction of the program and should be an outcome of the strategic planning process.[24]

Strategic planning should involve many individuals, including administrators, other allied health care providers, student-athletes, coaches, physicians, staff athletic trainers, parents, and community-based health leaders. Including many individuals in the planning process will help secure allies who are committed to seeing the program succeed.[35]

Strategic planning should be an ongoing process that takes a critical look at the strengths and weaknesses of the program and then takes immediate action to correct deficiencies. The *SWOT* analysis—which looks at Strengths, Weaknesses, Opportunities, and Threats underlying planning[33]—is a useful and effective technique in strategic planning for existing athletic health

SWOT analysis
• Strengths
• Weaknesses
• Opportunities
• Threats

care programs. Administrators should take a close look at a cost-effectiveness analysis of operating an athletic health care program to determine the value of the return on their investment.

Developing a Policies and Procedures Manual

Once the strategic planning process is complete and some consensus has been reached by those involved in the process, the next step is to create a detailed policies and procedures manual for use by everyone who is involved with providing some aspect of health care, including the athletic training staff, physicians, other allied health personnel, and administrators.[4] *Policies* are clear and accurate written statements that identify the basic rules and principles (the what and why) used to control and expedite decision making. Policies are essential for operating the athletic training clinic. *Procedures* describe the process by which something is done (the how). *Focus Box 2–1:* "Items to include in a policies and procedures manual" includes recommendations for topics to be included.

> Every athletic training program must develop policies and procedures that carefully delineate the daily routine of the program.

ISSUES SPECIFIC TO ATHLETIC TRAINING PROGRAM OPERATION IN THE SECONDARY-SCHOOL, COLLEGE, OR UNIVERSITY SETTING

It is imperative that every athletic program develop policies and procedures that carefully delineate the daily routine of the program.[20]

The Scope of the Athletic Training Program

A major consideration in any athletic training program is to determine who is to be served by the athletic training staff.[46] The individual athlete, the institution, and the community are considered.

The Athlete The athletic trainer must decide the extent to which the athlete will be served. For example, will prevention and care activities be extended to athletes for the entire year, including summer and other vacations, or only during the competitive season? Also, the athletic trainer must decide what care will be rendered. Will it extend to all systemic illnesses or just to musculoskeletal problems?

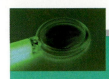

Items to include in a policies and procedures manual

Program Operation

- Goals and objectives
- Mission statement
- Organizational structure
- Scope of operation
- Hours of operation
- Patient scheduling
- Patient billing
- Patient referral
- Facility cleaning, sanitation, and hygiene
- Equipment use, maintenance, and repair
- Documentation and maintenance of medical records
- Release of medical records
- Budget and purchasing
  - Supplies
  - Equipment
- Emergency procedures
  - Fire

- Code (cardiac arrest)
- Emergency action plan
- Safety and security considerations
  - Access to facility
  - OSHA guidelines
- Inclement weather
- Incident reports

Human Resources Issues

- Job descriptions
- Hiring practices
- Quarterly and yearly employee evaluations
- Licensure
- Dress code
- Vacation policy
- Benefits
- Sexual harassment
- Termination policy
- Staff attendance

The Institution A policy must be established as to who, other than the athletes, will be served by the athletic training program. Often, legal concerns and the school liability insurance dictate who, beyond the athlete, is to be served. A policy should make it clear whether students other than athletes, athletes from other schools, faculty, and staff are to receive care. If so, how are they to be referred and medically directed? Also, it must be decided whether the athletic training program will act as a clinical setting for student athletic trainers.

The Community A decision must be made as to which, if any, outside group(s) or people in the community will be served by the athletic training staff. Again, legality and the institution's insurance program must be taken into consideration when making this decision. If a policy is not delineated in this matter, outside people may abuse the services of the athletic training clinic and staff.

Providing Coverage

Facility Personnel Coverage A major concern of any athletic department is whether proper personnel coverage is provided for the athletic training clinic and specific sports. If a school has a full-time athletic training staff, an athletic training clinic could, for example, operate from 6 A.M. to 11 P.M. Mornings are commonly reserved for treatments and exercise rehabilitation; early afternoons are for treatment, exercise rehabilitation and preparation for practice or a contest; and late afternoons and early evenings are spent in injury management. High schools with limited available supervision may be able to provide athletic training clinic coverage only in the afternoons and during vacation periods.

Sports Coverage Ideally, all sports should have a certified athletic trainer in attendance at all practices and contests, both at home and away. Many colleges and universities have sufficient personnel to provide coverage to a variety of sports simultaneously. At the secondary-school level, however, only one or occasionally two athletic trainers may be available to cover every sport that the high school offers. Thus, it is impossible for the athletic trainer to be in several places at one time. The athletic trainer in this difficult situation must make some decisions about where the greatest need for coverage is, based on the potential risk of a particular sport and the number of athletes involved.[31]

Hygiene and Sanitation

The practice of good hygiene and sanitation is of the utmost importance in an athletic training program. The prevention of infectious diseases is a direct responsibility of the athletic

> **Good hygiene and sanitation are essential for an athletic training program.**

trainer, whose duty it is to see that all athletes are surrounded by the most hygienic environment possible and that each individual is practicing sound health habits. Chapter 14 discusses the management of bloodborne pathogens. The athletic trainer must be aware of and adhere to guidelines for the operation of an athletic care facility as dictated by the Occupational Safety and Health Administration (OSHA).

The Athletic Training Clinic The athletic training clinic should be used only for the prevention and care of sports injuries.[20] Too often, the athletic training clinic becomes a meeting or club room for the coaches and athletes. Unless definite rules are established and practiced, cleanliness and sanitation become an impossible chore. Unsanitary practices or conditions must not be tolerated. The following are some important athletic training clinic policies:

1. No cleated shoes are allowed. Dirt and debris tend to cling to cleated shoes; therefore, athletes should remove cleated shoes before entering the athletic training clinic.
2. Game equipment is kept outside. Because game equipment, such as balls and bats, add to the sanitation problem, they should be kept out of the athletic training clinic. Coaches and athletes must be continually reminded that the athletic training clinic is not a storage room for sports equipment.
3. Shoes must be kept off treatment tables. Because of the tendency of shoes to contaminate treatment tables, they must be removed before any care is given to the patient.
4. Athletes should shower before receiving treatment. The athlete should make it a habit to shower before being treated if the treatment is not an emergency. This procedure helps keep tables and therapeutic modalities sanitary.
5. Roughhousing and profanity should not be allowed. Athletes must be continually reminded that the athletic training clinic is for injury care and prevention. Horseplay and foul language lower the basic purpose of the athletic training clinic.
6. No food or smokeless tobacco should be allowed.

General cleanliness of the athletic training clinic cannot be stressed enough. Through the athletic trainer's example, the athlete may develop an appreciation for cleanliness and in turn develop wholesome personal health habits. Cleaning responsibilities in most schools are divided between the athletic training staff and the maintenance crew. The custodial staff and the athletic training staff should work closely together to make certain that all duties relative to cleanliness are covered. Care of permanent building structures and trash disposal are usually the responsibilities of maintenance, whereas the upkeep of specialized equipment falls within the province of the athletic training staff.

The division of routine cleaning responsibilities may be generally organized as follows:

1. Maintenance crew
   a. Sweeps floors daily
   b. Cleans and disinfects sinks and built-in tubs daily
   c. Mops and disinfects hydrotherapy area twice a week
   d. Refills paper towel and drinking cup dispensers as needed
   e. Empties wastebaskets and disposes of trash daily
2. Athletic training staff
   a. Cleans and disinfects treatment tables daily
   b. Cleans and disinfects hydrotherapy modalities daily
   c. Cleans and polishes other therapeutic modalities weekly

The Gymnasium Maintaining a clean environment is a continual battle in the secondary-school, college, and university settings.[39] Practices such as passing a common towel to wipe off perspiration, using common water dispensers, and failing to change dirty clothing for clean are prevalent violations of sanitation in sports. The following is a suggested cleanliness checklist that may be used by the athletic trainer:

1. Facilities cleanliness
   a. Are the gymnasium floors swept daily?
   b. Are drinking fountains, showers, sinks, urinals, and toilets cleaned and disinfected daily?
   c. Are lockers aired and sanitized frequently?
   d. Are mats cleaned routinely (wrestling mats and wall mats cleaned daily)?
2. Equipment and clothing issuance
   a. Are equipment and clothing fitted to the athlete to avoid skin irritations?
   b. Is swapping of equipment and clothes prevented?
   c. Is clothing laundered and changed frequently?
   d. Is wet clothing allowed to dry thoroughly before the athlete wears it again?
   e. Is individual attention given to proper shoe fit and upkeep?
   f. Is protective clothing provided during inclement weather or when the athlete is waiting on the sidelines?
   g. Are clean, dry towels provided each day for each athlete?

The Athlete To promote good health among the athletes, the athletic trainer should encourage sound health habits. The following checklist may be a useful guide for coaches, athletic trainers, and athletes:

1. Does the athlete promptly report injuries, illnesses, and skin disorders to the coach or the athletic trainer?
2. Are good daily living habits of resting, sleeping, and proper nutrition practiced?
3. Do the athletes shower after practice?
4. Do they dry thoroughly and cool off before departing from the gymnasium?
5. Do they avoid drinking from a common water dispenser?
6. Do they avoid using a common towel?
7. Do they avoid exchanging gym clothes with teammates?
8. Do they practice good foot hygiene?
9. Do they avoid contact with teammates who have a contagious disease or infection?
10. Do they understand the role exercise can play in maintaining a healthy lifestyle and preventing chronic disease?

Emergency Telephones

The installation or availability of an emergency telephone adjacent to all activity areas or the availability of a cell phone is a must. It should be possible to use this phone to call outside for emergency aid or to contact the athletic training facilities when additional assistance is required. Occasionally, wireless service may be interrupted. Also, it is important to know that in certain calling areas outside of the wireless area code, 911 calls are routed back to the originating service area code, which does no good in an emergency situation. Walkie-talkies are also useful when practices or games occur at several different facilities simultaneously. These devices can greatly enhance communication without incurring tremendous expense.

Budgetary Concerns

One of the major problems athletic trainers face is to obtain a budget of sufficient size to permit them to perform a creditable job of athletic training.

> A major problem facing many athletic trainers is a budget of insufficient size.

Most secondary schools provide only limited budgetary provisions for athletic training, except for the purchase of tape, ankle wraps, and an athletic training kit that contains a minimum amount of supplies.[7] Many fail to provide a room and any of the special facilities that are needed to establish an effective athletic training program. Some school boards and administrators fail to recognize that the functions performed in the athletic training clinic are an essential component of the athletic

program and that, even if no specialist is used, the facilities are necessary.[7] Colleges and universities face similar problems, but not to the extent of secondary schools. By and large, athletic training at the college level is recognized as an important aspect of the athletic program.

Budgetary needs vary considerably within programs; some require only a few thousand dollars, whereas others spend hundreds of thousands of dollars. The amount spent on building and equipping an athletic training clinic, of course, is entirely a matter of local option. In purchasing equipment, immediate needs and the availability of personnel to operate specialized equipment should be kept in mind.

Budgeting should be a continuous process involving prioritizing, planning, documenting, and evaluating the goals of the athletic training program and formulating a plan for how available resources can be utilized and expended during the next budget period.[33]

Budget records should be kept on file, so that they are available for use in projecting the following year's budgetary needs. The records present a picture of the distribution of current funds and substantiate future budgetary requests.

Supplies The supplies that the athletic trainer uses to carry out daily tasks may be classified as either expendable or nonexpendable. Some athletic trainers spend much of their budget on expendable supplies, which cannot be reused.

> Supplies may be expendable or nonexpendable.

Supplies that are expendable are used for injury prevention, first aid, and management. Examples of expendable supplies are adhesive tape, adhesive bandages, and hydrogen peroxide. Nonexpendable supplies are those that can be reused. Examples are compression wraps, scissors, and neoprene sleeves. An annual inventory must be conducted at the end of the year or before supplies are ordered. Accurate records must be kept to justify future requests.

Equipment The term *equipment* refers to items that may be used in the athletic training clinic for a number of years. Equipment may be further divided into nonconsumable capital and capital equipment. Nonconsumable capital equipment is not usually removed from the athletic training

> Equipment may be nonconsumable capital or capital.

clinic. Examples of nonconsumable capital equipment are ice machines, treatment tables, isokinetic machines, and electrical therapeutic modalities. Capital equipment includes crutches, coolers, and athletic training kits.

Purchasing Systems The purchase of supplies and equipment must be done through either direct buy or competitive bid. For expensive purchases, an in-stitutional purchasing agent is sent out to competing vendors, who quote a price on specified supplies or equipment. Orders are generally placed with the lowest bidder. Smaller purchases and emergency purchases may be made directly from a single vendor.[7]

> Purchasing may be done through direct buy or competitive bid.

An alternative to purchasing expensive equipment is to lease it. Many manufacturers and distributors are willing to lease equipment on a monthly or yearly basis. Over the long run, purchasing equipment is less costly. In the short term, however, if a large capital expenditure is not possible, a leasing agreement should be considered.[33]

Additional Budget Considerations In addition to supplies and equipment, the athletic trainer must also consider other costs included in the operation of an athletic training program; these include telephone and postage, utilities, contracts with physicians or clinics for services, professional liability insurance, memberships in professional organizations, professional journals or textbooks, travel and expenses for attending professional meetings, and clothing to be worn in the athletic training clinic.[33,35]

2–1 Clinical Application Exercise

The principal at All-American High School has received a mandate from the school board to develop a risk management plan for the athletic program. The principal asks the athletic trainer to chair a committee to develop this plan.

? What considerations are important for inclusion in this risk management plan?

Developing a Risk Management Plan

The athletic trainer, working in conjunction with the appropriate administrative personnel, must be responsible for developing a risk management plan that covers security issues, fire safety, electrical and equipment safety, and emergency action plans.[3,4,12,42,43]

Security Issues The athletic trainer must decide who will have access to the athletic training clinic. In addition to the staff athletic trainers, the team physician must have keys to access the athletic training clinic. Athletic training students may also be given keys as necessary at the collegiate level; at the secondary-school level, however, athletic training students should be in the athletic training clinic only when directly supervised. At the collegiate level, coaches do not need to have access to the athletic training clinic; however, at the secondary-school level, coaches might need to have a key to get into the clinic at times when the athletic trainer is not available. Access to areas of the building other than the athletic training clinic should be strictly limited.

Fire Safety The athletic trainer should establish and clearly post a plan for evacuating the athletic training clinic, should a fire occur. Smoke detectors and fire alarm systems must be tested periodically and inspected to make certain that they are functioning normally.

Electrical Equipment Safety Electrical safety in the athletic training setting should be of primary concern to the athletic trainer. Accidents can be avoided by taking some basic precautions and acquiring some understanding of the power distribution system and electrical grounds. *Focus Box 2–2:* "Safety when using electrical equipment" lists considerations for electrical safety.

Emergency Action Plan In cooperation with existing community-based emergency health care delivery systems, the athletic trainer should develop a systematic plan for accessing the emergency medical system and subsequent transportation of injured athletes to an emergency care facility.[5] Meetings should be scheduled periodically with EMTs or paramedics who work in the community to make certain that they understand the role of the athletic trainer as a provider of emergency health care. It is important to communicate the special considerations for dealing with athletic equipment issues before an emergency arises. Chapter 12 discusses the emergency action plan in detail.

Accessing Community-Based Health Services

In addition to the community-based emergency medical services personnel, the athletic trainer should become familiar with existing local and regional community health services and agencies that may be accessed, should a need arise to refer an athlete for psychological or sociological services. Referrals should be made with input and assistance from the team physician. The family of an athlete requiring referral for psychological or sociological counseling must be informed of the existing problems, particularly when the athlete is a minor.

2–2 Clinical Application Exercise

State University has an opening for an assistant athletic trainer in its Department of Athletics. The athletic director has asked the head athletic trainer to be in charge of the recruitment and hiring process for the new position.

? What factors must be considered in hiring a new employee?

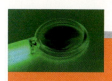
Safety when using electrical equipment

- The entire electrical system of the building or athletic training clinic should be designed or evaluated by a qualified electrician.
- Problems with the electrical system may exist in older buildings or in situations in which rooms have been modified to accommodate therapeutic devices (e.g., putting a whirlpool in a locker room in which the concrete floor is always wet or damp).
- It should not be assumed that all three-pronged wall outlets are grounded. The ground must be checked. Ground fault interrupters (GFIs) should be installed, particularly in those areas in which water is present (e.g., whirlpools).
- The athletic trainer should become very familiar with the equipment being used and with any problems that exist or may develop. Any defective equipment should be removed immediately from the clinic. The plug should not be jerked out of the wall by pulling on the cable.
- Extension cords or multiple adapters should never be used.
- Equipment should be reevaluated on a yearly basis and should conform to *National Electrical Code* guidelines. A clinic that is not in compliance with this code has no legal protection in a lawsuit.
- Common sense should always be exercised when using electrotherapeutic devices. A situation that appears to be potentially dangerous may, in fact, result in injury or death.

Human Resources and Personnel Issues

Putting together the appropriate personnel to accomplish program goals and objectives is critical to success. Any program is only as good as the group of individuals who make up the team. Recruiting, hiring, and retaining the most qualified personnel is essential if the athletic training program is to be effective.

- Specific policies dealing with recruitment, hiring and firing, performance evaluations, and promotions are mandated by federal law (Equal Employment Opportunity Commission). The policies for recruitment and hiring clearly mandate that all qualified applicants should receive equal consideration regardless of their race, gender, religion, or nationality. Athletic trainers who are in a position to hire new staff must strictly adhere to these mandates.[17]
- Once an individual has been hired, it is important for everyone to understand what his or her roles and responsibilities are. Individual job descriptions and job specifications that describe qualifications, accountability, a code of conduct, and the scope of that position should be written. A well-defined organizational chart should be created to show the chain of command.[35]
- The head athletic trainer must serve as a supervisor for the staff assistants, graduate students, and undergraduate athletic training students.[23] The supervisor should strive to improve the job performance and enhance the professional development of those being supervised. *Focus Box 2–3:* "Models

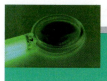
Models of supervision for the head athletic trainer*

Clinical supervision—Involves direct observation of the assistant trainers in the performance of their written job responsibilities, followed by an analysis of strengths and weaknesses and a collaborative effort to correct weaknesses

Developmental supervision—A mentoring approach in which the head athletic trainer works in a collaborative manner with the assistants, helping them develop professionally while meeting the needs of the day-to-day athletic training program

Inspection production supervision—An authoritative management style in which the head athletic trainer demands that lines of authority be strictly maintained to accomplish the stated goals of the athletic training program

*These models should not be confused with the models of clinical supervision established by the Education Council for Students.

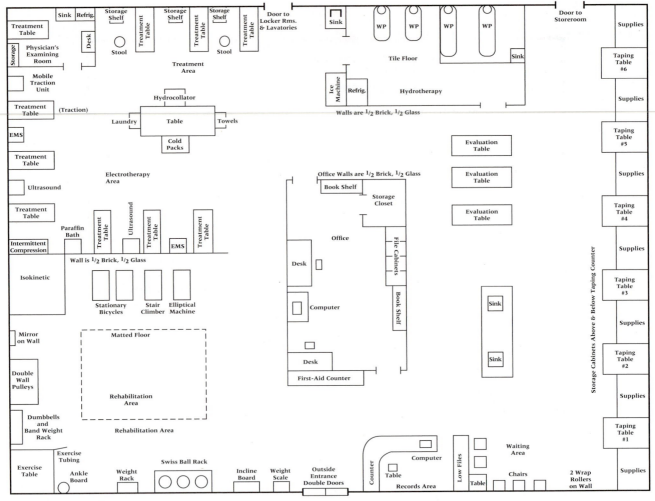

A

FIGURE 2–1　The ideal athletic training clinic should be well designed to maximize its use. A, Larger athletic training clinic at a college or university.

Continued

of supervision for the head athletic trainer" defines supervisory models.[35]

- Performance evaluations should be done at regularly scheduled intervals to analyze the quality of the work being performed. Evaluations should focus first on the positive aspects of job performance and then on any weaknesses.[23]

Each of these policies relative to personnel issues should be included in the policies and procedures manual.

Designing an Athletic Training Clinic

Maximizing the use of facilities and effectively using equipment and supplies are essential to the function of any athletic program.[34] The athletic training clinic must be designed to meet the many requirements of the athletic training program (Figure 2–1).[29,37] The size and layout of the athletic training clinic will depend on the scope of the athletic training program, including the size and number of teams and athletes and what sports are offered.[31] The clinical setting has a much broader patient population than a secondary-school or university program, and thus the requirements for equipment and supplies are somewhat different.[29] To accommodate the various functions of an athletic training program, the athletic training clinic must serve as a health care center for athletes.[10]

> The athletic training clinic is a multipurpose area used for first aid, therapy and rehabilitation, injury prevention, medical procedures (such as physical examinations), and athletic training administration.

Size　The size of the athletic training clinic can range anywhere from a large storage closet in some secondary schools to 15,000 + square-foot (1,394 sq. m) sports medicine complexes in some universities. Certainly, the size of the clinic can have a major impact on how the athletic training program is managed. But the most important consideration is to

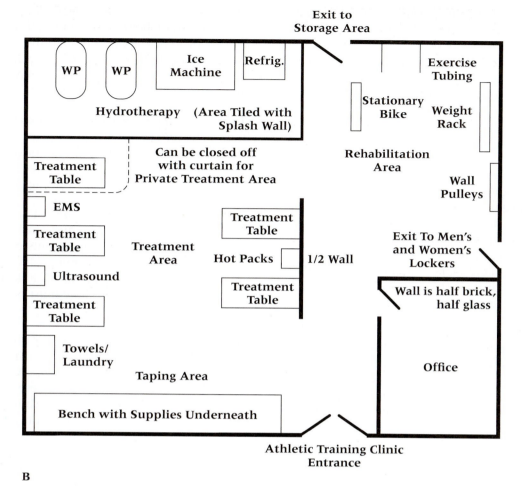

B

FIGURE 2–1 **continued,** Small athletic training clinic at a high school.

organize the athletic training program in a manner that most efficiently takes advantage of the space available. When designing a new athletic training clinic, the athletic trainer should work closely with design architects to communicate the specific needs of the institution and the number of athletes who will be served.[36]

Location The athletic training clinic should have an outside entrance from the athletic field or court. This arrangement makes it unnecessary to take injured athletes in through the building and possibly through several doors; it also permits access when the rest of the building is not in use. A double door at each entrance is preferable to allow easy passage of a wheelchair or a stretcher. A ramp at the outside entrance is safer and far more functional than are stairs.

The athletic training clinic should be near the locker rooms if possible, so that showers are readily available to athletes going in for treatment following practice. Toilet facilities should be located adjacent to the athletic training clinic and should be readily accessible through a door in the athletic training clinic.

Because the athletic training clinic is where emergency treatment is given, its light, heat, and water sources should be independent from those for the rest of the building.

Illumination The athletic training clinic should be well lighted throughout. Lighting should be planned with the advice of a technical lighting engineer. Obviously, certain areas need to be better lit than others. For example, the wound care and taping areas need better lighting than is necessary in the rehabilitation area. Ceilings and walls act as reflective surfaces to help provide an equitable distribution and balance of light. Natural lighting through windows or skylights can be helpful.

Special Service Areas Apart from the storage and office space, a portion of the athletic training clinic should be divided into special sections, preferably by half walls or partial glass walls. Space, however, may not permit a separate area for each service section, and an overlapping of functions may be required.

Treatment Area The treatment area should include a minimum of four treatment tables, preferably of adjustable height, that can be used during the application of ice packs or hydrocollator packs or for manual therapy techniques, such as massage, mobilization, or proprioceptive neuromuscular facilitation (PNF). Three or four adjustable stools on rollers should also be readily available. The hydrocollator unit and ice bags should be easily accessible to this area.

Electrotherapy Area The electrotherapy area is used for treatment by ultrasound, diathermy, or electrical stimulating units. Equipment should include at least two treatment tables, several wooden chairs, one or two dispensing tables for holding supplies, shelves, and a storage cabinet for supplies and equipment. The area should contain a sufficient number of grounded outlets, preferably in the walls and several feet above the floor. It is advisable to place rubber mats or runners on each side of the treatment tables as a precautionary measure. This area must be under supervision at all times, and the storage cabinet should be kept locked when not in use.

Hydrotherapy Area In the hydrotherapy area, the floor should slope toward a centrally located drain to prevent standing water. Equipment should include two or three whirlpool baths (one permitting complete immersion of the body), several lavatories, and storage shelves. Because some of this equipment is electrically operated, many precautions must be taken. All electrical outlets should be placed 4 to 5 feet (1.2 to 1.5 m) above the floor and should have spring-locked covers and water spray deflectors. All cords and wires must be kept clear of the floor to eliminate any possibility of electrical shock. To prevent water from entering the other areas, a slightly raised, rounded curb should be built at the entrance to the area. When an athletic training clinic is planned, ample outlets must be provided; under no circumstances should two or more devices be operated from the same outlet. All outlets must be properly grounded using ground fault interrupters (GFIs).[28]

Exercise Rehabilitation Area Ideally, an athletic training clinic should accommodate injury reconditioning under the strict supervision of the athletic trainer. Selected pieces of resistance equipment should be made available. Depending on the existing space, dumbbells and free weights; exercise machines for knee, ankle, shoulder, hip, and so forth; isokinetic equipment; devices for balance and proprioception; and space for using exercise tubing may all be available for use.

Taping, Bandaging, and Orthotics Area Each athletic training clinic should provide a place in which taping, bandaging, and applying orthotic devices can be executed. This area should have three or four taping tables adjacent to a sink and a storage cabinet.

Physician's Examination Room In most colleges and universities, the team physician has a room in which examinations and treatments may be given. This room contains an examining table, a sink, locking storage cabinets, and a small desk with a telephone. At all times, this clinic must be kept locked to outsiders.

Records Area Some space, either in the office or at the entrance to the athletic training clinic, should be devoted to record keeping. Record-keeping facilities range from a filing system to a more sophisticated computer-based system. Records should be accessible to sports medicine personnel only.

Storage Facilities Many athletic training clinics lack ample storage space. Often, storage facilities are located a considerable distance away, which is extremely inconvenient. In addition to the storage cabinets and shelves provided in each of the three special service areas, a small storage closet should be placed in the athletic trainer's office. All these cabinets should be used for the storage of general supplies as well as for the small, specialized equipment used in the respective areas. A large walk-in closet, 80 to 100 square feet (7.4 to 9.3 sq. m) in area, is a necessity for the storage of bulky equipment, medical supplies, adhesive tape, bandages, and protective devices (Figure 2–2). A refrigerator for the storage of frozen water in styrofoam cups for ice massage and other necessities is also an important piece of equipment. In small sports programs, a large refrigerator is probably sufficient for all ice needs. If at all possible, an ice-making

> It is essential to have adequate storage space available for supplies and equipment.

A clinical athletic trainer is approached by the community recreation department with a request to use the clinic to treat its community-based recreational football and basketball league participants who are injured.

? How should the athletic trainer deal with this request?

2–4 Clinical Application Exercise

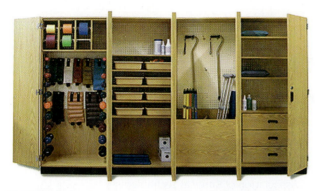

FIGURE 2–2 An effective athletic training program must have appropriate storage facilities that are highly organized. (Courtesy Thera-Wall)

machine should be installed in an auxiliary area to provide an ample and continuous supply of ice for treatment purposes.

There should also be storage spaces provided for patients in which to place their belongings (e.g., book bags, clothes) while they are being treated.

Athletic Trainer's Office A space at least 10 feet by 12 feet (3 by 3.6 m) is ample for the athletic trainer's office. The office should be located so that all areas of the athletic training clinic can be well supervised without the athletic trainer having to leave the office. Glass partitions on two sides permit the athletic trainer to observe all activities even while seated at the desk. A desk, a computer chair, a tackboard for clippings and other information, telephones, and a record file are the basic equipment. The office should have an independent lock-and-key system so that it is accessible only to authorized personnel.

Additional Areas If space is available, several other areas could be included as part of an athletic training clinic.

Pharmacy Area A separate room that can be secured for storing and administering medications is helpful. All medications, including over-the-counter drugs, should be kept under lock and key. If prescription medications are kept in the athletic training clinic, only the team physician or pharmacist from a campus health center should have access to the storage cabinet. Records for administering medications to patients should be kept in this area. It is essential to adhere to state regulations regarding the storage and administration of medications (see Chapter 17).

Rehabilitation Pool If the clinic has the space and the institution can afford one, a pool can be an extremely useful rehabilitation tool. The pool should be accessible to individuals with various types of injuries. It should have a graduated depth to at least 7 feet (2.1 m), the deck should have a nonslip surface, and the filter system should be in a separate room.[33]

Restrooms There should be at least one restroom available in the athletic training clinic. Requirements for the number of restrooms are usually dictated by the occupancy limits assigned to that facility.

ISSUES SPECIFIC TO ATHLETIC TRAINING PROGRAM OPERATION IN THE CLINIC, HOSPITAL, CORPORATE, OR INDUSTRIAL SETTING

As is the case for those working in secondary schools and colleges or universities, athletic trainers working in clinical, hospital, corporate, and industrial settings must be competent in preventing and recognizing injuries and supervising injury rehabilitation programs. However, staff athletic trainers working in these settings treat and rehabilitate a wider range of patients in terms of age and physical condition. The athletic trainer may provide care to pediatric, adolescent, young adult, adult, and geriatric patients. The patients have physical ailments that may or may not be related to physical activity. In addition, athletic trainers who work in clinical, corporate, or industrial facilities may find themselves in the role of an entrepreneur who owns a clinic facility or practice; an administrator who oversees the day-to-day operations; a marketing director; or a community outreach coordinator. They must also be knowledgeable regarding administrative and management skills, marketing, fiscal responsibilities, reimbursement, documentation, and outcomes assessment.[23]

Scope of Practice

Athletic trainers who work in a clinic or in a hospital or an ambulatory care center will likely see a patient population that is diverse not only in age but also in the variety of injuries, illnesses, and conditions. Athletic trainers in hospitals may be involved in inpatient, outpatient, or ambulatory care.

For the most part, the owner of an outpatient clinic or its chief administrator will dictate the patient population that the clinic will treat (i.e., orthopedic, sports, occupational, cardiac, etc.). Athletic trainers working in either a privately owned clinic or a corporate/industrial setting may be involved in individual patient care, working in on-site employee fitness centers, working in ergonomic and occupational work hardening safety programs, supervising employee drug-testing programs, overseeing wellness programs, or overseeing and engaging in outreach programs and athletic event coverage, which essentially helps market the clinic to the community.

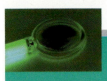

Additional certifications for athletic trainers working in a clinic or hospital

Certification	Association/Organization
Orthopedic technologist (OT)	National Association of Orthopedic Technologists
Orthotics and prosthetics (ABC)	American Board for Certification in Orthotics and Prosthetics
Certified surgical technologist (CST)	Association of Surgical Technologists
Certified professional ergonomist (CPE)	Board of Certification for Professional Ergonomists
Certified strength and conditioning specialist (CSCS)	National Strength and Conditioning Association
Performance enhancement specialist (PES)	National Academy of Sports Medicine
Corrective exercise specialist (CES)	National Academy of Sports Medicine
Certified clinical research associate (CRA)	Association of Clinical Research Professionals

Regardless of the setting, limitations and restrictions on what an athletic trainer can do and who can be treated are in large part determined by the regulatory statutes governing professional practice in individual states. It is the responsibility of both the administrator and the athletic trainer to know the limits of practice.

Location of the Clinic Because most privately owned clinics are in business to make a profit, it is essential to build a patient base. Certainly, the location of the facility is a key to attracting patients and making it a successful business.[29] Several other factors may determine whether the chosen location is good:

- What are the zoning laws in the area?
- Is there any type of traffic problem that would create an accessibility issue for potential patients?
- Are there doctors in the area who will refer patients to this clinic?
- Will these doctors use an athletic trainer to treat their patients?
- Are there businesses in the area for which this clinic could provide industrial rehabilitation or on-site workplace assessment?
- Are there schools in the area that could use sports medicine coverage by an athletic trainer?
- Are there any other clinics or hospitals that provide similar services that may directly or indirectly compete with the new business?

Hours of Operation To most effectively meet the scheduling needs of potential patients, the clinic must be open at times that do not conflict with normal working hours. This means that the clinic must be open early in the morning and remain open at least into the early evening, so patients can get to the facility either before or immediately after work. Also, it is important to maintain hours of operation at least one day over the weekend.[29]

Clinic Personnel and Human Resources Issues

The athletic trainer must work with a number of different health care providers in the clinical or corporate setting, including physicians, physician's assistants, physical therapists, physical therapy assistants, occupational therapists, occupational therapy assistants, nutritionists, and nurses. Additionally, if the clinic is in a hospital, respiratory therapists, speech therapists, recreational therapists, and pharmacists may also be involved in patient care. Each of these individuals should have a formal, specific job description developed by human resources personnel. The most effective treatment models seem to involve a team approach and require communication and cooperation on the part of all involved in providing some aspect of health care.

Athletic trainers who work in a clinical or hospital setting may seek additional certifications that can expand the scope of their roles and responsibilities. *Focus Box 2–4: "Additional certifications for athletic trainers working in a clinic or hospital"* lists those certifications.

Potential Athletic Training Duties

Ergonomic Assessment Ergonomics is the science of designing products, machines, and systems to maximize the comfort, efficiency, and safety of the people who use them.[47] Ergonomics is based on the principles of anthropometry (the science of human measurement) and biomechanics (the study of muscular activity) applied to industrial engineering to adapt or alter the design of products and workplaces to an individual's physical strengths, limitations, size, and shape.

One of the primary goals of ergonomics is the prevention of accidents and injuries in the workplace by attempting to minimize risk factors, such as repetition, vibration, force, and awkward/static postures as they relate to musculoskeletal disorders.[47] Ergonomists work to eliminate these problems by designing workplaces, such as assembly lines, computer workstations and to prevent injuries. They position machinery and tools to be accessible without twisting, reaching, or bending. They design adjustable desks, chairs, and workbenches to comfortably accommodate workers of many different sizes, preventing the need to continuously lean or overextend the arms.

An athletic trainer may work with an occupational therapist or an ergonomist to provide an ergonomic assessment, an evaluation of a workstation and the physical environment and its interaction with the employee.[41] This assessment involves not only adjusting and making recommendations regarding the employee's workstation but also providing instruction on injury prevention techniques, including suitable stretches, strengthening exercises, and suggested rest breaks. An ergonomic assessment report outlines the results of the assessment and is forwarded to the injured employee, workplace manager or administrator, medical practitioner, and other involved parties.[47] A follow-up review may be conducted to ensure that the recommendations have been implemented (Figure 2–3).

Work Hardening/Conditioning Programs Athletic trainers may supervise or participate in work hardening or conditioning programs that involve intensive outpatient therapy for individuals injured on the job. The goal is to regain functionality and return to work in a full-duty capacity. The starting point for these patients is a musculoskeletal evaluation of their strength, posture, flexibility, gait, sensation, and reflexes.[41] This is followed by a functional capacity evaluation to determine skill deficits as measured against physical job requirements. The following skills may be evaluated in a functional capacity evaluation:[41]

- Tolerance for prolonged sitting and standing
- Hand grip strength and coordination
- Repetitive lifting capacity at various levels
- Repetitive push, pull, and carrying capacities
- Repetitive squat
- Prolonged trunk flexion or rotation in sitting and standing
- Prolonged crawling, kneeling, and crouch positions
- Maximum walking, stairs, and stepladder capacity
- Balance

The athletic trainer then discusses the results and recommendations of these evaluations with the patient. This collective information is used to develop a rehabilitation plan to allow the patient to return to work at the appropriate level of performance.

Work conditioning refers to intensive rehabilitation offered 3 hours a day for 3 days a week, whereas *work hardening* refers to intensive therapy offered 8 hours a day for 5 days a week. Treatments may involve simulated work, education about avoiding reinjury, and job site analysis to assist the employer in making appropriate equipment modifications for an employee returning to work after an injury (Figure 2–4).

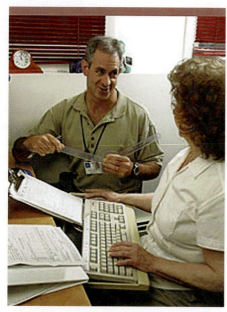

FIGURE 2–3   Ergonomic assessment.

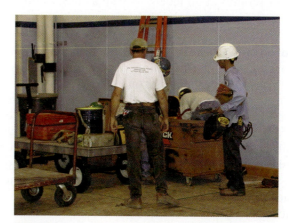

FIGURE 2–4   Work hardening.

Wellness Center Athletic trainers may supervise a wellness center and assume responsibility for organizing wellness screenings, workshops, and employee health fairs. Worksite health screenings may be offered for asthma, hypertension, diabetes, cholesterol, osteoporosis, prostate cancer, skin cancer, glaucoma, and stroke. Early detection can save both the employees and a company the emotional and financial costs of medical conditions that have advanced because they went undetected. Results may be given directly to employees or sent to their homes with a detailed explanation.

Wellness workshops raise employees' awareness about their health, help them understand their susceptibility to disease, and motivate them to seek medical consultation or make important changes that will reduce their risks and enhance the quality of their lives. Workshop topics might include nutrition, men's health, women's health, skin care, fitness and exercise, family and personal development, and workplace health and safety.

Health fairs are an effective and enjoyable means of educating employees about various health issues. In addition to offering multiple screening services at various booths, employees can obtain health education materials at information tables while learning from and interacting with health professionals.

Community Outreach and Marketing When employed by some clinics or occasionally a hospital, athletic trainers may see patients or have other in-house responsibilities during part of the day. But in the afternoons or evenings they may be assigned to provide athletic training coverage for an athletic program at a local secondary school or small college. They may also cover single athletic events in the community. These outreach programs not only provide a valuable service to athletes in the community but also serve as an effective marketing tool to promote and advertise the clinic. This marketing strategy helps provide visibility for the clinic to physicians, other health care providers, parents, and other schools at all levels, as well as other potential patients from throughout the community.

Corporate Fitness Programs Athletic trainers working in corporate settings are commonly charged with the responsibility of overseeing in-house employee fitness programs.[24] Physical fitness offers a variety of proven health benefits, including a decreased risk of heart disease and heart attack. Physically fit employees can also handle physical work tasks better and deal with stressful situations more easily, and they tend to be less susceptible to illness and injuries. Corporations offer fitness programs to their employees to reduce health costs, increase productivity, reduce absenteeism, decrease turnover,

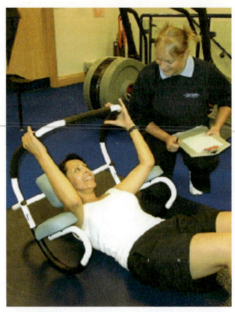

FIGURE 2–5 A corporate fitness program.

improve morale, lower health care expenditures, and reduce sick leave (Figure 2–5).

After an initial consultation, the athletic trainer administers fitness evaluations for all participating employees to determine their baseline fitness levels for cardiorespiratory endurance, body composition, flexibility, muscle strength, and endurance. Based on information from the initial consultation and fitness evaluation, an individual exercise prescription may be developed for each participating employee. Typical exercise sessions may include warm-up activities, aerobic conditioning, strength training, flexibility exercises, and cool-down. Training sessions should teach safe, effective exercise techniques and educate employees on training intensity, frequency, and progression to maximize results and reduce injuries. By following these guidelines, employees can meet their fitness goals, while the corporation benefits from a healthier workforce.[26]

Drug-Testing Programs An athletic trainer working in a corporate or a clinic setting may be asked to oversee a drug-testing program for employees. A drug-testing program can deter employees from coming to work unfit for duty. It also discourages drug abusers from applying to a company in the first place. A corporation may require a full-service testing program to comply with federal requirements or a simple preemployment screening program. Legal defensibility is the most important aspect of any drug-testing program. The corporation should use federally certified laboratories and confirm and verify all positive results through a medical review department.

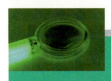

FOCUS 2-5 Focus on Organizational and Professional Health and Well-Being

Information contained in medical records

Medical History

Family history
Social history
Habits
Immunization history
Growth chart and developmental history
Substance abuse inquiry
   Surgical history
   Obstetric history

Medical Encounters

Chief complaint
History of the present illness
   Complete physical examination
   Assessment and plan

Orders and Prescriptions

Progress Notes

Results of Previous Diagnostic Tests

Fiscal Management

When an athletic trainer is employed by a for-profit business, such as a clinic or a hospital, he or she must have some understanding of basic business practices and fiscal management.[35] Certainly, if the athletic trainer is an administrator or an owner of a clinic, it is even more critical to understand how to run a profitable business.

For the most part in the health care industry, businesses rely on billing a patient's insurance company and being reimbursed for services provided to that patient. Third-party reimbursement and issues with managed care are discussed in detail in Chapter 3. Maintaining a positive accounts payable to accounts receivable (AP/AR) ratio, in which more money is being collected than must be paid out in expenses, is the goal of every successful business. Other responsibilities include financial planning, which assesses the goals and objectives of the company; establishing contractual obligations with payors and providers; developing an efficient billing and collection system; formulating a budget, which requires the coordination of resources and expenditures; and deciding on expenditures for necessary equipment and supplies.

RECORD KEEPING

Record keeping is a major responsibility of the athletic trainer. Some athletic trainers object to keeping records and filling out forms, stating that they have neither the time nor the inclination to be bookkeepers. Nevertheless, because lawsuits are the rule rather than the exception, accurate and up-to-date records are an absolute necessity. Medical records are also critical for accurate and

> **Keeping adequate records is critical for any athletic trainer.**

timely assessment and evaluation of practices and for documentation of practices and activities to ensure that responsibilities and expectations are being met. *Focus Box 2-5* lists the type of information usually found in standard medical records. Medical records, injury reports, treatment logs, personal information cards, injury evaluations and progress notes, supply and equipment inventories, and annual reports are essential records that should be maintained by the athletic trainer.

Electronic Versus Paper Medical Records

Paper records are still the most common method for recording and maintaining patient information in health care. However, the transition to electronic medical records is rapidly occurring. Compared to digital records, paper records and imaging films require a significant amount of storage space. This can become problematic because in most states medical records are required to be maintained for at least 7 years. Additionally, if paper records on the same individual are stored in different places, collating them in a central location may prove to be a difficult task. Electronic medical records can certainly simplify the process for any health care provider who may need to review a complete medical record for an individual patient eliminating the need for faxing, copying, and transporting these records between facilities. It seems fairly clear that using electronic medical records improves overall efficiency, reduces errors, and reduces costs. The downside to using electronic medical records is that the improved portability and accessibility creates security issues that threaten patient privacy. Nevertheless, in the not too distant future, electronic medical records will be routinely used by all healthcare practitioners regardless of the setting where they practice.

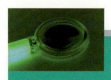

Patient files management

The athletic trainer should look for the following features when using a patient file management system:
- A forms engine that replaces paper forms
- Effective document organization that looks like paper document files
- Security features that control access and user rights on documents
- Multitask features to access and use several patient charts simultaneously
- Ability to name and classify documents with templates
- A user-friendly interface to optimize usability

Patient File Management Systems

Effective management of patient records and supporting documents is a critical factor in the efficiency of operation an athletic training program. Optimally, athletic trainers should use some type of comprehensive patient-file management system for appropriate chart documentation, risk management, outcomes, and billing. *Focus Box 2-6:* "Patient Files Management" lists the advantages that come from using document management systems.

Maintaining Confidentiality in Record Keeping

Release of Medical Records The athletic trainer may not release a patient's medical records to anyone without written consent. If the patient wishes to have medical records released to professional sports organizations, insurance companies, the news media, or any other group or individual, the athlete must sign a waiver that specifies which information is to be released. The only exception to this is the appropriate disclosure of information among those professionals who are involved in providing health care to the injured individual.

Health Insurance Portability and Accountability Act (HIPAA) The Health Insurance Portability and Accountability Act (HIPAA) regulates how athletic trainers, physicians, administrators, and other allied health personnel with private health information (PHI) about patients can share that information with others.[19] The regulation guarantees that patients have access to their medical records, gives them more control over how their protected health information is used and disclosed, and provides a clear avenue of recourse if their medical privacy is compromised.[30] Authorization by a patient to release medical information is not necessary on a per-injury basis.[18] A written blanket authorization signed by the patient at the beginning of the year will suffice for all injuries and treatments during the course of participation

for that year. These one-time, blanket authorizations must indicate what information may be released, to whom, and for what length of time.[18] *Focus Box 2–7:* "HIPAA authorization" is a list of core elements that must be present for the authorization to be valid.

Family Educational Rights and Privacy Act (FERPA) The Family Educational Rights and Privacy Act (FERPA) protects the privacy of student educational records. It has been suggested that in some instances medical records should be kept along with a student's educational records; thus, the right to privacy of medical records would be protected under FERPA instead of HIPAA.[19] FERPA gives parents certain rights with respect to their children's educational records. These rights transfer to the student when he or she reaches the age of 18 or attends a school beyond the high-school level. Students to whom the rights have been transferred are "eligible students." Parents and eligible students have the right to inspect and review the student's educational records maintained by the school. Parents and eligible students have the right to request that a school correct records that they believe to be inaccurate or misleading. Schools must have written permission from the parent or eligible student to release any information from a student's educational records.

Administering Preparticipation Examinations

The first piece of information that the athletic trainer should collect on each athlete is obtained from an initial preparticipation examination before the start of practice.[22] The primary purpose of the preparticipation exam is to identify an

Preparticipation health examination:
- Medical history
- Physical examination
- Cardiovascular screening
- Maturity assessment
- Orthopedic screening
- Wellness screening

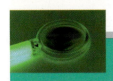
HIPAA authorization

Following is a list of core elements that must be present for a disclosure authorization to be valid:

- A description of the information to be used or disclosed
- Identification of the persons or class of persons authorized to make use of or disclosure of the protected health information
- Identification of the persons or class of persons to whom the covered entity is authorized to provide or disclose information

- A description of each purpose of the use or disclosure
- An expiration date or event
- The individual's signature and date
- If signed by a personal representative, a description of his or her authority to act for the individual

---

athlete who may be at risk before he or she participates in a specific sport.[1] The preparticipation examination should consist of a medical history, a physical examination, a cardiovascular screening, a maturity assessment, a brief orthopedic screening, and, in some situations, a wellness screening.[32] Information obtained during this examination establishes a baseline to which comparisons may be made after injury. It may also reveal conditions that could warrant disqualification from certain sports.[22] The examination also satisfies insurance and liability issues. The preparticipation exam may be administered on an individual basis by a personal physician, or it may be done using a station examination system with a team of examiners.[45]

Examination by a personal physician has the advantage of yielding an in-depth history and an ideal physician-patient relationship. A disadvantage of this type of examination is that it may not be directed to the detection of the factors that predispose the athlete to a sports injury.[6]

The most thorough and sport-specific type of preparticipation examination is the station examination.[6] This method can provide the athlete with a detailed examination in a short period of time. A team of nine people is needed to examine 30 or more athletes. The team should include two physicians, two medically trained nonphysicians (nurse, athletic trainer, physical therapist, or physician's assistant), and five managers, athletic training students, or assistant coaches (Table 2–1).[6]

Medical History A medical history form should be completed before the physical examination and orthopedic screening; its purpose is to identify any past or existing medical problems.[1] This form should be updated for each individual every year. Medical histories should be closely reviewed by both the physician and the athletic trainer, so that personnel can be prepared, should a medical emergency arise. Necessary participation release forms and insurance information should be collected along with the medical history (Figure 2–6).[25]

Physical Examination The physical examination should include an assessment of height, weight, body composition, blood pressure, pulse, vision, skin, teeth, ear, nose, throat, heart and lung function, abdomen, lymphatics, genitalia (males only), maturation index, urinalysis, and blood work (Figure 2–7).[25]

Cardiovascular Screening In 1996, the American Heart Association (AHA) published recommendations concerning the cardiovascular component of the preparticipation exam in competitive athletes.[40] The critical task of

---

2-5 Clinical Application Exercise

A sports medicine clinic has agreed to organize and conduct preparticipation exams for All-American High School, which offers 18 sports—6 in the fall, 6 in the winter, and 6 in the spring. There are a total of approximately 500 athletes, and approximately 200 of them are involved in the fall sports. The athletic trainer who works in the clinic is charged with arranging and administering preparticipation examinations so that each athlete can be cleared for competition.

❓ How can the athletic trainer most efficiently set up the preparticipation exams to clear 200 athletes for competition in the fall sports?

Potentially lethal cardiovascular conditions:

- Hypertrophic cardiomyopathy
- Aortic stenosis
- Marfan's syndrome

TABLE 2-1	Suggested Components of a Preparticipation Physical Examination	
Station	**Points Noted**	**Personnel**
1. Individual history (reviewed); height, weight, body composition, body mass index (BMI)	"Yes" answers are probed in depth; height and weight relationships	Physician, nurse, or athletic trainer
2. Snellen test, vision	Upper limits of visual acuity—20/40	Athletic training student
3. Oral (mouth), ears, nose, throat	Dental prosthesis or caries; abnormalities of the ears, nose, throat	Physician, nurse, or athletic trainer
4. Chest, heart, lungs	Heart abnormalities, blood pressure, pulse, murmurs, clarity of lungs	Physician
5. Abdomen	Masses, tenderness, organomegaly	Physician or physician's assistant
6. Genitalia (male only)	Abnormalities of genitalia, hernia	Physician or physician's assistant
7. Skin	Suspicious rashes or lesions	Physician or physician's assistant
8. Musculoskeletal	Postural asymmetry, decreased range of motion or strength, abnormal joint laxity	Physician, athletic trainer, or nurse practitioner
9. Urinalysis	Lab test for sugar and protein	Athletic training student or manager
10. Blood work	Lab test to determine hematocrit	Nurse or physician
Review	History and physical examination reports are evaluated and the following decisions are made: (a) No sports participation (b) Limited participation (no participation in specific sports, such as football or ice hockey) (c) Clearance withheld until certain conditions are met (e.g., additional tests taken, rehabilitation completed) (d) Full, unlimited participation allowed	Physician and athletic trainer

the preparticipation cardiac examination is identifying life-threatening conditions. Although the cardiac examination need not involve complex tests, it must permit the recognition of abnormal heart sounds and other signs of pathology.

The vast majority of exams are negative, but the physician should be alert to such potentially lethal conditions as hypertrophic cardiomyopathy, aortic stenosis, and Marfan's syndrome. A history of symptoms during exertion, certain features of physical appearance, and clinical findings require referral to a cardiologist.[40]

Maturity Assessment Maturity assessment should be part of the physical examination as a means of protecting the young, physically developing athlete.[27] The most commonly used methods are circumpubertal (sexual maturity), skeletal, and dental assessments. Of the three, Tanner's five stages of maturity assessment, indicating the maturity of secondary sexual characteristics, is the most expedient for use in the station method of examination.[44] The Tanner approach evaluates pubic hair and genitalia development in boys and pubic hair and breast development in girls (Figure 2–8). Other indicators are facial and axillary hair. Stage 1 indicates that puberty is not evident, and stage 5 indicates full development. The crucial stage in terms of collision and high-intensity noncontact sports is stage 3, in which the fastest bone growth occurs. In this stage, the growth plates are two to five times weaker than the joint capsule and tendon attachments.[26] Young athletes in grades 7 through 12 must be matched by maturity, not age.[44]

Orthopedic Screening Orthopedic screening may be done as part of the physical examination or separately by the athletic trainer. A quick orthopedic

DATE OF EXAM_____

Name_____	Sex_____ Age_____ Date of birth_____
Grade____ School_____ Sport(s)_____	
Address_____ Phone_____	
Personal physician_____	

In case of emergency, contact

Name_____ Relationship_____ Phone (H)_____ (W)_____

Explain "Yes" answers below.
Circle questions you don't know the answers to.

	Yes	No
1. Has a doctor ever denied or restricted your participation in sports for any reason?	☐	☐
2. Do you have an ongoing medical condition (like diabetes or asthma)?	☐	☐
3. Are you currently taking any prescription or nonprescription (over-the-counter) medicine or pills?	☐	☐
4. Do you have allergies to medicines, pollens, foods, or stinging insects?	☐	☐
5. Have you ever passed out or nearly passed out DURING exercise?	☐	☐
6. Have you ever passed out or nearly passed out AFTER exercise?	☐	☐
7. Have you ever had discomfort, pain, or pressure in your chest during exercise?	☐	☐
8. Does your heart race or skip beats during exercise?	☐	☐
9. Has a doctor ever told you that you have (check all that apply):		

☐ High blood pressure ☐ A heart murmur
☐ High cholesterol ☐ A heart infection

	Yes	No
10. Has a doctor ever ordered a test for your heart? (for example, ECG, echocardiogram)	☐	☐
11. Has anyone in your family died for no apparent reason?	☐	☐
12. Does anyone in your family have a heart problem?	☐	☐
13. Has any family member or relative died of heart problems or of sudden death before age 50?	☐	☐
14. Does anyone in your family have Marfan syndrome?	☐	☐
15. Have you ever spent the night in a hospital?	☐	☐
16. Have you ever had surgery?	☐	☐

	Yes	No
17. Have you ever had an injury, like a sprain, muscle or ligament tear, or tendonitis, that caused you to miss a practice or game? If yes, circle affected area below:	☐	☐
18. Have you had any broken or fractured bones or dislocated joints? If yes, circle below:	☐	☐
19. Have you had a bone or joint injury that required x-rays, MRI, CT, surgery, injections, rehabilitation, physical therapy, a brace, a cast, or crutches? If yes, circle below:	☐	☐

Head	Neck	Shoulder	Upper arm	Elbow	Forearm	Hand/fingers	Chest
Upper back	Lower back	Hip	Thigh	Knee	Calf/shin	Ankle	Foot/toes

	Yes	No
20. Have you ever had a stress fracture?	☐	☐
21. Have you been told that you have or have you had an x-ray for atlantoaxial (neck) instability?	☐	☐
22. Do you regularly use a brace or assistive device?	☐	☐
23. Has a doctor ever told you that you have asthma or allergies?	☐	☐

	Yes	No
24. Do you cough, wheeze, or have difficulty breathing during or after exercise?	☐	☐
25. Is there anyone in your family who has asthma?	☐	☐
26. Have you ever used an inhaler or taken asthma medicine?	☐	☐
27. Were you born without or are you missing a kidney, an eye, a testicle, or any other organ?	☐	☐
28. Have you had infectious mononucleosis (mono) within the last month?	☐	☐
29. Do you have any rashes, pressure sores, or other skin problems?	☐	☐
30. Have you had a herpes skin infection?	☐	☐
31. Have you ever had a head injury or concussion?	☐	☐
32. Have you been hit in the head and been confused or lost your memory?	☐	☐
33. Have you ever had a seizure?	☐	☐
34. Do you have headaches with exercise?	☐	☐
35. Have you ever had numbness, tingling, or weakness in your arms or legs after being hit or falling?	☐	☐
36. Have you ever been unable to move your arms or legs after being hit or falling?	☐	☐
37. When exercising in the heat, do you have severe muscle cramps or become ill?	☐	☐
38. Has a doctor told you that you or someone in your family has sickle cell trait or sickle cell disease?	☐	☐
39. Have you had any problems with your eyes or vision?	☐	☐
40. Do you wear glasses or contact lenses?	☐	☐
41. Do you wear protective eyewear, such as goggles or a face shield?	☐	☐
42. Are you happy with your weight?	☐	☐
43. Are you trying to gain or lose weight?	☐	☐
44. Has anyone recommended you change your weight or eating habits?	☐	☐
45. Do you limit or carefully control what you eat?	☐	☐
46. Do you have any concerns that you would like to discuss with a doctor?	☐	☐

FEMALES ONLY

	Yes	No
47. Have you ever had a menstrual period?	☐	☐

48. How old were you when you had your first menstrual period? _____
49. How many periods have you had in the last 12 months? _____

Explain "Yes" answers here: _____

_____

_____

_____

_____

_____

_____

_____

I hereby state that, to the best of my knowledge, my answers to the above questions are complete and correct.

Signature of athlete_____ Signature of parent/guardian_____ Date_____

Used with permission from ©2004 American Academy of Family Physicians, American Academy of Pediatrics, American College of Sports Medicine, American Medical Society for Sports Medicine, American Orthopedic Society for Sports Medicine, and American Osteopathic Academy of Sports Medicine.

FIGURE 2–6 Sample medical history form.

PHYSICAL EXAMINATION FORM

Name _____ Date of birth _____

Grade _____ Weight _____ % Body fat (optional) _____ Pulse _____ BP ___/_____ (___/____, ___/____)

Vision R 20 /_____ L 20 /_____   Corrected: Y N   Pupils: Equal _____ Unequal _____

Follow-Up Questions on More Sensitive Issues	Yes	No
1. Do you feel stressed out or under a lot of pressure?	☐	☐
2. Do you ever feel so sad or hopeless that you stop doing some of your usual activities for more than a few days?	☐	☐
3. Do you feel safe?	☐	☐
4. Have you ever tried cigarette smoking, even 1 or 2 puffs? Do you currently smoke?	☐	☐
5. During the past 30 days, did you use chewing tobacco, snuff, or dip?	☐	☐
6. During the past 30 days, have you had at least 1 drink of alcohol?	☐	☐
7. Have you ever taken steroid pills or shots without a doctor's prescription?	☐	☐
8. Have you ever taken any supplements to help you gain or lose weight or improve your performance?	☐	☐
9. Questions from the Youth Risk Behavior Survey (http://www.cdc.gov/HealthyYouth/yrbs/index.htm) on guns, seatbelts, unprotected sex, domestic violence, drugs, etc.	☐	☐

Notes: _____
_____
_____

	NORMAL	ABNORMAL FINDINGS	INITIALS*
MEDICAL			
Appearance			
Eyes/ears/nose/throat			
Hearing			
Lymph nodes			
Heart			
Murmurs			
Pulses			
Lungs			
Abdomen			
Genitourinary (males only)†			
Skin			
MUSCULOSKELETAL			
Neck			
Back			
Shoulder/arm			
Elbow/forearm			
Wrist/hand/fingers			
Hip/thigh			
Knee			
Leg/ankle			
Foot/toes			

*Multiple-examiner set-up only.
†Having a third party present is recommended for the genitourinary examination.

Notes: _____
_____

Name of physician (print/type) _____ Date _____

Address _____ Phone _____

Signature of physician _____, MD or DO

Used with permission from ©2004 American Academy of Family Physicians, American Academy of Pediatrics, American College of Sports Medicine, American Medical Society for Sports Medicine, American Orthopedic Society for Sports Medicine, and American Osteopathic Academy of Sports Medicine.

FIGURE 2–7 Sample physical examination form.

Males

Stage 1. **No evidence of pubic hair.**
Stage 2. **Slightly pigmented hair laterally at the base of the penis. Usually straight.**
Stage 3. **Hair becomes darker and coarser, begins to curl, and spreads over the pubic region.**
Stage 4. **Hair is adult in type but does not extend onto thighs.**
Stage 5. **Hair extends onto the thighs and frequently up the linea alba.**

Females

Stage 1. **No evidence of pubic hair.**
Stage 2. **Long, slightly pigmented, downy hair along the edges of the labia.**
Stage 3. **Darker, coarser, slightly curled hair spread sparsely over the mons pubis.**
Stage 4. **Adult type of hair but it does not extend onto thighs.**
Stage 5. **Adult distribution, including spread along the medial aspects of the thighs.**

FIGURE 2–8   Tanner's five stages of maturity.[44]

Orthopedic Screening Examination

Activity and Instruction	To Determine
Stand facing examiner	Acromioclavicular joints; general habitus
Look at ceiling, floor, over both shoulders; touch ears to shoulders	Cervical spine motion
Shrug shoulders (examiner resists)	Trapezius strength
Abduct shoulders 90° (examiner resists at 90°)	Deltoid strength
Full external rotation of arms	Shoulder motion
Flex and extend elbows	Elbow motion
Arms at sides, elbows 90° flexed; pronate and supinate wrists	Elbow and wrist motion
Spread fingers; make fist	Hand or finger motion and deformities
Tighten (contract) quadriceps; relax quadriceps	Symmetry and knee effusion; ankle effusion
"Duck walk" four steps (away from examiner with buttocks on heels)	Hip, knee, and ankle motion
Stand with back to examiner	Shoulder symmetry; scoliosis
Knees straight, touch toes	Scoliosis, hip motion, hamstring tightness
Raise up on toes; raise heels	Calf symmetry, leg strength

FIGURE 2–9   Orthopedic screening. Equipment that may be needed includes reflex hammer, tape measure, pin, and examining table.

screening usually takes about 90 seconds (Figure 2–9).[8] A more detailed orthopedic examination may be conducted to assess strength, range of motion, and stability at various joints (Figure 2–10).

Wellness Screening Some preparticipation exams include a screening for wellness. The purpose is to determine whether the athlete is engaging in healthy lifestyle behaviors and should include questions about diet, rest, exercise, and weight control, as well as questions about lifestyle habits that pose a threat to wellness such as alcohol, drug, and tobacco use, and stress. A number of wellness screening tools are available. Figure 2–11 provides an example of a wellness screening questionnaire.

Health Maintenance and Personal Hygiene Screening A screening tool for assessing the general principles of health maintenance and personal hygiene, should include questions about skin care, dental hygiene and dental care, sanitation, immunizations, avoiding infectious and contagious diseases, and sleep habits.

Sickle Cell Trait Screening In 2010, the NCAA instituted mandatory testing for sickle cell trait for all athletes in Division I. Students are given a blood test to screen for the sickle cell trait prior to the first season that they are eligible to compete. Under the current rules, athletes can avoid testing by proving they have previously been tested or by signing a waiver

ORTHOPEDIC SCREENING FORM

Name: _____ SS #: _____

FLEXIBILITY		CHECK IF NORMAL
Shoulder:		Abduction
		Adduction
		Flexion
		Extension
		Internal rot.
		External rot.
Hip:		Ext. (flex knee)
		Flex. (flex knee)
		Ext. (str. leg)
		Flex. (str. leg)
		Abduction
		Adduction
Knee:		Flexion
		Extension
Ankle:		Dorsiflexion
		Plantar flexion
Trunk:		Flexion
		Extension
		Rotation
		Lat. flexion
JOINT STABILITY		
Knee:		Lachman
		Pivot shift
		Anterior drawer
		Posterior drawer
		Valgus
		Varus
		McMurray
		Apley's grind
Ankle:		Anterior drawer
		Talor tilt
LEG LENGTH		
Posture:		Pelvis height
		Shoulder height
		Spine
PREVIOUS INJURY:		

Comments: _____

_____

_____

FIGURE 2–10 Sample of a detailed orthopedic screening form.

Note
1. Circle the appropriate response for each question.
2. Add the total number of points for each section.

BEHAVIOR	Almost Always	Sometimes	Almost Never
TOBACCO USE			
If you never smoke or use tobacco products, enter a score of 10 for this section and go to the next section on Alcohol and Drugs.			
1. I avoid smoking cigarettes and chewing tobacco.	2	1	0
2. I smoke only low-tar and low-nicotine cigarettes, or I smoke a pipe or cigars.	2	1	0
			Tobacco Use Score: _____
ALCOHOL AND DRUGS			
1. I avoid drinking alcoholic beverages or I drink no more than one or two a day.	4	1	0
2. I avoid using alcohol or other drugs (especially illegal drugs) as a way of handling stressful situations or problems in my life.	2	1	0
3. I am careful not to drink alcohol when taking certain medicines (e.g., medicine for sleeping, pain, colds, and allergies) or when pregnant.	2	1	0
4. I read and follow the label directions when using prescribed and over-the-counter drugs.	2	1	0
			Alcohol and Drug Score: _____
EATING HABITS			
1. I eat a variety of foods each day, such as fruits and vegetables, whole-grain breads and cereals, lean meats, dairy products, dry peas and beans, and nuts and seeds.	4	1	0
2. I limit my intake of fat, saturated fat, and cholesterol (including fat in meats, eggs, butter and other dairy products, shortenings, and organ meats, such as liver).	2	1	0
3. I limit the amount of salt I eat by cooking with only small amounts, not adding salt at the table, and avoiding salty snacks.	2	1	0
4. I avoid eating too much sugar (especially frequent snacks of sticky candy or soft drinks).	2	1	0
			Eating Habits Score: _____
EXERCISE/FITNESS HABITS			
1. I maintain a desired weight, avoiding overweight and underweight.	3	1	0
2. I do vigorous exercises for 15–30 minutes at least three times a week (examples include running, swimming, and brisk walking).	3	1	0
3. I do exercises that enhance my muscle tone for 15–30 minutes at least three times a week (examples include yoga and calisthenics).	2	1	0
4. I use part of my leisure time participating in individual, family, or team activities that increase my level of fitness (such as gardening, bowling, golf, and baseball).	2	1	0
			Exercise/Fitness Score: _____

	Almost Always	Sometimes	Almost Never
STRESS CONTROL			
1. I have a job or do other work that I enjoy.	2	1	0
2. I find it easy to relax and to express my feelings freely.	2	1	0
3. I anticipate and prepare for events or situations likely to be stressful for me.	2	1	0
4. I have close friends, relatives, or others with whom I can discuss personal matters and call on for help when needed.	2	1	0
5. I participate in group activities (such as church and community organizations) or hobbies that I enjoy.	2	1	0
			Stress Control Score: _____
SAFETY			
1. I wear a seat belt when riding in a car.	2	1	0
2. I avoid driving while under the influence of alcohol and other drugs.	2	1	0
3. I obey traffic rules and the speed limit when driving.	2	1	0
4. I am careful when using potentially harmful products or substances (such as household cleaners, poisons, and electrical devices).	2	1	0
5. I avoid smoking in bed.	2	1	0
6. I am not sexually active or I have sex with only one mutually faithful, uninfected partner, or I always engage in safe sex (using condoms), and I do not share needles to inject drugs.	2	1	0
			Safety Score: _____

WHAT YOUR SCORES MEAN

Scores of 9 and 10: Excellent. Your answers show that you are aware of the importance of this area to your health.

Scores of 6 to 8: Good. Your health practices in this area are good, but there is room for improvement.

Scores of 3 to 5: Fair. Your health risks are showing.

Scores of 0 to 2: Poor. Your answers show that you may be taking serious and unnecessary risks with your health. Perhaps you are not aware of the risks and what to do about them. You can easily get the information and help you need to improve, if you wish.

If you have questions or concerns, you should consult your athletic trainers for advice.

FIGURE 2–11 Wellness screening questionnaire.

releasing the NCAA and their university from liability. The NATA has published a consensus statement, "Sickle Cell Trait and the Athlete" (http://www.nata.org/sites/default/files/SickleCellTraitAndTheAthlete.pdf) that provides guidelines and precautions for modifying workouts in athletes with sickle cell trait.

Sport Disqualification

As discussed previously, sports participation involves risks. Certain injuries and conditions warrant concern on the part of both the athlete and sports medicine personnel about continued participation in sport activities. Table 2–2 lists those conditions.[2] Sports medicine physicians can only recommend that an athlete voluntarily retire from participation. The Americans with Disabilities Act of 1990 dictates that the individual athlete is the only person who can make the final decision. Most conditions that potentially warrant disqualification should be identified by a preparticipation examination and noted in the medical history.[1]

Personal Information Card

Always on file in the athletic trainer's office is the athlete's personal information card. This card is completed by the athlete at the time of the health examination and serves as a means of contacting the athlete's family, personal physician, and insurance company in case of emergency.

TABLE 2–2	Recommendations for Participation in Competitive Sports				
	Contact		**Noncontact**		
	Contact/ Collision	Limited Contact/ Collision	Strenuous	Moderately Strenuous	Nonstrenuous
Atlantoaxial instability	No	No	Yes*	Yes	Yes
*Swimming: no butterfly, breast stroke, or diving starts					
Acute illnesses	*	*	*	*	*
*Needs individual assessment (e.g., contagiousness to others, risk of worsening illness)					
Cardiovascular					
Carditis	No	No	No	No	No
Hypertension					
Mild	Yes	Yes	Yes	Yes	Yes
Moderate	*	*	*	*	*
Severe	*	*	*	*	*
Congenital heart disease	†	†	†	†	†
*Needs individual assessment					
†Patients with mild forms can be allowed a full range of physical activities; patients with moderate or severe forms or who are postoperative should be evaluated by a cardiologist before athletic participation.					
Eyes					
Absence or loss of function of eye	*	*	*	*	*
Detached retina	†	†	†	†	†
*Availability of American Society for Testing and Materials (ASTM)–approved eye guards may allow competitor to participate in most sports, but this must be judged on an individual basis.					
†Consult ophthalmologist.					
Inguinal hernia	Yes	Yes	Yes	Yes	Yes
Kidney: absence of one	No	Yes	Yes	Yes	Yes
Liver: enlarged	No	No	Yes	Yes	Yes
Musculoskeletal disorders	*	*	*	*	*
*Needs individual assessment					
Neurological status					
History of serious head or spine trauma, repeated concussions, or craniotomy	*	*	Yes	Yes	Yes
Convulsive disorder					
Well controlled	Yes	Yes	Yes	Yes	Yes
Poorly controlled	No	No	Yes†	Yes	Yes††
*Needs individual assessment					
†No swimming or weight lifting					
††No archery or riflery					
Ovary: absence of one	Yes	Yes	Yes	Yes	Yes
Respiratory status					
Pulmonary insufficiency	*	*	*	*	Yes
Asthma	Yes	Yes	Yes	Yes	Yes
*May be allowed to compete if oxygenation remains satisfactory during a graded stress test					
Sickle-cell trait	Yes	Yes	Yes	Yes	Yes
Skin: Boils, herpes, impetigo, scabies	*	*	Yes	Yes	Yes
*No gymnastics with mats, martial arts, wrestling, or contact sports until not contagious					
Spleen: enlarged	No	No	No	Yes	Yes
Testicle: absent or undescended	Yes*	Yes*	Yes	Yes	Yes
*Certain sports may require protective cup.					

Name _____ **Sport** _____ **Date:** ___ /___ /___ **Time:** _____ **Injury number:** _____

Player I.D. _____ **Age:** _____ **Location:** _____ **Intercollegiate—nonintercollegiate**

Initial injury   **Recheck**   **Reinjury**   **Preseason—Practice—Game**   **Incurred while participating in sport: yes ___ no ___**

Description: How did it happen? _____
_____

Initial impression: _____
_____
_____

SITE OF INJURY	BODY PART		STRUCTURE	Treatment
1 Right	1 Head	25 MP joint	1 Skin	
2 Left	2 Face	26 PIP joint	2 Muscle	
3 Proximal	3 Eye	27 Abdomen	3 Fascia	
4 Distal	4 Nose	28 Hip	4 Bone	
5 Anterior	5 Ear	29 Thigh	5 Nerve	
6 Posterior	6 Mouth	30 Knee	6 Fat pad	
7 Medial	7 Neck	31 Patella	7 Tendon	
8 Lateral	8 Thorax	32 Lower leg	8 Ligament	
9 Other	9 Ribs	33 Ankle	9 Cartilage	
	10 Sternum	34 Achilles tendon	10 Capsule	
	11 Upper back	35 Foot	11 Compartment	
SITE OF EVALUATION	12 Lower back	36 Toes	12 Dental	
1 SHS	13 Shoulder	37 Other	13 _____	
2 Athletic Trn Rm.	14 Rotator cuff			Medication
3 Site-Competition	15 AC joint			
4 _____	16 Glenohumeral			
	17 Sternoclavicular	NONTRAUMATIC	NATURE OF INJURY	
PROCEDURES	18 Upper arm	1 Dermatological	1 Contusion	
1 Physical exam	19 Elbow	2 Allergy	2 Strain	
2 X-ray	20 Forearm	3 Influenza	3 Sprain	
3 Splint	21 Wrist	4 URI	4 Fracture	
4 Wrap	22 Hand	5 GU	5 Rupture	
5 Cast	23 Thumb	6 Systemic infect.	6 Tendonitis	
6 Aspiration	24 Finger	7 Local infect.	7 Bursitis	
7 Other		8 Other	8 Myositis	Prescription dispensed
			9 Laceration	1 Antibiotics 5 Muscle relaxant
			10 Concussion	2 Antiinflammatory 6 Enzyme
			11 Avulsion	3 Decongestant 7 _____
			12 Abrasion	4 Analgesic
		DISPOSITION OF INJURY	13 _____	INJECTIONS
DISPOSITION	REFERRAL	1 No part.		
1 SHS	1 Arthrogram	2 Part part.		1 Steroids
2 Trainer	2 Neurological	3 Full part.	Degree	2 Antibiotics
3 Hospital	3 Int. Med.		1 2 3	3 Steroids-xylo
4 H.D.	4 Orthropedic			4 _____
5 Other	5 EENT			
	6 Dentist			
	7 Other			

Previous injury _____

FIGURE 2–12   Athletic injury record form.

Injury Reports and Injury Disposition

An injury report serves as a record for future reference (Figure 2–12). If the emergency procedures followed are questioned at a later date, an athletic trainer's memory of the details may be somewhat hazy, but a report completed on the spot provides specific information. In a litigation situation, an athletic trainer may be asked questions about an injury that occurred three years in the past. All injury reports should be filed in the athletic trainer's office. One is well advised to make the reports out in triplicate, retaining one copy and sending copies to the school health office and the physician.

Patient Treatment Log

Each athletic training clinic should maintain individual daily treatment logs for each patient who receives any service. Emphasis is placed on recording the treatments for the patient who is receiving daily therapy for an injury. Like accident records and injury dispositions, these records often have the status of legal documents and are used to establish certain facts in a civil litigation, an insurance action, or a criminal action after injury.

Injury Evaluation and Progress Notes Injuries should be evaluated by the athletic trainer, who must record information obtained in some consistent format. The SOAP format (*S*ubjective, *O*bjective, *A*ssessment, *P*lan for treatment) is a concise method of recording the initial evaluation and progress notes for the injured athlete and is discussed in detail in Chapter 13. The subjective portion of the SOAP note refers to what the patient tells the athletic trainer about the injury relative to the history or what he or she felt. The objective portion documents information that the athletic trainer gathers during the evaluation, such as range of motion, strength levels, patterns of pain, and so forth. The assessment records the athletic trainer's professional opinion about the injury based on the information obtained during the subjective and objective portions. The plan for treatment indicates how the injury will be managed and includes short- and long-term goals for rehabilitation.

Supply and Equipment Inventory

The athletic trainer is responsible for managing a budget, most of which is spent on equipment and supplies. Every year an inventory must be conducted and recorded on such items as new equipment needed, equipment that needs to be replaced or repaired, and the expendable supplies that need replenishing.

Annual or Seasonal Reports

Both clinic administrators and athletic administrators require an annual or seasonal report on the functions of the athletic training program. This report serves as a means for making program changes and improvements. It commonly includes the number of patients served,

a survey of the number and types of injuries, an analysis of the program, and recommendations for future improvements.

COMPUTERS AND TABLETS AS TOOLS FOR THE ATHLETIC TRAINER

As is the case in all of our society, computers and tablets have become indispensable tools for the athletic trainer and have completely revolutionized the way information is managed. A great deal of information can be efficiently located and stored for immediate and future use because of constant improvement in storage and retrieval capacities. Software packages are available to help store and retrieve any type of relevant records or information.[15]

The first step in integrating computers and tablets into an athletic training program is to decide exactly how and for what purposes they will be used. Most athletic trainers do not have an extensive background in or understanding of computer or tablet hardware. It is essential to seek advice from expert professionals or consultants prior to purchasing a system to ensure that the hardware and corresponding operating system are capable of supporting the software that will make them useful information management and communication tools.

> **Computers facilitate the record-keeping process.**

Thousands of software programs are available that will allow the user to store, manipulate, and retrieve information; create written documents through word processing; analyze data statistically; and communicate with many individuals in a variety of forms.

Record keeping is a time-consuming but essential chore for all athletic trainers regardless of whether they work at a college or university, at a high school, in the clinical setting, or in industry. Several software packages are available specifically for managing injury records in the athletic training setting. A problem that athletic trainers must address is ensuring security and protecting the confidentiality of medical records stored on a computer or tablet. Databases that contain such information must be accessible only to the athletic trainer or team physician and must be protected by a password.

Besides record keeping, software can also be used for budgeting; managing a personal schedule or calendar; and creating a database or a spreadsheet from which injury data can be organized, retrieved, or related to specific injury situations or other injury records for statistical analysis. Other software can analyze and provide information about nutrition, body composition, and injury risk profiles based on other anthropometric measures and can be used to record isokinetic evaluation and exercise.[28]

The use of educational software to assist in teaching and the academic preparation of athletic training students has become an integral component in the majority of athletic training educational programs. New instructional and educational software with interactive capabilities of eBooks has made the multimedia presentation of instructional material, and thus learning, more interesting and effective for the student athletic trainer.

The Internet and the World Wide Web have impacted and changed all of our lives. We live in a world where virtually any kind of information is immediately accessible to anyone who knows how to use the system. The sports medicine community in general and the athletic trainer specifically can access Web sites that have direct application to clinical practice, to the education of athletic training students, and to the general base of knowledge that is relevant to the field.

COLLECTING INJURY DATA

Because of the vast number of physically active individuals involved with organized and recreational sports, some knowledge relative to the number and types of injuries sustained during participation in these activities is essential.[38] Although methods are much improved over the past, many weaknesses exist in systematic data collection and analysis of sports injuries.[21]

The Incidence of Injuries

An **accident** is an unplanned event capable of resulting in loss of time, property damage, injury, disablement, or even death.[48] An **injury** may be defined as damage to the body that restricts activity or causes disability to such an extent that the patient is not able to practice or compete the next day.[48]

Injury data may be analyzed by looking at several factors. The *incidence* of injury analyzes the risk of sustaining an injury during some specified time period (i.e., practice, games). Injury *prevalence* analyzes the total number of injuries in a specific population. *Incidence rate* is the number of new injuries that occur in a particular population during a specified time period. Injury *exposure rates* look at the incidence of injuries per the number of individual athlete exposures during a specific time period. Risk factors that might potentially contribute to the incidence of injury can be analyzed using outcome studies to determine the strength of their relevance and whether modifying these risk factors is effective in reducing injury rates.

There is little doubt that a *case study* approach, which looks at one incidence of an injury, can yield some critical information about the cause and subsequent efficacy of treatment for that injury. However, an approach that analyzes a large number of similar injuries can provide the greatest amount of information. In general, the incidence of sports injuries can be studied epidemiologically from many points of view—in terms of age at occurrence, gender, body regions that sustain injuries, or the occurrence in different sports.[49] Sports are usually classified according to the risk, or chances, of injuries occurring under similar circumstances and are broadly divided into contact or collision, limited contact, or noncontact[2] (Table 2–3).

Athletes in all sports, recreational and organized, who participate in sports in the span of one year face a 50 percent chance of sustaining some injury. Of the 50 million estimated sports injuries per year, 50 percent require only minor care and no restriction of activity.[21] Approximately 90 percent of injuries are muscle contusions, ligament sprains, and muscle strains; however, 10 percent of these injuries lead to microtrauma complications and eventually to a severe, chronic condition in later life.

Of the sports injuries that must be medically treated, sprains or strains, fractures, dislocations, and contusions are the most common.[21] In terms of the body regions most often injured, the knee has the highest incidence, with the ankle second and the upper limb third. For both males and

accident An unplanned event capable of resulting in loss of time, property damage, injury, disablement, or even death.

injury Damage to the body that restricts activity or causes disability.

The epidemiological approach toward injury data collection provides the most information.

Risk of injury is determined by the type of sport—contact or collision, limited contact, or noncontact.

TABLE 2-3	Classification of Sports*		
Contact or Collision	**Limited Contact**		**Noncontact**
Basketball	Baseball		Archery
Boxing	Bicycling		Badminton
Diving	Cheerleading		Bodybuilding
Field hockey	Canoeing or kayaking (white water)		Bowling
Football (tackle)	Fencing		Canoeing or kayaking (flat water)
Ice hockey	Field events		Crew or rowing
Lacrosse	High jump		Curling
Martial arts	Pole vault		Dancing (ballet, modern, Jazz)
Rodeo	Floor hockey		Field events
Rugby	Football (flag)		Discus
Ski jumping	Gymnastics		Javelin
Soccer	Handball		Shot put
Team handball	Horseback riding		Golf
Water polo	Racquetball		Orienteering
Wrestling	Skating (ice, in-line, roller)		Power lifting
	Skiing (cross-country, downhill, water)		Race walking
	Skateboarding		Riflery
	Snowboarding		Rope jumping
	Softball		Running
	Squash		Sailing
	Ultimate Frisbee		Scuba diving
	Volleyball		Swimming
	Windsurfing or surfing		Table tennis
			Tennis
			Track
			Weight lifting

*From the American Academy of Pediatrics Committee on Sports Medicine and Fitness: Medical conditions affecting sports participation, *Pediatrics* 107(5):1205, 2001.

females the most commonly injured body part is the knee, followed by the ankle; however, males have a much higher incidence of shoulder and upper-arm injuries than do females.

Catastrophic Injuries

Although millions of individuals participate in organized and recreational sports, there is a relatively low incidence of fatalities or catastrophic injuries. Ninety-eight percent of individuals with injuries requiring hospital emergency room medical attention are treated and released.[9] Deaths have been attributed to chest or trunk impact with thrown objects, other players, or nonyielding objects (e.g., goalposts). Deaths have occurred when players were struck in the head by sports implements (bats, golf clubs, hockey sticks) or by missiles (baseballs, soccer balls, golf balls, hockey pucks). Death has also resulted when an individual received a direct blow to the head from another player or the ground. On record are a number of sports deaths in which a playing structure, such as a goalpost or backstop, fell on a participant.

The highest incidence of indirect sports death stems from heatstroke. Less common indirect causes include cardiovascular and respiratory problems or congenital conditions not previously known. Catastrophic injuries leading to cervical injury and quadriplegia are seen mainly in American football. Although the incidence is low for the number of players involved, it could be lowered even further if more precautions were taken.[30]

In most popular organized and recreational sports activities, the legs and arms have the highest risk factor for injury, with the head and face next. Muscle strains, joint sprains, contusions, and abrasions are the most frequent injuries sustained by the active sports participant. The major goal of this text is to provide the reader with the fundamental principles necessary for preventing and managing illnesses and injuries common to the athlete.

Current National Injury Data-Gathering Systems

The state of the art of sports injury surveillance is unsatisfactory.[48] Currently, most local, state, and federal systems are concerned with the accident or injury only after it has happened, and they focus on injuries requiring medical assistance or those that cause time loss or restricted activity.

The ideal system takes an epidemiological approach.[48] **Epidemiology** is the scientific study of factors affecting the health and illness of individuals and populations. Epidemiology takes an evidence-based approach for identifying risk factors for injury and determining optimal treatment methods in clinical practice. It serves as the foundation for interventions made in the interest of public health and preventive medicine. When considering the risks inherent in a particular sport, both extrinsic and intrinsic factors must be studied.[33] Thus, information is gleaned from both epidemiological data and the individual measurements of the athlete. The term *extrinsic factor* refers to the type of activity that is performed, the amount of exposure to injury, factors in the environment, and the equipment. The term *intrinsic factor* refers directly to the athlete and includes age, gender, neuromuscular aspects, structural aspects, performance aspects, and mental and psychological aspects.

> **epidemiology** Study of factors affecting the health and illness of individuals and populations.

Over the years, a number of athletic injury surveillance systems have been implemented; most have collected data for a few years and then ceased to exist. The currently active systems that are most often mentioned are the National Safety Council, the Annual Survey of Football Injury Research, the National Center for Catastrophic Sports Injury Research, the NCAA Injury Surveillance System, the National Electronic Injury Surveillance System (NEISS), and the National High School Sports-Related Injury Surveillance Study.

National Safety Council The National Safety Council* is a nongovernmental, nonprofit public service organization. It draws sports injury data from a variety of sources, including educational institutions.

Annual Survey of Football Injury Research In 1931, the American Football Coaches Association (AFCA) conducted its first Annual Survey of Football Fatalities. Since 1965, this research has been conducted at the University of North Carolina. In 1980, the survey's title was changed to the Annual Survey of Football Injury Research. Every year, with the exception of 1942, data have been collected about public school, college, professional, and sandlot football. Information is gathered through personal contact interviews and questionnaires. The sponsoring organizations of this survey are the AFCA, the NCAA, and the National Federation of State High School Associations (NFHS).

*National Safety Council, Itasca, IL.

This survey classifies football fatalities as direct or indirect. Direct fatalities are those resulting directly from participation in football. Indirect fatalities are produced by systemic failure caused by the exertion of playing football or by a complication that arose from a nonfatal football injury.

National Center for Catastrophic Sports Injury Research In 1977, the NCAA initiated the National Survey of Catastrophic Football Injuries. As a result of the injury data collected from this organization, several significant rule changes have been incorporated into collegiate football. Because of the success of this football project, the research was expanded to all sports for both men and women, and a National Center for Catastrophic Sports Injury Research was established at the University of North Carolina. With support from the NCAA, the NFHS, the AFCA, and the Section on Sports Medicine of the American Association of Neurological Sciences, this center compiles data on catastrophic injuries at all levels of sport.[9]

NCAA Injury Surveillance System The NCAA Injury Surveillance System (ISS) was established in 1982 primarily for the purpose of studying the incidence of football injuries, so that rule change recommendations could be made to reduce the injury rate.[14] Since that time, this system has been greatly expanded and now collects data on most major sports. For the most part, athletic trainers are primarily involved in the collection and transmission of injury data.

The ISS has relied on the willingness of athletic trainers to submit paper forms reporting injuries in various NCAA-sponsored sports. In Fall 2004, the ISS fully converted to a Web-based data-collection system that can compile far more data than ever before, providing member institutions with a low-cost means of tracking medical information and analyzing injury trends.

National Electronic Injury Surveillance System In 1972, the federal government established the Consumer Product Safety Act (CPSA), which created and granted broad authority to the Consumer Product Safety Commission to enforce the safety standards for more than 10,000 products that may be risky to the consumer.[48] To perform this mission, the National Electronic Injury Surveillance System

---

2–8 Clinical Application Exercise

A collegiate athletic trainer is approached by the school administration to determine the potential risk of injury to their football team.

? What approach is best suited to gather this information?

(NEISS)[†] was established. Data on injuries related to consumer products are monitored 24 hours a day from a selected sample of 5,000 hospital emergency rooms nationwide. Sports injuries represent 25 percent of all injuries reported by NEISS. It should be noted that a product may be related to an injury, but not be the direct cause of that injury.[48]

Once a product is considered hazardous, the commission can seize the product or create standards to decrease the risk. Also, manufacturers and distributors of sports recreational equipment must report to the commission any product that is potentially hazardous or defective. The commission can also research the reasons that a sports or recreational product is hazardous.

National High School Sports-Related Injury Surveillance Study

The National High School Sports-Related Injury Surveillance Study, administered through the Center for Injury Research and Policy, was first implemented in 2005 and has collected data annually since then.

[†]National Electronic Injury Surveillance System, U.S. Consumer Product Safety Commission, Directorate for Epidemiology, National Injury Information Clearinghouse, Washington, DC.

It was first established as the high-school version of the NCAA Injury Surveillance System. Known as High School RIO™, it is an Internet-based data collection tool that looks at time-loss injuries in a national sample of U.S. high-school athletes. This system collects data weekly on athlete exposure, injury type, and the injury event, using certified athletic trainers to provide data.[47] The data collected meets the needs of the high-school sports community that includes student-athletes, parents, pediatric sports medicine clinicians, high-school athletic directors, local/state high-school athletic associations/administrators, and the NFHS (National Federation of State High School Associations).[13]

Using Injury Data

Valid, reliable sports injury data can materially help decrease injuries. If properly interpreted, the data can be used to modify rules, assist coaches and players in understanding risks, and help manufacturers evaluate their products against the overall market. The public, especially parents, should understand the risks inherent in a particular sport, and insurance companies that insure athletes must know risks in order to set reasonable costs.

SUMMARY

- The administration of a program of health care demands a significant portion of the athletic trainer's time and effort. The efficiency and success of the athletic training program depend in large part on the administrative abilities of the athletic trainer in addition to the clinical skills required to treat the injured patient.
- The athletic training health care program may best serve the athlete; the hospital, clinic, or corporation; and the community by establishing specific policies, procedures, and regulations governing the use of available services.
- An athletic training program in secondary schools, colleges, and universities should decide whom the program will serve and how coverage will be provided, establish rules for hygiene and sanitation of the facility, develop a budget, develop a risk management plan, and address human resources and personnel issues.
- The athletic training program can be enhanced by designing or renovating a facility to maximize the potential use of the space available. Space designed for injury treatment, rehabilitation, modality use, office space, physician examination, record keeping, and storage of supplies should be designated within each facility.
- An athletic training program in the hospital, clinical, corporate, or industrial setting must decide

what type of patients will be treated in that facility; how that facility can best serve that patient population; how to resolve clinic personnel and human resources issues; exactly what an athletic trainer might be responsible for in the day-to-day operation of that facility; and the fiscal management issues in a for-profit clinic.
- Preparticipation exams must be given to athletes and should include a medical history, a general physical examination, and orthopedic screenings.
- The athletic trainer must maintain accurate and up-to-date medical records in addition to the other paperwork that is necessary for the operation of the athletic training program in all settings in which an athletic trainer may work.
- Computers and tablets are extremely useful tools that enable athletic trainers to retrieve and store a variety of records.
- A number of data-collection systems tabulate the incidence of sports injuries. The systems mentioned most often are the National Safety Council, the Annual Survey of Football Injury Research, the National Electronic Injury Surveillance System, the NCAA Injury Surveillance System, the National Center for Catastrophic Sports Injury Research, and the National High School Sports-Related Injury Surveillance Study.

SOLUTIONS TO CLINICAL APPLICATION EXERCISES

2–1 The athletic trainer should work in conjunction with the appropriate administrative personnel to develop a risk management plan that includes security issues, fire safety, electrical and equipment safety, and emergency injury management.

2–2 Federal law mandates specific policies for recruitment, hiring, and firing. All qualified applicants should receive equal consideration regardless of their race, gender, religion, or nationality. The head athletic trainer must strictly adhere to these mandates.

2–3 The athletic training clinic should have specific areas designated for taping and preparation, treatment and rehabilitation, and hydrotherapy. It should have an office for the athletic trainer and adequate storage facilities positioned within the space to allow for an efficient traffic flow. Equipment purchases might include four or five treatment tables and two or three taping tables (these could be made in-house, if possible), a large-capacity ice machine, a combination ultrasound/electrical stimulating unit, a whirlpool, and various free weights and exercise tubing.

2–4 The athletic trainer should take this request to the clinic administrator to have it approved. They must decide on a fee for treating these patients and hours for treatment. A decision should also be made about personnel for game and event coverage. A budget should also be developed for supplies and equipment.

2–5 The preparticipation examination should consist of a medical history, a physical examination, and a brief orthopedic screening. The preparticipation physical may be effectively administered using a station examination system with a team of examiners. A station examination can provide the athlete with a detailed examination in a short period of time. A team of people is needed to examine this many individuals. The team should include several physicians, medically trained nonphysicians (nurses, athletic trainers, physical therapists, or physician's assistants), and managers, athletic training students, or assistant coaches.

2–6 The athletic trainer should explain that the computer can be used for maintaining medical records, word processing, planning a budget, managing a personal schedule or calendar, and creating a database containing injury data that can be organized, retrieved, or related to specific injury situations or to other injury records for analysis. Additional software can provide the athletic trainer with analysis and information about nutrition, body composition, and injury risk profiles.

2–7 The athletic trainer should do a simple study in which one-half of the players are randomly placed in the ankle braces while the other half continue to play in their high-top shoes. By comparing the number of ankle injuries in the group wearing the braces with those in the group without the braces, the athletic trainer can make a decision as to the effectiveness of the braces in preventing ankle injuries. Collecting and analyzing injury data is helpful in determining the efficacy of many of the techniques used by the athletic trainer.

2–8 The NCAA Injury Surveillance System would best suit this purpose. This system of information can also be used to prevent injuries by presenting information to coaches, referees, and administrators to enforce necessary changes to the football program.

REVIEW QUESTIONS AND CLASS ACTIVITIES

1. What are the major administrative functions that an athletic trainer must perform?
2. Design two athletic training clinics—one for a secondary school and one for a large university.
3. Observe the activities in the athletic training clinic. Pick both a slow time and a busy time to observe.
4. Why do hygiene and sanitation play an important role in athletic training? How should the athletic training clinic be maintained?
5. Fully equip a new medium-size high-school, college, or clinical athletic training clinic. Pick equipment from current catalogs.
6. Establish a reasonable budget for a small secondary school, a large high school, and a large college or university.
7. Identify the groups or individuals to be served in a collegiate athletic training clinic.
8. What job duties and responsibilities might an athletic trainer be assigned when working in a clinic, hospital, corporate, or industrial setting?
9. Help organize a preparticipation health examination for ninety football players.
10. Record keeping is a major function in athletic training. What records are necessary to keep? How can a computer help?
11. Debate what conditions constitute good grounds for medical disqualification from a sport.
12. Discuss the epidemiological approach to recording sports injury data.

REFERENCES

1. American Academy of Family Physicians: *Preparticipation physical evaluation*, ed 3, Minneapolis, 2005, McGraw-Hill Healthcare Information.
2. American Academy of Pediatrics Committee on Sports Medicine and Fitness: Medical conditions affecting sports participation, *Pediatrics* 107(5):1205, 2001.
3. Ammon R, Southall R: *Sport facility management: Organizing events and mitigating risks*, Morgantown, WV, 2010. Fitness Information Technology.
4. Anderson B: Policies and philosophies related to risk management in the athletic setting, *Athletic Therapy Today*, 11(1):10, 2006.
5. Anderson J, Courson R, Kleiner D, McLoda T: National Athletic Trainers' Association Position Statement: Emergency planning in athletics, *J Athl Train* 37(1):99, 2002.
6. Armsey T, Hosey R: Medical aspects of sports: Epidemiology of injuries, preparticipation physical examination, and drugs in sports, *Clin Sports Med* 23 (2):255–79, 2004.
7. Bagnall D: Budget planning key in secondary schools, *NATA News*, January 15, 2001.
8. Bernhardt D, Roberts W: *PPE: Preparticipation physical evaluation*, Elk Grove Village, IL 2010, American Academy of Pediatrics.
9. Boden BP, Pasquina P, Johnson J, Mueller FO: Catastrophic injuries in pole-vaulters, *Am J Sports Med* 29(1):50, 2001.
10. Brown J: Athletic training facilities. In Sawyer T, editor: *Facilities planning for health, fitness, physical activity, recreation & sports*, Champaign, IL, 2009, Sagamore Publishing.
11. Claiborne T, Su-I H, Cappaert T: 2007. Certified athletic trainers provide effective care in the high school setting, *Athletic Therapy Today* 12(2):34.
12. Curtis N: Risk management, *Athletic Therapy Today* 11(1):34, 2006.
13. Darrow C, Collins C, Yard E: Epidemiology of severe injuries among United States high school athletes 2005–2007, *American Journal of Sports Medicine* 37(9):1798–1805, 2009.
14. Dick R: NCAA injury surveillance system: A tool for health and safety risk management, *Athletic Therapy Today* 11(1):42, 2006.
15. Eng J: Computerizing clinical documentation, *Phys Ther* 14(6):36, 2006.
16. Fried G: *Managing sport facilities*. Champaign, Human Kinetics, 2009.
17. Jonas J: Ethics in injury management, *Athletic Therapy Today* 11(1):28, 2006.
18. Jones D: HIPAA: Friend or foe to athletic trainers? *Athletic Therapy Today* 8(2):17, 2003.

19. Keil J: HIPAA and FERPA: Competing or collaborating? *Journal of Allied Health* 39(4):161–65, 2010.

20. Knight KL: Athletic training clinic operations. In Knight K, editor: *Developing clinical proficiency in athletic training,* ed 3, Champaign, IL, Human Kinetics, pp. 14–19, 2009.

21. Knowles S, Marshall S, Guskiewicz K: Issues in estimating risks and rates in sports injury research, *J Athl Train* 41(2):207, 2006.

22. Koester M, Amundson C: Preparticipation screening of high school athletes: Are recommendations enough? *Physician Sportsmed* 31(8):330, 2003.

23. Konin J, Donley P: The athletic trainer as a personnel manager. In Konin J, editor: *The clinical athletic trainer,* Gaithersburg, MD, 1997, Slack.

24. Kurtz M: Leadership in athletic training: Implications for practice and education in allied health care, *Journal of Allied Health,* 39(4):265–79, 2010.

25. Landry G, Bernhardt D: Preparticipation physical examination. In Landry G, editor: *Essentials of primary care sports medicine,* Champaign, IL, 2003, Human Kinetics.

26. Marshall AL: Challenges and opportunities for promoting physical activity in the workplace, *Journal of Science and Medicine in Sport* 7(1 Supplement):60, 2004.

27. Mirwald R, Baxter J, Bailey D: An assessment of maturity from anthropometric measurements. *Med Sci Sports Exerc* 34(4):689, 2002.

28. Moss RI: Facilities and foibles, *Athletic Therapy Today* 7(1):22, 2002.

29. Moyer-Knowles J: Planning a new athletic facility. In Konin J, editor: *The clinical athletic trainer,* Gaithersburg, MD, 1997, Slack.

30. Mueller F, Casa D: Fatal and catastrophic injuries in athletics: Epidemiological data and challenging circumstances. In Casa D, editor: *Preventing sudden death in sport and physical activity,* Sudbury, MA, 2012, Jones and Bartlett.

31. Peterson E: Insult to injury: Feeling understaffed, underequipped and undervalued, athletic trainers say minimum of space and equipment will yield extensive benefits, *Athletic Business* 23(1):57, 1999.

32. *Physician and sportsmedicine: Preparticipation physical evaluation monograph,* ed 3; New York, 2004, McGraw-Hill.

33. Rankin J, Ingersoll C: *Athletic training management: Concepts and applications,* St. Louis, 2006, McGraw-Hill.

34. Ray R: Where athletic trainers work: Facility design and planning. In Ray R, Konin J, editors: *Management strategies in athletic training,* ed 4, Champaign, IL, 2011, Human Kinetics.

35. Ray R, Konin J, editors: *Management strategies in athletic training,* ed 4, Champaign, IL, 2011, Human Kinetics.

36. Sabo J: *Athletic training room design and layout.* In Proceedings, National Athletic Trainers' Association 50th Annual Meeting and Clinical Symposium, June 16–19, 1999, Kansas City, MO, Human Kinetics, 1999.

37. Sabo J: Design and construction of an athletic training facility, *NATA News,* May 10, 2001.

38. Schiff M: Soccer injuries in female youth players: Comparison of injury surveillance by certified athletic trainers and Internet, *J Athl Train.* 45(3):238–42, 2010.

39. Schwartz E: *Sport facility operations management.* St. Louis, 2010, Elsevier.

40. Shappy J: Preparticipation exam to identify risk for sudden cardiac death, *Athletic Training and Therapy,* 14(6):13–16, 2009.

41. Shephard RJ, Bonneau J: Supervision of occupational fitness assessments, *Canadian Journal of Applied Physiology* 28(2):225, 2003.

42. Streator S: Risk management in athletic training, *Athletic Therapy Today* 6(2):55, 2001.

43. Swann E, Carr D: Managing risk in an athletic training education program, *Athletic Therapy Today* 11(1):17, 2006.

44. Tanner M: *Growth of adolescence,* ed 2, Oxford, England, 1962, Blackwell Scientific.

45. Von Fange T, Wirth J: The preparticipation physical exam. In Hoffman R, editor: *Common musculoskeletal problems,* New York, 2010, Springer.

46. Wham G, Saunders R, Mensch J: Key factors for providing appropriate medical care in secondary school athletics: Athletic training services and budget, *J Athl Train* 45(1):75–86, 2010.

47. Wilson A, Boyling J: *Effective management of musculoskeletal injury: A clinical ergonomics approach to prevention, treatment, and rehabilitation,* Philadelphia, 2002, Churchill Livingstone.

48. Yard E, Collins C, Comstock D: A comparison of high school sports injury surveillance data reporting by certified athletic trainers and coaches, *J Athl Train,* 44(6):645–52, 2009.

49. Zemper E, Dick R: Epidemiology of athletic injuries. In McKeag DB, Moeller JL, editors: *ACSM's primary care sports medicine,* Philadelphia, 2007. Lippincott, Williams & Wilkins.

ANNOTATED BIBLIOGRAPHY

Harrelson G, Gardner G, Winterstein A: *Administrative topics in athletic training: Concepts to practice,* Thoroughfare, NJ, 2009, Slack Incorporated.

Addresses important administrative issues and procedures as well as fundamental concepts, strategies, and techniques related to the management of all aspects of an athletic training health care delivery system.

Karwowski W, Marras W: *Occupational ergonomics: engineering and administrative controls,* Boca Raton, FL, 2003, CRC Press.

Focuses on prevention of work-related musculoskeletal disorders with an emphasis on engineering and administrative controls.

Konin J: *The clinical athletic trainer,* Gaithersburg, MD, 1997, Slack.

A unique, practical book that specifically addresses the administration of a health care program for athletic trainers working in a clinical setting.

Konin J, Frederick M: *Documentation for athletic training,* Thorofare, NJ, 2011, Slack.

Presents the basic principles of medical documentation, various styles of writing, legal considerations, documentation for reimbursement, and many types of written documentation, including evaluations, injury reports, medical releases, and the like.

Mueller F, Cantu R: *Football fatalities and catastrophic injuries 1931–2008,* Durham, NC, 2011, Carolina Academic Press.

This text summarizes the epidemiologic data that has been collected on catastrophic injuries in football and other sports that has been collected over the past 70+ years.

Occupational Safety and Health Administration: Ergonomic for the prevention of Musculoskeletal disorders, Washington, D.C., 2011, U.S. Department of Labor.

Provides recommendations for industrial facilities to reduce the number and severity of work-related musculoskeletal disorders.

Rankin J, Ingersoll C: *Athletic training management: concepts and applications,* St. Louis, 2006, McGraw-Hill.

Designed for upper-division undergraduate or graduate students interested in all aspects of organization and administration of an athletic training program.

Ray R, Konin J: *Management strategies in athletic training,* Champaign, IL, 2011. Human Kinetics.

The first text that covered the principles of organization and administration as they apply to many different employment settings in athletic training; contains many examples and case studies based on principles of administration presented in the text.

Wilson A, Boyling J: *Effective management of musculoskeletal injury: a clinical ergonomics approach to prevention, treatment, and rehabilitation,* Philadelphia, 2002, Churchill Livingstone.

A practical guide designed to help clinicians understand the workplace and lifestyle factors that contribute to musculoskeletal injuries. Examines ergonomic causes as well as personal and psychosocial factors, in addition to discussing cumulative and chronic types of injury.

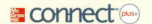

Legal Concerns and Insurance Issues

3

Key Terms

liability   malfeasance
negligence   misfeasance
duty of care   sovereign immunity
torts   Good Samaritan law
nonfeasance   assumption of risk

Connect Highlights **Mc Graw Hill** **connect** (plus+)

Visit connect.mcgraw-hill.com for further exercises to apply your knowledge:

- Clinical application scenarios covering chances of litigation, legal considerations, and insurance
- Click-and-drag questions covering legal considerations and insurance nomenclature
- Multiple-choice questions covering legal concepts and considerations, litigation, and insurance
- Selection questions covering chances of litigation

LEGAL CONCERNS FOR THE ATHLETIC TRAINER

Ours is a litigious society in which legal actions and subsequent lawsuits have become the rule rather than the exception.[33,39] Nowhere is this more true than in our health care system. Ironically, athletic trainers, like all health care providers, are constantly held accountable both for things they do and things they don't do when treating patients. The potential always exists that techniques and procedures athletic trainers use in providing health care will result in some legal action regarding issues of liability and negligence, regardless of the setting in which they practice. **Liability** means being legally responsible for the harm one causes another person.[25] A great deal of care must be taken in following athletic training procedures to reduce the risk of being sued by an athlete and being found liable for negligence.[3,11,18,30]

liability The state of being legally responsible for the harm one causes another person.

The Standard of Reasonable Care

Negligence is the failure to use ordinary or reasonable care—care that persons would normally exercise to avoid injury to themselves or to others under similar circumstances.[12] The *standard of reasonable care* assumes that an individual is neither exceptionally skillful nor extraordinarily cautious but is a person of reasonable and ordinary prudence. Put another way, it is expected that an individual will bring a common-sense approach to the situation at hand and will exercise due care in its handling. In most cases in which someone has been sued for negligence, the actions of a hypothetical, reasonably prudent person are compared with the actions of the defendant to ascertain whether the course of action the defendant followed was in conformity with the judgment exercised by such a reasonably prudent person.[26]

negligence The failure to use ordinary or reasonable care.

The standard of reasonable care requires that an athletic trainer act according to the standard of care of an individual with similar educational background or training.[14] An athletic trainer who is well educated in his or her field and who is certified and/or licensed must act in accordance with those qualifications.

To establish negligence, an individual making the complaint must establish four things: (1) a **duty of care** existed between the person injured and the person responsible for that injury; (2) conduct of the defendant fell short of the standard of care; (3) the defendant caused the injury to occur; and (4) personal, property, or punitive damages resulted.[24]

duty of care Part of an official job description.

Torts

Torts are legal wrongs committed against the person or property of another.[32] All individuals are expected to conduct themselves without injuring others. When they do so, either intentionally or by negligence, they can be required by a court to pay money to the injured party ("damages"), so that ultimately they will suffer some pain caused by their action. A tort also serves as a deterrent by sending a message to the community as to what is unacceptable conduct.

torts Legal wrongs committed against a person.

Such wrongs may emanate from **nonfeasance** (also referred to as an *act of omission*), wherein the individual fails to perform a legal duty; from **malfeasance** (also referred to as an *act of commission*), wherein an individual commits an act that is not legally his or hers to perform; or from **misfeasance,** wherein an individual improperly does something that he or she has the legal right to do. In any instance, if injury results, the person can be held liable. In the case of nonfeasance, an athletic trainer may fail to refer a seriously injured patient for the proper medical attention. In the case of malfeasance, the athletic trainer may perform a therapeutic treatment that violates the practice of another licensed health care professional and as a result serious medical complications develop. In a case of misfeasance, the athletic trainer may incorrectly administer a treatment technique procedure he or she has been trained to perform.

nonfeasance When an individual fails to perform a legal duty.

malfeasance An individual commits an act that is not legally his or hers to perform.

misfeasance An individual improperly does something he or she has the legal right to do.

Negligence When an athletic trainer is sued, the complaint typically is for the tort of negligence. Negligence is alleged when an individual (1) does something that a reasonably prudent person would not do or (2) fails to do something that a reasonably prudent person would do under circumstances similar to those shown by the evidence.[23] To be successful in a suit for negligence, an individual must prove that (1) the athletic trainer had a *duty* to exercise reasonable care, (2) that the athletic trainer *breached* that duty by failing to use reasonable care, and (3) that there is a reasonable connection between the failure to use reasonable care and the injury the individual suffered, or that the athletic trainer's action made the injury worse. If the athletic trainer breaches a duty to exercise reasonable care, but there is no reasonable connection between the failure to use reasonable care and the injury suffered, the suit for negligence will not succeed.

A baseball batter was struck with a pitched ball directly in the orbit of the right eye and fell immediately to the ground. The athletic trainer ran to the player to examine the eye. There was some immediate swelling and discoloration around the orbit, but the eye appeared to be normal. The player insisted that he was fine and told the athletic trainer he could continue to bat. After the game the athletic trainer told the patient to go back to his room, put ice on his eye, and check in tomorrow. That night the baseball player began to hemorrhage into the anterior chamber of the eye and suffered irreparable damage to his eye. An ophthalmologist stated that if the patient's eye had been examined immediately after the injury, the bleeding could have been controlled and there would not have been any damage to his vision.

? If the patient brings a lawsuit against the athletic trainer, what must the patient prove if he is to win a judgment?

sovereign immunity Neither the government nor any individual who is employed by the government can be held liable for negligence.

An example of negligence is when an athletic trainer, through improper or careless handling of a therapeutic agent, seriously burns a patient. Another illustration, occurring all too often in sports, is one in which a coach or some other individual moves a possibly seriously injured athlete from the field of play to permit competition or practice to continue and does so either in an improper manner or before consulting those qualified to know the proper course of action. Should a serious or disabling injury result, the individual who made the decision may be found liable.[23]

Athletic trainers employed by an institution have a duty to provide athletic training care to individuals at that institution. An athletic trainer who is employed by the public schools or by a state-funded college or university may be protected by the legal doctrine of **sovereign immunity,** which essentially states that neither the government nor any individual who is employed by the government can be held liable for negligence. However, it should be made clear that the level of protection afforded by sovereign immunity may vary significantly from state to state. Clinical athletic trainers have a greater choice than institutional athletic trainers of whom they may choose to treat as a patient. Once the athletic trainer assumes the duty of caring for a patient, the athletic trainer has an obligation to make sure that appropriate care is given. It should be made clear that the athletic trainer, or any other person, is not obligated to provide first-aid care for an injured person outside his or her scope of employment. However, if the athletic trainer chooses to become involved as a caregiver for an injured person, he or she is expected to provide reasonable care consistent with his or her level of training. The **Good Samaritan law** has been enacted in most states to provide limited protection against legal liability to any individual who voluntarily chooses to provide first aid, should something go wrong. As long as the first-aid provider does not overstep the limits of his or her professional training and exercises what would be considered reasonable care in the situation, the provider will not be held liable.

A person possessing more training in a given field or area is expected to possess a correspondingly higher level of competence than is a student.[13] An individual will therefore be judged in terms of his or her performance in any situation in which legal liability may be assessed. It must be recognized that liability per se in all its various aspects is not assessed at the same level nationally, but varies in interpretation from state to state and from area to area. Athletic trainers therefore should know and acquire the level of competence expected in their particular area. In essence, negligence is conduct that results in the creation of an unreasonable risk of harm to others.[9]

Good Samaritan law Provides limited protection against legal liability to any person who chooses to provide first aid. However, it does not apply to someone who has a duty to act as dictated by the nature of his or her job.

Statutes of Limitation

A *statute of limitation* sets a specific length of time that individuals may sue for damages from negligence. The length of time to bring suit varies from state to state, but in general plaintiffs have between one and five years to file suit for negligence. The statute of limitations begins to run on a plaintiff's time to file a lawsuit for negligence either from the time of the negligent act or omission that gives rise to the suit or from the time of the discovery of an injury caused by the negligent act or omission. Some states permit an injured minor to file suit up to three years after the minor reaches the age of 18.[6] Therefore, an injured minor's cause of action for negligence against an athletic trainer remains valid for many years after the negligent act or omission occurred or after the discovery of an injury caused by the negligent act or omission.[6]

? How should the first-aid care provided by a certified athletic trainer working in a health club differ from the care that may be provided by a lay person?

Assumption of Risk

An athlete assumes the risk of participating in an activity when he or she knows of and understands the dangers of that activity and voluntarily chooses to be exposed to those dangers. An assumption of risk can be expressed in the form of a waiver signed by an athlete or his or her parents or guardian or can be implied from the conduct of an athlete under the circumstances of his or her participation in an activity.[6]

assumption of risk The individual, through express or implied agreement, assumes that some risk or danger is involved in the particular undertaking. In other words, a person takes his or her own chances.

Assumption of risk may be asserted as a defense to a negligence suit. The athletic trainer bears the burden of proving that an individual assumed the risk by producing the document signed by that individual or his or her parents or guardian or by proving that the risk of the activity was known, understood, and voluntarily accepted.[6]

Assumption of risk, however, is subject to many and varied interpretations by courts, especially when a minor is involved, because he or she is not considered able to render a mature judgment about the risks inherent in the situation. Although individuals participating in a sports program are considered to assume a normal risk, this assumption in no way excuses those in charge from exercising reasonable care and prudence in the conduct of such activities, or from foreseeing and taking precautionary measures against accident-provoking circumstances.[8,15] In general, courts have been fairly consistent in upholding waivers and releases of liability for adults unless there is evidence of fraud, misrepresentation, or duress.[7]

Reducing the Risk of Litigation

The athletic trainer can significantly decrease the risk of litigation by paying attention to a number of important guidelines:

3-3 Clinical Application Exercise

An athletic trainer is cleaning out a filing cabinet in a rehabilitation clinic and decides to throw some older medical files away. Concern is expressed, however, about how long these files should be maintained for legal purposes.

? What is the statute of limitations for an adult patient to file suit?

1. Work to establish good personal relationships with athletes, parents, patients, clients, and coworkers.
2. Establish specific policies and guidelines for the operation of an athletic training facility or clinic, and maintain qualified and adequate supervision of the facility, its environs, facilities, and equipment at all times.
3. Develop, review annually, and carefully follow an emergency action plan.
4. Become familiar with the health status and medical history of the individuals under his or her care (see Chapter 2) so as to be aware of problems that could present a need for additional care or caution.
5. Keep factually accurate and timely records that document all injuries and rehabilitation steps, and set up a record retention policy that allows records to be kept and used in defense of litigation that may be brought by a patient. A record retention system needs to keep records long enough to defend against suits brought by patients after they reach the age of 18.
6. Document efforts to create a safe rehabilitation or training environment.
7. Have a detailed job description in writing.
8. Obtain, from parents or guardians when minors are involved, written consent for providing health care (see Chapter 2).
9. Maintain the confidentiality of medical records (see Chapter 2).
10. Exercise extreme caution in the administration, if allowed by law, of nonprescription medications; athletic trainers may not dispense prescription drugs.
11. Use only those therapeutic methods that he or she is qualified to use and that the law states may be used.
12. Do not use or permit the presence of faulty or hazardous equipment.
13. Work cooperatively with the coach and the team physician in the selection and use of sports protective equipment, and insist that the best equipment be obtained, properly fitted, and properly maintained.
14. Do not permit injured players to participate unless cleared by the team physician.
15. Develop an understanding with the coaches that an injured patient will not be allowed to reenter competition until, in the opinion of the team physician or the athletic trainer, he or she is psychologically and physically able. Athletic trainers should not allow themselves to be pressured to clear a patient until he or she is fully cleared by the physician.
16. Follow the express orders of the physician at all times.
17. Purchase professional liability insurance that provides adequate financial coverage, and be aware of the limitations of the policy.
18. Know the limitations of his or her expertise as well as the applicable state regulations and restrictions that limit the athletic trainer's scope of practice.
19. Use common sense in making decisions about a patient's health and safety.

In the case of an injury, the athletic trainer must use reasonable care to prevent additional injury until further medical care is obtained.[28] (See Chapter 12 for additional comments.)

Product Liability

Product liability is the liability of any or all parties along the chain of manufacture of any product for damage caused by that product.[17] This includes the manufacturer of component parts, an assembling manufacturer, the wholesaler, and the retail store owner. Products containing inherent defects that cause harm to a consumer of the product, or someone to whom the product was loaned or given, are the subjects of product liability suits. Product liability claims can be based on negligence, strict liability, or breach of warranty of fitness, depending on the jurisdiction within which the claim is based. Many states have enacted comprehensive product liability statutes, and these statutory provisions can be very diverse. There is no federal product liability law.

Manufacturers of athletic and rehabilitation equipment have a duty to design and produce equipment that will not cause injury as long as it is used as intended.[22] If the product is not used correctly by the consumer, the manufacturer cannot be held liable. Manufacturers are strictly liable for defects in the design and production of equipment that produces injury. This does not excuse the athletic trainer who misuses the equipment, only equipment that is faulty. An athletic trainer must not alter the equipment in any way. To do so invalidates the manufacturer's warranty and places liability solely on the athletic trainer. An express warranty is the manufacturer's written statement that a product is safe. For example, warning labels on football helmets inform the player of possible dangers inherent in using the product. Individuals must read and sign a form indicating that they have read and understand the warning. The National Operating Committee on Standards for Athletic Equipment (NOCSAE) establishes minimum standards for football helmets that must be met to ensure their safety.

INSURANCE CONSIDERATIONS

During the past 40 years, the insurance industry has undergone a significant evolutionary process. Health care reform initiated in the 1990s focused on the concept of *managed care*, in which the costs of a health care provider's medical care are closely monitored and scrutinized by insurance carriers. Often, preapproval is required prior to health care delivery.

More recently the highly controversial Patient Protection and Affordable Care Act, passed in 2010, asserts more federal control over health care benefits and financing. The effects of this Act on insurance coverage cannot be determined because there are many legal challenges to this legislation.

Since 1971, there has been a significant, steady increase in the number of lawsuits filed. The costs of insurance have also significantly increased during this period. More lawsuits and much higher medical costs are causing a crisis in the insurance industry.[29] Medical insurance is a contract between an insurance company and a policyholder in which the insurance company agrees to reimburse a portion of the total medical bill after some deductible has been paid by the policyholder. The major types of insurance about which individuals concerned with athletic training and sports medicine should have some understanding are general health insurance, accident insurance, professional liability insurance, and catastrophic insurance, as well as insurance for errors and omissions. There is a need to protect adequately all who are concerned with health and safety. *Focus Box 3–1:* "Common insurance terminology" lists some of the more common insurance terms.

General Health Insurance

Every person should have a *general health insurance* policy that covers illness, hospitalization, and emergency care. Some institutions offer primary insurance coverage in which all medical expenses are

> Every person should have a general health insurance policy that covers illness, hospitalization, and emergency care.

paid for by the institution. The institutions pay an extremely high premium for this type of coverage. Most institutions offer *secondary insurance* coverage, which pays the remaining medical bills once the personal insurance company has made its payment. Secondary insurance always includes a deductible that is not covered by the plan.

Many people are covered under some type of *family health insurance* policy. However, the institution or corporation must make certain that personal health insurance is arranged for or purchased by individuals not covered under family policies.[34] A form letter directed to the parents of all minors should be completed and returned to the institution to make certain that appropriate coverage is provided (Figure 3–1). Some so-called comprehensive plans do not cover every health need. For example, they may cover physicians' care but not hospital charges. Many of these plans require large prepayments before the insurance takes effect. Supplemental policies, such as accident insurance and catastrophic insurance, are designed to take over where general health insurance stops.

Accident Insurance

Besides general health insurance, low-cost *accident insurance* is available. It often covers accidents on

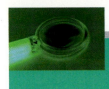

Common insurance terminology[10]

Allowable charge: the maximum amount, according to the individual policy, that insurance will pay for each procedure or service performed.

Beneficiary: a person eligible to receive the benefits of a specific policy or program.

Benefits: services that an insurer, a government agency, or a health care plan offers to pay for an insured individual.

Case management services: the process in which the attending physician or agent coordinates the care given to a patient by other health care providers and/or community organizations.

Claim: a form sent to an insurance company, requesting payment for covered medical expenses; information includes the insured's name and address, procedure codes, diagnostic codes, charges, and date of service.

Clean claim: a filed claim with all the necessary information that may be immediately processed.

Coinsurance: also referred to as copayment; the insurer and the insured split the cost of health care at a specified percentage, usually either 80/20 or 70/30.

Contract: a legally binding agreement between an insurance company and a physician describing the duties of both parties.

Copayment: a provision in an insurance policy requiring the policyholder to pay a specified percentage of each medical claim.

Customary fees: the average fee charged for a specified service or procedure in a defined geographical area.

Deductible: the amount owed by the insured on a yearly basis before the insurance company will begin to pay for services rendered.

Dependent: a person legally eligible for benefits based on his or her relationship with the policyholder.

Exclusions: specified medical services, disorders, treatments, diseases, and durable medical equipment that are listed as uncovered or not reimbursable in an insurance policy.

Explanation of benefits (EOB): an insurance report accompanying all claim payments that explains how the insurance company processed a claim.

Fee schedule: a comprehensive listing of the maximum payment amount that an insurance company will allow for specified medical procedures performed on a beneficiary of the plan.

Gatekeeper: the primary care physician assigned by the insurer who oversees the medical care rendered to a patient and initiates all specialty and ancillary services.

Participating provider: a health care provider who has entered into a contract with an insurance company to provide medical services to the beneficiaries of a plan; the provider agrees to accept the insurance company's approved fee and will only bill the patient for the deductible, the copayment, and uncovered services.

Policyholder: the person who takes out the medical insurance policy.

Premium: a periodic payment made to an insurance company by an individual policyholder.

Third-party administrator: an independent organization that collects premiums, pays claims, and provides administrative services within a health care plan.

UCR allowable charge: usual, customary, and reasonable charge that represents the maximum amount an insurance company will pay for a given service based on geographical averages.

---

school grounds while the student is in attendance or accidents that occur in the workplace. The purposes of this insurance are to protect against financial loss from medical and hospital bills, encourage an injured patient to receive prompt medical care, encourage prompt reporting of injuries, and relieve an institution or a corporation of financial responsibility.[38]

General insurance may be limited; thus, accident insurance for a specific activity may be needed to provide additional protection.[20] This type of coverage is limited and does not require knowledge of fault, and the amount it pays is limited. For serious injuries requiring surgery and lengthy rehabilitation, accident insurance is usually not adequate. This inadequacy can put families with limited budgets into a financial bind. Of particular concern is insurance that does not adequately cover catastrophic injuries.

Catastrophic Insurance

Although catastrophic injuries are relatively uncommon, when they do occur, the consequences to the individual, family, and institution, as well as to society, can be staggering.[34] In the past when available funds have been completely diminished, the family was forced to seek funding elsewhere,

3–4 Clinical Application Exercise

An athletic trainer who recently became certified is planning on working summer camps for an area high school before he starts his full-time employment in the fall.

? What should the athletic trainer do to protect himself from liability?

Emergency and Insurance Information on Student Athletes

Student's Name _____ Date of Birth _____ Sport _____

Home Address _____

Home Phone _____

Cell Phone/Pager _____

Social Security or Student ID Number _____ Sex: M ___ F ___

Family Doctor _____ Phone _____

Address _____

Policyholder _____ Relation to Student _____

Employer _____

Address _____

Home Phone _____ Work Phone _____

Name of Primary Insurance Company _____

Address of Primary Insurance Company _____

Certificate Number _____ Group _____ Type _____

Is preauthorization required for medical procedures? _____ _____

                                                              Yes   No

Name of Secondary Insurance Company _____

Address of Secondary Insurance Company _____

Certificate Number _____ Group_____Type _____

Policyholder _____ Relationship to Student _____

Employer of Policyholder _____

Is preauthorization required for medical procedures? _____ _____

                                                             Yes   No

Should my son/daughter require services beyond those covered by the Sports Medicine Program, I give permission to the Division of Sports Medicine to file a claim for such services with the above health insurer.

I understand that any insurance payments I receive must be returned to be placed on my child's account.

Parent/Guardian's Signature _____ Date _____

FIGURE 3–1   Sample emergency and insurance information form.

usually through a lawsuit. For example, in athletics, organizations such as the National Collegiate Athletic Association (NCAA) and National Association of Intercollegiate Athletics (NAIA) provide plans for the athlete who requires a lifetime of extensive medical and rehabilitative care because of a permanent disability.[4] Benefits begin when expenses have reached $25,000 and are then extended for a lifetime. A program at the secondary-school level is offered to districts by the National Federation of State High School Associations (NFHS). This plan provides medical, rehabilitation, and transportation costs in excess of $10,000 not covered by other insurance benefits.[34] Costs for catastrophic insurance are based on the number of sports and the number of hazardous sports offered by the institution.

To offset the shotgun approach of lawsuits and to cover what is not covered by a general liability policy, *errors and omissions liability insurance* has evolved. It is designed to cover school employees, officers, and the district against suits claiming malpractice, wrongful actions, errors and omissions, and acts of negligence.[34] Even when working in a program that has good liability coverage, each person within that program who works directly with students

3–5 Clinical Application Exercise

During a state gymnastics meet, a gymnast fell off the uneven parallel bars and landed on her forearm. The athletic trainer suspected a fracture and decided an X-ray was needed. The gymnast's parents had general health insurance through a PPO, but because the gymnast was in severe pain, she was sent to the nearest emergency room to be treated. Unfortunately, the emergency facility was not on the list of preferred providers, and the insurance company denied the claim. The athletic trainer assured the parents that the meet organizers would take care of whatever medical costs were not covered by their insurance policy.

? Because the PPO denied the claim, what type of insurance policy should the meet organizers carry to cover the medical costs?

must have his or her own personal liability insurance.

Insurance that covers an individual's health and safety can be complex. The athletic trainer must ensure that every individual is adequately covered by a reliable insurance company. In some employment settings, filing claims becomes the responsibility of the athletic trainer. This task can be highly time-consuming, taking the athletic trainer away from his or her major role of working directly with the patient. Because of the intricacies and time involved with claim filing and follow-up communications with patients, parents, doctors, and vendors, a staff person other than the athletic trainer should be assigned this responsibility.

Professional Liability Insurance

Most employers have general liability insurance to protect against damages that may arise from injuries occurring on their property. Liability

> **Because of the amount of litigation for alleged negligence, all professionals should be fully protected by professional liability insurance.**

insurance covers claims of negligence on the part of individuals.[8] Its major concern is whether supervision was reasonable and if unreasonable risk of harm was perceived by the individual who was injured.[36]

Because of the amount of litigation based on alleged negligence, premiums have become almost prohibitive. Typically, a victim's lawsuit has taken a shotgun approach, suing the employer athletic trainer, physician, administrator, and company or school district. If a piece of equipment is involved, the product manufacturer is also sued.

All athletic trainers should carry *professional liability insurance* and must clearly understand the limits of its coverage. Liability insurance typically covers negligence in a civil case. If a criminal complaint is filed, however, liability insurance will not cover the athletic trainer.

THIRD-PARTY REIMBURSEMENT

Third-party reimbursement is the primary mechanism of payment for medical services in the United States.[19] The policyholder's insurance company reimburses health care professionals for services performed. Medical insurance companies may provide group

> **Third-party reimbursement involves reimbursement by the policyholder's insurance company for services performed by health care professionals.**

and individual coverage for employees and dependents.[19] Managed care involves a prearranged system for delivering health care that is designed to control costs while continuing to provide quality care. To cut payout costs, many insurance companies pay for preventive care (to reduce the need for hospitalization) and limit where the individual can go for care. A number of health care systems have been developed to contain costs.[21]

Health Maintenance Organizations

Health maintenance organizations (HMOs) provide preventive measures and limit where the individual can receive care. Except in emergencies, permission must be obtained before the individual can go to another provider. HMOs generally pay 100 percent of the medical costs as long as care is rendered at an HMO facility. Many supplemental policies do not cover the medical costs that would normally be paid by the general policy. Therefore, an athlete treated outside the HMO

> **Third-party payers:**
> - HMO
> - PPO
> - POS
> - EPO
> - PHO
> - TPA
> - Medicare
> - Medicaid
> - Workers compensation
> - Indemnity plans
> - Capitation

may be ineligible for any insurance benefits. Many HMOs determine fees using a capitation system, which limits the amount that will be reimbursed for a specific service. It is essential that the athletic trainer understand the limits of and restrictions on coverage at his or her institution or company.

Preferred Provider Organizations

Preferred provider organizations (PPOs) provide discount health care but also limit where a person can go for treatment of an illness. The athletic trainer must be apprised in advance as to where the ill patient should be sent. Patients sent to a facility that is not on the approved list may be required to pay for care, whereas, if they are sent to a preferred facility, all costs are paid.[1] PPOs may provide added services, such as physical therapy, more easily and at no cost or at a much lower cost than would another insurance policy. PPOs pay on a fee-for-service basis.

Point of Service Plan

The point of service (POS) plan is a combination of the HMO and PPO plans. It is based on an HMO structure, yet it allows members to go outside the HMO to obtain services. This flexibility is allowed only with certain conditions and under special circumstances.

Exclusive Provider Organizations

Exclusive provider organizations (EPOs) are also a combination of the HMO and PPO plans. They are restrictive in the number and types of providers they have and consequently are more like an HMO. Most will not pay anything if you use out-of-network providers.

Physician Hospital Organization

Physician hospital organizations (PHOs) involve a major hospital or hospital chain and its physicians. A PHO organization contracts directly with employers to provide services and/or contracts with a managed care organization.

Third-Party Administrators

Third-party administrators (TPAs) are frequently used to administer services and to pay claims for self-insured group plans and thus function as pseudo insurance companies. They perform member services, such as enrollment and billing, and assist with controlling utilization without the financial risk.

Medicare

Medicare is the federal health insurance program for the aged and disabled. Most people at retirement age qualify for Medicare benefits. There are four parts, or sections, to Medicare. Part A, the hospital portion, is normally premium-free at retirement to the beneficiary. Part B, the physician portion, has a monthly premium charge to the beneficiary.

Part C is a program that allows a person to choose among several types of health care plans, including medical savings accounts, managed care plans, and private fee-for-service plans.

Part D, a federal program to subsidize the costs of prescription drugs for Medicare beneficiaries, went into effect in 2006. Beneficiaries can either join a Prescription Drug Plan (PDP) for drug coverage only, or they can join a Medicare Advantage (MA) plan that covers both medical services and prescription drugs.

Medicaid

Medicaid is a health insurance program for people with low incomes and limited resources. Medicaid is funded by both the federal government and individual states, with the states responsible for handling the administration of the program. Individual states administer Medicaid; thus, benefits vary by state.

Workers Compensation

Workers compensation laws and benefits for injured workers are mandated by the states. Employers pay the premiums, and the claims are settled by workers compensation insurance carriers whose goal is to return injured workers to the workforce as soon as possible.

Indemnity Plans

An indemnity plan is the most traditional form of billing for health care. It is a fee-for-service plan that allows the insured party to seek medical care without restrictions on utilization or cost. The provider charges the patient or a third-party payer for services provided. Charges are based on a set fee schedule.

Capitation

Capitation is a form of reimbursement used by managed care providers in which members make a standard payment each month regardless of how much service is rendered to the member by the provider.

Third-Party Reimbursement for Athletic Trainers

Athletic trainers have always been able to bill third-party payers for services rendered. For many years, most insurers were reluctant to reimburse the athletic trainer for the health care services provided. Throughout the 1990s and early 2000s, there was a significant increase in reimbursement from third-party payers for athletic trainers working in a variety of settings, including rehabilitation clinics, hospitals, physicians' offices, and college and university settings.[26] Most third-party payers view "licensed health care professionals" as the only reimbursable entities, and fortunately in most states this includes certified athletic trainers.

In 1995, NATA established the Reimbursement Advisory Group to monitor managed care changes and to help the athletic trainer secure

An athletic trainer working in a clinic is seeking third-party reimbursement for athletic training services performed. The athletic trainer is experiencing difficulty obtaining reimbursement from certain payers because of uncertainty about the effectiveness of the treatment program.

? What can the athletic trainer do to address the concerns of the third-party payers?

a place as a health care provider. Specifically, this group was charged with developing a model for approaching third-party payers for the reimbursement of athletic training services, of educating athletic trainers on issues related to reimbursement, and, perhaps most important, of designing and implementing a data-based clinical outcomes study.[5] In 1996, NATA initiated the Athletic Training Outcomes Assessment project designed to present supporting data that measure the results of interventions involving athletic training procedures. This three-year study was designed to provide data that focused on functional outcomes, including assessing the patients' perceptions of their functional capabilities and their overall satisfaction with their treatment program; assessing the physical, emotional, and social well-being of patients; assessing health care cost effectiveness relative to time lost from activity due to injury; and assessing the number of treatments.[10] The results of this study were critical in securing reimbursement for athletic training services, because the majority of third-party payers currently require outcomes research when evaluating a contract.[25]

Centers for Medicare & Medicaid Services (CMS) Ruling In 2005, the Centers for Medicare & Medicaid Services (CMS) issued a decision that has had and will continue to have a crippling effect on the ability of athletic trainers to receive reimbursement for health care services.[37] The ruling stated that they would "no longer pay for therapy 'incident to' a physician's services unless the provider is a physical therapist, occupational therapist or speech/language pathologist." Under this rule, physicians are not able to bill Medicare for treatment provided by athletic trainers. Though not bound by this ruling, there is little doubt that the majority of third-party payers tend to follow the lead of Medicare and Medicaid when deciding who will be reimbursed for health care services provided. With this ruling, it is clear that the federal government does not recognize athletic trainers as providers of rehabilitative services for Medicare patients, no matter what age.[37]

Certainly, this ruling directly and immediately affected reimbursement for athletic trainers working in clinics and hospitals or as physician extenders. It has also caused many clinical athletic trainers who also work in secondary schools to lose their jobs. It is likely that the CMS ruling will also negatively impact future state and national legislative efforts on behalf of athletic trainers. The NATA is currently exploring every means of legal recourse to have this ruling reversed or at least modified. In 2009, the Athletic Trainers' Equal Access to Medicare Act (bill HR 1137) was introduced in the United States House of Representatives. This act sought to ensure that Medicare beneficiaries would have better access to health care provided by state licensed or certified athletic trainers. Unfortunately, this bill did not make it out of the congressional committee level, and thus it never became a law. Certainly, securing third-party reimbursement for athletic training services must continue to be a priority, especially for the clinical athletic trainer.[35]

Insurance Billing

The athletic trainer must file insurance claims immediately and correctly.[36] Athletic trainers working in educational settings can facilitate this process by collecting insurance information on every individual at the beginning of the year. Letters should be drafted to the parents of all athletes, explaining the limits of the school insurance policy and what the parents must do to process a claim if injury does occur. Schools with secondary policies should stress that the parents must submit all bills to their insurance company before they submit the remainder to the school. In educational institutions, most claims will be filed with a single insurance company, which will pay for medical services provided by individual health care providers.

In most cases, when filing an insurance claim for a patient seen in a clinic or hospital, individuals other than health care providers are employed to make certain that a patient has provided current insurance information. The athletic trainer will likely not be the individual who is responsible for following up on insurance claims filed with third-party payers.[31]

Filing an Insurance Claim When filing an insurance claim to submit for reimbursement, athletic trainers will find that most carriers accept a standard form labeled HCFA-1500/HCFA-1450 (Blue Cross Blue Shield uses Form UB-92). These forms must be completed in detail with as much information as possible. Experience dictates that the more accurately and thoroughly these forms are completed, the quicker and higher the rate of reimbursement.

Athletic trainers working in the clinical setting should understand that the clinic must be able to collect reimbursement from third-party payers for services provided. The athletic trainer should request approval from insurance companies before treating patients.[35]

TABLE 3–1   Description of Billing Codes Used by Athletic Trainers

The following is a guide to procedure billing codes that may be used by athletic trainers when billing for athletic training services:

Code	Description
97005/97006	Athletic trainer evaluation and reevaluation (per visit)
97750	Physical performance test (each 15 minutes) treatment charges
97116	Gait training (each 15 minutes)
97110	Therapeutic exercise (each 15 minutes)
97112	Neuromuscular reeducation (each 15 minutes)
97530	Therapeutic activities (each 15 minutes)
97113	Aquatic therapeutic exercise (each 15 minutes)
97124	Massage (each 15 minutes)
97530	Body mechanics training (each 15 minutes)
97140	Manual therapy (each 15 minutes)
97504	Orthotics fitting and training (each 15 minutes)
97150	Therapeutic procedures—group (each visit)
97150	Supervised exercise (each visit)
11040	Debridement (each visit)
97139	Wound care (each 15 minutes)
97139	Taping (each visit)
95831	Manual muscle testing—extremity/trunk
95851	Range of motion (ROM) measurements
95852	ROM measurements of hand, with or without comparison with normal side
97545	Work hardening/conditioning (initial 2 hours)
97035	Ultrasound (each 15 minutes)
97035	Phonophoresis (each 15 minutes) (must bill for ultrasound if billing for this service)
97032	Electrical stimulation (each 15 minutes)
97033	Iontophoresis (each 15 minutes)
97032	Constant electrical stimulation (each 15 minutes)
97034	Contrast baths (each 15 minutes)
97014	Electric stimulation (application to one or more areas)
97022	Whirlpool (application to one or more areas)
97010	Hot packs (application to one or more areas)
97010	Cold packs/ice massage (application to one or more areas)
97012	Traction, mechanical (not time-based)
97016	Compression pump (application to one or more areas)

Two types of billing codes must be used when submitting a claim on standard HCFA-1500 or UB-92 forms to third-party payers: a *diagnostic code* and a *procedural code*.[16] A diagnostic code is required for all procedural billing, and they can be found in a book called the *International Classification of Diseases* (ICD-9-CM). This is a five-digit code that specifies the condition or injury that the athletic trainer or any other health care provider is treating.[31] For example, code 845.02 indicates that the patient has a sprain of the calcaneofibular ligament in the ankle.

The *Current Procedure Terminology Code* (CPT) was first developed by the American Medical Association in 1966. Each year, an annual publication designates changes corresponding to significant updates in medical technology and practice. The CPT code is used to identify specific medical procedures used in treating a patient.[31] Table 3–1 lists the current CPT codes most often used by the athletic trainer.

3–7 Clinical Application Exercise

? When filing an insurance claim for rehabilitation services following injury, what can an athletic trainer do to improve the reimbursement rate as well as to speed up the process?

3–8 Clinical Application Exercise

A sports medicine clinic is considering hiring an athletic trainer. However, the clinic administrator is concerned that the athletic trainer cannot bill third-party payers for services provided.

? What does the administrator need to be told about third-party reimbursement for athletic training services?

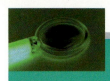

Guidelines for documentation*

When billing for and receiving reimbursement, the following points should be documented:

- Initial evaluation, including plan of treatment and goals (SOAP notes)
- Appropriate patient medical history
- Patient examination results
- Functional assessment
- Type of treatment and body parts to be treated
- Expected frequency and number of treatments
- Prognosis
- Functional, measurable, and time-based goals
- Precautions and contraindications
- A statement that the treatment plan and goals were discussed and understood by the patient and possibly by the guardian

- Daily treatment records
- A record of any changes in physical status, physician orders or treatment plan, or goals
- Weekly progress notes, especially on goals (SOAP or function-based)
- Copies of notes to or from the referring physician's office, whether by fax, e-mail, U.S. mail, or phone
- A prescription or other state-mandated documentation from a physician

*From the NATA Committee on Reimbursement.

Athletic trainers should never release medical records to third-party payers unless written authorization has been obtained from the patient, according to HIPAA and FERPA guidelines.[27] (See Chapter 2.) It is also essential when billing for and receiving reimbursement that the athletic trainer keep meticulous, accurate, and detailed documentation of all procedures, charges submitted, and payments received for services.[2] *Focus Box 3–2*: "Guidelines for documentation" identifies criteria that should be routinely followed when billing for charges.

National Provider Identifier (NPI) The National Provider Identifier (NPI) is a government-issued identification number for individual health care providers and provider organizations (i.e., clinics, hospitals, group practices). Covered health care providers and all health plans and health care clearinghouses must use the NPIs in administrative and financial transactions, according to the Health Insurance Portability and Accountability Act (HIPAA). The NPI is a 10-digit numeric identifier. As of 2007, any health care provider who uses standard electronic transactions, such as electronic claims, eligibility verifications, claims status inquiries, and claim attachments, is required by federal law to include NPIs on electronic transactions. To apply for an NPI, go to https://NPPES.cms.hhs.gov.

SUMMARY

- A great deal of care must be taken in following athletic training procedures that conform to the legal guidelines governing liability for negligence.
- Liability is the state of being legally responsible for the harm one causes another person. It assumes that an athletic trainer would act according to the standard of care of any individual with similar educational background and training.
- An athletic trainer who fails to use reasonable care—care that persons would normally exercise to avoid injury to themselves or to others under similar circumstances—may be found liable for negligence.
- Although athletes participating in a sports program are considered to assume a normal risk, this assumption in no way exempts those in charge from exercising reasonable care.
- Athletic trainers can significantly decrease the risk of litigation by making certain that they have done everything possible to provide a reasonable degree of care to the injured patient.

- The major types of insurance about which athletic trainers should have some understanding are general health insurance, accident insurance, professional liability insurance, catastrophic insurance, and insurance for errors and omissions.
- Third-party reimbursement is the primary mechanism of payment for medical services in the United States. A number of different health care systems have been developed to contain costs.
- It is essential that the athletic trainer file insurance claims immediately and correctly using appropriate forms and billing codes.

WEB SITES

Legal Information Institute at Cornell: http://topics.law.cornell.edu/wex/sports_law
This Web site is part of a series of legal information and specifically addresses law in sport; the information is rather technical in nature. The area relevant to sports medicine is addressed in the section titled "Torts."

Sports Lawyers Journal: www.law.tulane.edu/ tlsjournals/slj/index.aspx
Specialized academic and professional publication on legal aspects of sports.

Duhaime & Co. Legal Dictionary: www.duhaime.org/dictionary
This is a site that has put together an extensive list of legal terms with clear definitions and explanations.

SOLUTIONS TO CLINICAL APPLICATION EXERCISES

3–1 An athletic trainer who assumes the duty of caring for an athlete has an obligation to make sure that appropriate care is given. If the athletic trainer fails to provide an acceptable standard of care, there is a breach of duty on the part of the athletic trainer, and the athlete must then prove that this breach caused the injury or made the injury worse.

3–2 A person possessing more training in a given field or area is expected to possess a correspondingly higher level of competence than a layperson is. A certified athletic trainer will therefore be judged in terms of his or her performance in any situation in which legal liability may be assessed.

3–3 In personal injury cases, the individual would typically have between one and five years to file suit for negligence. The statute of limitations begins to run on a plaintiff's time to file a lawsuit for negligence either from the time of the negligent act or omission that gives rise to the suit or from the time of the discovery of an injury caused by the negligent act or omission.

3–4 The athletic trainer should purchase private professional liability insurance. In addition, the athletic trainer should keep proper records of injuries and keep those records in his or her possession.

3–5 Besides general health insurance, low-cost accident insurance often covers accidents on school grounds while the athlete is competing. The purposes of this insurance are to protect against financial loss from medical and hospital bills,

encourage an injured athlete to receive prompt medical care, encourage prompt reporting of injuries, and relieve a school of financial responsibility.

3–6 The athletic trainer could initiate an outcomes research project designed to present supporting data that measure the results of interventions involving athletic training procedures. This research project would assess the athletes' perceptions of their functional capabilities and overall satisfaction with their treatment program, the cost-effectiveness of the health care relative to time lost from activity due to injury, and the number of treatments. The majority of third-party payers currently require outcomes research when evaluating a contract.

3–7 The athletic trainer should file an insurance claim for reimbursement, using the standard form labeled HCFA-1500. The form should be completed in detail with as much information as possible. The athletic trainer who completes these forms accurately and thoroughly probably experiences a quicker and higher rate of reimbursement.

3–8 It should be pointed out that athletic trainers can bill third-party payers for services rendered to a patient. Whether the insurance company will reimburse the athletic trainer for services is up to the individual third-party payer. With the approval of the uniform billing code for athletic training services, it is more likely that the athletic trainer will be successfully reimbursed for treating patients.

REVIEW QUESTIONS AND CLASS ACTIVITIES

1. What are the athletic trainer's major legal concerns for negligence and for assumption of risk?
2. What measures can an athletic trainer take to minimize the chances of litigation, should an athlete be injured?
3. Invite an attorney who is familiar with sports litigation to class to discuss how athletic trainers can protect themselves from lawsuits.
4. Discuss what the athletic trainer must do to provide reasonable and prudent care in dealing with an injured patient.
5. Why is it necessary for an individual to have both general health insurance and accident insurance?
6. Briefly discuss the various methods of third-party reimbursement.
7. Why should an athletic trainer carry individual liability insurance?
8. What are the critical considerations for filing insurance claims?

REFERENCES

1. Albolm M, Campbell D, Konin J: *Reimbursement for athletic trainers,* Thorofare, NJ, 2001, Slack.
2. Altman S: Legal aspects of crisis-management communication: What to communicate, *Athletic Therapy Today* 10(3):6, 2005.
3. Appenzeller H: *Safe at first: A guide to help sports administrators reduce their liability,* Chapel Hill, NC, 1999, Carolina Academic Press.
4. Bill H, Belk J: *Health Insurance today: A practical approach,* St. Louis, 2010, Elsevier.
5. Campbell D: Workshop on third party reimbursement, *NATA News* 3:34, 1996.
6. Cotten DJ: 2005. Are you safe? Courts in an increasing number of states are enforcing liability waivers signed by parents on behalf of minors, *Athletic Business* 29(3):66–68; 70–72, 2005.
7. Cotten DJ: Waivers and releases can protect against liability, *Fitness management* 20(4):24, 2004.
8. Cotten DJ: What is covered by your liability insurance policy? A risk management essential, *Exercise Standard and Malpractice Reporter* 15(4):54, 2001.
9. Cozillio M, Levinstein M: 2007. *Sports law: Cases and materials,* Durham, NC, Carolina Academic Press.
10. De Carlo M: Reimbursement for health care services. In Konin J: *Clinical athletic training,* Thorofare, NJ, 1997, Slack.
11. Eickhoff-Shemek JAM, Evans JA: An investigation of law and legal liability content in masters academic programs in sports medicine and exercise science, *Journal of Legal Aspects of Sport* 10(3):172, 2000.
12. Frenkel DA: Medico-legal aspects in sport (abstract), *Exercise & Society Journal of Sport Science* (28):90, 2001.
13. Gallup E: *Law and the team physician,* Champaign, IL, 1995, Human Kinetics.
14. Gardiner S: *Sports Law,* New York, 2012, Routledge.
15. Gardiner S, Gray J: Training regimes and medical treatment of elite sports athletes: Issues of legal liability. (Abstract) *Journal of Science & Medicine in Sport* 7 (4 Supplement):111, 2004.
16. Garrison S: Fundamentals of coding, payment and documentation: Understanding their role and impact in healthcare, Chicago, 2011, American Medical Association.
17. Gorman L: Product liability in sports medicine. *Athletic Therapy Today* 4(4):36, 1999.
18. Grayson E: *Ethics, injuries and the law in sports medicine,* New York, 1999, Heinemann-Butterworth.
19. Green M, Rowell J: *Understanding health insurance: A guide to billing and reimbursement,* Albany, 2010, Delmar.
20. Harris D: *Contemporary issues in healthcare law and ethics,* Chicago, 2007, Health Administration Press.
21. Health Insurance Association of America: *Fundamentals of health insurance,* Washington, DC, 1997, HIAA.
22. Henderson J: *Products liability: Problems and process,* New York, 2008, Aspen Publishers.
23. Herbert D: *Legal aspects of sports medicine,* Canton, OH, 1995, Professional Reports Corporation.
24. Herbert DL, Herbert WG: *Legal aspects of preventive, rehabilitative and recreational exercise programs,* ed 4, Canton, OH, 2002, PRC.
25. Hertel J: Research training for clinicians: The crucial link between evidence-based practice and third-party reimbursement (editorial), *J Athl Train* 40(2):69, 2005.
26. Hunt V: Reimbursement efforts continue steady progress, *NATA News,* October:10–12, 2002.
27. Jones D: HIPAA: Friend or foe to athletic trainers? *Athletic Therapy Today* 8(2):17, 2003.
28. Kane S, White R: Medical malpractice and the sports medicine clinician, *Clinical Orthopedics and Related Research,* 467(2):412–19, 2009.
29. McClean S: Legal and ethical aspects of healthcare, New York, 2009, Cambridge University Press.
30. Mitten M, Mitten R: Legal considerations in treating the injured athlete, *J Orthop Sports Phys Ther* 21(1):38, 1995.
31. Moisio M: *Guide to health insurance billing,* Clifton Park, NY, 2006, Thompson Delmar Learning.
32. Pozgar G: *Legal aspects of health care administration,* 2011. Jones & Bartlett.
33. Quandt E, Mitten M: Legal liability in covering athletic events, *Sports Health: A Multidiciplinary Approach,* 1(1):84–90, 2009.
34. Rankin J, Ingersoll C: *Athletic training management: Concepts and applications,* New York, 2006, McGraw-Hill.
35. Ray R: Uniform billing code takes effect for ATCs, *NATA News,* Winter:20, 2000.
36. Ray R, Konin J: *Management strategies in athletic training,* Champaign, IL, 2011, Human Kinetics.
37. Rule change jeopardizes referrals to ATCs: *Physician Sportsmed* 33(7):10, 2005.
38. Vaughn E: *Fundamentals of risk and insurance,* New York, 2002, Wiley.
39. Wong G: *Essentials of sports law,* ed 4, Westport, CT, 2010, Greenwood Press.

ANNOTATED BIBLIOGRAPHY

Albolm M, Campbell D, Konin J: *Reimbursement for athletic trainers,* Thorofare, NJ, 2001, Slack.

Presents a "how to" approach for filing claims, appealing denials, and approaching payers. Covers all current trends in health care reimbursement as well as future directions for reimbursement.

Appenzeller H: *Youth sports and the law: A guide to legal issues,* Chapel Hill, NC, 2000, Carolina Academic Press.

Studies various court cases to understand the legal principles involved in sport participation. The objective of the book is to provide better and safer sporting experiences for today's children.

Gayson E: *Ethics injury and the law in sports medicine,* New York, 1999, Heinemann-Butterworth.

Provides a review of the status of sports medicine and the law. Addresses the key legal and ethical issues in sports and exercise medicine. For practitioners and students preparing for sport and exercise medicine exams.

Green RJ: *Understanding health insurance: A guide to billing and reimbursement,* Albany, 2010, Delmar.

A comprehensive resource for dealing with issues related to insurance.

Herbert D: *Legal aspects of sports medicine,* Canton, OH, 1995, Professional Reports Corporation.

A discussion of sports medicine, policies, procedures, responsibilities of the sports medicine team, informed consent, negligence, insurance and risk management, medication, drug testing, and other topics.

Moisio, M: *Guide to health insurance billing,* Clifton Park, NY, 2006, Thompson Delmar Learning.

All aspects of the billing process, from key terms to state and federal regulations, to guidelines for completing and submitting claims to health insurance programs.

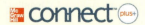

4

Fitness and Conditioning Techniques

■ Connect Highlights   connect plus+

Visit connect.mcgraw-hill.com for further exercises to apply your knowledge:

- Clinical application scenarios covering cardiorespiratory endurance, fitness training, conditioning and periodization
- Click-and-drag questions covering muscular endurance, cardiorespiratory fitness, and conditioning activities
- Multiple-choice questions covering warm-up, cool-down, muscular strength, roles of the athletic trainer in training athlete, and fitness testing
- Selection questions covering flexibility

Exercise is an essential factor in fitness conditioning, injury prevention, and injury rehabilitation. An athletic trainer working with an athletic population in secondary schools, in colleges and universities, or at the professional level

is well aware that to compete successfully at a high level, the athlete must be fit. An athlete who is not fit is more likely to sustain an injury. The athletic trainer should recognize that improper conditioning is one of the primary contributing factors to sports injuries. It is essential that the athlete engage in *conditioning exercises* that can minimize the possibility of injury while maximizing performance.[49]

> Lack of physical fitness is one of the primary causes of sports injury.

The basic principles of conditioning exercises also apply to techniques of therapeutic, rehabilitative, or reconditioning exercises that are specifically concerned with restoring normal body function following injury. Athletic trainers providing patient care in a clinic or hospital are more likely to apply these principles to reconditioning or rehabilitation of an injured patient. The term *therapeutic exercise* is perhaps most widely used to indicate exercises that are used in a rehabilitation program.

Regardless of whether the primary focus is making certain an athlete is fit or reconditioning an injured patient, the athletic trainer must understand the basic principles for improving cardiorespiratory endurance, muscle strength and endurance, and flexibility.

THE RELATIONSHIP BETWEEN ATHLETIC TRAINERS AND STRENGTH AND CONDITIONING COACHES

The responsibility for making certain that an athlete is fit for competition depends on the personnel who are available to oversee this aspect of the athletic program. At the professional level and at most colleges and universities, a full-time strength and conditioning coach is employed to conduct both team and individual training sessions. Many, but not all, strength coaches are certified by the National Strength and Conditioning Association. If a strength coach is involved, it is essential that both the athletic trainers and the team coaches communicate freely and work in close cooperation with the strength coach to ensure that the athletes achieve an optimal level of fitness.

The specific role of the athletic trainer is to critically review the training and conditioning program designed by the strength and conditioning coach and to be extremely familiar with what is expected of the athletes on a daily basis. The athletic trainer should feel free to offer suggestions and make recommendations that are in the best interest of the athletes' health and well-being. If it becomes apparent that a particular exercise or a specific training session seems to be causing an inordinate number of injuries, the athletic trainer should inform the strength and conditioning coach of the problem, so that some alternative exercise can be substituted.

If an athlete is injured and is undergoing a rehabilitation program, it should be the athletic trainer's responsibility to communicate to the strength and conditioning coach how the conditioning program should be limited and/or modified. The athletic trainer must respect the role of the strength and conditioning coach in getting the athlete fit. However, the responsibility for rehabilitating an injured patient clearly belongs to the athletic trainer.

In the majority of secondary-school settings, a strength and conditioning coach is not available; the responsibility for ensuring that the athlete gets fit lies with the athletic trainer and the team coaches. In this situation, the athletic trainer very often assumes the role of a strength and conditioning coach in addition to his or her athletic training responsibilities. The athletic trainer frequently finds it necessary not only to design training and conditioning programs but also to oversee the weight room and to educate young, inexperienced athletes about getting themselves fit to compete. The athletic trainer must demand the cooperation of the team coaches in supervising the training and conditioning program.

PRINCIPLES OF CONDITIONING

The following principles should be applied in all conditioning programs to minimize the likelihood of injury:

1. *Safety.* Make the conditioning environment safe. Take time to educate individuals regarding proper techniques, how they should feel during the workout, and when they should push harder or back off.[38]
2. *Warm-up/cool-down.* Take time to do an appropriate warm-up before engaging in any activity. Do not neglect the cool-down period after a training bout.
3. *Motivation.* Athletes are generally highly motivated to work hard because they want to be successful in their sport. Varying the training program and incorporating techniques of periodization can keep the program enjoyable rather than routine and boring. (See the discussion of periodization at the end of this chapter.)

4. *Overload.* To improve in any physiological component, the individual must work harder than he or she is accustomed to working. Logan and Wallis identified the **SAID principle,** which directly relates to the principle of overload.[61] SAID is an acronym for specific adaptation to imposed demands. The SAID principle states that, *when the body is subjected to stresses and overloads of varying intensities, it will gradually adapt over time to overcome whatever demands are placed on it.* For example, in weight training, as you progressively add more weight, the muscle tends to adapt to this increase in resistance by increasing in size and efficiency. Although overload is a critical factor in conditioning, the stress must not be great enough to produce damage or injury before the body has had a chance to adjust specifically to the increased demands.

> **SAID principle** Specific adaptation to imposed demands.

5. *Consistency.* An individual must engage in a conditioning program on a regularly scheduled basis if it is to be effective.

6. *Progression.* Increase the intensity of the conditioning program gradually and within the individual's ability to adapt to increasing workloads.

7. *Intensity.* Stress the intensity of the work rather than the quantity. Coaches and athletic trainers too often confuse working hard with working for long periods of time. They make the mistake of prolonging the workout rather than increasing tempo or workload. The tired athlete is prone to injury.

8. *Specificity.* Identify specific goals for the conditioning program. The program must be designed to address specific components of fitness (i.e., strength, flexibility, cardiorespiratory endurance) relative to the activity in which the individual is participating.

9. *Individuality.* The needs of different individuals vary considerably. The successful coach is one who recognizes these individual differences and adjusts or alters the conditioning program accordingly to best accommodate the individual.

10. *Minimal stress.* Expect that athletes will train as close to their physiological limits as they can. Push the athletes as far as possible, but consider other stressful aspects of their lives and allow them time to be away from the conditioning demands of their sport.

WARM-UP AND COOL-DOWN

Warm-Up

It is generally accepted that a period of warm-up exercises should take place before a training session begins, although a review of the evidence-based literature reveals little data-based research to support the efficacy of a warm-up. Nevertheless, most athletic trainers would agree empirically that a warm-up period is a precaution against unnecessary musculoskeletal injuries and possible muscle soreness.[30] A good warm-up may also improve certain aspects of performance.[3,88]

The function of the warm-up is to prepare the body physiologically for some upcoming physical work.[94] The purpose is to gradually stimulate the cardiorespiratory system to a moderate degree to increase the blood flow to working skeletal muscles and increase muscle temperature.[96]

Moderate activity speeds up the metabolic processes that produce an increase in core body temperature. An increase in the temperature of skeletal muscle alters the mechanical properties of the muscle. The elasticity of the muscle (the length to which the muscle can be stretched) is increased, and the viscosity (the rate at which the muscle can change shape) is decreased, which means that the muscle changes in shape more rapidly.

A good warm-up routine should begin with 2 or 3 minutes of slow walking, light jogging, or cycling to increase metabolism and warm up the muscles. Breaking into a light sweat is a good indication that muscle temperature has increased. Although research has indicated that increasing core temperature is effective in reducing injuries, there is little or no evidence that stretching during the warm-up reduces injury.[82] Empirically, many professionals feel that stretching should be a part of the warm-up, and they continue to recommend that flexibility exercises be included. There is also no evidence that stretching does any harm.

Dynamic Warm-Up For many years, the accepted technique was to perform a light jog followed by some static stretching. A more contemporary approach to the warm-up is to use an active, or "dynamic," warm-up to prepare for physical activity. A dynamic warm-up involves continuous movement using hopping, skipping, and bounding activities with several different footwork drills and patterns. It enhances coordination and motor ability as it revs up the nervous system. It prepares the muscles and joints in a more activity-specific manner than static stretching. The dynamic warm-up forces individuals to focus and concentrate. It should include exercises that address all the major muscle groups. The entire dynamic warm-up can be done in as little as 5 minutes or as long as 20 minutes, depending on the goals, age, and fitness level of the group.

> Warming up involves general body warming and warming specific body areas for the demands of the sport.

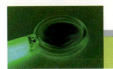
Dynamic warm-up routine

Two sets of cones are spaced 10 to 20 yards apart. The individual performs the following dynamic exercises between the cones, then jogs back to the start.

1. Jog forward
2. Jog backward
3. Walking calf stretch
4. Walking hamstring stretch
5. Hand-assisted knee stretch to chest
6. Hand-assisted knee stretch to opposite shoulder
7. Hand-assisted walking adductor stretch
8. Lateral shuffle moving to the right followed by the left
9. Walking lateral lunge to the right followed by the left
10. Skipping with low knees
11. Walking lunge, arms extended overhead
12. Walking lunge with rotation to each side
13. Walking quadriceps stretch
14. Jogging butt kicks
15. Open the gate exercise
16. Close the gate exercise
17. Carioca to the right followed by the left
18. Power high knees skipping
19. Prancing
20. High knees running
21. Back pedaling butt kicks
22. Forward sprint

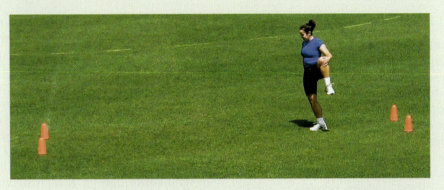

Focus Box 4–1: "Dynamic warm-up routine" lists a series of activities that can be included in a dynamic warm-up. Activity should begin immediately following the warm-up routine.

The individual should not wait longer than 15 minutes to begin the main sports activity after the warm-up, although the effects may last up to about 45 minutes.[74]

Cool-Down

Following a workout or training session, a cool-down period may be beneficial. The cool-down period enables the body to cool and return to a resting state. Such a period should last about 5 to 10 minutes. An example of a cool-down activity would be to have the individual jog and progressively decrease the pace to a walk to allow the metabolism to return to resting levels. This would be followed by stretching activities.

Although the warm-up period is common, the importance of a cool-down period afterward is often ignored. Again, experience and observation indicate that persons who stretch during the cool-down period tend to have fewer problems with muscle soreness after strenuous activity.[68]

CARDIORESPIRATORY ENDURANCE

Cardiorespiratory endurance is the ability to perform whole-body, large-muscle activities for extended periods of time. The cardiorespiratory system provides a means by which oxygen is supplied to the various tissues of the body.[60] For anyone who engages in exercise, cardiorespiratory endurance is critical both for performance and for preventing undue fatigue that may predispose the person to injury.

> **cardiorespiratory endurance** The ability to perform whole-body, large-muscle activities for extended periods of time.

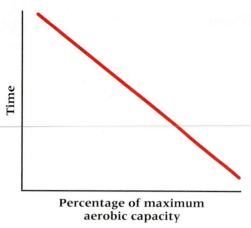

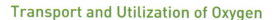

FIGURE 4–1 The greater the percentage of maximum aerobic capacity required during an activity, the less time the activity may be performed.

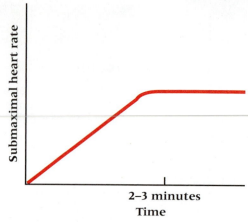

FIGURE 4–2 Two to 3 minutes are required for heart rate to plateau at a given workload.

Transport and Utilization of Oxygen

Basically, transport of oxygen throughout the body involves the coordinated function of four components: heart, lungs, blood vessels, and blood. The improvement of cardiorespiratory endurance through training occurs because of the increased capability of each of these four elements to provide necessary oxygen to the working tissues. The greatest rate at which oxygen can be taken in and used during exercise is referred to as *maximum aerobic capacity* ($\dot{V}O_2$max).[58] The performance of any activity requires a certain rate of oxygen consumption that is about the same for all persons, depending on the level of fitness. Generally, the greater the rate or intensity of the performance of an activity, the greater the oxygen consumption. Each person has his or her own maximal rate of oxygen consumption. That person's ability to perform an activity (or to fatigue) is closely related to the amount of oxygen required by that activity and is limited by the person's maximal rate of oxygen consumption. The greater the percentage of maximum oxygen consumption required during an activity, the less time the activity may be sustained (Figure 4–1).[67]

The maximal rate at which oxygen can be used is a genetically determined characteristic; a person inherits a certain range of maximum aerobic capacity, and the more active that person is, the higher the existing maximum aerobic capacity will be in that range.[33] A conditioning program allows an individual to increase maximum aerobic capacity to its highest limit within that person's range. Maximum aerobic capacity is most often presented in terms of the volume of oxygen used relative to body weight per unit of time (ml/kg/min). A normal maximum aerobic capacity for most college-age athletes would fall in the range of 45 to 60 ml/kg/min.[84] A world-class male marathon runner may have a maximum aerobic capacity in the 70 to 80 ml/kg/min range.

Three factors determine the maximal rate at which oxygen can be used: external respiration involving the ventilatory process or pulmonary function; gas transport, which is accomplished by the cardiovascular system (i.e., the heart, blood vessels, and blood); and internal respiration, which involves the use of oxygen by the cells to produce energy. Of these three factors, the most limiting is generally the ability to transport oxygen through the system; thus, the cardiovascular system limits the overall rate of oxygen consumption. A high maximum aerobic capacity within an individual's inherited range indicates that all three systems are working well.

Effects on the Heart

The heart is the main pumping mechanism, circulating oxygenated blood throughout the body to the working tissues. As the body begins to exercise, the muscles use oxygen at a much higher rate, and the heart must pump more oxygenated blood to meet this increased demand. The heart is capable of adapting to this increased demand through several mechanisms. Heart rate shows a gradual adaptation to an increased workload by increasing proportionally to the intensity of the exercise and will plateau at a given level after about 2 to 3 minutes (Figure 4–2).

Monitoring heart rate is an indirect method of estimating oxygen consumption. In general, heart rate and oxygen consumption have a linear relationship, although at very low intensities and at high intensities this linear relationship breaks down (Figure 4–3).[14] During higher-intensity activities, maximal heart rate may be achieved before maximal oxygen consumption, which will continue to rise.[54] The greater the intensity of the exercise, the higher the heart rate. Because of these existing relationships, it should become apparent that the rate of oxygen consumption can be estimated by taking heart rate.[20]

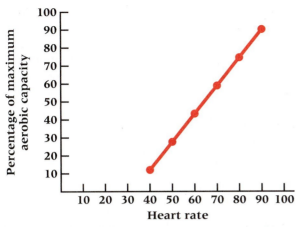

FIGURE 4–3 Maximal heart rate is achieved at about the same time as maximum aerobic capacity.

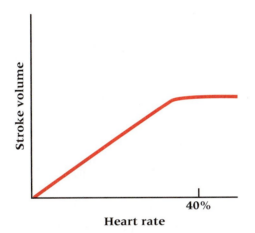

FIGURE 4–4 Stroke volume plateaus at 40 percent of maximal heart rate.

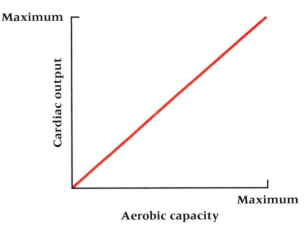

FIGURE 4–5 Cardiac output limits maximum aerobic capacity.

A second mechanism by which the heart is able to adapt to increased demands during exercise is to increase the *stroke volume*—the volume of blood being pumped out with each beat.[17] The heart pumps out approximately 70 ml of blood per beat. Stroke volume can continue to increase only to the point at which there is simply not enough time between beats for the heart to fill up. This point occurs at about 40 percent of maximal heart rate, and above this level increases in the volume of blood being pumped out per unit of time must be caused entirely by increases in heart rate (Figure 4–4).[66]

Stroke volume and heart rate together determine the volume of blood being pumped through the heart in a given unit of time. This is referred to as the *cardiac output,* which indicates how much blood the heart is capable of pumping in exactly 1 minute.[60] Approximately 5 L of blood are pumped through the heart during each minute at rest. Thus, cardiac output is the primary determinant of the maximal rate of oxygen consumption possible (Figure 4–5). During exercise, cardiac output increases to approximately four times that experienced during

rest in the normal individual and may increase as much as six times in the elite endurance athlete.

A **training effect** occurs with regard to cardiac output of the heart—the stroke volume increases while exercise heart rate is reduced at a given standard exercise load. The heart becomes more efficient because it is capable of pumping more blood with each stroke. Because the heart is a muscle, it will hypertrophy to some extent, but this hypertrophy is in no way a negative effect of training.

> **training effect** Stroke volume increases while heart rate is reduced at a given exercise load.

$$\begin{array}{ccc} \text{Cardiac} \\ \text{output} \end{array} = \begin{array}{c} \text{Increased} \\ \text{stroke volume} \end{array} \times \begin{array}{c} \text{Decreased} \\ \text{heart rate} \end{array}$$

Effects on Work Ability

Cardiorespiratory endurance plays a critical role in an individual's ability to resist fatigue. Fatigue is closely related to the percentage of maximum aerobic capacity that a particular workload demands.[74] For example, Figure 4–6 presents two individuals,

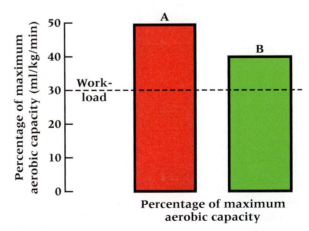

FIGURE 4–6 Person A should be able to work longer than Person B as a result of lower utilization of maximum aerobic capacity.

A and B. A has a maximum aerobic capacity of 50 ml/kg/min, whereas B has a maximum aerobic capacity of only 40 ml/kg/min. If A and B are both exercising at the same intensity, A will be working at a much lower percentage of maximum aerobic capacity than B. Consequently, A should be able to sustain his or her activity over a much longer period of time. Performance may be impaired if the ability to use oxygen efficiently is impaired. Thus, improvement of cardiorespiratory endurance should be an essential component of any conditioning program.

The Energy Systems

Various sports activities involve specific demands for energy. For example, sprinting and jumping are high-energy activities, requiring a relatively large production of energy for a short time. Long-distance running and swimming, on the other hand, are mostly low-energy activities per unit of time, requiring energy production for a prolonged time. Other physical activities demand a blend of both high- and low-energy output. These various energy demands can be met by the different processes in which energy can be supplied to the skeletal muscles.

ATP: The Immediate Energy Source Energy is produced from the breakdown of nutrient foodstuffs.[66] This energy is used to produce *adenosine triphosphate (ATP)*, which is the ultimate usable form of energy for muscular activity. ATP is produced in the muscle tissue from blood glucose or glycogen. Glucose is derived from the breakdown of dietary carbohydrates. Glucose not needed immediately is stored as glycogen in the resting muscle and liver. Stored glycogen in the liver can later be converted back to glucose and transferred to the blood to meet the body's energy needs. Fats and proteins can also be metabolized to generate ATP.

Once much of the muscle and liver glycogen is depleted, the body relies more heavily on fats stored in adipose tissue to meet its energy needs. The longer the duration of an activity, the greater the amount of fat that is used, especially during the later stages of endurance events. During rest and submaximal exertion, both fat and carbohydrates are used as energy substrate in approximately a 60 percent to 40 percent ratio.[66]

Regardless of the nutrient source that produces ATP, it is always available in the cell as an immediate energy source. When all available sources of ATP are depleted, more must be regenerated for muscular contraction to continue.

Aerobic versus Anaerobic Metabolism Three energy-generating systems function in muscle tissue to produce ATP: the ATP, glycolytic, and oxidative systems. During sudden outbursts of activity in intensive, short-term exercise, ATP can be rapidly metabolized to meet energy needs. However, after a few seconds of intensive exercise, the small stores of ATP are used up. The body then turns to stored glycogen as an energy source. Glycogen is broken down to supply glucose, which is then metabolized within the muscle cells to generate ATP for muscle contractions without the need for oxygen. This breakdown also produces a byproduct called lactic acid, or *lactate*, which seeps out of the muscle cells into the blood to be used elsewhere. This energy system is referred to as *anaerobic metabolism*.[11]

As exercise continues, the body has to rely on a more complex form of carbohydrate and fat metabolism to generate ATP. This energy system requires oxygen and is therefore referred to as *aerobic metabolism*. The aerobic system burns the lactate using oxygen, thus removing it and creating far more ATP than the anaerobic system. Normally, it takes about 20 minutes to clear the lactate from the system. Training to improve endurance helps an individual get rid of the lactic acid before it can build to the point where it causes muscle fatigue.[5]

In most activities, both aerobic and anaerobic systems function simultaneously.[66] The degree to which the two are involved is determined by the intensity and duration of the activity. If the intensity of the activity is such that sufficient oxygen can be supplied to meet the demands of working tissues, the activity is considered to be aerobic. Conversely, if the activity is of high enough intensity or the duration is such that there is insufficient oxygen available to meet energy demands, the activity becomes anaerobic. Consequently, an oxygen debt is incurred, which must be paid back during the recovery period. For example, short bursts of muscle contraction, as in running or swimming sprints, use predominantly the anaerobic system. However, endurance events depend a great deal on the aerobic

TABLE 4–1 Comparison of Aerobic versus Anaerobic Activities

	Mode	Relative Intensity	Performance	Frequency	Duration	Miscellaneous
Aerobic activities	Continuous, long-duration, sustained activities	Less intense	60% to 90% of maximum range	At least three but not more than six times per week	20 to 60 min	Less risk to sedentary or older individuals
Anaerobic activities	Explosive, short-duration, burst-type activities	More intense	90% to 100% of maximum range	Three to four times per week	10 sec to 2 min	Used in sport and team activities

system. Most activities use a combination of anaerobic and aerobic metabolism (Table 4–1).

Training Techniques for Improving Cardiorespiratory Endurance

Cardiorespiratory endurance may be improved through a number of methods.[57] Largely, the amount of improvement possible will be determined by an individual's initial levels of cardiorespiratory endurance.

Continuous Training Continuous training involves four considerations:

- *Frequency* of the activity
- *Intensity* of the activity
- *Type* of activity
- *Time* of the activity

Frequency To see at least minimal improvement in cardiorespiratory endurance, it is necessary for the average person to engage in no fewer than three sessions per week.[5] If possible, an individual should aim for four or five sessions per week. A competitive athlete should be prepared to train as often as six times per week. Everyone should take at least one day per week off to allow for both psychological and physiological rest.

Intensity Of the four factors being considered, the most critical factor is the intensity of training, even though recommendations regarding training intensities vary. Intensity is particularly critical in the early stages of training, when the body is forced to make a lot of adjustments to increase workload demands.

Because heart rate is linearly related to the intensity of the exercise and to the rate of oxygen consumption, it becomes a relatively simple process to identify a specific workload (pace) that will make the heart rate plateau at the desired level. By monitoring heart rate, we know whether the pace is too fast or too slow to get the heart rate into a target range.[5]

Several formulas identify a training target heart rate.[5] To calculate a specific target heart rate, maximal heart rate must be determined. Exact determination of maximal heart rate (HR) involves exercising an individual at a maximal level and monitoring the HR using an electrocardiogram. This is a difficult process outside of a laboratory. An approximate estimate of maximal HR is thought to be about 220 beats per minute. However, maximal HR decreases with age. Thus, a relatively simple estimate of maximal HR in adults would be $HR_{max} = 220 - Age$. For a 20-year-old individual, maximal heart rate would be about 200 beats per minute ($220 - 20 = 200$). Heart rate reserve is used to determine exercise heart rates. Heart rate reserve (HRR) is the difference between resting heart rate (HR_{rest}) and maximal heart rate (HR_{max}):[48]

$$HRR = HR_{max} - HR_{rest}$$

The greater the difference, the larger the heart rate reserve and the greater the range of potential training heart rate intensities. The Karvonen equation is used to calculate exercise heart rate at a given percentage of training intensity. To use the Karvonen formula, the individual's HR_{max} and HR_{rest} must be known:[47]

Exercise HR = % of target intensity ($HR_{max} - HR_{rest}$) + HR_{rest}

When using estimated HR_{max} or/and HR_{rest} the values are always predictions. Thus, in a 20-year-old with a resting heart rate of 70 beats per minute, the heart rate reserve is 130 ($200 - 70 = 130$).

The heart works in a range between the lower limit and an upper limit. The lower limit is calculated by taking 60 percent of the heart rate reserve and adding the resting heart rate, which would be 148 beats per minute $((130 \times 0.6) + 70 = 148)$. The upper limit is calculated by taking 85 percent of the heart rate reserve and adding the resting heart rate $((130 \times 0.85) + 70 = 180.5)$.

Regardless of the formula used, to see minimal improvement in cardiorespiratory endurance, the heart rate should be elevated to at least 70 percent of its maximal rate.[20] A well-conditioned individual should be able to sustain a heart rate at the 85 percent level.

Type The type of activity used in continuous training must be aerobic.[20] Aerobic activities are those that elevate the heart rate and maintain it at that level for an extended time. Aerobic activities generally involve repetitive, whole-body, large-muscle movements performed over an extended time. Examples of aerobic activities are running, jogging, walking, cycling, swimming, rope skipping, stair climbing, and cross-country skiing. The advantage of these aerobic activities as opposed to more intermittent activities, such as racquetball, squash, basketball, or tennis, is that aerobic activities are easy to regulate by either speeding up or slowing down the pace. Because the given intensity of the workload elicits a given heart rate, these aerobic activities allow athletes to maintain heart rate at a specified or target level. Intermittent activities involve variable speeds and intensities that cause the heart rate to fluctuate considerably. Although these intermittent activities improve cardiorespiratory endurance, their intensity is much more difficult to monitor.

Time For minimal improvement to occur, an individual must participate in at least 20 minutes of continuous activity with the heart rate elevated to its working level.[5] Recent evidence suggests that even shorter exercise bouts of as little as 12 minutes may be sufficient to show improvement. Generally, the greater the duration of the workout, the greater the improvement in cardiorespiratory endurance. The competitive athlete should train for at least 45 minutes with the heart rate elevated to training levels.

Interval Training Unlike continuous training, interval training involves more intermittent activities.

interval training
Alternating periods of work with active recovery.

Interval training consists of alternating periods of relatively intense work and active recovery. It allows for performance of much more work at a more intense workload over a longer period of time than does working continuously.[62]

It is most desirable in continuous training to work at an intensity of about 60 percent to 80 percent of maximal heart rate. Obviously, sustaining activity at a relatively high intensity over a 20-minute period would be extremely difficult. The advantage of interval training is that it allows work at this 80 percent or higher level for a short period of time followed by an active period of recovery during which an individual may be working at only 30 percent to 45 percent of maximal heart rate.[15] Thus, the intensity of the workout and its duration can be greater than with continuous training.

Most sports are anaerobic, involving short bursts of intense activity followed by some type of active recovery period (for example, football, basketball, soccer, and tennis). Conditioning with the interval technique allows the athlete to be more sport-specific during the workout. With interval training, the overload principle is applied by making the training period much more intense.

There are several important considerations in interval training. The conditioning period is the amount of time that continuous activity is actually being performed, and the recovery period is the time between training periods. A set is a group of combined training and recovery periods, and repetitions are the number of training and recovery periods per set. Training time or distance is the rate or distance of the training period. The training-recovery ratio indicates a time ratio for training versus recovery.

An example of interval training is a soccer player running sprints. An interval workout would involve running ten 120-yard sprints with a 45-second walking recovery period between sprints. During this conditioning session, the soccer player's heart rate would probably increase to 85 percent to 90 percent of maximal level during the dash and should fall to the 30 percent to 45 percent level during the recovery period.

Speed Play Speed play is a training technique that is a type of cross-country running, originally referred to "fartlek." It is similar to interval training in that the individual must run for a specified period of time; however, pace and speed are not specified. The course for a speed play workout should be some type of varied terrain with some level running, some uphill and downhill running, and some running through obstacles, such as trees or rocks. The object is to put surges into a running workout, varying the length of the surges according to individual purposes. One advantage of this type of conditioning is that, because the terrain is always changing, the course may prevent boredom and may actually be relaxing.

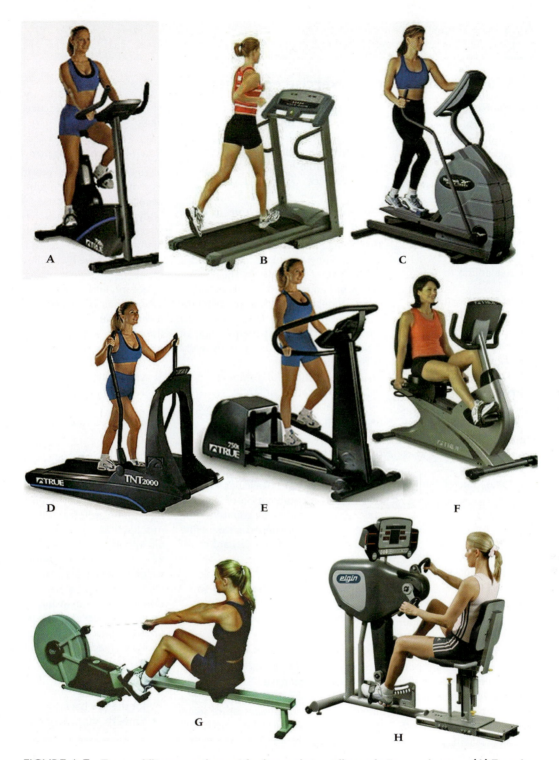

FIGURE 4–7   Types of fitness equipment for improving cardiorespiratory endurance. **(A)** Exercise bicycle. **(B)** Treadmill. **(C)** Stair climber. **(D)** Cross-country ski machine. **(E)** Elliptical trainer. **(F)** Recumbent bicycle. **(G)** Rowing machine. **(H)** Upper-body ergometer. (Courtesy Sports Authority (www.thesportsauthority.com).)

To improve cardiorespiratory endurance, speed play must elevate the heart rate to at least minimal training levels. Speed play may be utilized best as an off-season conditioning activity or as a change-of-pace activity to counteract the boredom of conditioning using the same activity day after day.

Equipment for Improving Cardiorespiratory Endurance

The extent and variety of fitness and exercise equipment available to the consumer are at times mind boggling (Figure 4–7). Prices of equipment

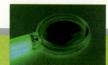
Guidelines for choosing aerobic exercise equipment

Exercise bicycle (Figure 4–7A)

Most models work only the lower body, but some have pumping handlebars for arms and shoulders. Some can be programmed for various workouts, such as climbing hills. Some models let you pedal backward, which enhances the work on your hamstring muscles. Look for these features:

- Smooth pedaling motion
- A comfortable seat
- Handlebars that adjust to your height
- Pedal straps to keep your feet from slipping and to make your legs work on the upstroke, too
- Easy-to-adjust workload
- Solid construction

Treadmill (Figure 4–7B)

Some machines have adjustable inclines to simulate hills and make workouts more strenuous. Some can be programmed for various preset workouts. Look for the following:

- Easily adjustable speed and incline
- A running surface that is wide and long enough for your stride and that absorbs shock well
- A strong motor that can handle high speeds and a heavy load

Stair climber (Figure 4–7C)

Some larger models simulate real stair climbing. But most home models have pedals that work against your weight as you pump your legs; this feature puts less strain on your knees because you don't take real steps. Some people prefer pedals that remain parallel to the floor; others like pivoting pedals. Models with independent pedals provide a more natural stepping motion. Look for these features:

- Smooth stepping action
- Large, comfortable pedals with no wobble
- Easily adjustable resistance
- Comfortable handlebars or rails for balance

Cross-country ski machine (Figure 4–7D)

These machines work most muscle groups. They simulate the outdoor sport: Your feet slide in the tracks, and your hands pull on cords or poles, either independently or in synchronized movements. Machines with cords rather than poles may provide an especially strenuous upper-body workout. Look for

- A base that is long enough to accommodate your stride
- Adjustable leg and arm resistance
- Smooth action

Elliptical trainer (Figure 4–7E)

An elliptical exercise machine allows for a no-impact cardiovascular workout that mimics a combination of walking, stair climbing, and cross-country skiing using an elliptical-shaped stride while standing upright using a forward or reverse motion. Look for

- An electronically adjustable ramp that allows the incline to be raised or lowered
- Resistance that can be adjusted

Recumbent Bike (Figure 4–7F)

A recumbent is, for the most part, similar to a regular exercise bike, except the individual is in a semireclined position rather than sitting straight-up or leaning slightly forward while pedaling. The advantage of this position is that it takes pressure off the lumbar area of the spine—in particular, the lumbar disks.

Rowing machine (Figure 4–7G)

A rowing machine provides a fuller workout than does running or cycling because it tones muscles in the upper-body. Most machines have hydraulic pistons to provide variable resistance; many larger models use a flywheel. Piston models have hydraulic arms and are cheaper and more compact than are flywheel models, which have a smoother action that is usually more like real rowing. One new model actually has a flywheel in a water tank to mimic real rowing. Look for these components:

- Seats and oars that move smoothly
- Footrests that pivot

Upper-body ergometer (UBE) (Figure 4–7H)

An upper-body ergometer is essentially a stationary bicycle that you pedal with the arms rather than the legs. These machines are most often used to help maintain cardiorespiratory endurance in rehabilitation programs for individuals with injuries to the lower extremities who, for whatever reason, cannot use weight-bearing activities. A UBE may also be used as a training and conditioning tool to help increase muscular endurance for the upper extremities. Look for these features:

- Easily adjustable speed and resistance
- A comfortable seat that provides some support and stabilization for the low back
- Smooth, quiet action

can range from $2 for a jump rope to $60,000 for certain computer-driven isokinetic devices. It is certainly not necessary to purchase expensive exercise equipment to see good results. Many of the same physiological benefits can be achieved from using a $2 jump rope as from running on a $10,000 treadmill. *Focus Box 4–2: "Guidelines for choosing aerobic exercise equipment"* identifies and discusses some of the more widely used pieces of exercise equipment.

THE IMPORTANCE OF MUSCULAR STRENGTH, ENDURANCE, AND POWER

The development of **muscular strength** is an essential component of a conditioning program for every athlete. Strength is the ability of a muscle to generate force against some resistance. Most movements in sports are explosive and must include elements of both strength and speed if they are to be effective. If a large amount of force is generated quickly, the movement can be referred to as a **power** movement. Without the ability to generate power, an athlete is limited in his or her performance capabilities.[74]

Muscular strength is closely associated with muscular endurance. **Muscular endurance** is the ability to perform repetitive muscular contractions against some resistance for an extended period of time. As muscular strength increases, there tends to be a corresponding increase in endurance.[55,90] For example, an individual can lift a weight 25 times. If muscular strength is increased by 10 percent through weight training, it is likely that the maximum number of repetitions will be increased because it is easier for the individual to lift the weight.

> **muscular strength** The maximum force that can be applied by a muscle during a single maximum contraction.
>
> **power** The ability to generate force rapidly.
>
> **muscular endurance** The ability to perform repetitive muscular contractions against some resistance.

A college swimmer has been engaged in an off-season weight-training program to increase her muscular strength and endurance. Although she has seen some improvement in her strength, she is concerned that she also seems to be losing flexibility in her shoulders, which she feels is critical to her performance as a swimmer. She has also noticed that her muscles are hypertrophying to some degree and is worried that this may be causing her to lose flexibility. She has just about decided to abandon her weight-training program altogether.

? What can the athletic trainer recommend to her that will allow her to continue to improve her muscular strength and endurance while maintaining or perhaps even improving her flexibility?

4–4 Clinical Application Exercise

Physiological and Biomechanical Factors That Determine Levels of Muscular Strength

Muscular strength is proportional to the cross-sectional diameter of the muscle fibers. The greater the cross-sectional diameter or the bigger a particular muscle, the stronger it is, and thus the more force it is capable of generating. The size of a muscle tends to increase in cross-sectional diameter with weight training. This increase in muscle size is referred to as **hypertrophy**.[53] Conversely, a decrease in the size of a muscle is referred to as **atrophy**.

Size of the Muscle Strength is a function of the number and diameter of muscle fibers composing a given muscle. The number of fibers is an inherited characteristic; thus, an individual with a large number of muscle fibers to begin with has the potential to hypertrophy to a much greater degree than does someone with relatively fewer fibers.[53]

> **hypertrophy** Enlargement of a muscle caused by an increase in the size of its cells in response to training.
>
> **atrophy** Decrease of a muscle caused by a decrease in the size of its cells because of inactivity.

Explanations for Muscle Hypertrophy A number of theories have been proposed to explain why a muscle hypertrophies in response to strength training.[66] Some evidence exists that the number of muscle fibers increases because fibers split in response to training.[36] However, this research has been conducted in animals and should not be generalized to humans. It is generally accepted that the number of fibers is genetically determined and does not seem to increase with training.

Another hypothesis is that because the muscle is working harder in weight training, more blood is required to supply that muscle with oxygen and other nutrients. Thus, the number of capillaries is increased. This hypothesis is only partially correct; few new capillaries are formed during strength training, but a number of dormant capillaries may become filled with blood to meet the increased demand for blood supply.

A third theory to explain this increase in muscle size seems the most credible. Muscle fibers are composed primarily of small protein filaments, called myofilaments, which are the contractile elements in muscle. These myofilaments increase in both size and number as a result of strength training, causing the individual muscle fibers themselves to increase in cross-sectional diameter.[36] This increase is particularly true in men, although women also see some increase in muscle size.[1] More research is needed to further clarify and determine the specific causes of muscle hypertrophy.

Improved Neuromuscular Efficiency Typically with weight training, an individual sees some remarkable gains in strength initially, even though muscle bulk does not necessarily increase. This gain in strength must be attributed to something other than muscle hypertrophy. For a muscle to contract, an impulse

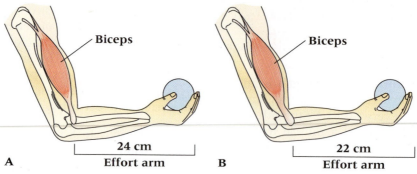

A 24 cm **Effort arm**   **B** 22 cm **Effort arm**

FIGURE 4–8 The position of attachment of the muscle tendon on the arm can affect the ability of that muscle to generate force. Person B should be able to generate greater force than person A because the tendon attachment is closer to the resistance.

must be transmitted from the nervous system to the muscle. Each muscle fiber is innervated by a specific motor unit. By overloading a particular muscle, as in weight training, the muscle is forced to work efficiently. Efficiency is achieved by getting more motor units to fire, causing a stronger contraction of the muscle.[92] Consequently, it is not uncommon to see extremely rapid gains in strength when a weight-training program is first begun due to an improvement in neuromuscular function.[53]

Other Physiological Adaptations to Resistance Exercise In addition to muscle hypertrophy, there are a number of other physiological adaptations to resistance training.[11] The strength of noncontractile structures, including tendons and ligaments, is increased. The mineral content of bone is increased, making the bone stronger and more resistant to fracture. Maximal oxygen uptake is improved when resistance training is of sufficient intensity to elicit heart rates at or above training levels. Several enzymes important in aerobic and anaerobic metabolism also increase.[20,66]

Biomechanical Factors Strength in a given muscle is determined not only by the physical properties of the muscle itself but also by biomechanical factors that dictate how much force can be generated through a system of levers to an external object.[42] If we think of the elbow joint as one of these lever systems, we would have the biceps muscle producing flexion of this joint (Figure 4–8). The position of attachment of the biceps muscle on the lever arm—in this case, the forearm—will largely determine how

much force this muscle is capable of generating.[39] If there are two persons, A and B, and person B has a biceps attachment that is farther from the center of the joint than is person A's, then person B should be able to lift heavier weights because the muscle force acts through a longer lever (moment) arm and thus can produce greater torque around the joint.

The length of a muscle determines the tension that can be generated.[42] By varying the length of a muscle, different tensions may be produced. This *length-tension* relationship is illustrated in Figure 4–9. At position B in the curve, the interaction of the crossbridges between the actin and myosin myofilaments within the sarcomere is at a maximum. Setting a muscle at this length will produce the greatest amount of tension. At position A the muscle is shortened, and at position C the muscle is lengthened. In either case, the interaction between the actin and myosin myofilaments through the crossbridges is greatly reduced, and the muscle is not capable of generating significant tension.

Overtraining Overtraining can have a negative effect on the development of muscular strength. Overtraining

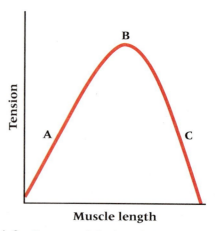

FIGURE 4–9 Because of the length-tension relation in muscle, the greatest tension is developed at point B, with less tension developed at points A and C.

can result in psychological breakdown (staleness) or physiological breakdown, which may involve musculoskeletal injury, fatigue, or sickness. Engaging in proper and efficient resistance training, eating a proper diet, and getting appropriate rest can minimize the potential negative effects of overtraining.

Reversibility If strength training is discontinued or interrupted, the muscle will atrophy, decreasing in both strength and mass. Adaptations in skeletal muscle that occur in response to resistance training may begin to reverse in as little as 48 hours. It does appear that consistent exercise of a muscle is essential to prevent loss of the hypertrophy that occurs due to strength training.

Fast-Twitch versus Slow-Twitch Fibers and Muscular Endurance

Skeletal muscle fibers in a particular motor unit are either *slow-twitch* or *fast-twitch* fibers, each of which has distinctive metabolic and contractile capabilities.

Four basic types of muscle fibers:
• Slow-twitch, or type I
• Fast-twitch type IIa
• Fast-twitch type IIb
• Fast-twitch type IIx

Slow-twitch (ST) fibers, also referred to as type I or slow oxidative (SO) fibers, are dense with capillaries and are rich in mitochondria and myoglobin, giving the muscle tissue its characteristic red color. They can carry more oxygen and thus are more resistant to fatigue than are fast-twitch fibers.[43] Slow-twitch fibers are associated primarily with long-duration, aerobic-type activities.[66]

Fast-twitch (FT) fibers are referred to as type II or fast oxidative glycolytic (FOG) fibers. They are capable of producing quick, forceful contractions but have a tendency to fatigue more rapidly than do slow-twitch fibers. Fast-twitch fibers are useful in short-term, high-intensity activities, which mainly involve the anaerobic system. Fast-twitch fibers are capable of producing powerful contractions, whereas slow-twitch fibers produce a long-endurance type of force.

Fast-twitch fibers can be subdivided into three groups, although all three types are capable of rapid contraction. Type IIa fibers, like slow-twitch muscle fibers, are moderately resistant to fatigue. Type IIx, also known as fast glycolytic (FG) and occasionally type IId, are less dense in mitochondria and myoglobin than type IIa. This is the fastest muscle type in humans and it can contract more quickly and with a greater amount of force than type IIa. But these fibers can sustain only short, anaerobic bursts of acitivity before muscle contraction becomes painful. Type IIb fibers are less dense in mitochondria and myoglobin and fatigue rapidly. They are white in color and are considered the "true" fast-twitch fibers.[66]

Any given muscle contains all types of fibers, and the ratio in an individual muscle varies with each person.[54] Those muscles whose primary function is to maintain posture against gravity require more endurance and have a higher percentage of slow-twitch fibers. Muscles that produce powerful, rapid, explosive strength movements tend to have a much greater percentage of fast-twitch fibers. Because this ratio is genetically determined, it may play a large role in determining ability for a given sport activity. Sprinters and weight lifters, for example, have a large percentage of fast-twitch fibers in relation to slow-twitch fibers.[20] Conversely, marathon runners generally have a higher percentage of slow-twitch fibers.

The metabolic capabilities of both fast-twitch and slow-twitch fibers may be improved through specific strength and endurance training. It appears that there can be an almost complete change from slow-twitch to fast-twitch and from fast-twitch to slow-twitch fiber types in response to training.[66] Fibers that are in the process of transitioning from one fiber type to another share some properties of both type I and type II fibers and are referred to as "hybrid" fibers.

Skeletal Muscle Contractions

Skeletal muscle is capable of three types of contraction: *isometric contraction, concentric contraction,* and *eccentric contraction.*[26] An isometric contraction occurs when the muscle contracts to increase tension but there

Skeletal muscle is capable of three types of contraction:
• Isometric
• Concentric
• Eccentric

is no change in the length of the muscle. Considerable force can be generated against some immovable resistance even though no movement occurs. In concentric contraction, the muscle shortens in length as a contraction is developed to overcome or move some resistance. In eccentric contraction, the resistance is greater than the muscular force being produced, and the muscle lengthens while continuing to contract. Concentric and eccentric contractions are both considered to be dynamic movements.[26]

It is critical to understand that functional movements involve acceleration, deceleration, and stabilization in all three planes of motion simultaneously. Functional movements are controlled by neuromuscular mechanoreceptors located within the muscle.[26]

Techniques of Resistance Training

There are a number of techniques of resistance training for strength improvement, including functional strength-training exercises, core stability training, isometric exercise, progressive resistance exercise, isokinetic exercise, circuit training, calisthenic strengthening exercises, and plyometric exercise. Regardless of which of these techniques is used, one basic principle of training is extremely important. For a muscle to improve in strength, it must be forced to work at a higher level than it is accustomed to working. In other words, the muscle must be *overloaded*. Without overload, the muscle will be able to maintain strength as long as training is continued against a resistance the muscle is accustomed to. To most effectively build muscular strength, weight training requires a consistent, increasing effort against progressively increasing resistance.[34] If this principle of overload is applied, all eight conditioning techniques can produce improvement in muscular strength over a period of time.

Functional Strength Training For many years, the strength-training techniques in conditioning or rehabilitation programs have focused on isolated, single-plane exercises used to elicit muscle hypertrophy in a specific muscle. These exercises have a very low neuromuscular demand because they are performed primarily with the rest of the body artificially stabilized on stable pieces of equipment.[26] The central nervous system controls the ability to integrate the proprioceptive function of a number of individual muscles that must act collectively to produce a specific movement pattern that occurs in three planes of motion. If the body is designed to move in three planes of motion, then isolated training does little to improve functional ability. When strength training using isolated, single-plane, artificially stabilized exercises, the entire body is not being prepared to deal with the imposed demands of normal daily activities (walking up or down stairs, getting groceries out of the trunk, etc.).[26] Functional strength training provides a unique approach that may revolutionize the way the sports medicine community thinks about strength training.

To understand the approach to functional strength training, the athletic trainer must understand the concept of the *kinetic chain* and must realize that the entire kinetic chain is an integrated functional unit. The kinetic chain is composed of not only muscle, tendons, fasciae, and ligaments but also the articular system and the neural system. All of these systems function simultaneously as an integrated unit to allow for structural and functional efficiency. If any system within the kinetic chain is not working efficiently, the other systems are forced to adapt and compensate; this can lead to tissue overload, decreased performance, and predictable patterns of injury. The functional integration of the systems allows for optimal neuromuscular efficiency during functional activities.[26,95]

During functional movements, some muscles contract concentrically (shorten) to produce movement, others contract eccentrically (lengthen) to allow movement to occur, and still other muscles contract isometrically to create a stable base on which the functional movement occurs. These functional movements occur in three planes. Functional strength training uses integrated exercises designed to improve functional movement patterns in terms of not only increased strength and improved neuromuscular control but also high levels of stabilization strength and dynamic flexibility.[18]

Unlike traditional strength-training techniques, which use barbells, dumbbells, or exercise machines and single-plane exercises day after day, a primary principle of functional strength training is to make use of training variations to force constant neural adaptations instead of concentrating solely on morphological changes. Exercise variables that can be changed include the plane of motion, body position, base of support, upper- or lower-extremity symmetry, the type of balance modality, and the type of external resistance.[26] Table 4–2 lists these exercise training variables. Figure 4–10 provides examples of functional strengthening exercises.

Core Stability Training A core stabilization training program is designed to help an individual gain strength, neuromuscular control, power, and muscle endurance of the muscles in the lumbar spine, in the abdomen, and around the hips and pelvis. These muscles are collectively referred to as the **core**.[27] The concept of core stability training is essential. A weak core is a fundamental problem of inefficient movements that lead to injury.[51] If the muscles in the extremities are strong and the core is weak, the force required for efficient movements cannot be produced. Core stability training should be an important component of all comprehensive

> **core** Muscles of the lumbar spine, abdomen, hips, and pelvis.

TABLE 4–2 | Exercise Training Variables

Plane of Motion	Body Position	Base of Support	Upper-Extremity Symmetry	Lower-Extremity Symmetry	Balance Modality	External Resistance
▪ Sagittal	▪ Supine	▪ Exercise bench	▪ 2 arms	▪ 2 legs	▪ Floor	▪ Barbell
▪ Frontal	▪ Prone	▪ Stability ball	▪ Alternate arms	▪ Staggered stance	▪ Sport beam	▪ Dumbbell
▪ Transverse	▪ Side-lying	▪ Balance modality	▪ 1 arm	▪ 1 leg	▪ ½ foam roll	▪ Cable machines
▪ Combination	▪ Sitting	▪ Other	▪ 1 arm w/ rotation	▪ 2-leg unstable	▪ Airex pad	▪ Tubing
	▪ Kneeling			▪ Staggered stance unstable	▪ Dyna disc	▪ Medicine balls
	▪ Half kneeling			▪ 1-leg unstable	▪ BOSU	▪ Power balls
	▪ Standing				▪ Proprio shoes	▪ Bodyblade
					▪ Sand	▪ Other

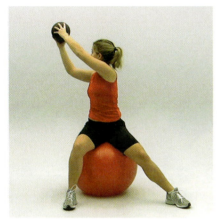

A

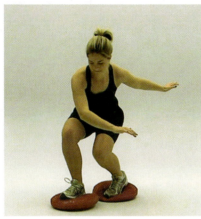

B

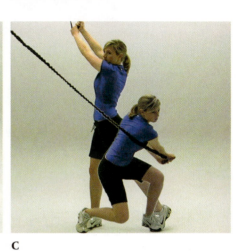

C

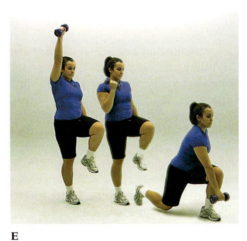

D

E

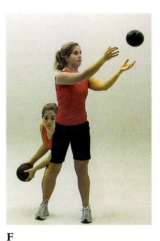

F

FIGURE 4–10 Functional strengthening exercises use simultaneous movements (concentric, eccentric, and isometric contractions) in three planes on both stable and unstable surfaces. **(A)** Stability ball diagonal rotations with weighted ball. **(B)** Tandem stance on Dyna disc with trunk rotation. **(C)** Standing diagonal rotations with cable or tubing reistance. **(D)** Weight-resisted multiplanar lunges. **(E)** Front lunge balance to one-arm press. **(F)** Weighted-ball double arm rotation toss from squat.

strengthening programs.[21,32,65] Dynamic core stabilization programs and exercises are discussed in detail in Chapters 16 and 25. Figure 4–11 shows several examples of exercises that may be used to improve core stability.

Isometric Exercise An **isometric exercise** involves a muscle contraction in which the length of the muscle remains constant while tension

isometric exercise
Contracts the muscle statically without changing its length.

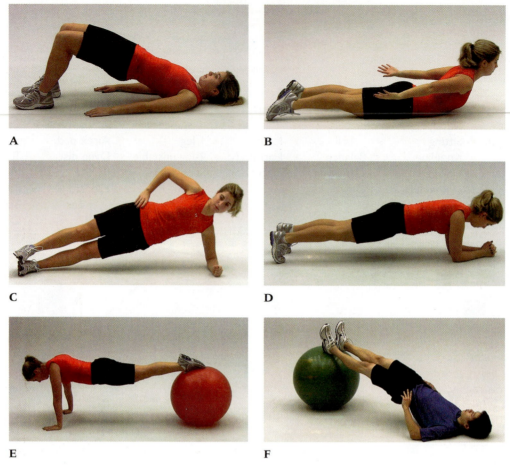

FIGURE 4–11   Core stability exercises.
(A) Bridging. **(B)** Prone cobra. **(C)** Side-lying isolated abdominal. **(D)** Human arrow.
(E) Stability ball push-up. **(F)** Hip-ups on stability ball.

develops toward a maximal force against an immovable resistance.[9] The muscle should generate a maximal force for 10 seconds at a time, and this contraction should be repeated 5 to 10 times per day. Isometric exercises are capable of increasing muscular strength; unfortunately, strength gains are specific to the joint angle at which training is performed. At other angles, the strength curve drops off dramatically because of a lack of motor activity at that angle.

Another major disadvantage of isometric exercises is that they tend to produce a spike in systolic blood pressure, which can result in potentially life-threatening cardiovascular accidents.[74] This sharp increase in blood pressure results from an individual holding his or her breath and increasing intrathoracic pressure. Consequently, the blood pressure the heart experiences is increased significantly. This phenomenon has been referred to as the Valsalva effect. To avoid or minimize this increase in pressure, it is recommended that breathing be continued during the maximal contraction.

Isometric exercises are useful in the rehabilitation of certain injuries; this use is discussed in the rehabilitation sections in Chapters 18 through 26.

Progressive Resistance Exercise   A third technique of resistance training is perhaps the most commonly used and the most popular technique for improving muscular strength. *Progressive resistance exercise (PRE)* strengthens muscles through a contraction that overcomes some fixed resistance produced by equipment, such as dumbbells, barbells, or various weight machines (Figure 4–12). Progressive resistance exercise uses isotonic contractions that generate force while the muscle is changing in length.[34]

Isotonic Contractions   Isotonic contractions may be either concentric or eccentric. An individual who is performing a biceps curl offers a good example of an isotonic contraction. To lift the weight from the starting position, the biceps muscle must contract and shorten in length. This shortening contraction is referred to as a **concentric,** or **positive, contraction.** If the biceps muscle does not remain contracted when the weight is

concentric (positive) contraction The muscle shortens while contracting against resistance.

eccentric (negative) contraction The muscle lengthens while contracting against resistance.

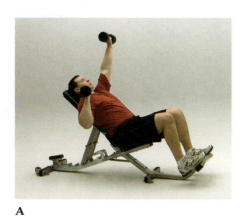 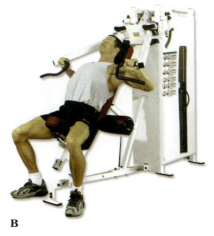

A   B

FIGURE 4–12 **(A)** Barbells and dumbbells are free weights that assist in developing isotonic strength. **(B)** Many machine exercise systems provide a variety of exercise possibilities.

being lowered, gravity will cause the weight to simply fall back to the starting position. Thus, to control the weight as it is being lowered, the biceps muscle must continue to contract while gradually lengthening. A contraction in which the muscle is lengthening while still applying force is called an **eccentric,** or **negative, contraction.**[46]

Eccentric Contractions versus Concentric Contractions It is possible to generate greater amounts of force against resistance with an eccentric contraction than with a concentric contraction. This greater force occurs because eccentric contractions require a much lower level of motor unit activity to achieve a certain force than do concentric contractions. Because fewer motor units are firing to produce a specific force, additional motor units may be recruited to generate increased force. In addition, oxygen utilization is much lower during eccentric exercise than during comparable concentric exercise. Thus, eccentric contractions are more resistant to fatigue than are concentric contractions. The mechanical efficiency of eccentric exercise may be several times higher than that of concentric exercise.[46]

Concentric contractions accelerate movement, whereas eccentric contractions decelerate motion. For example, the hamstrings must contract eccentrically to decelerate the angular velocity of the lower leg during running. Likewise, the external rotators in the rotator cuff muscles surrounding the shoulder contract eccentrically to decelerate the internally rotating humerus during throwing. Because of the excessive forces involved with these eccentric contractions, injury to the muscles is quite common. Thus, eccentric exercise must be routinely incorporated into the strength-training program to prevent injury to those muscles that act to decelerate movement.

Free Weights versus Machine Weights Various types of exercise equipment can be used with progressive resistance exercise, including free weights (barbells and dumbbells) or exercise machines, such as those made by Universal, Nautilus, Cybex, Eagle, and Body Master. Dumbbells and barbells require the use of iron plates of varying weights that can be changed easily by adding or subtracting equal amounts of weight to both sides of the bar. The exercise machines have a stack of weights that are lifted through a series of levers or pulleys. The stack of weights slides up and down on a pair of bars that restrict the movement to only one plane. Weight can be increased or decreased simply by changing the position of a weight key.

Both free weights and exercise machines have advantages and disadvantages. The exercise machines are relatively safe to use compared with free weights. It is also a simple process to increase or decrease the weight on exercise machines by moving a single weight key, although changes can generally be made only in increments of 10 or 15 pounds. The iron plates used with free weights must be added or removed from each side of the barbell or dumbbell.

Figure 4–13 shows examples of different isotonic strengthening exercises.

Spotting for free weight exercises When training with free weights, it is essential that the lifter have a partner who can assist in performing a particular exercise. This assistance is particularly critical when the weights to be lifted are extremely heavy. A *spotter* has three functions: to protect the lifter from injury, to make recommendations on proper lifting technique, and to help motivate the lifter. *Focus Box 4–3:* "Proper spotting techniques" provides some guidelines for correct spotting techniques.

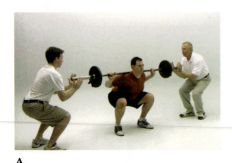

A

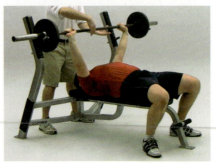

B

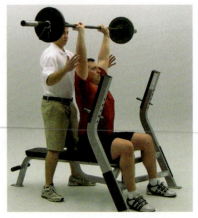

C

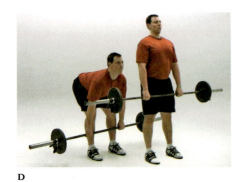

D

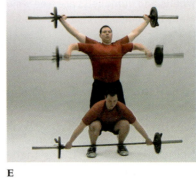

E

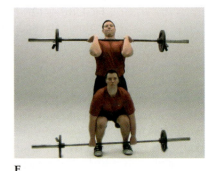

F

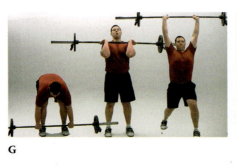

G

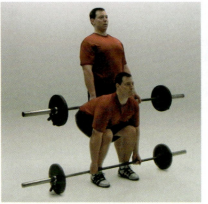

H

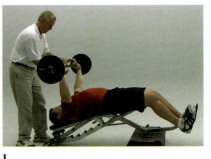

I

FIGURE 4–13 Examples of isotonic strengthening exercises using barbells, shown with appropriate spotting techniques where required **(A)** Squat. **(B)** Bench press. **(C)** Military press. **(D)** Romanian dead lift. **(E)** Snatch. **(F)** Power clean. **(G)** Clean and jerk. **(H)** Dead lift. **(I)** Decline press. **(J)** Incline press. **(K)** Standing bicep curl.

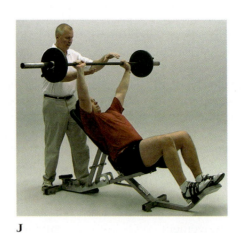

J

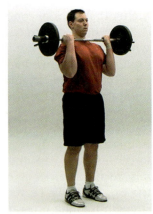

K

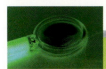

FOCUS 4–3 Focus on Treatment and Rehabilitation

Proper spotting techniques

- Make sure the lifter understands how to get out of the way of missed attempts, particularly with overhead techniques.
- Check to see that the lifter is in a safe, stable position.
- Communicate with the lifter to know how many reps are to be done, whether a liftoff is needed, and how much help the lifter wants in completing a rep.
- Stand behind the lifter.
- When spotting dumbbell exercises, spot as close to the dumbbells as possible above the elbow joint.

- If heavy weights exceed the limits of your ability to control the weight, use a second spotter.
- Make sure the lifter uses the proper grip.
- Make sure the lifter inhales and exhales during the lift.
- Make sure the lifter moves through a complete range of motion at the appropriate speed.
- Always be in a position to protect both the lifter and yourself from injury.

Isotonic Training Regardless of which type of equipment is used, the same principles of **isotonic exercise** may be applied. In progressive resistance exercise, it

isotonic exercise
Shortens and lengthens the muscle through a complete range of motion.

is essential to incorporate both concentric and eccentric contractions. Research has clearly demonstrated that the muscle should be overloaded and fatigued both concentrically and eccentrically for the greatest strength improvement to occur.[54,66]

When an individual is weight training specifically to develop muscular strength, the concentric, or positive, portion of the exercise should require 1 to 2 seconds, and the eccentric, or negative, portion of the lift should require 2 to 4 seconds. The ratio of negative to positive should be approximately one to two. Physiologically, the muscle will fatigue much more rapidly concentrically than eccentrically.

Individuals who have weight trained with both free weights and machines realize the difference in the amount of weight that can be lifted. Unlike the machines, free weights have no restricted motion and can thus move in many different directions, depending on the forces applied. With free weights, an element of muscular control on the part of the lifter to prevent the weight from moving in any direction other than vertical will usually decrease the amount of weight that can be lifted.[43]

One problem often mentioned in relation to isotonic training is that the amount of force necessary to move a weight through a range of motion changes according to the angle of pull of the contracting muscle. The amount of force is greatest when the angle of pull is approximately 90 degrees. In addition, once the inertia of the weight has been overcome and momentum has been established, the force required to move the resistance varies according to the force that the muscle can produce through the range of motion. Thus, it has been argued that a disadvantage

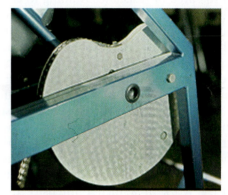

FIGURE 4–14 The cam system on the Nautilus equipment is designed to equalize the resistance throughout the full range of motion.

of any type of isotonic exercise is that the force required to move the resistance is constantly changing throughout the range of movement.

Certain exercise machines are designed to minimize this change in resistance by using a cam system (Figure 4–14). The cam has been individually designed for each piece of equipment so that the resistance is variable throughout the movement. The cam system attempts to alter resistance so that the muscle can handle a greater load—at the points at which the joint angle or muscle length is at a mechanical disadvantage, the cam reduces the resistance to muscle movement. Whether this design does what it claims is debatable. This change in resistance at different points in the range is called **accommodating resistance,** or variable resistance.

accommodating resistance Change in resistance at different points in the range.

PRE Techniques Perhaps the single most confusing aspect of progressive resistance exercise is the terminology used to describe specific programs. The following list of terms and their operational definitions may help clarify the confusion:

- Repetitions—the number of times a specific movement is repeated.
- Repetitions maximum (RM)—the maximum number of repetitions at a given weight.
- One repetition maximum (1 RM)—the maximum amount of weight that can be lifted one time.
- Set—a particular number of repetitions.
- Intensity—the amount of weight or resistance lifted.
- Recovery period—the rest interval between sets.
- Frequency—the number of times an exercise is done in 1 week.

A considerable amount of research has been done in the area of resistance training to determine optimal techniques in terms of the intensity or the amount of weight to be used, the number of repetitions, the number of sets, the recovery period, and the frequency of training. It is important to realize that there are many different effective techniques and training regimens. Regardless of specific techniques used, it is certain that to improve strength the muscle must be overloaded in a progressive manner.[57] This overload is the basis of progressive resistance exercise. The amount of weight used and the number of repetitions must be enough to make the muscle work at a higher intensity than it is used to working at. This overload is the single most critical factor in any strength-training program. The strength-training program must also be designed to meet the specific needs of the individual.

There is no such thing as an optimal strength-training program. Achieving total agreement on a program of resistance training—with specific recommendations about repetitions, sets, intensity, recovery time, and frequency—among researchers or other experts in resistance training is impossible. However, the following general recommendations will provide an effective resistance-training program.

In adults, for any given exercise, the amount of weight selected should be sufficient to allow six to eight repetitions maximum (RM) in each of three sets with a recovery period of 60 to 90 seconds between sets.[13] Initial selection of a starting weight may require some trial and error to achieve this six to eight RM range. If at least three sets of six repetitions cannot be completed, the weight is too heavy and should be reduced. If it is possible to do more than three sets of eight repetitions, the weight is too light and should be increased.[10] Progression to heavier weights is determined by the ability to perform at least eight RM in each of three sets. An increase of about 10 percent of the current weight being lifted should still allow at least six RM in each of three sets.[13]

Occasionally, athletes may be tested at 1 RM to determine the greatest amount of weight that can be lifted one time. Extreme caution should be exercised when trying to determine 1 RM. Attention should be directed toward making sure the athlete has had ample opportunity to warm up and that the lifting technique is correct before attempting a maximum lift. Determining 1 RM should be done very gradually to minimize the chances of injuring the muscle.

A particular muscle or muscle group should be exercised consistently every other day.[13] Thus, the frequency of weight training should be at least three times per week but no more than four times per week. It is common for serious weight trainers to lift every day; however, they exercise different muscle groups on successive days. For example, Monday, Wednesday, and Friday may be used for upper-body muscles, whereas Tuesday, Thursday, and Saturday are used for lower-body muscles.

Training for Muscular Strength versus Endurance Muscular endurance is the ability to perform repeated muscle contractions against resistance for an extended period of time. Most weight-training experts believe that muscular strength and muscular endurance are closely related.[74] As one improves, the other tends to improve also.

When weight training for strength, use heavier weights with a lower number of repetitions. Conversely, endurance training uses relatively lighter weights with a greater number of repetitions.

Endurance training should consist of three sets of 10 to 15 repetitions, using the same criteria for weight selection, progression, and frequency as recommended for progressive resistance exercise.[9] Thus, suggested training regimens for muscular strength and endurance are similar in terms of sets and numbers of repetitions. Persons who possess great levels of strength also tend to exhibit greater muscular endurance when asked to perform repeated contractions against resistance.

Isokinetic Exercise An **isokinetic exercise** involves a muscle contraction in which the length of the muscle is changing while the contraction is performed at a constant velocity.[73] In theory, maximal resistance is provided throughout the range of motion by the machine.

isokinetic exercise
Exercise at a fixed velocity of movement with accommodating resistance.

The resistance provided by the machine will move only at some preset speed regardless of the force applied to it by the individual.[1] Thus, the key to isokinetic exercise is not the resistance, but the speed at which the resistance can be moved.[1,73]

Currently, only one isokinetic device is available commercially—Biodex (Figure 4–15). Isokinetic

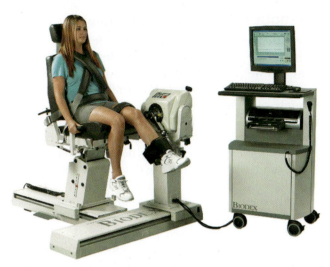

FIGURE 4–15 During isokinetic exercise, the speed of movement is constant regardless of the force applied by the athlete.

devices rely on hydraulic, pneumatic, or mechanical pressure systems to produce constant velocity of motion. Isokinetic devices are capable of resisting both concentric and eccentric contractions at a fixed speed to exercise a muscle.

A major disadvantage of an isokinetic unit is its cost. The unit comes with a computer and printing device and is used primarily as a diagnostic and rehabilitative tool in the treatment of various injuries.

Isokinetic devices are designed so that, regardless of the amount of force applied, the resistance can be moved only at a certain speed. That speed will be the same whether maximal force or only half the maximal force is applied. Consequently, when training isokinetically, it is absolutely necessary to exert as much force against the resistance as possible (maximal effort) for maximal strength gains to occur. This need for maximal effort is one of the major problems with an isokinetic strength-training program.

Anyone who has been involved in a weight-training program knows that on some days it is difficult to find the motivation to work out. Because isokinetic training does not require a maximal effort, it is easy to "cheat" and not go through the workout at a high level of intensity. In a progressive resistance exercise program, the individual knows how much weight has to be lifted with how many repetitions.[49] Thus, isokinetic training is often more effective if a partner system is used as a means of motivation toward a maximal effort.

When isokinetic training is done properly with a maximal effort, it is theoretically possible that maximal strength gains are best achieved through the isokinetic training method in which the velocity and force of the resistance are equal throughout the range of motion.[1] However, there is no conclusive evidence-based research to support this theory. Whether changing force capability is, in fact, a deterrent to improving the ability to generate force against some resistance is debatable.

In the athletic training setting, isokinetics are perhaps best used as a rehabilitative and diagnostic tool rather than as a conditioning device.[1]

Circuit Training **Circuit training** employs a series of exercise stations that consist of various combinations of weight training, flexibility, calisthenics, and brief aerobic exercises. Circuit training is used in the majority of fitness centers in corporate and health club settings. Circuits may be designed to accomplish many different training goals. With circuit training, the individual moves rapidly from one station to the next and performs whatever exercise is to be done at that station within a specified time period. A typical circuit consists of 8 to 12 stations, and the entire circuit is repeated three times.

> **circuit training**
> Exercise stations that consist of various combinations of weight training, flexibility, calisthenics, and aerobic exercises.

Circuit training is definitely an effective technique for improving strength and flexibility. Certainly, if the pace or the time interval between stations is rapid and if workload is maintained at a high level of intensity with heart rate at or above target training levels, the cardiorespiratory system may benefit from this circuit. However, little research evidence exists to show that circuit training is effective in improving cardiorespiratory endurance. It should be, and is most often, used as a technique for developing and improving muscular strength and endurance.

Calisthenic Strengthening Exercises Calisthenics, or free exercise, is one of the more easily available means of developing strength. Isotonic movement exercises can be graded according to intensity by using gravity as an aid, by ruling gravity out, by moving against gravity, or by using the body or a body part as a resistance against gravity. Most calisthenics require the individual to support the body or move the total body against the force of gravity. Push-ups are a good example of a vigorous antigravity free exercise. Calisthenic-like exercises are used in functional strength training, discussed earlier. To be considered maximally effective, the isotonic calisthenic exercise, like all types of exercise, must be performed in an exacting manner and in full range of motion. In most cases, 10 or more repetitions are performed for each exercise and are repeated in sets of two or three.

Some free exercises use an isometric, or holding, phase instead of a full range of motion. Examples of these exercises are back extensions and sit-ups. When the exercise produces maximum muscle tension, it is held between 6 and 10 seconds and then repeated one to three times.

Plyometric Exercise Plyometric exercise is a technique that includes specific exercises that encompass a rapid stretch of a muscle eccentrically,

| plyometric exercise Type of exercise that takes advantage of the stretch-shortening cycle. |

followed immediately by a rapid concentric contraction of that muscle to facilitate and develop a forceful, explosive movement over a short period of time.[2,25] This effect requires that the time between eccentric contraction and concentric contraction be very short. It is theorized that this extra power is due to the muscle gaining potential energy. This energy dissipates rapidly, so the action must be quick. The process is frequently referred to as the *stretch-shortening* cycle and is the underlying mechanism of plyometric training. The greater the stretch put on the muscle from its resting length immediately before the concentric contraction, the greater the resistance the muscle can overcome. Plyometric exercises emphasize the speed of the eccentric phase.[24] The rate of the stretch is more critical than the magnitude of the stretch.

All movements involve repeated stretch-shortening cycles. Picture a jumping athlete preparing to transfer forward energy to upward energy. As the final step is taken before jumping, the loaded leg must stop the forward momentum and change it into an upward direction. As this happens, the muscle undergoes a lengthening eccentric contraction to decelerate the movement and prestretch the muscle. This prestretch energy is then immediately released in an equal and opposite reaction, thereby producing kinetic energy. The neuromuscular system must react quickly to produce the concentric shortening contraction to prevent falling and produce the upward change in direction. Consequently, specific functional exercises to emphasize this rapid change of direction must be used. Because plyometric exercises train specific movements in a biomechanically accurate manner, the muscles, tendons, and ligaments are all strengthened in a functional manner.

An advantage of plyometric exercises is that they can help develop eccentric control in dynamic movements.[76] Plyometric exercises involve hops, bounds, and depth jumping for the lower extremities and use medicine balls and other types of weighted equipment for the upper extremities (Figure 4–16). Depth jumping is an example of a plyometric exercise in which an individual jumps to the ground from a specified height and then quickly jumps again as soon as ground contact is made.[25] Plyometrics place a great deal of stress on the musculoskeletal system. The learning and perfection of specific jumping skills and other plyometric exercises must be technically correct and specific to the individual's age, activity, physical development, and skill development.[70]

Strength Training for the Female

Strength training is critical for the female. Significant muscle hypertrophy in the female is dependent on the presence of the hormone testosterone. Testosterone is considered a male hormone, although all females possess some testosterone in their systems. Females with higher testosterone levels tend to have more masculine characteristics, such as increased facial and body hair, a deeper voice, and the potential to develop a little more muscle bulk.[62]

Both males and females experience initial rapid gains in strength due to an increase in neuromuscular efficiency, as discussed previously.[92] However, in the female, these rapid initial strength gains tend to plateau after 3 to 4 weeks. Minimal improvement in muscular strength will be realized during a continuing strength-training program because the muscle will not continue to hypertrophy to any significant degree.

Perhaps the most critical difference between males and females regarding physical performance is the ratio of strength to body weight. The reduced *strength-to-body-weight ratio* in females is the result of their higher percentage of body fat. The strength-to-body-weight ratio may be significantly improved through weight training by decreasing the percentage of body fat while increasing lean weight.[40]

Strength Training in Prepubescents and Adolescents

The principles of resistance training discussed previously may be applied to younger individuals. A number of sociological questions regarding the advantages and disadvantages of younger—in particular, prepubescent—individuals engaging in rigorous strength-training programs emerge, however. From a physiological perspective, experts have for years debated the value of strength training in young individuals. Recently, a number of studies have indicated that, if properly supervised, prepubescents and adolescents can improve strength, power, endurance, balance, and proprioception; develop a positive body image; improve sport performance; and prevent injuries.[5] A prepubescent child can experience gains in levels of muscle strength without significant muscle hypertrophy.[38]

An athletic trainer supervising a conditioning program for a young athlete should certainly incorporate resistive exercise into the program. However, close supervision, proper instruction, and appropriate modification of progression and intensity based on the extent of physical maturation of the individual are critical to the effectiveness of the resistive exercises.[69] A functional strengthening program that uses calisthenic strengthening exercises with body weight as resistance should be encouraged.

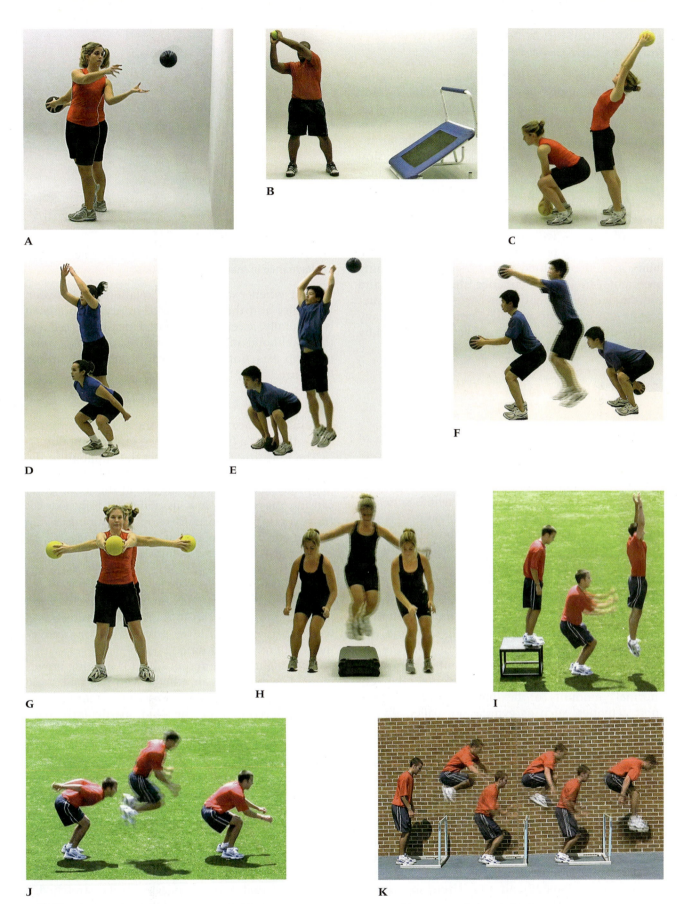

FIGURE 4–16   Plyometric exercises. **(A)** Weighted ball double-arm rotation toss. **(B)** Plyback two-arm toss with rotation. **(C)** Weighted ball squat to stand extension. **(D)** Squat jumps. **(E)** Overhead weighted ball throw. **(F)** Weighted ball forward jump from squat. **(G)** Weighted ball standing rotations. **(H)** Double-leg lateral hop overs. **(I)** Depth jump to vertical jump. **(J)** Repeat two-leg standing long jump. **(K)** Three-hurdle jumps.

The Relationship between Strength and Flexibility

It is often said that strength training has a negative effect on flexibility.[79] For example, we tend to think of individuals who have highly developed muscles as having lost much of their ability to move freely through a full range of motion. Occasionally, an individual develops so much bulk that the physical size of the muscle prevents a normal range of motion. It is certainly true that strength training that is not properly done can impair movement; however, weight training, if done properly through a full range of motion, will not impair flexibility. Proper strength training probably improves dynamic flexibility and, if combined with a rigorous stretching program, can greatly enhance the powerful and coordinated movements that are essential for success in many athletic activities. In all cases, a heavy weight-training program should be accompanied by a strong flexibility program.

IMPROVING AND MAINTAINING FLEXIBILITY

Flexibility is the ability to move a joint or series of joints smoothly and easily through a full range of motion.[4] Flexibility can be discussed in relation to movement involving only one joint, such as the knees, or movement involving a whole series of joints, such as the spinal vertebral joints, which must all move together to allow smooth bending or rotation of the trunk.

The Importance of Flexibility

Maintaining a full, nonrestricted range of motion has long been recognized as essential to normal daily living. Lack of flexibility can also create uncoordinated or awkward movement patterns resulting from lost neuromuscular control.[16] In most individuals, functional activities require relatively "normal" amounts of flexibility. However, some sport activities, such as gymnastics, ballet, diving, and karate, require increased flexibility for superior performance (Figure 4–17).[6]

Flexibility is generally seen as essential for improving performance in physical activities. However, a review of the evidence-based information in the literature looking at the relationship between flexibility and improved performance is at best conflicting and inconclusive.[82,87] Although many studies done over the years have suggested that stretching improves performance,[19,51,71] several recent studies have found that stretching causes decreases in performance parameters, such as strength, endurance, power, joint position sense, and reaction times.[12,29,37,50,64,81,84,93] The same can

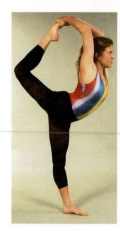

FIGURE 4–17 Good flexibility is essential to successful performance in many sport activities.

be said when examining the relationship between flexibility and the incidence of injury. Although it is generally accepted that good flexibility reduces the likelihood of injury, a true cause-effect relationship has not been clearly established in the literature.[7,8,23,71,93]

Factors That Limit Flexibility

A number of factors may limit the ability of a joint to move through a full, unrestricted range of motion.

The *bony structure* may restrict the endpoint in the range. An elbow that has been fractured through the joint may deposit excess calcium in the joint space, causing the joint to lose its ability to fully extend. However, in many instances bony prominences stop movements at normal endpoints in the range.

Excessive *fat* may also limit the ability to move through a full range of motion. An athlete who has a large amount of fat on the abdomen may have severely restricted trunk flexion when asked to bend forward and touch the toes. The fat may act as a wedge between two lever arms, restricting movement wherever it is found.

Skin might also be responsible for limiting movement. For example, an athlete who has had some type of injury or surgery involving a tearing incision or laceration of the skin, particularly over a joint, will have inelastic scar tissue at that site. This scar tissue is incapable of stretching with joint movement.

Muscles and their tendons, along with their surrounding fascial sheaths, are most often responsible for limiting range of motion. An individual who performs stretching exercises to improve flexibility about a particular joint is attempting to take advantage of the highly elastic properties of a muscle. Over time, it is possible to increase the elasticity, or the length that a given muscle can be stretched.[77] Individuals who have a good deal of movement at a particular joint tend to have highly elastic and flexible muscles.

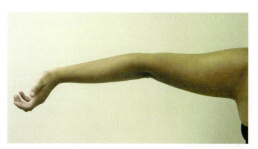

FIGURE 4–18 Excessive joint motion, or hypermobility, can predispose an individual to injury.

Connective tissue surrounding the joint, such as ligaments on the joint capsule, may be subject to contractures. Ligaments and joint capsules do have some elasticity; however, if a joint is immobilized for a period of time, these structures tend to lose some elasticity and shorten. This condition is most commonly seen after surgical repair of an unstable joint, but it can also result from long periods of inactivity.

Neural tissue tightness resulting from acute compression, chronic repetitive microtrauma, muscle imbalances, joint dysfunction, or poor posture can create morphological changes in neural tissues that may result in irritation, inflammation, and pain. Pain causes muscle guarding to protect inflamed and irritated neural structures, and this alters normal movement patterns. Over time neural fibrosis results, decreasing the elasticity of neural tissue and preventing normal movement of surrounding tissues.

It is also possible for an individual to have relatively slack ligaments and joint capsules. These individuals are generally referred to as being hypermobile. An example of hypermobility is an elbow or a knee that hyperextends beyond 180 degrees (Figure 4–18). Frequently, the instability associated with hypermobility presents as great a problem in movement as ligamentous or capsular contractures.

The elasticity of skin contractures caused by scarring, ligaments, joint capsules, and musculotendinous units can be improved to varying degrees over time through stretching. With the exception of bony structure, age, and gender, all the other factors that limit flexibility also may be altered to increase range of joint motion.

Agonist versus Antagonist Muscles

Understanding flexibility requires defining the terms *agonist* and *antagonist*. Most joints in the body are capable of more than one movement. The knee joint, for example, is capable of flexion and extension. Contraction of the quadriceps group of muscles on the front of the thigh causes knee extension, whereas contraction of the hamstring muscles on the back of the thigh produces knee flexion.

To achieve knee extension, the quadriceps group contracts while the hamstring muscles relax and stretch. The muscle that contracts to produce a movement—in this case, the quadriceps—is referred to as the **agonist** muscle. The muscle being stretched in response to contraction of the agonist muscle is called the **antagonist** muscle. In knee extension, the antagonist muscle is the hamstring group. Some degree of balance in strength between agonist and antagonist muscle groups is necessary to produce normal, smooth, coordinated movement and to reduce the likelihood of muscle strain caused by muscular imbalance.[59]

> **agonist** Muscle contracting to cause movement.
>
> **antagonist** Muscle being stretched.

Active and Passive Range of Motion

Active range of motion, also called *dynamic flexibility*, is the degree to which a joint can be moved by a muscle contraction, usually through the midrange of movement.[89] Dynamic flexibility is not necessarily a good indicator of the stiffness or looseness of a joint because it applies to the ability to move a joint efficiently, with little resistance to motion.[80]

Passive range of motion, sometimes called *static flexibility*, is the degree to which a joint may be passively moved to the endpoints in the range of motion. No muscle contraction is involved to move a joint through a passive range.

When a muscle actively contracts, it produces a joint movement through a specific range of motion. However, if passive pressure is applied to an extremity, it is capable of moving farther in the range of motion. It is essential in sport activities that an extremity be capable of moving through a nonrestricted range of motion. For example, a hurdler who cannot fully extend the knee joint in a normal stride is at a considerable disadvantage because stride length and thus speed will be reduced significantly.

Passive range of motion is important for injury prevention. In many sports situations, a muscle is forced to stretch beyond its normal active limits. If the muscle does not have enough elasticity to compensate for this additional stretch, the musculotendinous unit will likely be injured.

Mechanisms for Improving Flexibility

For many years the efficacy of stretching in improving range of motion has been theoretically attributed to neurophysiological phenomena involving the stretch reflex.[22] However, a more recent study that extensively reviewed the existing literature has suggested that improvements in range of motion resulting from stretching must be explained by mechanisms other than the stretch reflex.[23] Studies

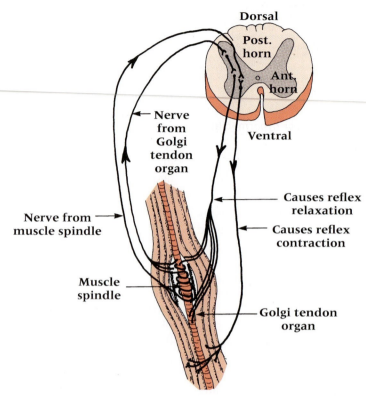

FIGURE 4–19 Stretch reflex. The muscle spindle produces a reflex resistance to stretch, and the Golgi tendon organ causes a reflex relaxation of the muscle in response to stretch.

reviewed indicate that changes in the ability to tolerate stretch and/or the viscoelastic properties of the stretched muscle are possible mechanisms.

Neurophysiological Basis of Stretching Every muscle in the body contains various types of mechanoreceptors that, when stimulated, inform the central nervous system of what is happening with that muscle. Two of these mechanoreceptors are important in the stretch reflex: the *muscle spindle* and the *Golgi tendon organ* (Figure 4–19). Both types of receptors are sensitive to changes in muscle length. The Golgi tendon organs are also affected by changes in muscle tension.

When a muscle is stretched, both the muscle spindles and the Golgi tendon organs immediately begin sending a volley of sensory impulses to the spinal cord. Initially, impulses coming from the muscle spindles inform the central nervous system that the muscle is being stretched. Impulses return to the muscle from the spinal cord, causing the muscle to reflexively contract, thus resisting the stretch.[63] The Golgi tendon organs respond to the change in length and the increase in tension by firing off sensory impulses of their own to the spinal

cord. If the stretch of the muscle continues for an extended period of time (at least 6 seconds), impulses from the Golgi tendon organs begin to override muscle spindle impulses. The impulses from the Golgi tendon organs, unlike the signals from the muscle spindle, cause a reflex relaxation of the antagonist muscle. This reflex relaxation serves as a protective mechanism that will allow the muscle to stretch through relaxation without exceeding the extensibility limits, which could damage the muscle fibers.[10] This relaxation of the antagonist muscle during contractions is referred to as **autogenic inhibition.**

In any synergistic muscle group, a contraction of the agonist causes a reflex relaxation in the antagonist muscle, allowing it to stretch and protecting it from injury. This phenomenon is referred to as *reciprocal inhibition* (Figure 4–20).[82]

The Effects of Stretching on the Physical and Mechanical Properties of Muscle The neurophysiological mechanisms of both autogenic and reciprocal inhibition result in reflex relaxation with subsequent lengthening of a muscle. Thus, the

> **autogenic inhibition** Relaxation of the antagonist muscle during contractions.

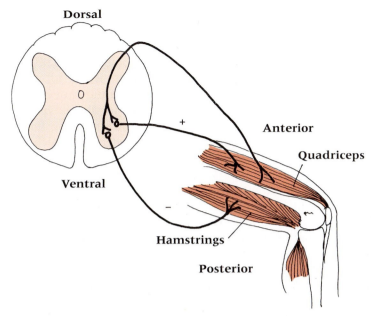

FIGURE 4–20   Reciprocal inhibition. A contraction of the agonist will produce relaxation in the antagonist.

mechanical properties of that muscle that physically allow lengthening to occur are dictated via neural input.

Both muscle and tendon are composed largely of noncontractile collagen and elastin fibers. Collagen enables a tissue to resist mechanical forces and deformation, whereas elastin composes highly elastic tissues that assist in recovery from deformation.[86]

Unlike tendon, muscle also has active contractile components, which are the actin and myosin myofilaments. Collectively, the contractile and noncontractile elements determine the muscle's capability of deforming and recovering from deformation.[56]

Both the contractile and the noncontractile components appear to resist deformation when a muscle is stretched or lengthened. The percentage of their individual contribution to resisting deformation depends on the degree to which the muscle is stretched or deformed and on the velocity of deformation. The noncontractile elements are primarily resistant to the degree of lengthening, while the contractile elements limit high-velocity deformation. The greater the stretch, the more the noncontractile components contribute.[86]

Lengthening of a muscle via stretching allows for viscoelastic and plastic changes to occur in the collagen and elastin fibers. The viscoelastic changes that allow slow deformation with imperfect recovery are not permanent. However, plastic changes, although difficult to achieve, result in residual or permanent change in length due to deformation created by long periods of stretching.

The greater the velocity of deformation, the greater the chance for exceeding that tissue's capability to undergo viscoelastic and plastic change.[56]

Stretching Techniques

The maintenance of a full, nonrestricted range of motion has long been recognized as critical to injury prevention and as an essential component of a conditioning program.[8] The goal of any effective flexibility program should be to improve the range of motion at a given articulation by altering the extensibility of the neuromusculotendinous structures that produce movement at that joint.[33,41] Exercises that stretch these neuromusculotendinous structures over several months increase the range of motion possible at a given joint.[79]

Ballistic Stretching Ballistic stretching involves a bouncing movement in which repetitive contractions of the agonist muscle are used to produce quick stretches of the antagonist muscle. The ballistic stretching technique, although apparently effective in improving range of motion, has been criticized in the past because increased range of motion is achieved through a series of jerks or pulls on the resistant muscle tissue.[4] The concern was that, if the forces generated by the jerks are greater than the tissues' extensibility, muscle injury may result.

> **ballistic stretching**
> Older stretching technique that uses repetitive bouncing motions.

Dynamic Stretching Certainly, successive, forceful contractions of the agonist muscle that result in stretching of the antagonist muscle may cause muscle soreness. For example, forcefully kicking a soccer ball 50 times may result in muscle soreness of the hamstrings (antagonist muscle) as a result of eccentric contraction of the hamstrings to control the dynamic movement of the quadriceps (agonist muscle). Stretching that is controlled usually does not cause muscle soreness.[63] This is the difference between ballistic stretching and dynamic stretching. In fact, in the athletic population, **dynamic stretching** has become the stretching technique of choice. The argument has been that dynamic stretching exercises are more closely related to the types of activities that athletes engage in and should be considered more functional.[31,63] Thus, dynamic stretching exercises are routinely recommended for athletes prior to beginning an activity (Figure 4–21A).

dynamic stretching
Controlled stretches recommended prior to beginning an activity.

Static Stretching The **static stretching** technique is a widely used and effective technique of stretching. This technique involves passively stretching a given antagonist muscle by placing it in a maximal position of stretch and holding it there for an extended time (Figure 4–21B). Recommendations for the optimal time for holding this stretched position vary from as short as 3 seconds to as long as 60 seconds.[44] Recent data indicate that 30 seconds may be an optimal time to hold the stretch. The static stretch of each muscle should be repeated three or four times.[10]

static stretching
Passively stretching an antagonist muscle by placing it in a maximal stretch and holding it there.

Much research has been done comparing ballistic and static stretching techniques for the improvement of flexibility. It has been shown that both static and ballistic stretching are effective in increasing flexibility and that there is no significant difference between the two. However, static stretching offers less danger of exceeding the extensibility limits of the involved joints because the stretch is more controlled. Ballistic stretching is apt to cause muscle soreness, whereas static stretching generally does not and is commonly used in injury rehabilitation of sore or strained muscles.[4,52]

Static stretching is certainly a much safer stretching technique, especially for sedentary or untrained individuals. However, many physical activities involve dynamic movement. Thus, stretching as a warm-up for these types of activities should begin with static stretching followed by ballistic and dynamic stretching, which more closely resemble the dynamic activity.

PNF Stretching Techniques Proprioceptive neuromuscular facilitation (PNF) techniques were first used by physical therapists for treating patients who had various types of neuromuscular paralysis.[75] More recently, PNF exercises have been used as a stretching technique for increasing flexibility.

A number of different PNF techniques are currently being used for stretching, including slow-reversal-hold-relax, contract-relax, and hold-relax techniques. All involve some combination of alternating contraction and relaxation of both agonist and antagonist muscles. All three techniques use a 10-second active push phase followed by a 10-second passive relax phase repeated three times for a total of 60 seconds.

proprioceptive neuromuscular facilitation (PNF)
Stretching techniques that involve combinations of alternating contractions and stretches.

Using a hamstring stretching technique as an example (Figure 4–21C), the slow-reversal-hold-relax technique would be done as follows:[75]

- With the patient lying supine with the knee extended and the ankle flexed to 90 degrees, the athletic trainer passively flexes the hip joint to the point at which there is slight discomfort in the muscle.
- At this point, the patient begins actively pushing against the athletic trainer's resistance by contracting the hamstring muscle.
- After actively pushing for 10 seconds, the hamstring muscles are relaxed and the agonist quadriceps muscle is actively contracted while the athletic trainer applies passive pressure to further stretch the antagonist hamstrings. This action should move the leg so that there is increased hip joint flexion.
- The relaxing phase lasts for 10 seconds, after which the patient again actively pushes against the athletic trainer's resistance, beginning at this new position of increased hip flexion.
- This push-relax sequence is repeated at least three times.

The contract-relax and hold-relax techniques are variations on the slow-reversal-hold-relax method. In the contract-relax method, the hamstrings are

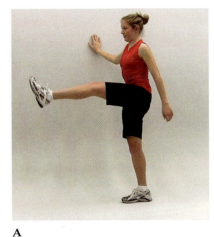

A

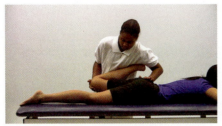

B

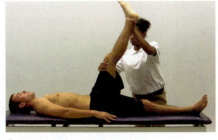

C

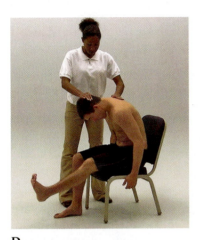

D

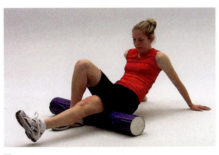

E

FIGURE 4–21   Stretching techniques. **(A)** Dynamic stretch for hip flexors and extensors. **(B)** Static stretch for knee extensors. **(C)** Slow-reversal-hold-relax PNF techniques for hamstrings. **(D)** Slump-stretch for sciatic nerve. **(E)** Myofascial stretching for hamstrings.

isotonically contracted so that the leg actually moves toward the floor during the push phase. The hold-relax method involves an isometric hamstring contraction against immovable resistance during the push phase. During the relax phase, both techniques involve the relaxation of hamstrings and quadriceps while the hamstrings are passively stretched. The same basic PNF technique can be used to stretch any muscle in the body. The PNF stretching techniques are perhaps best performed with a partner, although they may also be done using a wall as resistance (see Chapter 16).[75]

Comparing Techniques   Although all four stretching techniques have been demonstrated to improve flexibility, there is still considerable debate as to which technique produces the greatest increases in range of motion. In the past, the ballistic technique has not been recommended because of the potential for causing muscle soreness. However, most sport activities are dynamic in nature (e.g., kicking, running), and those activities use the stretch reflex to enhance performance.[31] In highly trained individuals, it is unlikely

that dynamic stretching will result in muscle soreness. Static stretching is perhaps the most widely used technique. It is a simple technique and does not require a partner. A fully nonrestricted range of motion can be attained through static stretching over time.[35]

The PNF stretching techniques can produce dramatic increases in range of motion during one stretching session. Studies comparing static and PNF stretching suggest that PNF stretching can produce greater improvement in flexibility over an extended training period.[44,75] The major disadvantage of PNF stretching is that it requires a partner for stretching, although stretching with a partner may have some motivational advantages. *Focus Box 4–4:* "Guidelines and precautions for stretching" provides recommendations for various stretching techniques.

Stretching Neural Structures

The athletic trainer should be able to differentiate between tightness in the musculotendinous unit and abnormal neural tension. When an individual performs both active and passive multiplanar movements,

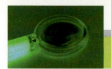

Guidelines and precautions for stretching

The following guidelines and precautions should be incorporated into a sound stretching program:

- Warm up using a slow jog or fast walk before stretching vigorously.
- To increase flexibility, the muscle must be stretched within pain tolerances and tissue healing limitations to attain functional or normal range of motion.
- Stretch only to the point where you feel tightness or resistance to stretch or perhaps some discomfort. Stretching should not be painful.
- Increases in range of motion are specific to whatever joint is being stretched.
- Exercise caution when stretching muscles that surround painful joints. Pain is an indication that something is wrong and should not be ignored.
- Avoid overstretching the ligaments and capsules that surround joints, beyond their limits of extensibility.
- Exercise caution when stretching the lower back and neck. Exercises that compress the vertebrae and their disks may cause damage.

- Stretching from a seated position rather than a standing position takes stress off the low back and decreases the chances of back injury.
- Stretch those muscles that are tight and inflexible.
- Strengthen those muscles that are weak and loose.
- Be sure to continue normal breathing during a stretch. Do not hold your breath.
- Static, dynamic, and PNF techniques are most often recommended for individuals who want to improve their range of motion.
- Ballistic stretching should be done only by those who are already flexible or are accustomed to stretching and should be done only after static stretching.
- Stretching should be done at least three times per week to see minimal improvement. Stretching five or six times per week is recommended to see maximum results.

---

tension is created in the neural structures that exacerbates pain, limits range of motion, and increases radiating neural symptoms, including numbness and tingling. For example, the slump stretch position is used to detect an increase in nerve/root tension in the sciatic nerve and stretching should be done to assist in relieving tension (Figure 4–21D).

Stretching Fascia

Tight fascia, the connective tissue that surrounds the musculotendinous unit, can significantly limit motion. Damage to the fascia due to injury, disease, or inflammation creates pain and motion restriction. Thus, it may be necessary to release tightness in the area of injury. Stretching of tight fascia can either be done manually or by using a firm foam roller (Figure 4–21E). Myofascial release as a treatment technique is discussed in detail in Chapter 16.

Alternative Stretching Techniques

The Pilates Method of Stretching The Pilates method is a somewhat different approach to stretching for improving flexibility. This method has become extremely popular and widely used among personal fitness trainers and physical therapists. Pilates is an exercise technique devised by German-born Joseph Pilates, who established the first Pilates studio in the United States before World War II. The Pilates method is a conditioning program that improves muscle control, flexibility, coordination, strength,

and tone. The basic principles of Pilates exercise are to make people more aware of their bodies as single, integrated units; to improve body alignment and breathing; and to increase efficiency of movement.[72] Unlike other exercise programs, the Pilates method does not require the repetition of exercises but instead consists of a sequence of carefully performed movements, some of which are carried out on specially designed equipment (Figures 4–22 and 4–23).

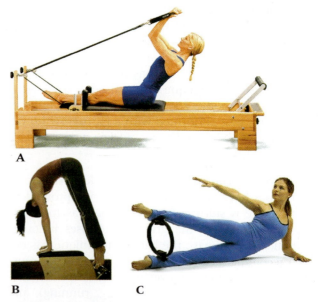

FIGURE 4–22 Pilates techniques using equipment. **(A)** Reformer. **(B)** Wunda chair. **(C)** Magic ring.

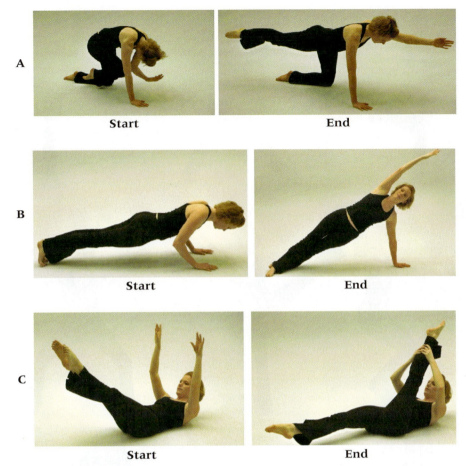

	Start	End
A		
B		
C		

FIGURE 4–23 Pilates floor exercises.
(A) Alternating arm, opposite leg extensions. **(B)** Push-up to a side plank.
(C) Alternating legs scissors.

Each exercise is designed to stretch and strengthen the muscles involved. There is a specific breathing pattern for each exercise to help direct energy to the areas being worked, while relaxing the rest of the body. The Pilates method works many of the deeper muscles together, improving coordination and balance, to achieve efficient and graceful movement. Instead of seeking an ideal or perfect body, the goal is for the practitioner to develop a healthy self-image through the attainment of better posture, proper coordination, and improved flexibility. This method concentrates on correcting body alignment, lengthening all the muscles of the body into a balanced whole, and building endurance and strength without putting undue stress on the lungs and heart.[72] Pilates instructors believe that problems such as soft-tissue injuries can cause bad posture, which can lead to pain and discomfort. Pilates exercises aim to correct this.

Normally, a beginner sees a Pilates instructor on a one-to-one basis for the first session. The instructor assesses the client's physical condition and asks the client about any problems and about the client's lifestyle. The client is then shown a series of exercises that work joints and muscles through a range of motion appropriate for the client's needs.

A class in a studio might involve working on specially designed equipment that primarily uses resistance against tensioned springs to isolate and develop specific muscle groups. Mat work classes involve a repertoire of exercises on a floor mat only. This type of class has become very popular in health clubs and gyms and is often compared to other forms of body conditioning. In fact, the Pilates mat exercises are generally less strenuous than mat exercises in most other conditioning classes.

Yoga Yoga originated in India approximately 6,000 years ago. Its basic philosophy is that most illness is related to poor mental attitudes, posture, and diet. Practitioners of yoga maintain that stress can be reduced through combined mental and physical approaches. Yoga can help an individual cope with stress-induced behaviors and conditions, such as overeating, hypertension, and smoking. Yoga's meditative aspects are believed to help alleviate psychosomatic illnesses. Yoga aims to unite the body and mind to reduce stress. For example, Dr. Chandra Patel, a yoga expert, has found that persons who practice yoga can reduce their blood pressure indefinitely as long as they continue to practice

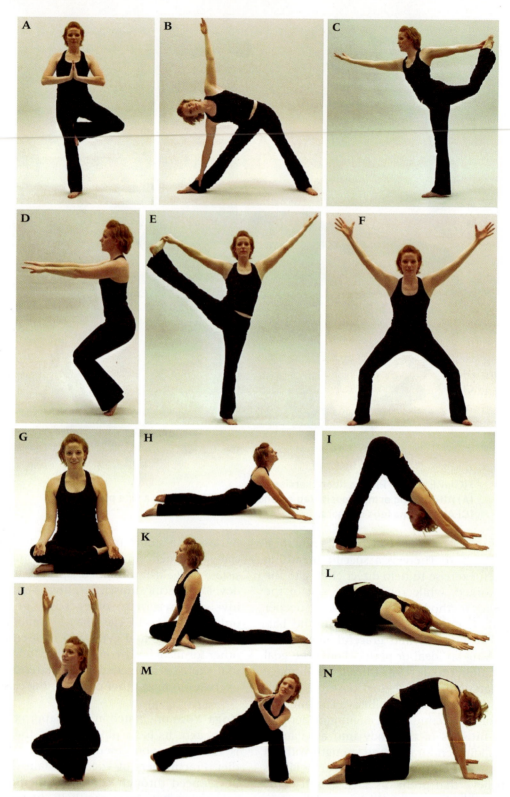

FIGURE 4–24   Yoga positions.
(A) Tree. (B) Triangle. (C) Dancer. (D) Chair. (E) Extended hand to big toe. (F) Big mountain.
(G) Lotus. (H) Cobra. (I) Downward facing dog. (J) Static squat. (K) Pigeon. (L) Child.
(M) Runner's lunge with twist. (N) Cat.

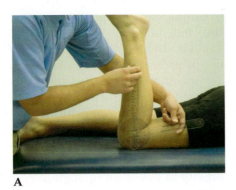
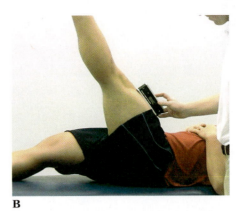

FIGURE 4–25 A goniometer can be used to measure joint angles and range of motion. **(A)** Universal goniometer. **(B)** Inclinometer.

yoga. Yoga consists of various body postures and breathing exercises. Hatha yoga uses a number of positions through which the practitioner may progress, beginning with the simplest and moving to the more complex (Figure 4–24).[78] The various positions are intended to increase mobility and flexibility. However, practitioners must use caution when performing yoga positions. Some can be dangerous, particularly for someone who is inexperienced in yoga technique.

Slow, deep, diaphragmatic breathing is an important part of yoga. Many people take shallow breaths; however, breathing deeply, fully expanding the chest when inhaling, helps lower blood pressure and heart rate.[78] Deep breathing has a calming effect on the body, and it increases production of endorphins.

Measuring Range of Motion

Accurate measurement of the range of joint motion takes some practice on the part of the clinician. Various devices have been designed to accommodate variations in the size of the joints and the complexity of movements in articulations that involve more than one joint.[45] Of these devices, the simplest and most widely used is the *goniometer* (Figure 4–25A). A goniometer is a large protractor with measurements in degrees. By aligning the two arms parallel to the longitudinal axis of the two segments involved in motion about a specific joint, it is possible to obtain relatively accurate measures of range of movement. The goniometer has its place in a rehabilitation setting, where it is essential to assess improvement in joint flexibility for the purpose of modifying injury rehabilitation programs.[83]

Some clinics use an *inclinometer* instead of a goniometer. An inclinometer is a more precise measuring instrument with high reliability that has most

often been used in research settings. However, inclinometers are affordable and can easily be used to accurately measure range of motion of all joints of the body, from complex movements of the spine to simpler movements of the large joints of the extremities, and the small joints of fingers and toes (Figure 4–25B).[83]

FITNESS ASSESSMENT

Fitness testing provides the athletic trainer or strength and conditioning coach with information about the effectiveness of the conditioning program for an individual. Testing may be done in a pretest/posttest format to determine significant improvement from some baseline measure. Tests may be used to assess flexibility, muscular strength, endurance, power, cardiorespiratory endurance, speed, balance, or agility, depending on the stated goals of the training and conditioning program. A variety of established tests can be used to assess these parameters. *Focus Box 4–5:* "Fitness testing" lists various tests that can be administered, along with recommended references to consult for specific testing procedures and for in-depth testing directions.

PERIODIZATION IN CONDITIONING

Serious athletes no longer engage only in preseason conditioning and in-season competition. Sports conditioning is a year-round endeavor. *Periodization* is an approach to conditioning that brings about peak performance while reducing injuries and overtraining in the athlete through a conditioning program that is followed throughout the various seasons.[85] Periodization takes into account that athletes have different conditioning needs during different

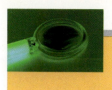

Fitness testing

Muscle strength, power, endurance

One-repetition maximum tests
Timed push-ups
Timed sit-ups
Chin-ups
Bar dips
Flexed arm hang
Vertical jump

Flexibility

Sit-and-reach test
Trunk extension test
Shoulder lift test

Cardiorespiratory endurance

Cooper's 12-minute walk/run
1.5-mile run
Harvard step test

Speed

6-second dash
10- to 60-yard dash

Agility

T-test
Edgren side step
SEMO agility test

Balance

Stork test

Fitness testing references

Baumgartner T, Jackson A: *Measurement for evaluation in physical education and exercise science*, Dubuque, IA, 1999, WCB/McGraw-Hill.

Prentice W: *Fitness and wellness for life*, ed 6, Dubuque, IA, 1999, WCB/McGraw-Hill.

Semenick D: Testing procedures and protocols. In Baechle T, editor: *Essentials of strength training and conditioning*, Champaign, IL, 1994, Human Kinetics.

seasons and modifies the program according to individual needs (Table 4–3).[28]

Macrocycle

Periodization organizes the conditioning program into cycles. The complete training period, which could be a year, in the case of seasonal sports, or 4 years, for an Olympic athlete, is referred to as a *macrocycle*. With seasonal sports, the macrocycle can be divided into a preseason, an in-season, and an off-season. Throughout the course of the macrocycle, intensity, volume, and specificity of conditioning are altered, so that an athlete can achieve peak levels of fitness for competition. As competition approaches, conditioning sessions change gradually and progressively from high-volume, low-intensity, non–sport-specific activity to low-volume, high-intensity, sport-specific training.[91]

> **Sports conditioning often falls into three seasons: preseason, in-season, and off-season.**

Mesocycles Within the macrocycle are a series of *mesocycles*, each of which may last for several weeks or even months. A mesocycle is further divided into *transition, preparatory,* and *competition* periods.[91]

Transition Period The transition period begins after the last competition and comprises the early part of the off-season. The transition period is generally unstructured, and the athlete is encouraged to participate in sport activities on a recreational basis. The idea is to allow the athlete to escape both physically and psychologically from the rigor of a highly organized training regimen.

Preparatory Period The preparatory period occurs primarily during the off-season, when there are no upcoming competitions. The preparatory period has three phases: the hypertrophy/endurance phase, the strength phase, and the power phase.

During the hypertrophy/endurance phase, which occurs in the early part of the off-season, conditioning is at a low intensity with a high volume of repetitions, using activities that may or may not be directly related to a specific sport. The goal is to develop a base of endurance on which more intense conditioning can occur. This phase may last from several weeks to 2 months.

During the strength phase, which also occurs during the off-season, the intensity and volume progress to moderate levels. Weight-training activities should become more specific to the sport or event.

The third phase, or power phase, occurs in the preseason. The athlete trains at a high intensity at or near the level of competition. The volume of training is decreased so that full recovery is allowed between sessions.

Competition Period In certain cases, the competition period lasts for only a week or less. With seasonal sports, however, the competition period may last for several months. In general, this period involves high-intensity conditioning at a low volume. As conditioning volume decreases, an increased

TABLE 4–3 Periodization Training

Season	Period/Phase	Type of Training Activity
Off-season	Transition period	Unstructured Recreational

	Preparatory period
	  Hypertrophy/endurance
	  phase
		Cross training
		Low intensity
		High volume
		Non–sport specific

	Strength phase	Moderate intensity Moderate volume More sport specific
Preseason	Power phase	High intensity Decreased volume Sport specific
In-season	Competition period	High intensity Low volume Skill training Strategy Maintenance of strength and power gained during the off-season

amount of time is spent on skill training or strategy sessions. During the competition period, it may be necessary to establish microcycles, which are periods lasting from 1 to 7 days. During a weekly microcycle, conditioning should be intense early in the week and should progress to moderate and finally to light training the day before a competition. The goal is to make sure that the athlete will be at peak levels of fitness and performance on days of competition.[17]

Cross Training

Cross training is an approach to training and conditioning for a specific sport that involves substituting alternative activities that have some carryover value to that sport. For example, a swimmer could engage in jogging, running, or aerobic exercise to maintain levels of cardiorespiratory conditioning. Cross training is particularly useful in both the transition and the early preparatory periods. It adds variety to the training regimen, thus keeping training during the off-season more interesting and exciting. However, although cross training can be effective in maintaining levels of cardiorespiratory endurance, it is not sport specific and thus should not be used during the preseason.

SUMMARY

- Proper physical conditioning for sports participation should prepare the athlete for high-level performance while helping prevent injuries inherent to that sport.
- Physical conditioning must follow the SAID principle, which is an acronym for specific adaptation to imposed demands. Conditioning must work toward making the body as lean as possible, commensurate with the athlete's sport.
- A proper warm-up should precede conditioning, and a proper cool-down should follow. It takes at least 15 to 30 minutes of gradual warm-up to bring the body to a state of readiness for vigorous sports training and participation. Warming up consists of a general, unrelated activity followed by a specific, related activity.
- Cardiorespiratory endurance is the ability to perform whole-body, large-muscle activities repeatedly for long periods of time. Maximal oxygen consumption is the greatest determinant of the level of cardiorespiratory endurance. Most sport activities involve some combination of both

aerobic and anaerobic metabolism. Improvement of cardiorespiratory endurance may be accomplished through continuous, interval, or speed play training.

- Strength is the capacity to exert a force or the ability to perform work against a resistance. There are many ways to develop strength, including functional strength training; core stability training; and isometric, isotonic, and isokinetic muscle contraction. Isometric exercise generates heat energy by forcefully contracting the muscle in a stable position that produces no change in the length of the muscle. Isotonic exercise involves shortening and lengthening a muscle through a complete range of motion. Isokinetic exercise allows resisted movement through a full range at a specific velocity. Circuit training uses a series of exercise stations to improve strength and flexibility. Plyometric training uses a quick, eccentric

contraction to facilitate a more explosive concentric contraction.

- Optimum flexibility is necessary for success in most sports. Too much flexibility can allow joint trauma to occur, and too little flexibility can result in muscle tears or strains. Ballistic stretching exercises should be avoided. The safest means of increasing flexibility are dynamic stretching, static stretching, and the proprioceptive neuromuscular facilitation (PNF) technique, consisting of slow-reversal-hold-relax, contract-relax, and hold-relax methods.
- Year-round conditioning is essential in most sports to assist in preventing injuries. Periodization is an approach to conditioning that attempts to bring about peak performance while reducing injuries and overtraining in the athlete by developing a training and conditioning program to be followed throughout the various seasons.

WEB SITES

Kaiser Permanente Health Reference:
    http://mydoctor.kaiserpermanente.org
    Click on Cardiovascular Exercise and find several topics, including how to start, target heart rate, and injuries.

National Academy of Sports Medicine:
    www.nasm.org
    This site provides educational opportunities and course work for athletic trainers and personal fitness trainers.

National Strength and Conditioning Association (NSCA): www.nsca-lift.org
    This is the Web site for an organization that focuses on strength and conditioning to support and disseminate research-based knowledge and its practical application and to improve athletic performance and fitness.

SOLUTIONS TO CLINICAL APPLICATION EXERCISES

4–1 The warm-up should begin with a 5- to 7-minute slow jog, during which the athlete should break into a light sweat. At that point, she should engage in stretching (using either static or PNF techniques), concentrating on quadriceps, hamstrings, groin, and hip abductor muscles. Each specific stretch should be repeated four times, and the stretch should be held for 15 to 20 seconds. Once the workout begins, the athlete should gradually and moderately increase the intensity of her activity. She may also find it effective to stretch during the cool-down period after the workout.

4–2 Although athletes should make every effort to maintain existing levels of fitness during the rehabilitation period, to improve their fitness to competitive levels, athletes in any sport must practice or engage in that specific activity. The football player must begin a heavy strength-training program for the upper body immediately in the postseason and must continue to progressively return to heavy lifting with the lower extremities as soon as the healing process will allow. It is essential for this player to progressively increase the intensity and variety of conditioning drills that specifically relate to performance at his position.

4–3 Because this athlete suffers from a lower-extremity injury in which weight bearing is limited, alternative activities, such as swimming or riding a stationary exercise bike, should be incorporated into her rehabilitation program immediately. If the pressure on her ankle when riding an exercise bike is too painful, she may find it helpful initially to use a bike that

incorporates upper-extremity exercise. The athletic trainer should recommend that this soccer player engage in a minimum of 30 minutes of continuous training as well as some higher-intensity interval training to maintain both aerobic and anaerobic fitness.

4–4 Weight training will not have a negative effect on flexibility as long as the lifting is done properly. Lifting the weight through a full range of motion will improve strength and simultaneously maintain range of motion. A female swimmer is not likely to bulk up to the point that muscle size affects range of motion. It is also important to recommend that this athlete continue to incorporate active stretching into her training regimen.

4–5 The athletic trainer can discuss the rationale for strength and conditioning with the athlete. Helping the athlete understand why it is important to increase strength and endurance can increase her motivation. In addition to improving performance and efficiency, muscular endurance and strength are also critical in preventing athletic injuries. The athletic trainer should work with the coaches to provide a periodization program that will keep the athlete's interest and prevent atrophy from occurring.

4–6 The shot put, like many other dynamic movements in sports, requires not only great strength but also the ability to generate that strength rapidly. To develop muscular power, this athlete must engage in dynamic, explosive training techniques that will help him develop his ability.

Power lifting techniques should be helpful. Plyometric exercises using weights for added resistance will help him improve his speed of muscular contraction against some resistive force.

4–7 The athletic trainer should recommend that the construction worker engage in a regular, consistent flexibility program using either static or PNF stretching techniques. Stretching should be done several times a day if possible. The worker should also be instructed to engage in full range of motion strength training for the hamstrings. The athletic trainer should also explain that when the construction worker feels tightness or discomfort during a training session, he should stop the activity immediately to avoid making a hamstring strain more severe.

4–8 During the early part of the preparatory period, training should be at a low intensity with a high volume of repetitions, using activities that may or may not be directly related to football. This phase may last from several weeks to 2 months. The intensity and volume of these activities should progress to moderate levels. Weight-training activities should eventually become more specific to football. Just before the preseason, the athlete should train at a high intensity, and the volume of training should decrease to allow full recovery between sessions.

REVIEW QUESTIONS AND CLASS ACTIVITIES

1. In terms of injury prevention, list as many advantages as you can for conditioning.
2. How does the SAID principle relate to sports conditioning and injury prevention?
3. What is the value of proper warm-up and cool-down to sports injury prevention?
4. Critically observe how a variety of sports use warm-up and cool-down procedures.
5. Discuss the relationships among maximal oxygen consumption, heart rate, stroke volume, and cardiac output.
6. Differentiate between aerobic and anaerobic training methods.
7. How is continuous training different from interval training?
8. How may increasing strength decrease susceptibility to injury?
9. Compare different techniques of increasing strength. How may each technique be an advantage or a disadvantage to the athlete in terms of injury prevention?
10. Compare ways to increase flexibility and how they may decrease or increase the athlete's susceptibility to injury.
11. Why is year-round conditioning so important for injury prevention?

REFERENCES

1. Akima H, Takahashi H, Kuno SY: Early phase adaptations of muscle use and strength to isokinetic training, *Med Sci Sports Exerc* 31(4):588, 1999.
2. Allerheiligen W: Speed development and plyometric training. In Baechle T, editor: *Essentials of strength training and conditioning,* Champaign, IL, 2008, Human Kinetics.
3. Allerheiligen W: Stretching and warm-up. In Baechle T, editor: *Essentials of strength training and conditioning,* Champaign, IL, 2008, Human Kinetics.
4. Alter M: *The science of flexibility,* Champaign, IL, 2004, Human Kinetics.
5. American College of Sports Medicine: *Guidelines for exercise testing and prescription,* Philadelphia, 2009, Lippincott, Williams and Wilkens.
6. Andersen JC: Flexibility in performance: Foundational concepts and practical issues, *Athletic Therapy Today* 11(3):9, 2006.
7. Andersen JC: Stretching before and after exercise: Effect on muscle soreness and injury risk, *J Athl Train* 40(3):218, 2005.
8. Armiger P: Preventing musculotendinous injuries: A focus on flexibility, *Athletic Therapy Today* 5(4):20, 2000.
9. Baker D, Wilson G, Carlyon B: Generality vs. specificity: A comparison of dynamic and isometric measures of strength and speed-strength, *Eur J Appl Physiol* 68:350, 1994.
10. Bandy WD, Irion JM, Briggler M: The effect of static stretch and dynamic range of motion training on the flexibility of the hamstring muscles, *J Orthop Sports Phys Ther* 27(4):295, 1998.
11. Bassett DR, Howley ET: Limiting factors for maximum oxygen uptake and determinants of endurance performance, *Med Sci Sports Exerc* 32(1):70, 2000.
12. Behm DG, Bambury A, Cahill F, Power K: Effect of acute static stretching on force, balance, reaction time, and movement time, *Med Sci Sports Exerc* 36(8):1397, 2004.
13. Berger R: *Conditioning for men,* Boston, 1973, Allyn & Bacon.
14. Bergh U, Ekblom B, Astrand PO: Maximal oxygen uptake "classical" versus "contemporary" viewpoints, *Med Sci Sports Exerc* 32(1):85, 2000.
15. Billat LV: Interval training for performance: A scientific and empirical practice. Special Recommendations for middle- and long distance running. Part I: Aerobic interval training. *Sports Med* 31(1):13, 2001.
16. Blanke D: Flexibility. In Mellion M, editor: *Sports medicine secrets,* Philadelphia, 2002, Hanley & Belfus.
17. Bompa TO: *Periodization: Theory and methodization of training,* Champaign, IL, 2010, Human Kinetics.
18. Boyle M: *Functional training for sports,* Champaign, IL, 2004, Human Kinetics.
19. Boyle P: The effect of static and dynamic stretching on muscle force production. *Journal of Sports Sciences* 22(3):273, 2004.
20. Brooks G, Fahey T, White T: *Exercise physiology: Human bioenergetics and its applications,* San Francisco, 2004, McGraw-Hill.
21. Brumitt J: *Core assessment and training* Champaign, IL, 2010, Human Kinetics.
22. Burke DG, Culligan CJ, Holt LE: The theoretical basis of proprioceptive neuromuscular facilitation, *Strength Cond* 14(4):496, 2000.
23. Chalmers G: Re-examination of the possible role of Golgi tendon organ and muscle spindle reflexes in proprioceptive neuromuscular facilitation muscle stretching, *Sports Biomechanics* 3(1):159, 2004.
24. Chimera N, Swanik K, Swanik C: Effects of plyometric training on muscle activation strategies and performance in female athletes, *J Athl Train* 39(1):24, 2004.
25. Chu DA: Plyometics in sports injury rehabilitation and training, *Athletic Therapy Today* 4(3):7, 1999.
26. Clark M: *Integrated training for the new millennium,* Calabasas, CA, 2001, National Academy of Sports Medicine.
27. Colston M: Core Stability, Part 1: Overview and the concept, *Athletic Therapy and Training,* 17(1):8–13, 2012.
28. Conroy M: The use of periodization in the high school setting, *Strength Cond* 21(1):52, 1999.
29. Cornwell AN: The acute effects of passive stretching on active musculotendinous stiffness. *Med Sci Sports Exer* 29(5):281, 1997.
30. Cross KM, Worrell TW: Effects of a static stretching program on the incidence of lower extremity musculotendinous strains, *J Athl Train* 34(1):11, 1999.
31. Curtis N: Stretching and functional flexibility, *Athletic Therapy Today* 11(3):30, 2006.
32. Dale B, Lawrence R: Principles of core stabilization for athletic populations, *Athletic Therapy Today* 10(4):13, 2005.

33. Decoster L, Cleland J, Altieri C: The effects of hamstring stretching on range of motion: A systematic literature review, *J Orthop Sports Phys Ther* 3(6):377, 2005.

34. DeLorme TL, Watkins AL: *Progressive resistance exercise*, New York, 1951, Appleton-Century-Crofts.

35. DePino GM, Webright WG, Arnold BL: Duration of maintained hamstring flexibility after cessation of an acute static stretching protocol, *J Athl Train* 35(1):56, 2000.

36. Fleck S, Kraemer W: *Designing resistance training programs*, Champaign, IL, 2003, Human Kinetics.

37. Fowles JR, Sale DG, MacDougall JD: Reduced strength after passive stretch of the human plantarflexors, *J App Physiol* 89(3):1179, 2000.

38. Gardner PJ: Youth strength training. *Athletic Therapy Today* 8(1):42, 2003.

39. Goldberg L: *Strength ball training*, Champaign, IL, 2006, Human Kinetics.

40. Gravelle BL, Blessing DL: Physiological adaptation in women concurrently training for strength and endurance, *J Strength Cond Res* 14(1):5, 2000.

41. Gribble P, Prentice W: Effects of static and hold-relax stretching on hamstring range of motion using the FlexAbility LE1000, *J Sport Rehabil* 8(3):195, 1999.

42. Harman E: The biomechanics of resistance exercise. In Baechle T, editor: *Essentials of strength training and conditioning*, Champaign, IL, 2008, Human Kinetics.

43. Hilbert S, Plisk SS: Free weights versus machines, *Strength Cond* 21(6):66, 1999.

44. Holcomb WR: Improved stretching with proprioceptive neuromuscular facilitation, *Strength Cond* 22(1):59, 2000.

45. Holt LE, Pelham TW, Burke DG: Modifications to the standard sit-and-reach flexibility protocol, *J Athl Train* 34(1):43, 1999.

46. Kaminski TW, Wabbersen CV, Murphy RM: Concentric versus enhanced eccentric hamstring strength training: Clinical implications, *J Athl Train* 33(3):216, 1998.

47. Karvonen MJ, Kentala E, Mustala O: The effects of training on heart rate: A longitudinal study, *Ann Med Exp Biol* 35:305, 1957.

48. Klinger T, McConnell T, Gardner J: Prescribing target heart rates without the use of a graded exercise test, *Clinical Exercise Physiology* 3(4):207, 2001.

49. Knight K, Ingersoll C, Bartholomew J: Isotonic contractions might not be more effective than isokinetic contractions in developing muscle strength, *J Sport Rehabil* 10(2):124, 2001.

50. Kokkonen J, Arnall DA: Acute stretching inhibits strength endurance, *Med Sci Sports Exerc* 35(5):11, 2001.

51. Kokkonen J, Caroline S, Nelson AG: Chronic stretching improves sport specific skills, *Med Sci Sports Exerc* 29(5):67, 1997.

52. Kovacs M: The argument against static stretching before sport and physical activity, *Athletic Therapy Today* 11(3):6, 2006.

53. Kraemer W: General adaptation to resistance and endurance training programs. In Baechle T, editor: *Essentials of strength training and conditioning*, Champaign, IL, 2008, Human Kinetics.

54. Kraemer W, Fleck S: *Strength training for young athletes*, Champaign, IL, 2004, Human Kinetics.

55. Kraemer W, Hakkinen K, Kraemer W: *Strength training for sport*, Cambridge, MA, 2002, Blackwell Science.

56. Kubo K, Kanehisa H, Fukunaga T: Effect of stretching training on the viscoelastic properties of human tendon structures in vivo, *J App Physiol* 92(2):595, 2002.

57. Kubukeli ZN, Noakes TD, Dennis SC: Training techniques to improve endurance exercise performances, *Sports Med* 32(8):489, 2002.

58. Laursen PB, Jenkins DG: The scientific basis for high-intensity interval training: Optimizing training programmes and maximizing performance in highly trained endurance athletes, *Sports Med* 32(1):53, 2002.

59. Leetun D, Ireland M, Wilson J: Core stability measures as risk factors for lower extremity injury in athletes, *Med Sci Sports Exerc* 36(6):926, 2005.

60. Lepretre P, Koralsztein J, Billat V: Effect of exercise intensity on relationship between $\dot{V}O_2max$ and cardiac output, *Med Sci Sports Exerc* 36(8):1357, 2004.

61. Logan GA, Wallis EL: Recent findings in learning and performance. Paper presented at the Southern Section Meeting, California Association for Health, Physical Education, and Recreation, Pasadena, 1960.

62. MacDougall D, Sale D: Continuous vs. interval training: A review for the athlete and coach, *Can J Appl Sport Sci* 6:93, 1981.

63. Mann D, Whedon C: Functional stretching: Implementing a dynamic stretching program, *Athletic Therapy Today* 6(3):10, 2001.

64. Marek S, Cramer J, Fincher L: Acute effects of static and proprioceptive neuromuscular facilitation stretching on muscle strength and power output, *J Athl Train* 40(2):94, 2005.

65. Marshall P, Murphy B: Core stability exercises on and off a Swiss ball, *Arch Phys Med Rehabil* 86(2):242, 2005.

66. McArdle W, Katch F, Katch V: *Exercise physiology, energy, nutrition, and human performance*, Philadelphia, 2006, Lippincott, Williams and Wilkins.

67. Merce J, Dufek J, Bates B: Analysis of peak oxygen consumption and heart rate during elliptical and treadmill exercise, *J Sport Rehabil* 10(1):48, 2001.

68. Middlesworth M: More than ergonomics: Warm-up and stretching key to injury prevention, *Athletic Therapy Today* 7(2):32, 2002.

69. Moreno A: The practicalities of adolescent resistance training, *Athletic Therapy Today* 8(3):26, 2003.

70. Moss RI: Physics, plyometrics, and injury prevention, *Athletic Therapy Today* 7(2):44, 2002.

71. Nelson, R: An update on flexibility. *Natl Strength Cond Assoc J* 27(1):10, 2005.

72. Owsley A: An introduction to clinical Pilates. *Athletic Therapy Today* 10(4):19, 2005.

73. Parr J, Yarrow J: Symptomatic and functional responses to concentric-eccentric isokinetic versus eccentric-only isotonic exercise, *J Athl Train*, 44(5): 462–68, 2009.

74. Prentice W: *Get fit stay fit*, ed 6, New York, 2011, McGraw-Hill.

75. Prentice W: Proprioceptive neuromuscular facilitation techniques. In Prentice W, editor: *Rehabilitation techniques in sports medicine and athletic training*, St. Louis, 2011, McGraw-Hill.

76. Radcliffe JC, Farentinos RC: *High-powered plyometrics*, Champaign, IL, 2005, Human Kinetics.

77. Rubley M, Brucker J, Knight K: Flexibility retention 3 weeks after a 5-day training regime, *J Sport Rehabil* 10(2):105, 2001.

78. Ryba T, Kaltenborn J: The benefits of yoga for athletes: The body, *Athletic Therapy Today* 11(2):32, 2006.

79. Schilling BK, Stone MH: Stretching: Acute effects on strength and power performance, *Strength Cond* 22(1):44, 2000.

80. Sexton P, Chambers J: The importance of flexibility for functional range of motion, *Athletic Therapy Today* 11(3):13, 2006.

81. Siatras T, Papadopoulos G, Maeletzi D, Gerodimos V, Kellis P: Static and dynamic acute stretching effect on gymnasts' speed in vaulting, *Ped Ex Sci* 15:383, 2004.

82. Small K: A systematic review into the efficacy of static stretching as part of a warm-up for the prevention of exercise-related injury. *Research in Sports Medicine* 16(3):213–31, 2008.

83. Soames R: *Joint motion: Clinical measurement and evaluation*, Philadelphia, 2002, Elsevier.

84. Swain D, Parrott J, Bennett A: Validation of a new method for estimating $\dot{V}O_2max$ based on $\dot{V}O_2$ reserve, *Med Sci Sports Exerc* 36(8):1421, 2004.

85. Swanson J: Periodization for the multisport athlete, *Strength Cond* 26(4):50, 2004.

86. Taylor DC, Brooks DE, Ryan JB: Viscoelastic characteristics of muscle: Passive stretching versus muscular contractions, *Med Sci Sports Exerc* 29(12):1619, 1997.

87. Thacker S, Gilchrist J, Stroup D: The impact of stretching on sports injury risk: A systematic review of the literature, *Med Sci Sports Exerc* 36(3):371, 2004.

88. Thomas M: The functional warm-up, *Strength Cond* 22(2):51, 2000.

89. Van Hatten B: Passive versus active stretching, *Phys Ther* 85(1):80, 2005.

90. Walker M, Sussman D, Tamburello M: Relationship between maximum strength and relative endurance for the empty-can exercise, *J Sport Rehabil* 12(1):31, 2003.

91. Wathen D: Periodization: Concepts and applications. In Baechle T, editor: *Essentials of strength training and conditioning*, Champaign, IL, 2008, Human Kinetics.

92. Wilkerson G, Colson M, Short N: Neuromuscular changes in female collegiate athletes resulting from a plyometric jump-training program, *J Athl Train* 39(1):17, 2004.

93. Winters MV, Blake CG, Trost JS: Passive versus active stretching of hip flexor muscles in subjects with limited hip extension: A randomized clinical trial, *Phys Ther* 84(9): 800, 2004.

94. Woods C: *A warm-up exercise regimen reduces risk of girls' soccer injuries*, American Academy of Pediatrics Grand Rounds, Elk Grove Willage, IL, 2009, AAP.

95. Zech A, et al.: Balance training for neuromuscular control and performance enhancement: A systematic review, *J Athl Train* 45(4): 392–403, 2010.

96. Zentz C: Warm up to perform up, *Athletic Therapy Today* 5(2):59, 2000.

ANNOTATED BIBLIOGRAPHY

Adler S, Beckers D, Buck M: *PNF in practice: an illustrated guide*, New York, 2008, Springer.

A heavily illustrated text that covers all aspects of PNF.

Alter M: *The science of flexibility*, Champaign, IL, 2004, Human Kinetics.

Explains the principles and techniques of stretching and details the anatomy and physiology of muscle and connective tissue. Includes guidelines for developing a flexibility program, illustrated stretching exercises, and warm-up drills.

Anderson B: *Stretching*, Bolinas, CA, 2010, Shelter.

An extremely comprehensive best-selling text on stretching exercises for the entire body.

Baechle T, editor: *Essentials of strength training and conditioning*, Champaign, IL, 2008, Human Kinetics.

A book from the National Strength Coaches Association that explains the science, theory, and practical application of various aspects of conditioning in a very concise, easily understood text.

Brooks G, Fahey T, White T: *Exercise physiology: human bioenergetics and its applications*, San Francisco, 2004, McGraw-Hill.

An advanced text in exercise physiology that contains a comprehensive listing of the journal articles relative to exercise physiology.

Chu D: *Jumping into plyometrics*, Champaign, IL, 1998, Human Kinetics.

Well-illustrated text that helps the athlete develop a safe plyometric training program with exercises designed to improve speed, upper-body strength, jumping ability, balance, and coordination.

Fleck S, Kraemer W: *Designing resistance training programs*, Champaign, IL, 2003, Human Kinetics.

A clear, readable, state-of-the-art guide to developing individualized training programs for both athletes and fitness enthusiasts.

Moran G, McGlynn G: *Dynamics of strength training*, St. Louis, 2000, McGraw-Hill.

A comprehensive resource using an individualized approach to strength training, including conditioning and cardiorespiratory fitness. Emphasizes the physiological basis of muscular strength and endurance. Illustrates the most efficient and effective training techniques.

Prentice W: *Fitness and wellness for life*, ed 7, Dubuque, IA, 1999, WCB/McGraw-Hill.

A comprehensive fitness text that covers all aspects of a training and conditioning program.

Verstegen M, Williams P: *Core performance: the revolutionary workout program to transform your body and your life*, Mountain View, CA, 2005, Rodale Press.

Concentrates primarily on core stabilization exercises to improve posture and improve performance in athletes.

Wiksten D, Peters C: *The athletic trainer's guide to strength and endurance training*, Thorofare, NJ, 2000, Slack.

Layout offers ease of reference, sport-specific programs, information on nutritional supplements, and illustrations on weight training and supplemental routines.

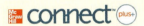

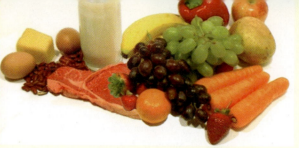

5

Nutrition and Supplements

■ Objectives

When you finish this chapter you should be able to

- Distinguish the six classes of nutrients and describe their major functions.
- Explain the importance of good nutrition in enhancing performance and preventing injuries.
- Assess the advantages and disadvantages of dietary supplements.
- Discuss popular eating and drinking practices.
- Discuss the advantages and disadvantages of consuming a pre-event meal.

- Differentiate between body weight and body composition.
- Explain the principle of caloric balance and how to assess it.
- Assess body composition using skinfold calipers.
- Evaluate methods for losing and gaining weight.
- Recognize the signs of bulimia nervosa and anorexia nervosa.

■ Outline

■ Key Terms

amino acids
osteoporosis
lactase deficiency
anemia
glycemic index (GI)

glycogen
supercompensation
obesity
adipose cell
body composition

■ Connect Highlights ＭｃＧｒａｗＨｉｌｌ connect plus+

Visit connect.mcgraw-hill.com for further exercises to apply your knowledge:

- Clinical application scenarios covering methods of losing and gaining weight, nutrition to enhance performance and prevent injury, dietary supplements, and caloric balance and how to assess it
- Click-and-drag questions covering vitamins, minerals, prevent meals, and body composition
- Multiple-choice questions covering nutrients, proper nutrition to enhance performance, dietary supplements, hydration, and eating disorders
- Selection questions covering nutrients and their major functions

The relation of nutrition, diet, and weight control to overall health and fitness should be an issue of critical importance to everyone. Individuals who practice sound nutritional habits reduce the likelihood of injury and illness by maintaining a higher standard of healthful living.[55] We know that eating a well-balanced diet can positively contribute to the development of strength, flexibility, and cardiorespiratory endurance.[33,71] Unfortunately, misconceptions, fads, and, in many cases, superstitions regarding nutrition have a significant impact on dietary habits.[41]

Many athletes associate successful performance with the consumption of special foods or supplements.[34] An athlete who is performing well may be reluctant to change dietary habits regardless of whether the diet is physiologically beneficial to overall health.[75] There is no question that the psychological aspect of allowing the athlete to eat whatever he or she is most comfortable with can greatly affect performance. The problem is that these eating habits tend to become accepted as beneficial and may become traditional when, in fact, they may be physiologically detrimental to athletic performance. Thus, many nutrition "experts" tend to disseminate nutritional information based on traditional rather than experimental information.[21] The athletic trainer must possess a strong knowledge of nutrition so that he or she may serve as an informational resource for the athlete.[39,57]

An athletic trainer working in the clinical, corporate, or industrial setting may be responsible for overseeing employee fitness or wellness programs. Providing direct nutritional counseling, organizing health fairs or workshops that focus on various aspects of nutrition, and serving as a resource in disseminating information related to diet and nutrition may all be part of the responsibilities of that position.

NUTRITION BASICS

Nutrition is the science of the substances in food that are essential to life. Nutrients have three major functions: the growth, repair, and maintenance of all tissues; the regulation of body processes; and the production of energy.[12]

The nutrients are categorized into six major classes: *carbohydrates, fats* (often called *lipids*), *proteins, water, vitamins,* and *minerals.* Carbohydrates, proteins, and fats are referred to as the *macronutrients:* the absorbable components of food, from which energy is derived. Vitamins, minerals, and water are considered to be *micronutrients,* which are necessary for regulating normal body functions. They do not provide energy, but without sufficient quantities of micronutrients, the energy from macronutrients cannot be utilized. For example, certain vitamins are necessary for other vitamins to be absorbed. Most foods are actually mixtures of these nutrients. Some nutrients can be made by the body, but an *essential nutrient* must be supplied by the diet.[75] Not all substances in food are considered nutrients. There is no such thing as the perfect food; that is, no single natural food contains all the nutrients needed for health. A summary of current percentages and recommended percentages of calories from protein, carbohydrate, and fat is shown in Figure 5–1.

> The six classes of nutrients are carbohydrates, fats, proteins, water, vitamins, and minerals.

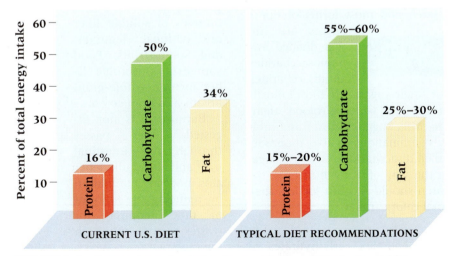

FIGURE 5–1 Comparison of calories from protein, carbohydrate, and fat.

It is recommended that the majority, about 55 to 60 percent, of the calories consumed be in the form of carbohydrates. Fat should account for between 25 to 30 percent of the total caloric intake. Only 15 to 20 percent of the caloric intake should be protein. For an athlete who requires additional energy during the course of a day, the extra calories consumed should be in the form of carbohydrates.

> **Dietary recommendations:**
> • Carbohydrate: 55%–60%
> • Fat: 25%–30%
> • Protein: 15%–20%

Nutrient-dense foods are those that supply adequate amounts of vitamins and minerals in relation to their caloric value. The so-called junk foods provide excessive amounts of calories from fat and sugar in relation to vitamins and minerals and therefore are not nutrient dense. However, many people live on junk foods that displace more nutrient-dense foods from their diet.[58] This behavior is not healthful in the long run.[74]

> **Nutrient-dense foods supply adequate amounts of vitamins and minerals in relation to caloric value.**

ENERGY SOURCES

Carbohydrates

Anyone who is physically active has increased energy needs. Carbohydrates are the body's most efficient source of energy and should be relied on to fill those needs.[43] Carbohydrate intake should account for 55 to 60 percent of total caloric intake. The following sections describe different forms of carbohydrates and their role in the production of energy and the maintenance of health.[12] It is important to understand that not all carbohydrates are digested and absorbed at the same rate.

Sugars Carbohydrates are classified as simple (sugars) or complex (starch and most forms of fiber). Sugars are further divided into monosaccharides and disaccharides.

> **Carbohydrates are sugars, starches, and fiber.**

Monosaccharides, or single sugars, are found mostly in fruits, syrups, and honey. Glucose (blood sugar) is a monosaccharide. Milk sugar (lactose) and table sugar (sucrose) are combinations of two monosaccharides and are called disaccharides. Because sugar contributes little in the way of other nutrients, the amount of sugar eaten should account for less than 15 percent of the total caloric intake.

Starches Starches are complex carbohydrates. A starch is made up of long chains of glucose units.

During the digestion process, the starch chain is broken down and the glucose units are free to be absorbed. Food sources of starch, such as rice, potatoes, and breads, often provide vitamins and minerals in addition to serving as the body's principal source of glucose. Many people believe that starchy foods contribute to obesity. However, most of these foods are eaten with fats from butter, margarine, sauces, and gravies that make the food more enjoyable but contribute an excess of calories.

The body cannot use starches and many sugars directly from food for energy. It must obtain the simple sugar glucose (blood sugar). During digestion and metabolism, starches and disaccharide sugars are broken down and converted to glucose. The glucose that is not needed for immediate energy is stored as glycogen in the liver and muscle cells. Glucose can be released from glycogen later if needed. The body, however, can store only a limited amount of glucose as glycogen. Any extra glucose is converted to body fat. When the body experiences an inadequate intake of dietary carbohydrate, it uses protein to make glucose, but the protein is then diverted from its own important functions. Therefore, a supply of glucose must be kept available to prevent the use of protein for energy. This is called the protein-sparing action of glucose.

> **Glycolysis is the process that breaks down glucose to produce energy.**

Fiber Fiber forms the structural parts of plants and is not digested by humans. Fiber is not found in animal sources of food. There are two kinds of dietary fiber: soluble and insoluble. Soluble fiber includes gums and pectins; cellulose is the primary insoluble form. Sources of soluble fiber are oatmeal, legumes, and some fruits. Food sources of insoluble fiber include whole-grain breads and bran cereals.

Because it is not digested, fiber passes through the intestinal tract and adds bulk. Fiber aids normal elimination by reducing the amount of time required for wastes to move through the digestive tract, which is believed to reduce the risk of colon cancer. Also, increased fiber intake is thought to reduce the risk of coronary artery disease. Soluble forms of fiber bind to cholesterol passing through the digestive tract and prevent its absorption, which can reduce blood cholesterol levels. Foods rich in saturated fats (meats, in particular) often take the place of fiber-rich foods in the diet, thus increasing cholesterol absorption and formation. Consumption of adequate amounts of fiber has been associated with lowered incidences of obesity, constipation, colitis, appendicitis, and diabetes.

The recommended amount of fiber in the diet is approximately 25 grams per day.[67] Unfortunately, the average person consumes only 10 to 15 grams per day. Fiber intake should be increased by increasing the amount of whole-grain cereal products and fruits and vegetables in the diet rather than by using fiber supplements. However, excessive consumption of fiber may cause intestinal discomfort as well as increased losses of calcium and iron.

Fats

Fats are an essential component of the diet. They are the most concentrated source of energy, providing more than twice the calories per gram when compared with carbohydrates or proteins. Fat is used as a primary source of energy. Some dietary fat is needed to make food more flavorful and for sources of the fat-soluble vitamins. Also, a minimal amount of fat is essential for normal growth and development.

Unfortunately, in the typical American diet, fat represents approximately 40 to 50 percent of the total caloric intake. This intake is believed to be too high and may contribute to the prevalence of obesity, certain cancers, and coronary artery disease. Intake should be limited to less than 30 percent of total calories.[73]

Saturated versus Unsaturated Fat Both plant and animal foods provide sources of dietary fat. About 95 percent of the fat consumed is in the form of triglycerides. De-

> **Fats may be saturated or unsaturated.**

pending on their chemical nature, fatty acids may be saturated or unsaturated. The unsaturated fatty acids can be subdivided into monounsaturates and polyunsaturates. Therefore, the terms *saturated, monounsaturated,* and *polyunsaturated* are used to describe the chemical nature of the fat in foods. The triglycerides that make up food fats are usually mixtures of saturated and unsaturated fatty acids but are classified according to the type that predominates. In general, fats containing more unsaturated fatty acids are from plants and are liquid at room temperature. Saturated fatty acids are derived mainly from animal sources.

Trans fatty acids (trans fat) have physical properties generally resembling saturated fatty acids, and their presence tends to harden oils. Found in many cookies crackers, dairy products, meats, potato chips, most junk foods, and fast foods, trans fatty acids increase the risk of heart disease by boosting levels of bad cholesterol. Because they are not essential and provide no known health benefit, there is no safe level of trans fatty acids in the blood, and people should eat as little of them as possible while consuming a nutritionally adequate diet.

Other Fats Phospholipids and sterols represent the remaining 5 percent of fats. One example of phospholipids is lecithin; cholesterol is the best known sterol. Cholesterol is consumed in animal foods; it is not supplied by plant sources of food. Generally, it is wise to avoid eating foods high in cholesterol. Although cholesterol is essential to many bodily functions, the body can manufacture cholesterol from carbohydrates, proteins, and especially saturated fat. Thus, there is little, if any, need to consume additional amounts of cholesterol in the diet. The American Heart Association recommends consuming less than 300 mg per day.

One type of unsaturated fatty acid seems to serve as a protective mechanism against certain disease processes. The omega-3 fatty acids apparently have the capability of reducing the likelihood of heart disease, stroke, and hypertension. These fatty acids are found in cold-water fish.

Fat Substitutes Fat-free products containing artificial fat substitutes, such as Simplese and Olean, are now available to the consumer. These products contain no cholesterol and 80 percent fewer calories than similar products made with fat. Despite Food and Drug Administration (FDA) approval of these fat substitutes, some individuals have reported abdominal cramping and diarrhea when using them.[8]

Proteins

Proteins make up the major structural components of the body. They are needed for the growth, maintenance, and repair of all body tissues. In addition, proteins are needed to make enzymes, many hormones, and antibodies that help fight infection. In general, the body prefers not to use much protein for energy; instead, it relies on fats and carbohydrates. Protein intake should be around 15 to 20 percent of total calories.

Amino Acids The basic units that make up proteins are smaller compounds called **amino acids.** Most of the body's proteins are made up of about 20 amino acids. Amino acids can be linked together in a wide variety of

> **amino acids** Basic units that make up proteins.

combinations, which is why there are so many different forms and uses of proteins. Most of the amino acids can be produced as needed in the body. The others cannot be made to any significant degree and therefore must be supplied by the diet. The amino acids obtained through food are referred to as the *essential amino acids*. The amount of protein and the levels of the individual essential amino acids are important for determining the quality of diet. A diet that contains large amounts of protein will not support growth, repair, and maintenance of tissues if the essential amino acids are not available in the proper proportions.[34]

Most of the proteins from animal foods contain all the essential amino acids that humans require and are called complete, or high-quality, proteins. Incomplete proteins—that is, proteins that do not contain all the essential amino acids—usually are from plant sources of food. Beans and legumes are a potential source of protein and iron for vegetarians.

> **Proteins are made up of amino acids.**

Protein Sources and Need Most people do not have difficulty meeting their protein needs because the typical diet is rich in protein. Many athletes consume more than twice the recommended amounts of protein. There is no advantage to consuming more protein, particularly in the form of protein supplements. If more protein is supplied than needed, the body must convert the excess to fat for storage. This conversion can create a situation in which excess water is removed from cells, leading to dehydration and possible damage to the kidneys or liver. Protein supplements may also create imbalances of the chemicals that make up proteins, the amino acids, which is not desirable. A condition of the bones, osteoporosis, has been linked to a diet that contains too much protein.[4]

Increased physical activity increases a person's need for energy, not necessarily for protein.[34] The increases in muscle mass that result from conditioning and training are associated with only a small increase in protein requirements, which can easily be met with the usual diet. Therefore, an athlete does not need protein supplements.

REGULATOR NUTRIENTS

Vitamins

Although vitamins are required in extremely small amounts when compared with water, proteins, carbohydrates, and fats, they perform essential functions, primarily as regulators of body processes.[4] Thirteen vitamins have specific roles in the body, many of which are still being explored. In the past, letters were assigned as names for vitamins. Today, most are known by their scientific names. Vitamins are classified into two groups: fat-soluble vitamins, which are dissolved in fats and stored in the body, and water-soluble vitamins, which are dissolved in watery solutions and are not stored. Table 5–1 lists the vitamins and indicates their primary functions.

Fat-Soluble Vitamins Vitamins A, D, E, and K are fat soluble. They are found in the fatty portions of foods and in oils. Because they are stored in the body's fat, it is possible to consume excess amounts and show the effects of vitamin poisoning.

> **Fat-soluble vitamins: A, D, E, and K.**

Water-Soluble Vitamins The water-soluble vitamins are vitamin C, known as ascorbic acid, and the B-complex vitamins thiamin, riboflavin, niacin, B_6, folate, B_{12}, biotin, and pantothenic acid. Although vitamins are not metabolized for energy, thiamin, riboflavin, niacin, biotin, and pantothenic acid are used to regulate the metabolism of carbohydrates, proteins, and fats to obtain energy. Vitamin B_6 regulates the body's use of amino acids. Folate and vitamin B_{12} are important in normal blood formation. Vitamin C is used for building bones and teeth, maintaining connective tissues, and strengthening the immune system. Unlike fat-soluble vitamins, water-soluble vitamins cannot be stored to any significant extent in the body and should be supplied in the diet each day.[4]

> **Water-soluble vitamins: C, thiamin, riboflavin, niacin, B_6, B_{12}, folate, biotin, and pantothenic acid.**

Antioxidants Certain nutrients, called antioxidants, may prevent premature aging, certain cancers, heart disease, and other health problems.[50] An antioxidant protects vital cell components from the destructive

> **Antioxidants: vitamin C, vitamin E, and beta-carotene.**

TABLE 5–1	Vitamins			
Vitamin	Major Function	Most Reliable Sources	Deficiency	Excess (toxicity)
A	Maintains skin and other cells that line the inside of the body, bone and tooth development, growth, vision in dim light	Liver, milk, egg yolk, deep green and yellow fruits and vegetables	Night blindness, dry skin, growth failure	Headaches, nausea, loss of hair, dry skin, diarrhea
D	Normal bone growth and development	Exposure to sunlight, fortified dairy products, eggs and fish liver oils	Rickets in children— defective bone formation leading to deformed bones	Appetite loss, weight loss, failure to grow
E	Prevents destruction of polyunsaturated fats caused by exposure to oxidizing agents, protects cell membranes from destruction	Vegetable oils, some in fruits and vegetables, whole grains	Breakage of red blood cells leading to anemia	Nausea and diarrhea, interferes with vitamin K absorption if vitamin D is also deficient, not as toxic as other fat-soluble vitamins
K	Production of blood-clotting substances	Green, leafy vegetables; normal bacteria that live in intestines	Increased bleeding time	
Thiamin	Needed for release of energy from carbohydrates, fats, and proteins	Cereal products, pork, peas, dried beans	Lack of energy, nerve problems	
Riboflavin	Energy from carbohydrates, fats, and proteins	Milk, liver, fruits and vegetables, enriched breads and cereals	Dry skin, cracked lips	
Niacin	Energy from carbohydrates, fats, and proteins	Liver, meat, poultry, peanut butter, legumes, enriched breads and cereals	Skin problems, diarrhea, mental depression, eventually death (rarely occurs in U.S.)	Skin flushing, intestinal upset, nervousness, intestinal ulcers
B_6	Metabolism of protein, production of hemoglobin	White meats, whole grains, liver, egg yolk, bananas	Poor growth, anemia	Severe loss of coordination from nerve damage
B_{12}	Production of genetic material, maintains central nervous system	Foods of animal origin	Neurological problems, anemia	
Folate (folic acid)	Production of genetic material	Wheat germ; liver; yeast; mushrooms; green, leafy vegetables; fruits	Anemia	
C (ascorbic acid)	Formation and maintenance of connective tissue, tooth and bone formation, immune function	Fruits and vegetables	Scurvy (rare), swollen joints, bleeding gums, fatigue, bruising	Kidney stones, diarrhea
Pantothenic acid	Energy from carbohydrates, fats, proteins	Widely found in foods	Not observed in humans under normal conditions	
Biotin	Use of fats	Widely found in foods	Rare under normal conditions	

effects of certain agents, including oxygen. Vitamin C, vitamin E, and beta-carotene are antioxidants. Beta-carotene is a plant pigment found in dark green, deep yellow, and orange fruits and vegetables. The body can convert beta-carotene to vitamin A. In the early 1980s, researchers reported that smokers who ate large quantities of fruits and vegetables rich in beta-carotene were less likely to develop lung cancer than were other smokers.[61] Since that time, more evidence has accumulated about the benefits of a diet rich in the antioxidant nutrients.[61]

Some experts believe that it is important to increase intake of antioxidants, even if it means taking supplements. Others are more cautious.[61] Excess beta-carotene pigments circulate throughout the body and may turn the skin yellow. However, the pigment is not believed to be toxic, like its nutrient cousin, vitamin A. On the other hand, increasing intake of vitamins C and E is not without some risk. Excess vitamin C is not well absorbed. The excess is irritating to the intestines and creates diarrhea. Although less toxic than vitamins A and D, too much vitamin E causes health problems.

Vitamin Deficiencies The illness that results from a lack of any nutrient, especially those nutrients, such as vitamins, that are needed only in small amounts, is referred to as a deficiency disease.[46] Vitamin deficiency diseases are rare. Adequate amounts of the vitamins, as with other nutrients, can be obtained if a wide variety of foods are eaten. Vitamin supplements can cause toxic effects if large enough quantities are taken. Table 5–1 describes some of vitamins' toxicity problems.

Minerals

More than 20 mineral elements have a role in body function and therefore must be supplied in the diet. The most essential minerals are listed in Table 5–2. Most minerals are stored in the body, especially in the liver and bones. Magnesium is needed in energy-supplying reactions; sodium and potassium are important for the transmission of nerve impulses. Iron plays a role in energy metabolism but is also combined with a protein to form hemoglobin, the compound that transports oxygen in red

TABLE 5–2	Minerals			
Mineral	**Major Role**	**Most Reliable Sources**	**Deficiency**	**Excess**
Calcium	Bone and tooth formation, blood clotting, muscle contraction, nerve function	Dairy products, calcium-enriched orange juice and bread	May lead to osteoporosis	Calcium deposits in soft tissues
Phosphorus	Skeletal development, tooth formation	Meats, dairy products, other protein-rich foods	Rarely seen	
Sodium	Maintenance of fluid balance	Salt (sodium chloride) added to foods and sodium-containing preservatives		May contribute to the development of hypertension
Iron	Formation of hemoglobin; energy from carbohydrates, fats, and proteins	Liver and red meats, enriched breads and cereals	Iron-deficiency anemia	Can cause death in children from supplement overdose
Copper	Formation of hemoglobin	Liver, nuts, shellfish, cherries, mushrooms, whole-grain breads and cereals	Anemia	Nausea, vomiting
Zinc	Normal growth and development	Seafood, meats	Skin problems, delayed development, growth problems	Interferes with copper use, may decrease high-density lipoprotein levels
Iodine	Production of the hormone thyroxin	Iodized salt, seafood	Mental and growth retardation, lack of energy	
Fluorine	Strengthens bones and teeth	Fluoridated water	Teeth are less resistant to decay	Damage to tooth enamel

blood cells. Calcium has many important functions: It is necessary for proper bone and teeth formation, blood clotting, and muscle contraction. In general, minerals have roles that are too numerous to detail. Eating a wide variety of foods is the best way to obtain the minerals needed in the proper concentrations.[6]

Water

Water is the most essential of all the nutrients and should be the nutrient of greatest concern to the athlete.[13] It is the most abundant nutrient in the body, accounting for approximately 60 percent of the body weight, although this varies considerably (+/−10%) among individuals due to age and percent of body fat. Water is essential for all the chemical processes that occur in the body, and an adequate supply of water is necessary for energy production and the normal digestion of other nutrients. Although water does not supply any energy (calories), an adequate amount of water is needed for energy production in all cells. Water also takes part in digestion and maintenance of the proper environment inside and outside cells. Water is also necessary for temperature control and for the elimination of waste products of nutrient and body metabolism. Too little water leads to dehydration, and severe dehydration can lead to death. The average adult requires a minimum of 2.5 liters, or about 10 glasses of water per day.

The body has a number of mechanisms designed to maintain body water at a near-normal level. Too little water leads to accumulation of solutes in the blood. These solutes signal the brain that the body is thirsty while signaling the kidneys to conserve water. Excessive water dilutes these solutes, which signals the brain to stop drinking and the kidneys to get rid of the excess water.

Water is the only nutrient that is of greater importance to the athlete than to those people who are more sedentary, especially when the athlete is engaging in prolonged exercise in a hot, humid environment.[31] Such a situation may cause excessive sweating and subsequent losses of large amounts of water. When the body burns carbohydrate and fat for energy, it produces a great deal of heat. During exercise, that heat is lost from the body primarily by sweating. Sweating is how the body uses water to keep itself from overheating. Restriction of water during this time results in dehydration. Symptoms of dehydration include fatigue, vomiting, nausea, exhaustion, fainting, and possibly death.

Electrolyte Requirements Electrolytes, including sodium, chloride, potassium, magnesium, and calcium, are electrically charged ions dissolved in body water. Among many other functions, electrolytes maintain the balance of water inside and outside the cell. In other words, electrolytes, especially sodium, are essential in helping the body rehydrate quickly.[3,11] Electrolyte replenishment may be needed when a person is not fit, suffers from extreme water loss, participates in a marathon, or has just completed an exercise period and is expected to perform at near-maximum effort within the next few hours. In most cases, electrolytes can be sufficiently replaced with a balanced diet, which can, if necessary, be salted slightly more than usual. Free access to water and sports drinks (ad libitum) before, during, and after activity should be the rule (see Chapter 6). In some people, electrolyte losses can produce muscle cramping and intolerance to heat. Sweating results not only in body water loss but in some electrolyte loss as well.[60] Chapter 6 discusses fluid and electrolyte replacement in great detail.

> **Electrolytes: sodium, chloride, potassium, magnesium, and calcium.**

> **Replacing fluid after heavy sweating is far more important than replacing electrolytes.**

NUTRIENT REQUIREMENTS AND RECOMMENDATIONS

A nutrient requirement is the amount of the nutrient that is needed to prevent the nutrient's deficiency disease. Nutrient needs vary among individuals within a population. A recommendation for a nutrient is different from the requirement for a nutrient. Scientists establish recommendations for nutrients and calories based on extensive scientific research and assessment of present dietary intakes.[17]

In the past, the *U.S. recommended dietary allowances (U.S. RDAs)* have served as the benchmark of nutritional adequacy in the United States. Over the past several years, new information has emerged about nutrient requirements that necessitated updating of the RDAs.[20] RDAs have been changed to *dietary reference intakes (DRIs)*, which are established using an expanded concept that includes indicators of good health and the prevention of chronic disease, as well as possible adverse effects of overconsumption.[17] The DRIs include not only recommended intakes (RDAs) intended to help individuals meet their daily nutritional requirements but also tolerable upper intake levels (ULs), which help individuals avoid harm from consuming too much of a nutrient; estimated average requirements (EARs), which are the average daily nutrient intake levels estimated to meet the requirements of half the healthy individuals in a particular age group; and adequate intake (AI), which is the recommended average daily intake level based on experimentally developed estimates of nutrient intake that are used when the RDA cannot be determined.[20] (A link to nutrient recommendations based on the latest DRIs can be found at www.mhhe.com/prentice15e.)

Food Labels

Food labels on packages help consumers make more informed food selections (Figure 5–2). Concern over the amount of fat, cholesterol, sodium, and fiber in the typical American diet led the drive for a more health-conscious label. For more than a decade, the U.S. RDAs appeared on nutrient labels. In 1994, the old food labels were replaced by a new format that presented the information in the form of percentages of daily values based on a standard 2,000-calorie diet.[16] The latest requirements for food labels were developed in 2009. The ingredients list, now added at the bottom of the label, tells you exactly what packaged food contains. Ingredients are listed in descending order of predominance. The first two or three ingredients are the ones that are the most predominant, whereas those at the bottom of the list may appear in only very tiny or trace amounts.

Although there are a few exceptions, most packaged supermarket foods must include nutritional labels.

MyPlate*

The USDA's new food icon MyPlate, introduced in 2011, replaces the MyPyramid icon which was introduced in 2005. MyPlate is now the government's primary food group symbol, designed to help consumers adopt healthy eating habits consistent with the 2010 Dietary Guidelines for Americans.[67] (See Figure 5–3.) The intent is to help consumers think about building a healthy diet, which consists of fruit, vegetable, grain, protein, and dairy food groups.

A new Web site, ChooseMyPlate.gov, has been developed to provide practical information to several groups, including individual Americans, health professionals, nutrition educators, and the food industry, to help these consumers build healthier diets. Resources and tools for dietary assessment, nutrition education, and other user-friendly nutrition information can also be found on this Web site. Because the American population is experiencing epidemic rates of overweight and obesity, the hope is that the online resources and tools can empower people to make healthier food choices for themselves, their families, and their children. Hopefully, this approach will help to eliminate consumer frustration over what they report as contradictory nutrition information.

The 2010 Dietary Guidelines for Americans form the basis of the federal government's nutrition education programs, federal nutrition assistance programs, and dietary advice provided by health and nutrition professionals. Action-oriented messages help professionals and the media understand and deliver relevant nutrition information to help people in their daily lives.

Nutrition Facts

Serving Size 1 cup (228g)
Servings Per Container 2

Amount Per Serving

Calories 250   Calories from Fat 110

	% Daily Value*
Total Fat 12g	**18%**
Saturated Fat 3g	**15%**
Trans Fat 3g	
Cholesterol 30mg	**10%**
Sodium 470mg	**20%**
Total Carbohydrate 31g	**10%**
Dietary Fiber 0g	**0%**
Sugars 5g	
Protein 5g	
Vitamin A	4%
Vitamin C	2%
Calcium	20%
Iron	4%

*Percent Daily Values are based on a 2,000 calorie diet. Your daily values may be higher or lower depending on your calorie needs.

	Calories:	2,000	2,500
Total Fat	Less than	65g	80g
Sat Fat	Less than	20g	25g
Cholesterol	Less than	300mg	300mg
Sodium	Less than	2,400mg	2,400mg
Total Carbohydrate		300g	375g
Dietary Fiber		25g	30g

INGREDIENTS: CORN, VEGETABLE OIL, (contains one or more of the following: CANOLA, CORN, CHEESES (CHEDDAR FROM COW'S MILK), SALT, BUTTERMILK, GARLIC POWDER, DEXTROSE, SUGAR)

FIGURE 5–2   Food label indicating nutrition information per serving.

*Modified from http://www.choosemyplate.gov

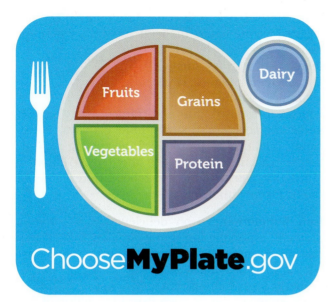

FIGURE 5–3 MyPlate Icon.

The Guidelines cover several actionable messages, including these:

Balance Calories

- Enjoy your food, but eat less.
- Avoid oversized portions.

Foods to Increase

- Make half your plate fruits and vegetables.
- Switch to fat-free or low-fat (1%) milk.
- Make at least half your grains whole grains.

Foods to Reduce

- Compare sodium (salt) in foods like soup, bread, and frozen meals, and choose foods with lower numbers.
- Drink water instead of sugary drinks.

DIETARY SUPPLEMENTS

Many people believe that exercise increases requirements for nutrients, such as proteins, vitamins, and minerals, and that it is possible and desirable to saturate the body with these nutrients.[22] There is no scientific basis for ingesting levels of these nutrients above DRI levels.[75] Exercise increases the need for energy, not for proteins, vitamins, and minerals.[12] Additionally, many athletes use nutritional supplements as ergogenic aids to improve various aspects of performance.[52,70] (The use of various supplements as ergogenic aids are discussed in Chapter 17.) Thus, it is necessary to

> **Vitamin requirements do not increase during exercise.**

explore some of the more common myths that surround the subject of nutrition's role in physical performance.

Vitamin Supplements

Many individuals believe that taking large amounts of vitamin supplements can lead to superior health and performance.[75] A megadose of a nutrient supplement is essentially an overdose; the amount ingested far exceeds the DRI levels.[12] The rationale used for such excessive intakes is that if taking a pill that contains the DRI for each vitamin and mineral makes a person healthy, taking a pill that has 10 times the DRI should make that individual 10 times healthier.[5]

> Since the majority of supplements are not regulated, these over-the-counter products may contain banned substances. Athletes should consult their athletic trainer or team physician prior to taking any supplement.

An example of a popular practice is to take megadoses of vitamin C. Such doses do not prevent the common cold or slow aging. They do cause diarrhea and possibly the development of painful kidney stones. There is no increased need for vitamin C. Fruits, juices, and vegetables are reliable sources of vitamin C that also supply other vitamins and minerals.[5]

Taking megadoses of vitamin E has become popular among people of all ages. The vitamin protects certain fatty acids in cell membranes from being damaged.[5] There is not much evidence to support the notion that this vitamin can extend life expectancy or enhance physical performance. Vitamin E does not enhance sexual ability, prevent graying hair, or cure muscular dystrophy. A person can obtain adequate amounts of vitamin E by consuming whole-grain products, vegetable oils, and nuts.

The B-complex vitamins that are involved in obtaining energy from carbohydrates, fats, and proteins are often abused by individuals who believe that vitamins provide energy. Any increased need for these nutrients is easily

> **5–3 Clinical Application Exercise**
>
> A rowing athlete complains of feeling tired lately and more exhausted than usual after workouts. She also states that she has noticed many bruises on her legs and arms. The bruises randomly appear in different places all over her body. When asked about her diet, she mentions she eats two meals a day and it is food she grabs on the run. She cannot remember the last time she had a meal with vegetables or quality meat.
>
> **?** What do you suspect might be wrong with her, and what is your suggested plan of action?

fulfilled when a person eats more nutritious foods while training.[70] If athletes do not increase their food consumption, they will lose weight because of their high level of caloric expenditure.

If an individual is not eating a well-balanced diet, taking a multiple vitamin once each day would be helpful and, in fact, is recommended by many physicians to make certain that minimum DRIs are met.

Mineral Supplements

Obtaining adequate levels of certain minerals can be a problem for some people.[5] Calcium and iron intakes may be low for those who do not include dairy products, red meats, or enriched breads and cereals in their diet. The following sections explore some minerals that can be deficient in the diet and some suggestions for improving the quality of the diet so that supplements are not necessary.

Calcium Supplements Calcium is the most abundant mineral in the body. It is essential for bones and teeth as well as for muscle contraction and the conduction of nerve impulses. However, the importance of obtaining adequate calcium supplies throughout life has become more recognized. If calcium intake is too low to meet needs, the body can remove calcium from the bones. Over time, bones become weakened and appear porous on X-rays. These bones are brittle and often break spontaneously.

osteoporosis A decrease in bone density.

This condition is called **osteoporosis** and is estimated to be eight times more common among women than men. It becomes a serious problem for women after menopause.[4] (See Chapter 29.)

The adequate intake (AI) for young adults is 1,000 mg (an 8-ounce glass of milk contains about 300 mg of calcium). Unfortunately, about 25 percent of all females in the United States consume less than 300 mg of calcium per day, well below the RDA. High-protein diets and alcohol consumption also increase calcium excretion from the body. Exercise causes calcium to be retained in bones, so physical activity is beneficial. However, younger females who exercise to extremes, so that their normal hormonal balance is upset, are prone to develop premature osteoporosis.[40] Calcium supplementation, preferably as calcium carbonate or citrate rather than phosphate, may be advisable for females who have a family history of osteoporosis.

Milk products are the most reliable sources of calcium. Many people complain that milk and other dairy products upset their stomach. They may lack an enzyme, called lactase, that is needed to digest the milk sugar lactose. This condition is referred to as lactose intolerance, or **lactase deficiency.**[12] The undigested lactose enters the large intestine, where the bacteria that normally reside there use it for energy. The bacteria produce large quantities of intestinal gas,

lactase deficiency Difficulty digesting dairy products.

which causes discomfort and cramps. Many lactose-intolerant people also suffer from diarrhea. Fortunately, scientists have produced the missing enzyme, lactase. Lactase is available without prescription in forms that can be added to foods before eating or can be taken with meals.

Iron Supplements Iron deficiency is a common problem, especially for young females. Lack of iron can result in iron-deficiency **anemia** (see Chapter 29).[47] Iron is needed to properly form hemoglobin.

anemia Lack of iron.

With anemia, the oxygen-carrying ability of the red blood cells is reduced, so muscles cannot obtain enough oxygen to generate energy.[15] Anemia leaves a person feeling tired and weak. Obviously, an athlete cannot compete at peak level while suffering from an iron deficiency. Excess intake of iron can be toxic, however, and may result in constipation.

Protein Supplements

Athletes often believe that more protein is needed to build bigger muscles.[35] It is true that athletes who are developing muscles in a conditioning program need a relatively small amount of extra protein. Many athletes, particularly those who are training with heavy weights or who are bodybuilders, routinely take protein supplements that are commercially produced and marketed.[34,35] To build muscle, athletes should consume 1 to 1.5 grams of extra protein per kilogram (0.5 to 0.7 gram per pound) of body weight every day. This range goes from slightly above to about double the protein RDA (0.8 gram per kilogram of desirable body weight). Anyone eating a variety of foods, but especially protein-rich foods, can easily meet the higher amounts. Thus, athletes do not need protein supplements, because their diets typically exceed even the most generous protein recommendations. An active adult most likely requires 0.6 gram per pound, or 66 percent more than the DRI.[17]

5-4 Clinical Application Exercise

A high-school football player has become interested in bodybuilding. He is most interested in seeing an increase in muscle mass. He is religious about his weight training but has heard that increasing protein intake causes the muscles to hypertrophy more quickly.

? What advice can the athletic trainer give him about taking commercially produced protein supplements?

Creatine Supplements

Creatine is a naturally occurring organic compound synthesized by the kidneys, liver, and pancreas. Free creatine can also be obtained from ingesting meat and fish that contain approximately 5 grams per kilogram. Creatine has an integral role in energy metabolism.[1]

There are two main types of creatine: free creatine and phosphocreatine. Phosphocreatine is stored in skeletal muscle and is used during anaerobic activity to produce ATP, with the assistance of the enzyme creatine kinase. With creatine supplementation, phosphocreatine depletion is delayed and performance is enhanced through the maintenance of the normal metabolic pathways.[65]

The positive physiological functions of creatine include increasing the resynthesis of ATP, thus allowing for increased intensity in a workout; acting as a lactic acid buffer, thus prolonging maximal effort and improving exercise recovery time during maximum-intensity activities; stimulating protein synthesis; decreasing total cholesterol while improving the HDL-to-LDL ratio; decreasing total triglycerides; and increasing fat-free mass.[1] Oral supplementation with creatine may enhance muscular performance during high-intensity resistance exercise.[65] It has been suggested that creatine supplementation may reduce the incidence of muscle cramps.[24] Side effects of creatine supplementation include weight gain, due primarily to an increase in total body water,[49] gastrointestinal disturbances, and renal dysfunction. There are apparently no other known long-term side effects.

It has been suggested that an initial *loading phase* should consist of ingesting approximately 0.3 gram of creatine per kilogram of body weight per day.[63] The dosage should be split over four or five times per day, with approximately 16 ounces of water per dose. The loading phase lasts for 5 days. A loading phase is not necessarily required, however. It has been shown that ingesting creatine at a much lower dose of 3 grams per day increases total muscle creatine to the same values observed with 5 days of 20 grams per day; however, this takes approximately 30 days.[65] Thus, the high "loading" dose is unnecessary to realize an increase in muscle creatine content. After completing the loading phase, one should take a maintenance dosage every day equal to about 0.03 gram of creatine per kilogram of body weight for a month. Then a "wash-out" phase should last for 1 month, during which there is no supplementation.[65]

In August 2000, the NCAA Committee on Competitive Safeguards and Medical Aspects of Sports banned the distribution of all muscle-building substances, including creatine, by NCAA member institutions. However the use of creatine itself is not necessarily banned by other organizations.

Herbal Supplements

The use of herbs as natural alternatives to drugs and medicines has clearly become a trend among American consumers. Most herbs, as edible plants, are safe to ingest as foods; as natural medicines, they are claimed to have few side effects, although occasionally a mild, allergic reaction may occur.[44] Those taking herbs should also be mindful of potential interactions.[38]

Herbs can offer the body nutrients that are reported to nourish the brain, glands, and hormones. Unlike vitamins, which work best when taken with food, herbs do not need to be taken with other foods, because they provide their own digestive enzymes.[18]

Herbs in their whole form are not drugs. As medicine, herbs are essentially body balancers that work with the body's functions so that it can heal and regulate itself. Herbal formulas can be general for overall strength and nutrient support or specific to a particular ailment or condition.

Hundreds of herbs are widely available at all quality levels. They are readily available at health food stores. However, unlike both food and medicine, no federal or governmental controls regulate the sale of herbs to ensure the quality of the products being sold.[19] The consumer of herbal products must exercise extreme caution.

Focus Box 5–1: "Commonly used herbs" lists the most popular and widely used herbal products sold in health food stores. Some additional potent and complex herbs, such as capsicum, lobelia, sassafras, mandrake tansy, canada snake root, wormwood, woodruff, poke root, and rue, may be useful in small amounts and as catalysts but should not be used alone.

Ephedrine Ephedrine is a stimulant that has been used as an ingredient in diet pills, illegal recreational drugs, and legitimate over-the-counter medications to treat congestion and asthma.[48] Ephedrine is similar to an amphetamine. In December 2003, the FDA banned the use of ephedrine as a dietary supplement. For several years the FDA has warned consumers about the potential dangers of using ephedrine. In recent years the NCAA, the National Football League, the National Basketball Association, minor league baseball, and the USOC have banned the use of ephedrine by their athletes. However some companies continue to sell dietary products that contain ephedrine or other stimulants despite the fact that these supplements have caused numerous problems. Ephedrine is known to produce the following adverse reactions: heart attack, stroke, tachycardia, paranoid psychosis, depression, convulsions, fever, coma, vomiting, palpitations, hypertension, and respiratory depression.[48,76]

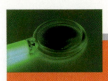
Commonly used herbs

The indications for using these herbs have at least minimal scientific basis in the literature. However, there is a substantial lack of strong evidence-based support for their use.

Cayenne (capsaicin)—pain control; may cause stomach irritation.

Cascara—used as a laxative; can cause dehydration.

Dong quai—weak evidence that it can be used to treat abnormal heart rhythm, prevent accumulation of platelets in blood vessels, protect the liver, promote urination, act as a mild laxative, promote sleep, and fight infection.

Echinacea—promotes wound healing and strengthens the immune system.

Feverfew—weak evidence that it prevents and relieves migraine headaches, arthritis, and PMS.

Garlic—weak evidence that it can be effective in treating atherosclerosis by reducing total blood cholesterol and triglyceride levels and raising HDL levels; also for use in treating hypertension, diabetes, the common cold, tuberculosis, and intestinal parasites.

Garcina cambagia—used to promote loss of fat.

Ginkgo biloba—weak evidence for its use in treating dementia and Alzheimer's disease, memory impairment, eye problems, intermittent claudication, and tinnitus.

Ginseng—used to prevent Alzheimer's disease, cancer, depression, diabetes, chronic respiratory disease, menopausal symptoms, and stress; has been shown to enhance cardiovascular health by raising HDL while reducing total cholesterol levels, fertility/sexual performance, immune system function, mental performance and mood, and physical endurance.

Guarana*—used as a stimulant because it contains large amounts of caffeine; often in weight-loss products.

Kava—used to reduce anxiety and insomnia; may cause rare cases of liver failure.

Ma huang*(ephedrine)—derived from the ephedra plant; has been used in China for medicinal purposes, including increased energy, appetite suppression, increased fat burning, and preservation of muscle tissue from breakdown; a central nervous system stimulant drug that was used in many diet pills; in 1995, the FDA revealed adverse reactions to ephedrine, such as heart attacks, strokes, paranoid psychosis, vomiting, fever, palpitations, convulsions, and comas; banned by the FDA in 2003.

Mate—central nervous system stimulant.

Saw palmetto—used to treat inflamed prostate; also used as a diuretic.

Senna—used as a laxative; can cause water and electrolyte loss.

St. John's wort—used as an antidepressant; also used to treat nervous disorders, depression, and seasonal affective disorder.

Valerian—used to treat insomnia, anxiety, and stress.

Vohimbe—used to increase libido and blood flow to sexual organs in the male.

*Banned by some athletic organizations and/or the FDA.

Glucose Supplements

Ingesting large quantities of glucose in the form of honey, candy bars, or pure sugar immediately before physical activity may have a significant impact on performance.[62] As carbohydrates are digested, large quantities of glucose enter the blood. This increase in blood sugar (glucose) levels stimulates the release of the hormone insulin. Insulin allows the cells to use the circulating glucose, so that blood glucose levels soon return to normal.[43] It was hypothesized that a decline in blood sugar levels was detrimental to performance and endurance. However, recent evidence indicates that the effect of eating large quantities of carbohydrates is beneficial rather than negative.[28,62]

Nevertheless, some athletes are sensitive to high-carbohydrate feedings and experience problems with increased levels of insulin. Also, some athletes cannot tolerate large amounts of the simple sugar fructose. For these individuals, too much fructose leads to intestinal upset and diarrhea. Athletes should test themselves with various high-carbohydrate foods to see whether they are affected (but not before a competitive event).[43]

EATING AND DRINKING PRACTICES

Caffeine Consumption

Caffeine is a central nervous system stimulant. Most people who consume caffeine in coffee, tea, or carbonated beverages are aware of its effect of increasing alertness and decreasing fatigue. Chocolate contains compounds that are related to caffeine and have the same stimulating effects. However, large amounts of caffeine cause nervousness, irritability, increased heart rate, and headaches.[12] Also, headaches are a withdrawal symptom experienced when a person tries to stop consuming caffeinated products.[46]

Although small amounts of caffeine do not appear to harm physical performance, cases of nausea and light-headedness have been reported. Caffeine enhances the use of fat during endurance exercise, thus delaying the depletion of glycogen stores.[40] This delay would help endurance performance. Caffeine also helps make calcium more available to muscles during contraction, allowing the muscles to work more efficiently. However, Olympic officials rightfully consider caffeine to be a drug. It should not be present in a drug test in levels greater than that resulting from drinking five or six cups of coffee.

Energy Drinks Over the last decade, consumption of energy drinks has increased dramatically, and there are now literally hundreds of energy drinks available to the consumer. Red Bull, Rockstar, AMP, Monster, and 5-hour Energy are just a few of the most common energy drinks. It must be clarified that energy drinks are different than sport drinks. Sports drinks contain no caffeine. Generally, the energy drinks contain caffeine in doses ranging anywhere from 50 mg to in excess of 500 mg, with the average between 70 and 80 mg per can or bottle. They are marketed for their performance-enhancing and stimulant drug effects. An obvious risk of caffeine intoxication exists when consuming a high amount of caffeine, which can cause adverse effects including nervousness, insomnia, headache, tachycardia (increased heart rate), and rarely seizure activity or occasionally death. Problems with caffeine dependence and withdrawal have also been reported.[54] Energy drinks also have a high concentration of carbohydrate, and most are carbonated.

There is currently little government regulation of energy drinks, including content labeling and health warnings. Of even greater concern is the combined use of caffeine and alcohol. Studies suggest that such combined use may increase the rate of alcohol-related injury.

Alcohol Consumption

Alcohol use is prevalent among athletes at all levels. It appears that alcohol consumption is higher among athletes when compared to non-athlete peers.[46] The depressant effects of alcohol on the central nervous system include decreased physical coordination, slowed reaction times, and decreased mental alertness. Also, this drug increases the production of urine, resulting in body water losses (diuretic effect). Alcohol does provide energy for the body; each gram of pure alcohol (ethanol) supplies seven calories. However, sources of alcohol provide little other nutritional value with regard to vitamins, minerals, and proteins. Therefore, the use of alcoholic beverages by the athlete is strongly discouraged before, during, and after physical activity.

Consumption of Organic, Natural, and Health Foods

Many people are concerned about the quality of the foods they eat—not just the nutritional value of the food but also its safety. Organic foods are grown without the use of synthetic fertilizers and pesticides. Those who advocate the use of organic farming methods claim that these foods are nutritionally superior and safer than the same products grown using chemicals, such as pesticides and synthetic fertilizers.[14]

Technically, the name *organic food* is meaningless. All foods (except water) are organic; that is, they contain the element carbon. Organically produced foods are often more expensive than the same foods that have been produced by conventional means. There is no advantage to consuming organic food products. They are not more nutritious than foods produced by conventional methods. Nevertheless, for some people the psychological benefit of believing that they are doing something good for their bodies justifies the extra cost.

Natural foods have been subjected to little processing and contain no additives, such as preservatives or artificial flavors.[72] Processing can protect nutritional value. Preservatives save food that would otherwise spoil and have to be destroyed. Both organic and natural foods can be described as health foods.

Vegetarianism

Vegetarianism is an alternative to the usual American diet. All vegetarians use plant foods to form the foundation of their diet; animal foods are either totally excluded or included in a variety of eating patterns.[22] People who choose to become vegetarians do so for economic, philosophical, religious, cultural, or health reasons. Vegetarianism is no longer considered to be a fad if it is practiced intelligently. However, the vegetarian diet may create deficiencies if nutrient needs are not carefully considered. Individuals who follow this eating pattern

> **Vegetarians: total vegetarians, lactovegetarians, ovolactovegetarians, and semivegetarians.**

must plan their diet carefully so that their caloric needs are met.[22] The types of vegetarian dietary patterns are categorized as follows.

Total vegetarians, or vegans—people who consume plant, but no animal foods; meat, fish, poultry,

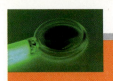
The pregame meal

- Try to achieve the largest possible storage of carbohydrates (glycogen) in both resting muscle and the liver. This storage is particularly important for endurance activities but may also be beneficial for intense, short-duration exercise.
- A stomach that is full of food during contact sports is subject to injury. Therefore, the type of food eaten should allow the stomach to empty quickly. Carbohydrates are easier to digest than are fats or proteins. A meal that contains plenty of carbohydrates leaves the stomach and is digested faster than a fatty meal. It would be wise to replace the traditional steak-and-eggs pre-event meal with a low-fat one containing a small amount of pasta, tomato sauce, and bread.
- Foods should not cause irritation or upset to the gastrointestinal tract. Foods high in cellulose and other forms of fiber, such as whole-grain products, fruits, and vegetables, increase the need for defecation. Highly spiced foods and gas-forming foods

(such as onions, baked beans, or peppers) must also be avoided because any type of disturbance in the gastrointestinal tract may be detrimental to performance. Carbonated beverages and chewing gum also contribute to the formation of gas.
- Liquids consumed should be easily absorbed and low in fat content and should not act as a laxative. Whole milk, coffee, and tea should be avoided. Water intake should be increased, particularly if the temperature is high.
- A meal should be eaten approximately 3 to 4 hours before the event or before exercising. This timing allows for adequate stomach emptying, but the individual will not feel hungry during activity.
- The athlete should not eat any food that he or she dislikes. Most important, the individual must feel psychologically satisfied by any pre-event meal. If not, performance may be impaired more by psychological factors than by physiological factors.

eggs, and dairy products are excluded from their diet. This diet is adequate for most adults if they give careful consideration to obtaining enough calories, vitamin B_{12}, and the minerals calcium, zinc, and iron.

Lactovegetarians—individuals who consume milk products along with plant foods; meat, fish, poultry, and eggs are excluded from their diet. Iron and zinc levels can be low in this form of vegetarianism.

Ovolactovegetarians—people who consume dairy products and eggs in their diet along with plant foods; meat, fish, and poultry are excluded. Again, obtaining sufficient iron can be a problem.

Semivegetarians—people who consume animal products but exclude red meats; plant products form an important part of the diet. This diet is usually adequate.

Pre-Event Nutrition

The importance and content of the pre-event meal has been heatedly debated among coaches, athletic trainers, and athletes.[26] The trend has been to ignore logical thinking about what should be eaten before competition and to upholding the tradition of "rewarding" the athlete for hard work by serving foods that may hamper performance. For example, the traditional steak-and-eggs meal before football games is great for coaches and athletic trainers; however, the athlete gains nothing from this

meal. The important point is that too often people are concerned primarily with the pre-event meal and fail to realize that the nutrients consumed over several days before competition are much more important than what is eaten 3 hours before an event. (See *Focus Box 5–2:* "The pregame meal.") The purpose of the pre-event meal should be to maximize carbohydrate stored in the muscles as well as blood glucose. It has been suggested that the athlete consume carbohydrates 3 to 4 hours before practice or competition. But it has also been suggested that consuming carbohydrates immediately before competition causes an increased release of insulin, which increases the rate at which muscles burn carbohydrate, thus lowering blood glucose levels (hypoglycemia). Different carbohydrates are digested and absorbed at different rates. The **glycemic index (GI)** is a scale that indicates how much different types of carbohydrate effect blood glucose levels.[73] Consuming foods

> **glycemic index (GI)**
> Indicates how much different types of carbohydrate effect blood glucose levels.

that have a low to medium GI prior to an event is recommended because they produce only small fluctuations in blood glucose and insulin levels and release energy more slowly over a longer time period. Ingesting carbohydrates that have a high GI within an hour of exercise may actually lower blood glucose. Figure 5–4 lists the glycemic index range for common foods.

Low Glycemic Index (<55)
Most fruits—grapefruit, apples, oranges
Whole-grain cereals, breads, pasta
Nuts
Beans and legumes
Green leafy vegetables
Yogurt, milk
Medium Glycemic Index (56–69)
Sweet potato
Spaghetti
Basmati rice
Bagel
Macaroni and cheese
Raisins
Ice cream
High Glycemic Index (>70)
White bread
White rice
Corn flakes
Baked potato
Watermelon
Popcorn

FIGURE 5–4 Glycemic Index Food Recommendations for Pre-Event Meals.

Additionally the foods selected should minimize gastrointestinal distress and should be foods that the individual athlete prefers. It is also critical to make certain that the athlete is appropriately hydrated.

Athletes should be encouraged to become conscious of their diets. However, no experimental evidence exists to indicate that performance may be enhanced by altering a diet that is basically sound. A nutritious diet may be achieved in many ways, and the diet that is optimal for one athlete may not be the best for another. In many instances, the individual is the best judge of what he or she should or should not eat in the pre-event meal or before exercising. It seems that a person's best guide is to eat whatever he or she is most comfortable with.

Liquid Food Supplements Liquid food supplements (e.g., Gatorade, Nutrition Shake, Exceed) have been recommended as effective pre-event meals and are being used by high-school, college, university, and professional teams with some indications of success.[53] These supplements supply from 225 to 400 calories per average serving. Athletes who have used these supplements report elimination of the usual pregame symptoms of dry mouth, abdominal cramps, leg cramps, nervous defecation, and nausea.

Under ordinary conditions, it usually takes approximately 4 hours for a full meal to pass through the stomach and the small intestine. Pregame emotional tension often delays the emptying of the stomach; therefore, the undigested food mass remains in the stomach and upper bowel for a prolonged time, even up to or through the actual period of competition, and frequently results in nausea, vomiting, and cramps. This unabsorbed food mass is of no value to the athlete. Team physicians who have experimented with the liquid food supplements say that a major advantage of the supplements is that they clear both the stomach and the upper bowel before game time, thus making available the caloric energy that would otherwise still be in an unassimilated state. There is merit in the use of such food supplements for pregame meals.[53]

Recommendations for Restoring Muscle Glycogen after Exercise

When the time period between exercise sessions is relatively short (less than 8 hours), the athlete should begin consuming carbohydrates to restore supplies of muscle glycogen as soon as possible after the workout to maximize recovery between sessions.[32] Ideally, the foods should have a high glycemic index. Given that complete muscle glycogen restoration takes at least 20 to 24 hours, athletes should not waste time. They should ingest approximately 0.45 to 0.55 grams of carbohydrate per pound of body weight for each of the first 4 hours after exercise or until they eat their next large meal. During this period, nutrient-rich carbohydrate foods, such as fruits and vegetables or a high-carbohydrate drink, are recommended.[32] Over a 24-hour period, carbohydrate intake should range from 2.3 grams to as much as 5.5 grams per pound of body weight, depending on the intensity of the activity.[32] Pasta, potatoes, oatmeal, and sports drinks are recommended. It has been suggested that adding protein to a carbohydrate supplement enhances aerobic endurance performance above that which occurs with carbohydrate alone, but the reason for this improvement in performance has not been established.[28] Most evidence supports a 4 to 1 carbohydrate to protein ratio, whereas others argue for a 1:1 or 3:1 ratio. Peanut butter and tuna are recommended as good sources of protein.

Eating Fast Foods

Eating fast food is a way of life in American society.[58] Athletes, especially young athletes, have for the most part grown up as fast-food junkies. Furthermore, travel budgets and tight schedules dictate that fast food is a frequent choice for coaches on road trips.[57] Aside from occasional problems with food flavor, the biggest concern in consuming fast foods, as can be seen in Table 5–3, is that 40 to 50 percent of the calories consumed are from fats. To compound this problem, these already sizable meals are often "supersized" at a more affordable price for those who want maximum fat, salt, and calories in a single sitting.[46]

TABLE 5–3 Fast-Food Choices and Nutritional Value

Food	Calories	Protein (g)	Carbohydrate (g)	Fat (g)	Calories from Fat (%)	Cholesterol (mg)	Sodium (mg)
Hamburgers							
McDonald's hamburger	263	12.4	28.3	11	38.6	29.1	506
Dairy Queen single hamburger w/cheese	410	24	33	20	43.9	50	790
Hardee's 1/4 pound cheeseburger	506	28	41	26	46.2	61	1,950
Wendy's double hamburger, white bun	560	4.1	24	34	54.6	125	575
McDonald's Big Mac	570	24.6	39.2	35	55.2	83	45
Burger King Whopper sandwich	640	27	42	41	57.6	94	842
Jack in the Box Jumbo Jack	485	26	38	26	48.2	64	905
Chicken							
Arby's chicken breast sandwich	592	28	56	27	41.0	57	1,340
Burger King chicken sandwich	688	26	56	40	52.3	82	1,423
Dairy Queen chicken sandwich	670	29	46	41	55.0	75	870
Church's Crispy Nuggets (one; regular)	55	3	4	3	49.0	—	125
Kentucky Fried Chicken Nuggets (one)	46	2.82	2.2	2.9	56.7	11.9	140
Fish							
Church's Southern fried catfish	67	4	4	4	53.7	—	151
Long John Silver's Fish & More	978	34	82	58	53.3	88	2,124
McDonald's Filet-O-Fish	435	14.7	35.9	25.7	53.1	45.2	799
Others							
Hardee's hot dog	346	11	26	22	57.2	42	744
Jack in the Box taco	191	8	1.6	11	51.8	21	406
Arby's roast beef sandwich (regular)	350	22	32	15	38.5	39	590
Hardee's roast beef sandwich	377	21	36	17	40.5	57	1,030
French fries							
Arby's french fries	211	2	33	8	34.1	6	30
McDonald's french fries (regular)	220	3	26.1	11.5	47.0	8.6	109
Wendy's french fries (regular)	280	40	35	14	45.0	15	95
Shakes							
Dairy Queen	710	14	120	19	24.0	50	260
McDonald's							
Vanilla	352	9.3	59.6	8.4	21.4	30.6	201
Chocolate	383	9.9	65.5	9	21.1	29.7	300
Strawberry	362	9	62.1	8.7	22.3	32.2	207
Soft drinks							
Coca-Cola	154	—	40	—	—	—	6
Diet Coke	0.9	—	0.3	—	—	—	16
Sprite	142	—	36	—	—	—	45
Tab	1	—	1	—	—	—	30
Diet Sprite	3	—	0	—	—	—	9
Mountain Dew	154	—	46	—	—	—	75
Pepsi	150	—	27	—	—	—	25
Diet Pepsi	0	—	0	—	—	—	37

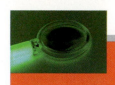
Tips for selecting fast foods

- Limit deep-fried foods, such as fish and chicken sandwiches and chicken nuggets, which are often higher in fat than plain burgers are. If you are having fried chicken, remove some of the breading before eating.
- Order roast beef, turkey, or grilled chicken, where available, for a lower-fat alternative to most burgers.
- Choose a small order of fries with your meal rather than a large one, and request no salt. Add a small amount of salt yourself if desired. If you are ordering a deep-fat-fried sandwich or one that is made with cheese and sauce, skip the fries altogether and try a plain baked potato (add butter and salt sparingly) or a dinner roll instead of a biscuit, or try a side salad to accompany your meal.
- Choose regular sandwiches instead of "double," "jumbo," "deluxe," or "ultimate" sandwiches. And order plain types rather than those with the works,

such as cheese, bacon, mayonnaise, and special sauce. Pickles, mustard, ketchup, and other condiments are high in sodium. Choose lettuce, tomatoes, and onions.

- At the salad bar, load up on fresh greens, fruits, and vegetables. Be careful of salad dressings, added toppings, and creamy salads (potato salad, macaroni salad, coleslaw). These can quickly push calories and fat to the level of other menu items or higher.
- Many fast-food items contain large amounts of sodium from salt and other ingredients. Try to balance the rest of your day's sodium choices after a fast-food meal.
- Alternate water, low-fat milk, or skim milk with a soda or a shake.
- For dessert, or a sweet-on-the-run, choose low-fat frozen yogurt where available.
- Remember to balance your fast-food choices with your food selections for the whole day.

On the positive side, fast-food restaurants have broadened their menus to include whole-wheat breads and rolls, salad bars, and low-fat milk products. Many of the larger fast-food restaurants provide nutritional information for consumers upon request or from well-stocked racks.[46] *Focus Box 5–3:* "Tips for selecting fast foods" provides suggestions for eating more healthfully at fast-food restaurants.

Low-Carbohydrate Diets

For many years, it was recommended that fat intake be limited as a means of controlling weight. More recently, the recommendation was to severely limit the intake of carbohydrate in the diet.[69] There are many versions of a low-carbohydrate diet, all of which recommend a strict reduction in the consumption of carbohydrates. Most "low-carb" diets replace carbohydrates with a high-fat and moderate-protein diet. The low-calorie and low-fat diets that have been recommended for years have failed to realize that dietary fat is not necessarily converted into body fat. However, carbohydrates are readily converted into fat. In a high-carbohydrate meal, the increased blood glucose stimulates insulin production by the pancreas. Insulin allows blood glucose to be used by the cells, but it also causes fat to be deposited, and it stimulates the brain to produce hunger signals. Thus, there is a tendency to eat more carbohydrates, and the cycle repeats. It has been shown that most overweight people became overweight

due to a condition called *hyperinsulinemia*—elevated insulin levels in the blood. Restricting carbohydrate intake halts this cycle by decreasing insulin levels. Carbohydrate restriction also increases the levels of *glucagon*, which is a hormone that causes body fat to be burned and aids in removing cholesterol deposits in the arteries. Severely restricting carbohydrate intake puts the body into a state of ketosis, in which blood glucose levels stabilize, insulin level drops, and because the body is burning fat, fairly rapid weight loss occurs.[69]

Glycogen Supercompensation

For endurance events, maximizing the amount of glycogen that can be stored, especially in muscles, may make the difference between finishing first or at the end of the pack. Athletes can increase glycogen supplies in muscle and liver by reducing the training program a few days before competing and by significantly increasing carbohydrate intake during the week before the event.[43] By reducing training for at least 48 hours before the competition, the athlete can eliminate any metabolic waste products that may hinder performance. The high-carbohydrate diet restores glycogen levels in muscle and the liver. This practice is called **glycogen supercompensation.** The basis for the practice is that the quantity of glycogen stored in muscle directly affects the endurance of that muscle.[43]

glycogen supercompensation
High-carbohydrate diet.

Glycogen supercompensation is accomplished over a 6-day period divided into three phases. In phase 1 (days 1 and 2), training should be hard and dietary intake of carbohydrates restricted. During phase 2 (days 3 through 5), training is cut back and the individual eats plenty of carbohydrates. Studies have indicated that glycogen stores may be increased from 50 to 100 percent, theoretically enhancing endurance during a long-term event. Phase 3 (day 6) is the day of the event, during which a normal diet must be consumed.

The effect of glycogen supercompensation in improving performance during endurance activities has not as yet been clearly demonstrated. It has been recommended that glycogen supercompensation not be done more than two or three times a year. Glycogen supercompensation is only of value in long-duration events that produce glycogen depletion, such as a marathon.[43]

5-5 Clinical Application Exercise

A recreational runner has been training to run his first marathon. He feels good about his level of conditioning but wants to make certain that he does everything that he can do to maximize his performance. He is concerned about eating the right type of foods both before and during the marathon to help ensure that he does not become excessively fatigued.

? What recommendations should the athletic trainer make regarding glycogen supercompensation, the pre-event meal, and food consumption during the event?

Fat Loading

Some endurance athletes have used fat loading in place of carbohydrate loading. Their intent was to have a better source of energy at their disposal. The deleterious effects of this procedure outweigh any benefits that may be derived. Associated with fat loading is cardiac protein and potassium depletion, causing arrhythmias and increased levels of serum cholesterol as a result of the ingestion of butter, cheese, cream, and marbled beef.

BODY COMPOSITION AND WEIGHT CONTROL

Gain or loss of weight often poses a problem because an individual's ingrained eating habits are difficult to change.[23] The athletic trainer's inability to adequately supervise the athlete's meal program in terms of balance and quantity further complicates the problem. An intelligent and conscientious approach to weight control requires that the athletic trainer, the coach, and the athlete have some knowledge of what is involved.[66] Such understanding allows individuals to better discipline themselves as to the quantity and kinds of foods they should eat.[25]

Body Composition

Ideal body weight is most often determined by consulting age-related height and weight charts, such as those published by life insurance companies. Unfortunately, these charts are inaccurate because they involve broad ranges and often fail to take individual body types into account. Health and performance, rather than body weight, may best be determined by body composition.[29]

Body composition refers to both the fat and nonfat components of the body. The portion of total body weight that is composed of fat tissue is referred to as the percentage of body fat. The total body weight that is composed of nonfat or lean tissue, which includes muscles, tendons, bones, and connective tissue, is referred to as lean body weight. Body composition measurements provide an accurate determination of precisely how much weight an individual may gain or lose.[43]

The average college-age female has between 20 and 25 percent body fat. The average college-age male has between 12 and 15 percent body fat. Male endurance athletes may get their fat percentage as low as 8 to 12 percent, and female endurance athletes may reach 10 to 18 percent. Body fat percentage should not go below 3 percent in males and 12 percent in females, because below these percentages the internal organs tend to lose their protective padding of essential fat, potentially subjecting them to injury.[9]

Being overweight and being obese are different conditions.[10] Being overweight implies having excess body weight relative to physical size and stature. Being overweight may not be a problem unless a person is also overfat, which means that the percentage of total body weight that is made up of fat is excessive. **Obesity** implies an excessive amount of body fat, much greater than what would be considered normal. Females with body fat above 30 percent and males with body fat above 20 percent are considered to be obese.[9]

obesity Excessive amount of body fat.

Two factors determine the amount of fat in the body: the number of fat, or adipose, cells and the size of each adipose cell. Proliferation, or hyperplagia, of adipose cells begins at birth and continues to

5-6 Clinical Application Exercise

A female softball player has a problem controlling her weight. Her body fat percentage has been measured at 25 percent and she asks the athletic trainer what she needs to do to be able to lose some weight quickly and then to maintain her body weight thereafter.

? How should the athletic trainer respond?

puberty. It is thought that after early adulthood the number of fat cells remains fixed, although some evidence suggests that the number of cells is not necessarily fixed.[43] Adipose cell size also increases gradually, or hypertrophies, to early adulthood and can increase or decrease as a function of caloric balance. In adults, weight loss or gain is primarily a function of the change in cell size, not cell number. Obese adults tend to exhibit a great deal of adipose cell hypertrophy.

The **adipose cell** stores triglyceride (a form of liquid fat). This liquid fat moves in and out of the cell according to the energy needs of the body, which are determined to some extent by activity type. The greatest amount of fat is used in activities of moderate intensity and long duration. The greater the amount of triglyceride contained in the adipose cell, the greater the amount of total body weight composed of fat.

adipose cell
Stores triglyceride.

One pound of body fat is made up of approximately 3,500 calories stored as triglyceride within the adipose cell.

Assessing Body Composition

Among the methods of assessing **body composition** are measurement of skinfold thickness;[11] hydrostatic, or underwater, weighing; and measurement of electrical impedance.

body composition
Percent body fat plus lean body weight.

Skinfold Measurements The method of measuring the thickness of skinfolds is based on the fact that about 50 percent of the fat in the body is contained in the subcutaneous fat layers and is closely related to total fat. The remainder of the fat in the body is found around organs and vessels and serves a shock-absorptive function. The skinfold technique measures the thickness of the subcutaneous fat layer with a skinfold caliper (Figure 5–5), at very specific

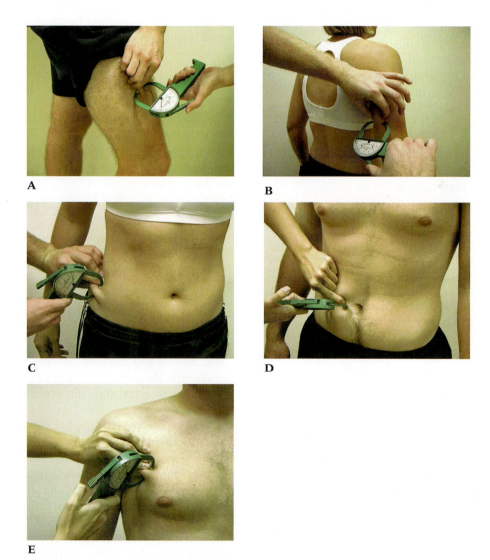

FIGURE 5–5 Sites and techniques for measuring body composition.
(A) Thigh. (B) Triceps. (C) Suprailiac. (D) Abdomen. (E) Chest.

locations, using a well-defined technique.[59] Its accuracy is relatively low; however, expertise in measurement is easily developed, and the time required for this technique is considerably less than for the others. It has been estimated that error in skinfold measurement is plus or minus 3 to 5 percent.[11]

Researchers have offered several different techniques for measuring body composition via skinfolds. A technique proposed by Jackson and Pollack,[32] which measures the thigh, triceps, suprailiac, abdomen, and chest skinfolds, is widely used.[46]

Hydrostatic Weighing

Hydrostatic (underwater) weighing involves placing a subject in a specially designed underwater tank to determine body density.[18] Fat tissue is less dense than lean tissue. Therefore, the more body fat present, the more the body floats (buoyancy) and the less it weighs in water. Body composition is calculated by comparing the weight of the submerged individual with the weight before entering the tank. If done properly, this technique is very accurate. Unfortunately, the tank and equipment are expensive and generally not available to most athletic trainers. In addition, this technique has other drawbacks. It is time-consuming (especially for large groups), and subjects must exhale completely and hold their breath while under water. Many individuals have fears about this aspect of the technique.

Bioelectrical Impedance

This technique involves the measurement of resistance to the flow of electrical current through the body between selected points.[1] It is based on the principle that electricity will choose to flow through the tissue that offers the least resistance, or impedance. Fat is generally a poor conductor of electrical energy, whereas lean tissue is a fairly good conductor. Thus, the higher the percentage of body fat, the greater the resistance to the passage of electrical energy. Very simply, this method predicts the percent body fat by measuring bioelectrical impedance.[30] Bioelectrical impedance measures can be affected by levels of hydration; if the body is dehydrated, the measurement will tend to overestimate percent body fat relative to measurements taken when there is normal hydration.[30] The equipment available for taking these measurements is fairly expensive and generally includes computer software.

Determining Body Mass Index

A relatively easy way to determine the extent of overweight or obesity is to use a person's body weight and height measurements to calculate body mass index (BMI).[43] BMI is a ratio of body weight to height. This technique represents a method for measuring health risks from obesity using height/weight measurements. Health problems associated with excess body fat tend to be associated with a BMI of more than 25. A BMI of 25 to 30 indicates that a person is overweight. A BMI of 30 or more indicates a state of obesity.[46] *Focus Box 5–4:* "Determining body mass index (BMI)" will help you calculate BMI.

Assessing Caloric Balance

Changes in body weight are almost entirely the result of changes in caloric balance.[36]

Caloric balance =
Number of calories consumed − Number of calories expended

If more calories are consumed than expended, this positive caloric balance results in weight gain. Conversely, weight loss results from a negative caloric balance, in which more calories are expended than are consumed. Caloric balance may be calculated by maintaining accurate records of both the number of calories consumed in the diet and the number of calories expended for metabolic needs and in activities performed during the day.

Caloric Consumption Caloric balance is determined by the number of calories consumed regardless of whether the calories are contained in fat, carbohydrate, or protein. There are differences in the caloric content of these foodstuffs:

> Positive caloric balance leads to weight gain; negative caloric balance leads to weight loss.

Carbohydrate = 4 calories per gram
Protein = 4 calories per gram
Fat = 9 calories per gram
Alcohol = 7 calories per gram

Estimations of caloric intake for college athletes range between 2,000 and 5,000 calories per day. Estimations of caloric expenditure range between 2,200 and 4,400 calories on average. Energy demands will be considerably higher in endurance-type athletes, who may require as many as 7,000 calories per day.[43]

Caloric Expenditure Calories may be expended by three processes: basal metabolism, work (any activity that requires more energy than sleeping), and excretion. When estimating caloric expenditure, it is first necessary to determine the amount of calories (energy) needed to support basal metabolism. This is the minimal amount of energy required to sustain the body's vital functions, such as respiration, heartbeat, circulation, and maintenance of body temperature during a 24-hour period. The basal metabolic

WEB SITES

The American Dietetic Association:
www.eatright.org
This site includes access to the journal published by the American Dietetic Association and provides informative nutritional tips as well as gateways to nutrition and related sites.

American Heart Association:
www.americanheart.org
Complete with comprehensive nutrition guidelines, the American Heart Association is a great resource for health practitioners and laypersons.

Athletes and Eating Disorders: www.eda.org
This site is part of the Eating Disorders Resources Web site; it gives some statistics from a recent NCAA study and has a section on the coaches' responsibility. The site also includes information about warning signs and the female athlete triad.

Center for Food Safety and Applied Nutrition—FDA:
http://cfsan.fda.com
Timely fact sheets and press releases are available from the Food and Drug Administration.

Food and Nutrition Information Center:
http://fnic.nal.usda.gov/
This site is part of the information centers at the National Agricultural Library and offers access to information
on healthy eating habits, food composition, and many additional resources.

Gatorade Sports Science Institute:
www.gssiweb.com
This Web site provides information for coaches, athletic trainers, physicians, nutritionists, and others in the field of sports medicine, sports nutrition, and exercise science.

Healthy Biz 2000: www.healthybiz2000.com
This site provides information about sports nutrition and nutritional supplements for fitness and weight loss.

MyPlate: http://www.choosemyplate.gov/
Government Web site designed to help consumers adopt healthy eating habits consistent with the 2010 Dietary Guidelines.

U.S. Dietary Guidelines:
http://health.gov/dietaryguidelines/
This site details the revised 2005 U.S. Dietary Guidelines for Americans.

Yahoo Health and Nutrition Information:
http://health.yahoo.net/healthyliving/nutrition
This site includes diet analysis information, nutritional facts, and links to many other informative sites.

SOLUTIONS TO CLINICAL APPLICATION EXERCISES

5–1 The important consideration for weight control is the total number of calories that are consumed relative to the total number of calories expended. It makes no difference whether the calories consumed are carbohydrates, fat, or protein. Fat contains more than twice the number of calories than either carbohydrates, or protein contains, so an athlete can eat significantly more food and still have about the same caloric intake if the diet is high in carbohydrates. This dancer should be told that it is also essential to consume at least some fat, which is necessary for the production of several enzymes and hormones.

5–2 For a person who is truly consuming anything close to a well-balanced diet, vitamin supplementation is generally not necessary. However, if taking a one-a-day type of vitamin supplement makes her feel better, there is no harm. Vitamins do not provide energy. Her tiredness could be related to a number of medical conditions (e.g., mononucleosis). An iron-deficiency anemia may be detected through a laboratory blood test. The athletic trainer should refer this individual to a physician for blood work.

5–3 This athlete should be referred to the team physician and nutritionist. From her history, the athletic trainer can assume she is not consuming enough iron by not eating meats or other nutritious foods. Iron is essential for hemoglobin formation and energy formation. In addition, since she is not eating vegetables in a well-balanced diet, she is not receiving an adequate amount of vitamin K, which is found in green, leafy vegetables. Vitamin K is important in blood coagulation.

5–4 A small amount of protein (slightly above to about double the protein DRI) is needed for developing muscles in a training program. However, an athlete can easily get these necessary higher amounts by eating a variety of foods, especially protein-rich foods. Thus, athletes do not need protein supplements, because their diets typically exceed protein recommendations.

5–5 The amount of glycogen that can be stored in the muscle and liver can be increased by reducing the training program a few days before competing and by significantly increasing carbohydrate intake during the week before the event. Nutrients consumed over several days before competition are much more important than what is eaten 3 hours before an event. The purpose of the pre-event meal should be to provide the competitor with sufficient nutrient energy and fluids for competition while taking into consideration the digestibility of the food. Glucose-rich drinks taken at regular intervals are beneficial for highly intense and prolonged events that severely deplete glycogen stores.

5–6 The athletic trainer should recommend that this athlete set a goal of 18 to 20 percent body fat. If the softball player needs to lose weight, she must consume fewer calories than she is burning off, and this is not something that can be achieved in a short period of time. It also must be explained that weight control is simply a matter of achieving caloric balance and making lifestyle changes in terms of eating and exercise habits to achieve caloric balance.

5–7 This athlete must understand the importance of adding lean tissue muscle mass rather than increasing his percentage of body fat. His caloric intake must be increased so that he is in a positive caloric balance of about 500 calories per day. Additional caloric intake should consist primarily of carbohydrates. Additional supplementation with protein is not necessary. It is absolutely essential that this athlete incorporate a weight-training program using heavy weights that will overload the muscle, forcing it to hypertrophy over a period of time.

5–8 Treating eating disorders is difficult even for health care professionals specifically trained to counsel these individuals. The athletic trainer should approach the individual, not with accusation but with support, showing concern about her weight loss and expressing a desire to help her secure appropriate counseling. Remember that the athlete must first be willing to admit that she has an eating disorder before treatment and counseling will be effective. Eliciting the support of close friends and family can help with treatment.

Chapter Five ■ Nutrition and Supplements

REVIEW QUESTIONS AND CLASS ACTIVITIES

1. What is the value of good nutrition in terms of performance and injury prevention?
2. Ask coaches of different sports about the type of diet they recommend for their athletes and their rationale behind the diet.
3. Have a nutritionist talk to the class about food myths and fallacies.
4. Have each member of the class prepare a week's food diary; then compare it with other class members' diaries.
5. What are the daily dietary requirements, according to MyPlate? Should the requirements of the typical athlete's diet differ from those requirements? If so, in what ways?
6. Debate the value of vitamin and mineral supplements.
7. Describe the advantages and disadvantages of supplementing iron and calcium.
8. Is there some advantage to pre-event nutrition?
9. Are there advantages or disadvantages in a vegetarian diet for the athlete?
10. What is the current thinking on the value of creatine as a nutritional supplement?
11. What is the primary concern of using herbs?
12. Discuss the importance of monitoring body composition.
13. Explain the most effective technique for losing weight.
14. Contrast the signs and symptoms of bulimia nervosa and anorexia nervosa. If an athletic trainer is aware of an individual who may have an eating disorder, what should he or she do?

REFERENCES

1. American College of Sports Medicine: The physiological and health effects of oral creatine supplementation, *Med Sci Sports Exerc* 32(3):706, 2000.
2. American College of Sports Medicine: Position stand on the appropriate intervention strategies for weight loss and prevention of weight regain for adults, *Med Sci Sports Exerc* 33(12):2145, 2001.
3. American College of Sports Medicine: Position stand on exercise and fluid replacement, *Medicine and Science in Sports and Exercise* 39(2):377–90, 2007.
4. Anderson J, Stender M, Rodando P: Nutrition and bone in physical activity and sport. In Wolinsky I, Hickson J, editors: *Nutrition in exercise and sport*, Boca Raton, FL, 1998, CRC Press.
5. Antonio J: *Essentials of Sports Nutrition and Supplements*, New York, 2008, Humana Press.
6. Beals K: *Disordered eating among athletes: A comprehensive guide for health professionals*, Champaign, IL, 2004, Human Kinetics.
7. Black D, Larkin L, Coster D: Physiologic screening test for eating disorders/disordered eating among female collegiate athletes, *J Athl Train* 38(4):286, 2003.
8. Blackburn H: Olestra and the FDA, *N Engl J Med* 334(15):984, 1996.
9. Bonci C, Bonci L, Granger, L: National Athletic Trainers' Association position statement: Preventing, detecting and managing disordered eating in athletes, *J Athl Train* 43(1):80, 2008.
10. Brownell K, Horgen K: *Food fight: The inside story of America's obesity crisis—and what we can do about it*, New York, 2003, McGraw-Hill.
11. Brzycki M: What's the most accurate way to measure body composition? *Fitness Management* 20(2):45, 2004.
12. Byrd-Bredbenner C, Bernig J: *Perspectives in nutrition*, New York, 2008, McGraw-Hill.
13. Casa D, Armstrong L, Hillman S: National Athletic Trainers' Association position statement: Fluid replacement for athletes, *J Athl Train* 35(2):212, 2000.
14. Coyle E: Highs and lows of carbohydrate diets, *Sports Science Exchange* 17(2):1, 2004.
15. Dubnov G, Constantini NW: Prevalence of iron depletion and anemia in top-level basketball players, *Int J Sport Nutr Exerc Metab* 14(1):30, 2004.

16. Food and Drug Administration: Guidance for industry: A food labeling guide, Office of Nutrition, Labeling, and Dietary Supplements, 2009, U.S. Department of Health and Human Services.
17. Food and Nutrition Board, National Academy of Sciences—National Research Council: *Recommended dietary allowances*, ed 12, Washington, DC, 1998, U.S. Government Printing Office.
18. Friedman-Kester K: The function of functional foods. *Athletic Therapy Today* 7(3):46, 2002.
19. Friedman-Kester K: Herbal remedies are drugs, too! *Athletic Therapy Today* 7(4):40, 2002.
20. Friedman-Kester K: RDAs, RDIs—R U confused? *Athletic Therapy Today* 6(3):56, 2001.
21. Froiland K, Koszewski W, Hingst J: Nutritional supplement use among college athletes and their sources of information, *Int J Sport Nutr Exerc Metab* 14(1):104, 2004.
22. Fuhrman J: Fueling the vegetarian athlete, *Current Sports Medicine Reports*, 9(4):233–41, 2010.
23. Gorinski R: In pursuit of the perfect body composition: Do dietary strategies make a difference? *Athletic Therapy Today* 6(6):54, 2001.
24. Greenwood M, Kreider R, Greenwood L: Cramping and injury incidence in collegiate football players are reduced by creatine supplementation, *J Athl Train* 38(3):216–19, 2003.
25. Gutgesell M, Moreau K, Thompson D: Weight concerns, problem eating behaviors, and problem drinking behaviors in female college athletes, *J Athl Train* 38(1):62, 2003.
26. Hale CW: The precompetition meal. *Athletic Therapy Today* 6(3):21, 2001.
27. Hostetter K: The need for qualified intervention for the female athlete triad syndrome patient, *Athletic Therapy and Training*, 15(3):29–33, 2010.
28. Ivy JL, Res PT, Sprague RC, Widzer MO: Effect of a carbohydrate-protein supplement on endurance performance during exercise of varying intensity, *Int J Sport Nutr Exerc Metab* 13(3):382, 2003.
29. Jackson AS, Pollack M: Generalized equations for predicting body density of women, *Med Sci Sports Exerc* 12:175, 1980.

30. Kemble D: Accuracy of bioelectrical impedence analyzers in college athletes: Does hydration matter? *Journal of Strength and Conditioning Research*, 24(1):1, 2010.
31. Kleiner S: Fluids for performance, *Athletic Therapy Today* 5(1):51, 2000.
32. Kleiner SM: Postexercise-recovery nutrition. *Athletic Therapy Today* 6(2):40, 2001.
33. Kleiner SM: *Power eating*, Champaign, IL, 2001, Human Kinetics.
34. Kleiner SM: Protein power. *Athletic Therapy Today* 7(1):24, 2002.
35. Kleiner SM: The scoop on protein supplements. *Athletic Therapy Today* 6(1):52, 2001.
36. Kleiner SM: Top-ten rules for healthy weight control. *Athletic Therapy Today* 7(2):38, 2002.
37. Litt A: Tactics for gaining weight. In Litt A, editor: *Fuel for young athletes*, Champaign, IL, 2004, Human Kinetics.
38. Martin M, Kishman M: Drug-herb interactions: Are your athletes at risk? *Athletic Therapy Today* 10(1):15, 2005.
39. Massad S, Headley S: Nutrition assessment: Considerations for athletes, *Athletic Therapy Today* 4(6):6, 1999.
40. Maughn R: Dietary supplements, *Journal of Sport Sciences* 22(1):95, 2004.
41. Maughn R: *Sports nutrition*, Malden, MA, 2002, Blackwell Scientific.
42. Mazzeo S, Espelage D: Association between childhood physical and emotional abuse and disordered eating behaviors in female undergraduates: An investigation of the mediating role of alexithymia and depression, *Journal of Counseling Psychology* 49(1):86, 2002.
43. McArdle W, Katch F, Katch V: *Sports and exercise nutrition*, Philadelphia, 2008, Lippincott, Williams and Wilkins.
44. McVicar J: *The complete herb book*. Westport, CT, 2008, Firefly Books.
45. Merrick MA: Osteoporosis and the female athlete, *Athletic Therapy Today* 6(3):42, 2001.
46. Payne W, Hahn D: *Focus on health*, ed 8, St. Louis, 2010, McGraw-Hill.
47. Peterson D: Athletes and iron deficiency: Is it true anemia or "sport anemia"? *Physician Sportsmed* 26(2):24, 1998.
48. Powers M: Ephedra and its application to sport performance: Another concern for the athletic trainer? *J Athl Train* 36(4):420, 2001.

49. Powers M, Arnold B, Weltman A: Creatine supplementation increases total body water without altering fluid distribution, *J Athl Train* 38(1):44, 2003.

50. Powers S, DeRuisseau K: Dietary antioxidants and exercise, *Journal of Sports Sciences* 22(1):81, 2004.

51. Rauh M, Nichols J: Relationships among injury and disordered eating, menstrual dysfunction, and low bone mineral density in high school athletes: A prospective study, *J Athl Train* 45(3):243–52, 2010.

52. Ray T, Flowers B: What you need to know about performance-enhancing supplements, *Athletic Therapy Today* 11(2):56, 2006.

53. Reimers K: The role of liquid supplements in weight gain, *Strength Cond* 17(1):64,1995.

54. Reissig C: Caffeinated energy drinks—A growing problem. *Drug and Alcohol Dependence* 99(1):1–10, 2009.

55. Rodriguez N: The role of nutrition in injury prevention and healing, *Athletic Therapy Today* 4(6):27, 1999.

56. Sanborn CF: Disordered eating and the female athlete triad, *Clin Sports Med* 19(2):199, 2000.

57. Sawyer TH, editor: *A guide to sport nutrition: For student-athletes, coaches, athletic trainers, and parents,* Champaign, IL, 2003, Sagamore.

58. Schlosser, E: *Fast food nation: The dark side of the all-American meal,* New York, 2005, Harper Perennial.

59. Selkow N, Pietrosimone B: Subcutaneous thigh fat assessment: A comparison of skin-fold calipers and ultrasound imaging, *J Athl Train* 46(1):50–54, 2011.

60. Shi X, Gisolfi CV: Fluid and carbohydrate replacement during intermittent exercise, *Sports Med* 25(3):157, 1998.

61. Snyder, M: The antioxidant counter: A pocket guide to the revolutionary ORAC acale for choosing healthy foods, Berkeley, 2011, Ulysses Press.

62. Spriet L, Gibala M: Nutritional strategies to influence adaptations to training, *Journal of Sports Sciences* 22(1):127, 2004.

63. Stout J., Antonia, J. *Essentials of creatine in sports and health.* Clifton, NJ, 2010, Humana Press.

64. Sundgot-Borgen J: Eating disorders in athletes. In Sundgot-Borgen J, editor: *Nutrition in sport,* Oxford, England, 2000, Blackwell.

65. Terjung R, Clarkson P, Eichner R: American College of Sports Medicine roundtable on the physicological and health effects of oral creatine supplementation, *Med Sci Sports Exerc* 32(3):706, 2000.

66. Turk JC, Prentice WE: Collegiate coaches' knowledge of eating disorders, *J Athl Train* 34(1):19, 1999.

67. U.S. Department of Agriculture. *Dietary guidelines for Americans 2010,* Washington DC, U.S. Government Printing Office.

68. Vaughn J, King K, Cottrell R: Collegiate athletic trainers confidence in helping female athletes with eating disorders, *J Athl Train* 39(1):71, 2004.

69. Vinci D: Navigating the low-carb craze, *Athletic Therapy Today* 10(1):20, 2005.

70. Vinci D: Negotiating the maze of nutritional ergogenic aids. *Athletic Therapy Today* 8(2):28, 2003.

71. Vinci, DM: The training room: Developing a sports-nutrition game plan, *Athletic Therapy Today* 7(5):52, 2002.

72. Vinci DM: What's for lunch? *Athletic Therapy Today* 8(1):50, 2003.

73. Weil A. 2008. *Eating well for optimal health: The essential guide to food, diet and nutrition,* 2008, London, Sphere.

74. Wilder N, Deivert R, Hagerman F: The effects of low-dose creatine supplementation versus creatine loading in collegiate football players, *J Athl Train* 36(2):124, 2001.

75. Williams M: *Nutrition for health, fitness and sports,* Boston, 2009, McGraw-Hill.

76. Winterstein A, Storrs C: Herbal supplements: Considerations for the athletic trainer, *J Athl Train* 36(4):425, 2001.

77. Zawila L, Steib C, Hoogenboom B: The female, collegiate, cross-country runner: Nutritional knowledge and attitudes, *J Athl Train* 38(1):67, 2003.

ANNOTATED BIBLIOGRAPHY

American Dietetic Association, Dyrugff R: *Complete food and nutrition guide,* ed 4, Minnetonka, MN, 2012, Chronimed.

An extensive text packed with information concerning every aspect of eating and food safety. Highly recommended for individuals who aspire to the highest understanding of healthful eating.

Bernadot D: *Advanced sports nutrition,* Champaign, IL, 2012, Human Kinetics.

Presents cutting-edge nutritional concepts tailored for application by athletes in any sport.

Clark N: *Sport nutrition guidebook: Eating to fuel your active lifestyle,* Champaign, IL, 2008, Human Kinetics.

Provides real-life case studies of nutritional advice given to athletes; also provides recommendations for pregame meals.

Hendler S, Rorvik D: *PDR for nutritional supplements,* Montvale, NJ, 2008, Medical Economics Company.

From the publishers of the Physicians, Desk Reference; gathers solid clinical evidence about the use of dietary supplements from the available medical literature and presents it in a unique and authoritative manner.

Sheldan M: *Wellness encyclopedia for food and nutrition,* New York, 2002, Rebus.

Covers every type of whole, fresh food found in supermarkets, specialty shops, and health-food stores. Also presents information on what makes up a healthy diet and the connection between diet and disease protection.

Wardlaw G: *Contemporary nutrition,* New York, 2010, McGraw-Hill.

Presents nutritional concepts tailored for application by athletes in any sport.

Weil A: *Eating well for optimum health: the essential guide to food, diet, and nutrition,* New York, 2008, Knopf.

A thorough rundown of nutritional basics and a primer on micronutrients, such as vitamins, minerals, and fiber.

Williams M: *Nutrition for fitness and sport,* Boston, 2009, McGraw-Hill.

Thorough coverage of the role nutrition plays in enhancing health, fitness, and sport performance. Current research and practical activities incorporated throughout.

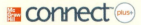

6

Environmental Considerations

■ Objectives

When you finish this chapter you should be able to

- Describe the physiology of hyperthermia.
- Recognize the clinical signs of heat stress and how they can be prevented.
- Identify the causes of hypothermia and the major cold disorders and how they can be prevented.
- Examine the problems that high altitude might present to the athlete, and explain how they can be managed.
- Review how an athlete should be protected from exposure to the sun.

- Describe precautions that should be taken in a lightning storm.
- List the problems that air pollution presents to the athlete and how they can be avoided.
- Discuss what effect circadian dysrhythmia can have on athletes and the best procedures for handling this problem.
- Compare the effect of synthetic versus natural turf on the incidence of injury.

■ Outline

■ Key Terms

hypothermia SPF
circadian dysrhythmia flash-to-bang
hyperthermia

■ Connect Highlights connect plus+

Visit connect.mcgraw-hill.com for further exercises to apply your knowledge:

- Clinical application scenarios covering physiology of hyperthermia, clinical signs of heat stress, high altitude management, circadian dysrhythmia, protection of exposure to the sun, precautions of inclement weather, and playing surfaces
- Click-and-drag questions covering heat conditions, clinical signs of heat stress and prevention, environmental conditions, and air quality
- Multiple-choice questions covering recognition and prevention of hyperthermia and heat illnesses, inclement weather, sun exposure, circadian dysrhythmia, and playing surfaces
- Selection questions covering hyponatremia, lightning safety, and prevention of heat illnesses

Environmental stress can adversely affect performance and in some instances can pose a serious health threat.[31,71] The environmental categories that are of major concern to athletic trainers, particularly those involved in outdoor sports, are hyperthermia, hypothermia, altitude, exposure to the sun, lightning storms, air pollution, and circadian dysrhythmia (jet lag).

HYPERTHERMIA

Hyperthermia is a condition in which, for one reason or another, body temperature is elevated. Over the years, hyperthermia has caused a number of deaths in athletes at the secondary-school, collegiate, and professional levels.[42]

hyperthermia Elevated body temperature.

It is vitally important that the athletic trainer and the coaching staff have knowledge about temperature and humidity factors to assist them in planning practice. The athletic trainer must clearly understand when environmental heat and humidity are at a dangerous level and must make recommendations to the coaches accordingly to prevent the occurrence of heat-related illnesses. In addition, the athletic trainer must recognize and properly manage the clinical signs and symptoms of heat-related illnesses.

Heat Stress

Regardless of the level of physical conditioning, athletes must take extreme caution when exercising in hot, humid weather. Prolonged exposure to extreme heat can result in heat illness.[12] Heat stress is preventable, but each year many athletes suffer illness and even death from a heat-related cause.[32] Anyone who engages in exercise in hot, humid environments is particularly vulnerable to heat stress.[20] Some athletes have medical conditions such as sickle-cell trait (see Chapter 29) which make them more susceptible to the dangers of exercising in hot humid conditions. Young athletes and elderly are particularly susceptible to heat stress.

Although heat-related illnesses most often occur in hot, humid, sunny conditions, an individual training or competing in a cold environment may also be susceptible if he or she becomes dehydrated or if protective equipment does not allow heat dissipation through the sweating mechanism.[17]

The physiological processes in the body will continue to function only as long as body temperature is maintained within a normal range.[15] The maintenance of normal temperature in a hot environment depends on the body's ability to dissipate heat. Body temperature can be affected by five factors, described in the following sections.

Metabolic Heat Production Normal metabolic function results in the production and radiation of heat. Consequently, metabolism always causes an increase in body heat that depends on the intensity of the physical activity. The higher the metabolic rate, the more heat produced.

Heat can be gained or lost through:
• Metabolic heat production
• Conductive heat exchange
• Convective heat exchange
• Radiant heat exchange
• Evaporative heat loss

Conductive Heat Exchange Physical contact with other objects can result in either a heat loss or a heat gain. A football player competing on artificial turf on a sunny August afternoon experiences an increase in body temperature simply by standing on synthetic turf.

Convective Heat Exchange Convection occurs when a mass of either air or water moves around an individual. Body heat can be either lost or gained, depending on the temperature of the circulating medium. A cool breeze tends to cool the body by removing heat from the body surface. Conversely, if the temperature of the circulating air is higher than the temperature of the skin, body heat increases.

Radiant Heat Exchange Radiant heat from sunshine causes an increase in body temperature. Obviously, the effects of this radiation are much greater in the sunshine than in the shade.[29] On a cloudy day, the body also emits radiant heat energy; thus, radiation may result in either heat loss or heat gain. During exercise the body attempts to dissipate heat produced by metabolism by dilating superficial arterial and venous vessels, thus channeling blood to the superficial capillaries in the skin.

Evaporative Heat Loss Sweat glands in the skin allow water to be transported to the surface, where it evaporates, taking large quantities of heat with it. When the temperature and radiant heat of the environment become higher than body temperature, the loss of body heat becomes highly dependent on the process of sweat evaporation.

The rate of sweating is critical for an athlete to dissipate heat. A normal person can sweat off about 1 quart of water per hour for about 2 hours. However, certain individuals can lose as much as 2 quarts of water (4 pounds) per hour.[62] *Focus Box 6–1:* "Variations in Sweat Rates" identifies the factors that influence sweat rates. Sweating does not cause heat loss. The sweat must evaporate for heat to be dissipated. But the air must be relatively free of water for evaporation to occur. Heat loss through evaporation is severely impaired when the relative humidity reaches 65 percent and virtually stops when the humidity reaches 75 percent.

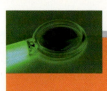

Variations in sweat rates

Sweat rates can vary considerably from one athlete to another and are determined by a number of factors:

- Athlete's height and weight (heavier athletes sweat more)
- Degree of acclimatization (well-acclimated athletes sweat earlier and more)
- Fitness level (fit athletes sweat more)
- Hydration status (athletes who begin activity well hydrated sweat earlier)
- Environmental conditions
- Clothing
- Intensity and duration of activity
- Heredity

Preventing Heat Illness

The athletic trainer should understand that heat illness is preventable if he or she exercises some common sense and caution. An athlete can only perform at an optimal level when dehydration and hyperthermia are minimized by the ingestion of ample volumes of fluid during exercise and when commonsense precautions are used to keep cool.[3,63] (See *Focus Box 6–2:* "NATA recommendations for preventing heat illness." The links to the NATA position statement "Exertional heat illnesses" (http://www.nata.org/sites/default/files/ExternalHeatIllnesses.pdf), and the consensus statement "Interassociation task force on exertional heat illness" (http://www.nata.org/sites/default/files/inter-association-task-force-exertional-heat-illness.pdf) can both be found at www.mhhe.com/prentice15e.) The following factors should be considered when planning a training or competitive program that is likely to take place during hot weather.

Prevention of hyperthermia:

- Appropriate hydration
- Unrestricted fluid and electrolyte replacement
- Gradual acclimatization
- Identification of susceptible individuals
- Appropriate uniforms
- Weight records
- Monitoring of the heat index

Hydration Athletes should always begin activities in a well-hydrated state.[12,21] It is essential that the athlete be aware of the importance of ingesting sufficient fluids throughout the 24-hour period preceding exercise, to make certain that he or she is appropriately hydrated. The best way to check this is to monitor the color of the urine. The urine should appear to be light yellow (the color of lemonade). If it is completely clear, this may indicate overhydration. Dark urine (the color of cider) indicates dehydration.

The hydration process should involve ingesting small quantities of fluid at regular intervals throughout the day rather than drinking a huge volume all at once.[46] It has been recommended that an athlete drink 17 to 20 fluid ounces of water or a sports drink 2 to 3 hours before exercise and drink another 7 to 10 fluid ounces of water or a sports drink 10 to 20 minutes before exercise.[63]

Dehydration An athlete who does not replenish fluids is likely to become dehydrated. Whenever an individual is exercising, some dehydration will occur, because it is difficult to balance fluid loss through sweating with fluid intake. An individual is said to have mild dehydration when fluids lost are less than 2 percent of normal body weight.[77] Even mild dehydration can impair cardiovascular and thermoregulatory response and can reduce the capacity for exercise and have a negative effect on performance.[47,63] Individuals who are becoming dehydrated may exhibit any or all of the following symptoms and signs: thirst, dry mouth, headache, dizziness, irritability, lethargy, excessive fatigue, and possibly cramps. Obviously, an athlete who is dehydrated needs to replace fluids and should be moved to a cool environment. The athlete should rehydrate with a sports drink that contains carbohydrates and electrolytes (particularly sodium and potassium) and should not return to full activity until he or she is symptom free and has returned to normal body weight.[28] It is important to note that fluid replacement should not exceed fluid loss. Again, individuals can determine when they have reached an appropriate level of hydration by monitoring the color of their urine.

> Mild dehydration is the loss of less than 2 percent of body weight.

> Fluid intake should equal fluid loss.

Fluid and Electrolyte Replacement During hot weather, it is essential that athletes continually replace fluids lost through evaporation by drinking large quantities of water or other beverages throughout the day.[37,78] The average adult doing minimal physical activity requires at least 2.5 liters, or about 10 glasses, of water a day. A normal sweat-loss rate for a person during an hour of exercise ranges between 0.8 and 3 liters, with an average of 1.5 liters

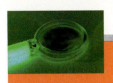

NATA recommendations for preventing heat illness[11]

- Ensure that appropriate medical care is available.
- Conduct a thorough physician-supervised preparticipation exam to identify susceptible individuals.
- Acclimatize athletes over 10 to 14 days.
- Educate athletes and coaches regarding the prevention, recognition, and treatment of heat illnesses.
- Educate athletes to balance fluid intake with sweat and urine losses to maintain adequate hydration.
- Encourage athletes to sleep 6 to 8 hours per night in a cool environment.
- Monitor environmental conditions and develop guidelines for altering practice sessions based on those conditions.

- Provide an adequate supply of water or sports drinks to maintain hydration.
- Weigh high-risk athletes before and after practice to make certain they are not dehydrated.
- Minimize the amount of equipment and clothing worn in hot, humid conditions.
- Minimize warm-up time in hot, humid conditions.
- Allow athletes to practice in shaded areas and use cooling fans when possible.
- Have appropriate emergency equipment available (e.g., fluids, ice, immersion tank, rectal thermometer, telephone or two-way radio).

per hour. Because water is so vital, the healthy body carefully manages its internal water levels.[72] When body weight drops by 1 to 2 percent (1.5 to 3 pounds in a 150-pound individual), he or she begins to feel thirsty.[63] Drinking water and other beverages eventually returns the internal water levels to normal. However, if thirst signals are ignored and body water continues to decrease, dehydration results. People who are dehydrated cannot generate enough energy, and they feel weak. Dehydration is more likely to occur when an individual is outdoors and is sweating heavily while engaging in some strenuous activity. To prevent dehydration, an athlete should make sure to replace the lost water by drinking plenty of fluids and not relying on thirst as a signal that it's time to have a drink. By the time thirst develops, the body is already slightly dehydrated. Many people ignore their thirst, or if they do heed it, they don't drink enough, especially during physical activity. Most people replace only about 50 percent of the water they lose through sweating.[63] For this reason, athletes should consciously consume fluids before, during, and after practice and competition.

Athletes must have unlimited access to fluids. There is no acceptable reason for allowing or causing an athlete to become hypohydrated.[64] Failure to permit ad libitum access to fluids not only undermine an athlete's performance but also may predispose the athlete to unnecessary heat-related illnesses (Figure 6–1).

A number of adverse physiological and potentially pathological effects can be caused by hypohydration, including reduced muscular strength and endurance, decreased blood and plasma volume, altered cardiac function, impaired thermoregulation, decreased kidney function, reduced glycogen stores, and loss of electrolytes.[64] Athletes who are taking creatine or using carbohydrate gels for

energy must make certain to consume sufficient fluids to stay appropriately hydrated.[6,83]

It has been shown that replacing lost fluids with an appropriately formulated sports drink is more effective than using water alone.[55] Research has shown that because of the flavor, an athlete is likely to drink more sports drinks than plain water. In addition, sports drinks replace both the fluids and the electrolytes that are lost

> **Sports drinks are more effective than water for fluid replacement.**

in sweat, and they provide energy in the form of carbohydrates to the working muscles. Water is a good thirst quencher, but it is not a good rehydrator because it actually "turns off" thirst before the body is completely rehydrated. Water also "turns on" the kidneys prematurely, so an individual loses fluid in the form of urine more quickly than when he or she is drinking a sports drink. The small

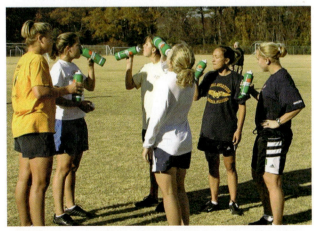

FIGURE 6–1 Athletes must have unlimited access to fluids, especially in hot weather.

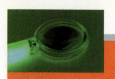

FOCUS 6–3 Focus on Injury/Illness Prevention and Wellness Protection

Recommendations for fluid replacement*

- Athletes should begin all exercise sessions well hydrated[77] (determined by light yellow color of urine).
- A hydration protocol for fluid replacement should be established.
- To ensure proper hydration, the athlete should consume 17 to 20 ounces of water or a sports drink 2 to 3 hours before exercise and then 7 to 10 ounces 10 to 20 minutes before exercise.
- Fluid replacement beverages should be easily accessible during activity and should be consumed at a minimal rate of 7 to 10 ounces every 10 to 20 minutes.
- During activity, the athlete should consume the maximal amount of fluid that can be tolerated, but it is important that fluid intake does not exceed fluid loss.
- A cool, flavored beverage at refrigerator temperature is recommended.

- The addition of proper amounts of carbohydrates and electrolytes to a fluid replacement solution is recommended for exercise events that last longer than 50 minutes or are intense.
- For vigorous exercise lasting less than 1 hour, the addition of carbohydrates and electrolytes does enhance physical performance.
- A 6 percent carbohydrate solution appears to be optimal (14 grams of carbohydrate per 8-ounce serving). A concentration greater than 8 percent slows gastric emptying.
- Adding a modest amount of sodium (0.3 to 0.7 gram per liter) is acceptable to stimulate thirst and increase fluid intake.

*Based on recommendations from the National Athletic Trainers' Association,[19] American College of Sports Medicine,[1] and Gatorade Sport Science Institute.[63]

---

amount of sodium in sports drinks allows the body to hold on to the fluid consumed rather than losing it through urine.[63]

Not all sports drinks are the same. How a sports drink is formulated dictates how well it works to provide rapid rehydration and energy. The optimal level of carbohydrate is 14 grams per 8 ounces of water (6 percent carbohydrate) for the quickest fluid absorption.[28] Sports drinks or even carbohydrate gels with greater than 6 percent carbohydrate, as well as sports drinks with too little carbohydrate, are absorbed more slowly. For this reason, appropriately formulated sports drinks should be used without diluting to maximize their rate of absorption. Most sports drinks contain no carbonation or artificial preservatives, so they are satisfying during exercise and cause no stomach bloating. Also, most sports drinks contain a minimal number of calories.

It has been clearly established that sports drinks are effective for enhancing long-term endurance exercise.[12,21,72] It has also been suggested that sports drinks are effective for improving performance during both endurance activities and short-term, high-intensity activities, such as soccer, basketball, and tennis, that last from 30 minutes to an hour.[28] *Focus Box 6–3:* "Recommendations for Fluid Replacement" provides some suggestions for using sports drinks. A link to the NATA position statement on "Fluid replacement for athletes" (http://www.nata.org/sites/default/files/FluidReplacementsForAthletes.pdf) can be found at www.mhhe.com/prentice15e.[15]

Gradual Acclimatization Gradual acclimatization is critical in avoiding heat stress. Acclimatization should involve not only becoming accustomed to heat but also becoming acclimatized to exercising in hot temperatures.[42] A good preseason conditioning program, started well before the advent of the competitive season and carefully graded as to intensity, is recommended.[20] Progressive exposure should occur over a 7- to 10-day period.[64] During the first 5 or 6 days, an 80 percent acclimatization can be achieved on the basis of a 2-hour practice period in the morning and a 2-hour practice period in the afternoon. Each practice period should be broken down into 20 minutes of work alternated with 20 minutes of rest in the shade. Equipment restrictions may help the athlete become gradually acclimated. *Focus Box 6–4:* "NCAA-mandated guidelines for acclimatization in preseason football practices" shows how the NCAA mandates the use of equipment in preseason football. A link to the NATA consensus statement "Preseason heat acclimatization guidelines for high school athletes" (http://www.nata.org/health-issues/heat-acclimatization) can be found at www.mhhe.com/prentice15e.

Identifying Susceptible Individuals Athletes with a large muscle mass are particularly prone to heat illness.[20] Body build must be considered when determining individual susceptibility to heat stress. Overweight individuals may have as much as 18 percent greater heat production than underweight individuals, because metabolic heat is produced

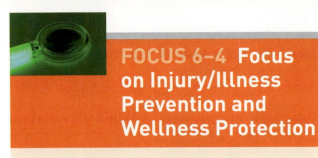

FOCUS 6-4 Focus on Injury/Illness Prevention and Wellness Protection

NCAA-mandated guidelines for acclimatization in preseason football practices[64]

Days 1–5	Only one practice per day—equipment use restricted
Days 1 and 2	Helmets only
Days 3 and 4	Helmets and shoulder pads only
Day 5	Full pads
After day 5	Twice-a-day practices every other day

proportionately to surface area. It has been found that heat illness victims tend to be overweight. Death from heatstroke increases at a ratio of approximately four to one as body weight increases.[19]

Women are apparently more physiologically efficient at body temperature regulation than are men. Although women possess as many heat-activated sweat glands as men do, they sweat less and manifest a higher heart rate when working in heat.[55] Although slight differences exist, the same precautionary measures apply to both genders.

Other individuals who are susceptible to heat stress include the young, the elderly, those with relatively poor fitness levels, those with a history of

heat illness, and anyone with a febrile condition.[64] A link to an NATA official statement "Youth football and heat related illness" (http://www.nata.org/sites/default/files/HeatRelatedIllness.pdf) can be found at www.mhhe.com/prentice15e.

Selecting Appropriate Uniforms Uniforms should be selected on the basis of temperature and humidity. Initial practices should be conducted in short-sleeved T-shirts, shorts, and socks, and athletes should be moved gradually into short-sleeved net jerseys, lightweight pants, and socks as acclimatization proceeds. All early-season practices and games should be conducted in lightweight uniforms with short-sleeved net jerseys and socks. The use of dark-colored clothing or uniforms should be discouraged. Rubberized suits should never be used.[64]

Maintaining Weight Records Careful weight records of all players must be kept. Weights should be measured both before and after practice for at least the first 2 weeks of practice or as long as hot, humid conditions persist. If a sudden increase in temperature or humidity occurs during the season, weight should be recorded again for a period of time. A loss of greater than 2 percent of body weight indicates that the athlete is severely dehydrated and should be held out of practice until normal body weight has returned.[86]

Monitoring the Heat Index The athletic trainer must exercise common sense when overseeing the health care of athletes who are training or competing in the heat. Obviously, when the combination of heat, humidity, and bright sunshine is present, extra caution is warranted (Figure 6–2). The universal

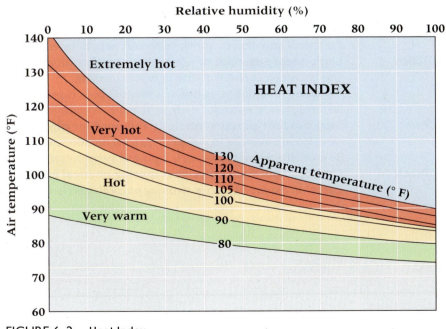

FIGURE 6–2   Heat Index

wet bulb globe temperature (WBGT) index provides the athletic trainer with an objective means for determining necessary precautions for practice and competition in hot weather.[14] The index incorporates readings from several different thermometers. The dry bulb temperature (DBT) is recorded from a standard mercury thermometer. The wet bulb temperature (WBT) uses a wet wick or piece of gauze wrapped around the end of a thermometer that is swung around in the air. Globe temperature (GT) measures the sun's radiation and has a black metal casing around the end of the thermometer. Once the three readings have been taken, the following formula is used to calculate the WBGT index:

$$WBGT = 0.1 \times DBT + 0.7 \times WBT + GT \times 0.2$$

If only web bulb and dry bulb temperatures are taken, the WBGT index is calculated using the following modified formula:

$$WBGT = 0.3 \times DBT + 0.7 \times WBT$$

Using this formula yields a universally accepted WBGT index (Table 6–1), on which recommendations relative to outdoor activity are based. Table 6–2 is a modification of the WBGT index that indicates activity restrictions for outdoor physical conditioning in hot weather.

The DBT and WBT can be measured easily using a *psychrometer*. It consists of two identical thermometers—the wet bulb thermometer and the dry bulb thermometer. When the cloth is soaked and the thermometers are properly ventilated, the wet

TABLE 6–1 Universal WBGT Index

Heat Category	WBGT °F	Easy Work Work/Rest*	Easy Work Water per Hour	Moderate Work Work/Rest*	Moderate Work Water per Hour	Hard Work Work/Rest*	Hard Work Water per Hour
1	78–81.9	No limit	1/2 qt	No limit	3/4 qt	40/20 min	3/4 qt
2	82–84.9	No limit	1/2 qt	50/10 min	3/4 qt	30/30 min	1 qt
3	85–87.9	No limit	3/4 qt	40/20 min	3/4 qt	30/30 min	1 qt
4	88–89.9	No limit	3/4 qt	30/30 min	3/4 qt	20/40 min	1 qt
5	≥90	50/10 min	1 qt	20/40 min	1 qt	10/50 min	1 qt

*Rest means minimal physical activity (sitting or standing) and should be accomplished in the shade if possible.

TABLE 6–2 Activity Restrictions for Outdoor Physical Conditioning in Hot Weather

WBGT* (° F)	Flag Color††	Guidance† for Nonacclimatized Personnel in Boldface / Guidance for Fully Acclimatized Personnel in Italics
<78.0° F	No flag	**Extreme exertion may precipitate heat illness.** *Normal activity*
78.0° F–82.0° F	Green	**Use discretion in planning intense exercise.** *Normal activity* Pay special attention to at-risk individuals in both cases.
82.1° F–86.0° F	Yellow	**Limit intense exercise to 1 hour; limit total outdoor exercise to 2.5 hours.** *Use discretion in planning intense physical activity.* Pay special attention to at-risk individuals in both cases. Be on high alert; watch for early signs and symptoms in both cases.
86.1° F–89.9° F	Red	**Stop outdoor practice sessions and outdoor physical conditioning.** *Limit intense exercise to 1 hour; limit total outdoor exercise to 4 hours.* Be on high alert; watch for early signs and symptoms throughout.
≥90° F	Black	**Cancel all outdoor exercise requiring physical exertion.** *Cancel all outdoor exercise involving physical exertion.*

Modified from Nunnelly SA, Reardon MJ: Prevention of heat illness. In Pandolf KB, Burr RE, editors: *Medical aspects of harsh environments: volume I,* Washington, DC, 2002, TMM.

*WGBT is wet bulb globe temperature.
Calculation of WBGT: $0.7 T_{wb} + 0.2 T_{bg} + 0.1 T_{db}$, where T_{wb} is wet bulb temperature; T_{bg} is black globe temperature; T_{db} is dry bulb temperature.
†Guidelines assume that athletes are wearing summer-weight clothing and that all activities are constantly supervised by an athletic trainer to assure early detection of problems. When equipment must be worn, as in football, please use guidelines one step below. For example, if WBGT is 86° F (yellow), then use the guidelines for red.
††Flag color indicates a warning flag, which is placed in a location visible from a practice field, that is used to notify everyone using that facility what the conditions are and the restrictions that should be applied.

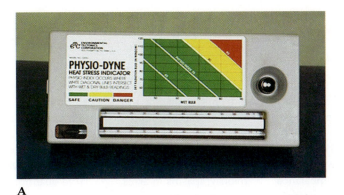

A

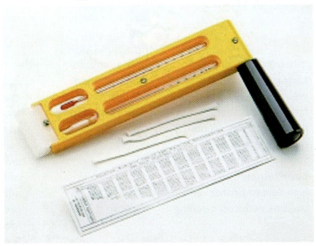

B

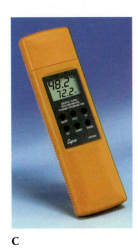

C

FIGURE 6–3   (A) Physio-Dyne. (B) Sling psychrometer. (C) Digital psychrometer.
All can be used to determine the WBGT heat index.

bulb temperature will be lower than the dry bulb temperature (actual air temperature) because of cooling due to the evaporation of water from the cloth. The drier the air is, the greater the evaporation, and thus the more wet bulb temperature is depressed. In some units, such as the Physio-Dyne, ventilation is provided by a suction fan (aspiration psychrometer) (Figure 6–3A) or thermometers at the end of a chain (sling psychrometer) (Figure 6–3B). Newer psychrometers use digital sensors (Figure 6–3C). Recording the temperature requires about 90 seconds. Either instrument is relatively inexpensive and easy to use, although it appears that the old sling psychrometer may have the greatest accuracy.[19]

Recognizing and Managing Exertional Heat Illnesses

In 2003, a consensus statement on exertional heat illnesses was prepared by an interassociation task force; the statement included input from experts representing 18 professional sports medicine organizations.[42] Exercising in a hot, humid environment can cause various forms of heat illness, including heat rash, heat syncope, exertional heat cramps, exertional heat exhaustion, exertional heatstroke, and exertional hyponatremia.[5,6,47]

Heat Rash Heat rash, also called prickly heat, is a benign condition associated with a red, raised rash accompanied by sensations of prickling and tingling during sweating. It usually occurs when the skin is continuously wet with unevaporated sweat. The rash is generally localized to areas of the body that are covered with clothing. Continually toweling the body can help prevent the rash from developing.[27]

Heat Syncope Heat syncope, or heat collapse, is associated with rapid physical fatigue during overexposure to heat. It is usually caused by standing in heat for long periods or by not being accustomed to exercising in the heat. It is caused by peripheral vasodilation of superficial vessels, hypotension, or a pooling of blood in the extremities, which results in dizziness, fainting, and nausea. Heat syncope is quickly relieved by laying the athlete down in a cool environment, elevating the lower extremities, and replacing fluids.[12]

Exertional Heat Cramps Heat cramps are extremely painful muscle spasms that occur most commonly in the calf and abdomen, although any muscle can be involved (Table 6–3). The occurrence

| | | **TABLE 6–3** | **Heat Disorders** | |

Disorder	Cause	Clinical Features and Diagnosis	Prevention	Treatment
Heat syncope	Rapid physical fatigue during overexposure to heat	Pooling of blood in extremities, leading to dizziness, fainting, and nausea	Gradually acclimatize to exercising in a hot, humid environment	Lying down in a cool environment, replenishing fluids
Exertional heat cramps	Hard work in heat, sweating heavily, imbalance between water and electrolytes (sodium)	Muscle twitching and cramps, usually after midday; spasms in arms, legs, and abdomen	Acclimatize athlete properly; provide large quantities of fluids; increase intake of calcium, sodium, and potassium slightly	Ingesting large amounts of fluid, mild stretching, ice massage of affected muscle
Exertional heat exhaustion	Prolonged sweating leading to dehydration and an inability to sustain adequate cardiac output	Excessive thirst, dry tongue and mouth, weight loss, fatigue, weakness, incoordination, mental dullness, low urine volume, slightly elevated body temperature, high serum protein and sodium, reduced swelling	Supply adequate fluids; provide adequate rest and opportunity for cooling	Bed rest in cool room, IV fluids if drinking is impaired; increase fluid intake to 6 to 8 L/day; sponge with cool water; keep records of body weight and fluid balance; provide semiliquid food until salination is normal
Exertional heatstroke	Thermoregulatory failure of sudden onset	Abrupt onset; CNS abnormalities, including headache, vertigo, and fatigue; flushed skin; relatively less sweating than seen with heat exhaustion; rapidly increasing pulse rate that may reach 160 to 180; increased respiration; blood pressure seldom rises; rapid rise in temperature to 104°F (40°C); athlete feels as if he or she is burning up; diarrhea, vomiting; can lead to permanent brain damage; circulatory collapse may produce death	Ensure proper acclimatization and proper hydration; educate those supervising activities conducted in the heat; adapt activities to the environment; screen participants with history of heat illness for malignant hyperthermia	Take immediate emergency measures to reduce temperature (e.g., immersion in ice-water bath or sponge cool water and air fan over body, massage limbs); remove to hospital as soon as possible
Exertional hyponatremia	Fluid/electrolyte disorder resulting in low concentration of sodium in the blood	Progressively worsening headache, nausea and vomiting, swelling in hands and feet, lethargy or apathy, low blood sodium, compromised central nervous system	Hydrate with sports drinks; increase sodium intake; make sure fluid intake equals fluid loss	Do not try to rehydrate; transport to medical facility; sodium levels must be increased and fluid levels decreased

of heat cramps is related to the excessive loss of water and several electrolytes or ions (sodium, chloride, potassium, magnesium, and calcium), but

> Heat cramps occur because of an imbalance between water and electrolytes.

especially sodium, that are essential elements in muscle contraction.

Profuse sweating involves losses of large amounts of water and small quantities of sodium, potassium,

> Heat cramps involve excessive loss of water and sodium.

magnesium, and calcium, thus destroying the balance in the

concentration of these elements within the body. This imbalance will ultimately result in painful muscle contractions and cramps.[44] The person most likely to get heat cramps is one who is in fairly good condition but who is not acclimatized to the heat.

Heat cramps may be prevented by adequate replacement of sodium, chloride, potassium, magnesium, calcium, and, most important, fluids.[7,11,35] Ingestion of salt tablets may help prevent cramps. Simply salting food a bit more heavily can replace sodium. Bananas are particularly high in potassium, and calcium is present in milk, cheese, and other dairy products. The immediate treatment for heat cramps is ingestion of large quantities of fluids, preferably a sports drink, and mild, prolonged stretching with ice massage of the muscle in spasm. An athlete who experiences heat cramps may have difficulty returning to practice or competition for the remainder of the day, because cramping is likely to reoccur with physical exertion.

Exertional Heat Exhaustion Exertional heat exhaustion is a more moderate form of heat illness that occurs from environmental heat stress and strenuous

> Exertional heat exhaustion results from dehydration.

physical exercise. In exertional heat exhaustion, an athlete becomes

dehydrated to the point that he or she is unable to sustain adequate cardiac output and thus cannot continue intense exercise. Mild hyperthermia is characteristic of heat exhaustion, with a rectal temperature of less

> Measuring rectal temperature is critical to differentiate heat exhaustion from heatstroke.

than 104°F and no evidence of central nervous system (CNS)

dysfunction.[39] Obtaining an accurate rectal temperature measurement is essential for the athletic trainer to differentiate between heat exhaustion and heatstroke. Rectal temperature is core temperature. Measuring temperature at any other site with any other type of thermometer will not provide a sufficiently accurate reading.[39,54,55] See *Focus Box 6–5:* "Measuring rectal

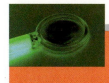

Measuring rectal temperature

Monitoring temperature with a thermometer inserted into the rectum is the most exact way of determining core temperature. Normal rectal temperature is 99.6°F (37.5°C).

- When using a glass thermometer shake the thermometer down to below the 97.8°F mark (36.18°C).
- Cover the tip of the glass thermometer or a flexible digital thermometer with lubricating or petroleum jelly.

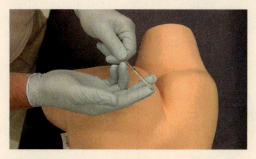

- Place the athlete on his or her stomach.
- Spread the buttocks and gently insert the thermometer 8–10 cm into the rectum. Never force it. Hold the buttocks together to keep the thermometer in place.
- If using a flexible digital thermometer tape can be used to secure it in place.

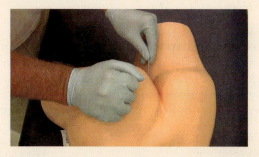

- Do not release your grip on a glass thermometer.
- Leave the thermometer in place for 3 minutes.
- To read the temperature on a glass thermometer, slowly turn the thermometer until you can see the line of mercury.
- Wash the thermometer carefully in soap and warm water after each use. Store in a safe place.

temperature" for a description of the procedure. An athlete who is experiencing heat exhaustion shows signs and symptoms of dehydration and/or electrolyte depletion, including pale skin; profuse sweating; stomach cramps with nausea, vomiting, or diarrhea; headache; persistent muscle cramps; and dizziness with loss of coordination.[12]

6–1 Clinical Application Exercise

A wrestler collapses during a match and exhibits signs of profuse sweating, pale skin, mildly elevated temperature (102° F), dizziness, hyperventilation, and rapid pulse. When questioned by the athletic trainer, the wrestler indicates that earlier in the day he took diuretic medication to facilitate water loss in an effort to help him make weight.

? What type of heat illness is the athlete experiencing, and what does the athletic trainer need to do to manage this situation appropriately?

An athlete who has exertional heat exhaustion must be immediately removed from play and taken to a shaded or air-conditioned area. Excess clothing or equipment should be removed, and the athlete should lie down with his or her legs elevated. Cooling efforts should continue until rectal temperature has lowered to 101°F. Rehydration should begin immediately with water or a sports drink as long as the athlete is not nauseated or vomiting. If the athlete cannot take fluids orally, intravenous fluid replacement should be initiated by a physician. The athletic trainer should continually monitor heart rate, blood pressure, and core temperature. If rapid improvement is not observed, the athlete must be transported to an emergency facility. Exertional heat exhaustion, if not properly managed, can progress to exertional heatstroke. Before returning to play, the athlete must be completely rehydrated and should be cleared by a physician.

Exertional Heatstroke Unlike heat cramps and exertional heat exhaustion, exertional heatstroke is a serious, life-threatening emergency (Table 6–3).[22,52] It is the most severe form of heat illness and is induced by strenuous physical exercise and increased environmental heat stress. It is characterized by CNS abnormalities and potential tissue damage resulting from a significantly elevated body temperature. As body temperature rises, extreme circulatory and metabolic stresses can produce damage and severe physiological dysfunction, which can ultimately result in death.[36]

Heatstroke can occur suddenly and without warning.[52] The specific cause of heatstroke is unknown. It is clinically characterized by sudden collapse with CNS dysfunction, such as altered consciousness, seizures, confusion, emotional instability, irrational behavior, or decreased mental acuity. Measured rectal temperature is 104°F or higher. Additionally, the victim is flushed and has hot skin, with sweating about 75 percent of the time, although about 25 percent of the cases have less sweating than would be seen with heat exhaustion. Other symptoms include shallow, fast breathing; a rapid, strong pulse; nausea, vomiting, or diarrhea; headache, dizziness, or weakness; decreased blood pressure; and dehydration. The heatstroke victim experiences a breakdown of the thermoregulatory mechanism due to excessively high body temperature, and the body loses the ability to dissipate heat through sweating.[60]

> **Heatstroke is a life-threatening emergency.**

The possibility of death from heatstroke can be significantly reduced if the victim's body temperature is lowered to normal as soon as possible. The longer that the body temperature is elevated to 104°F or higher, the higher the mortality rate. Thus, the key to managing this condition is aggressive and immediate whole-body cooling.[56,57] **Get the athlete into a cool environment, strip off all clothing, and immerse the athlete in a cold-water bath (35°F to 58°F)**.[18,25,40,67] If it is not possible to immerse the athlete in cold water, sponge him or her down with cool water and fan with a towel.[74] Also ice bags may be placed at the neck, and over other major arterial vessels.[76] Try to lower rectal temperature to 101°F. Call the rescue squad. It is imperative that the victim be transported to a hospital as quickly as possible; however, it is recommended that the victim be cooled down first and then transported if onsite rapid cooling and adequate medical supervision are available.[53] If rescue squad transport is delayed, it may be necessary to transport the victim in whatever vehicle happens to be available. Following exertional heatstroke, the athlete should avoid exercise for a minimum of 1 week and gradually return to full practice after being completely asymptomatic and cleared by a physician.

Malignant Hyperthermia Malignant hyperthermia is a rare, genetically inherited muscle disorder that causes hypersensitivity to anesthesia and extreme exercise in hot environments.[15] It is characterized by muscle breakdown.[48] This disorder causes muscle temperatures to increase faster than core temperature, and its symptoms are similar to those of heatstroke. The athlete complains of muscle pain after exercise, and rectal temperature remains elevated

6–2 Clinical Application Exercise

A high-school football team is doing conditioning outside. The temperature is 80°F with 85 percent humidity. The players have their helmets on and are running 100-yard sprints. One player looks like he is becoming fatigued and slightly disoriented. Thirty yards into the sprint, the athlete collapses.

? What is the immediate course of action to treat this athlete? What is wrong with the athlete?

for 10 to 15 minutes after exercise. During this period, muscle tissue is destroyed and products of muscle breakdown may damage the kidneys and cause acute renal failure.[61] The condition may be fatal if not treated immediately. Muscle biopsy is necessary for diagnosis. Athletes with malignant hyperthermia should be disqualified from competing in hot, humid environments.[48]

Acute Exertional Rhabdomyolysis Acute exertional rhabdomyolysis is a syndrome characterized by sudden catabolic destruction and degeneration of skeletal muscle accompanied by leakage of myoglobin (muscle protein) and muscle enzymes into the vascular system.[8] It can occur in healthy individuals during intense exercise in extremely hot and humid environmental conditions. It can result in the gradual onset of muscle weakness, swelling, and pain and the presence of darkened urine and renal dysfunction; in severe cases, the individual experiences sudden collapse, renal failure, and death. Rhabdomyolysis has been associated with individuals with sickle-cell trait.[15] If rhabdomyolysis is suspected, the athlete should be referred to a physician immediately.

Exertional Hyponatremia Hyponatremia is a condition involving a fluid/electrolyte disorder that results in an abnormally low concentration of sodium in the blood.[12]

> **Hyponatremia occurs with low blood sodium levels.**

It is most often caused by ingesting so much fluid before, during, and after exercise that the concentration of sodium is decreased.[73] It can also occur due to too little sodium in the diet or in ingested fluids over a period of prolonged exercise.[59] An individual with a high rate of sweating and a significant loss of sodium, who continues to ingest large quantities of fluid over a several-hour period of exercise (as in a marathon or triathlon), is particularly vulnerable to developing hyponatremia. Hyponatremia can be avoided completely by making certain that fluid intake during exercise does not exceed fluid loss and that sodium intake is adequate.[59]

The signs and symptoms of exertional hyponatremia are a progressively worsening headache; nausea and vomiting; swelling of the hands and feet; lethargy, apathy, or agitation; and low blood sodium (<130 mmol/L). Ultimately, a very low concentration of sodium can compromise the central nervous system, creating a life-threatening situation.[42]

If the athletic trainer suspects exertional hyponatremia and blood sodium levels cannot be determined on-site, measures to rehydrate the athlete should be delayed and the athlete should be transported immediately to a medical facility.[24] At the medical facility, the delivery of sodium, certain diuretics, or intravenous solutions may be necessary. A physician should clear the athlete before he or she is allowed to return to play.

Clinical Indications and Treatment

Focus Box 6–6: "Environmental conduct of sports, particularly football" lists the clinical symptoms of the various hyperthermia conditions and the indications for treatment. Although the Focus Box calls particular attention to some of the procedures for football, the precautions in general apply to all sports. Because of the specialized equipment worn by the players, football requires special consideration. Many football uniforms are heat traps, compounding the environmental heat problem, which is not true of lighter uniforms.[7]

Guidelines for Athletes Who Intentionally Lose Weight

Wrestlers or other athletes who purposely dehydrate themselves as a means of making weight are predisposing themselves to heat-related illness and may, in fact, be creating a potentially life-threatening situation. Weight loss to make a predetermined weight limit should not be accomplished through dehydration. The process must be gradual over a period of several weeks, or even months, and should result from a reduction in the percentage of body fat relative to lean body mass. The NCAA and many state high-school federations have established guidelines for weight loss and set policies for how and when a wrestler can weigh in officially.[64]

HYPOTHERMIA

Cold weather is a frequent adjunct to many outdoor sports in which the sport itself does not require heavy, protective clothing; consequently, the weather becomes a pertinent factor in injury susceptibility.[57] In most instances, the activity itself enables the athlete to increase the metabolic rate sufficiently to function physically in

> **hypothermia**
> Abnormally low body temperature.

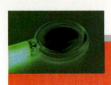

Environmental conduct of sports, particularly football

I. General warning
  A. Most adverse reactions to environmental heat and humidity occur during the first few days of training.
  B. It is necessary to become thoroughly acclimatized to heat to successfully compete in hot or humid environments.
  C. Occurrence of a heat injury indicates poor supervision of the sports program.

II. Athletes who are most susceptible to heat injury
  A. Individuals unaccustomed to working in the heat
  B. Overweight individuals, particularly large linemen
  C. Eager athletes who constantly compete at capacity
  D. Ill athletes who have an infection, a fever, or a gastrointestinal disturbance
  E. Athletes who receive immunization injections and subsequently develop temperature elevations

III. Prevention of heat injury
  A. Take a complete medical history and provide a physical examination.
    1. Include a history of previous heat illnesses or fainting in the heat.
    2. Include an inquiry about sweating and peripheral vascular defects.
  B. Evaluate general physical condition and type and duration of training activities for previous month.
    1. Extent of work in the heat
    2. General training activities
  C. Measure temperature and humidity on the practice or playing fields (WBGT index).
    1. Make measurements before and during training or competitive sessions.
    2. Adjust activity level to environmental conditions.
      a. Decrease activity if hot or humid.
      b. Eliminate unnecessary clothing when hot or humid.
  D. Acclimatize athletes to heat gradually.
    1. Acclimatization to heat requires work in the heat.
      a. Use recommended type and variety of warm-weather workouts for preseason training.
      b. Provide graduated training program for first 7 to 10 days and on other abnormally hot or humid days.
    2. Adequate rest intervals and fluid replacement should be provided during the acclimatization period.
  E. Monitor body weight loss during activity in the heat.
    1. Body fluid should be replaced as it is lost.
      a. Allow additional fluid as desired by players.
      b. Provide salt on training tables (no salt tablets should be taken).
      c. Weigh athletes each day before and after training or competition.
        (1) Treat athlete who loses excessive weight each day.
        (2) Treat well-conditioned athlete who continues to lose weight for several days.
  F. Monitor clothing and uniforms.
    1. Provide lightweight clothing that is loose-fitting at the neck, waist, and sleeves; use shorts and T-shirt at beginning of training.
    2. Avoid excessive padding and taping.
    3. Avoid the use of long stockings, long sleeves, double jerseys, and other excess clothing.
    4. Avoid the use of rubberized clothing or sweatsuits.
    5. Provide clean clothing daily—all items.
  G. Provide rest periods to dissipate accumulated body heat.
    1. Rest athletes in cool, shaded area with some air movement.
    2. Avoid hot brick walls and hot benches.
    3. Instruct athletes to loosen or remove jerseys or other garments.
    4. Provide fluids during the rest period.
    5. Remove helmets or other headgear.

IV. Trouble signs: Stop activity!

Headache	Visual	Unsteadiness	Diarrhea	Weak, rapid	Faintness
Nausea	disturbance	Collapse	Cramps	pulse	Chill
Mental slowness	Fatigue	Unconsciousness	Seizures	Pallor	Cyanotic
Incoherence	Weakness	Vomiting	Rigidity	Flush	appearance

a normal manner and dissipate the resulting heat and perspiration through the usual physiological mechanisms.[13] An athlete may fail to warm up sufficiently or may become chilled because of relative inactivity for varying periods of time demanded by the sport, during either competition or training; consequently, the athlete is exceedingly prone to injury.[16] Low temperatures alone can pose some problems, but when such temperatures are further accentuated by wind, the chill factor becomes critical (Figure 6–4).[57] For example, a runner proceeding at a pace of 10 mph directly into a wind of 5 mph creates a chill factor equivalent to a 15 mph headwind.

A third factor, dampness or wetness, further increases the risk of hypothermia. Air at a temperature of 50°F is relatively comfortable, but water at the same temperature is intolerable. The combination of cold, wind, and dampness creates an environment that easily predisposes the athlete to hypothermia.[69]

> **Low temperatures accentuated by wind and dampness can pose major problems for athletes.**

Sixty-five percent of the heat produced by the body is lost through radiation. This loss occurs most often from the warm, vascular areas of the head and neck, which may account for as much as 50 percent of total heat loss.[65] Twenty percent of heat loss is through evaporation, of which two-thirds is through the skin and one-third is through the respiratory tract.[13]

As an athlete's muscular fatigue builds up during strenuous physical activity in cold weather, the rate of exercise begins to drop and may reach a level at which the body heat loss to the environment exceeds the metabolic heat production, resulting in definite impairment of neuromuscular responses and exhaustion.[13] A relatively small drop in body core temperature can induce shivering sufficient to materially affect an athlete's neuromuscular coordination. Shivering ceases below a body temperature of 85°F to 90°F (29.4°C to 32.2°C). Death is imminent if the core temperature drops to between 77°F and 85°F (25°C and 29°C).

Prevention

Apparel for competitors must be geared to the weather.[4] The functions of such apparel are to provide a semitropical microclimate for the body and to prevent chilling. Several fabrics available on the market are waterproof and windproof but permit the passage of heat and allow sweat to evaporate. The clothing should not restrict movement, should be as lightweight as possible, and should consist of material that will permit the free passage of sweat and body heat that would otherwise accumulate on the skin or the clothing and provide a chilling factor when activity ceases. An individual should routinely dress in thin layers of clothing that can easily be added or removed as the temperature decreases or increases.[65] Continuous adjustment of these layers will reduce sweating and the likelihood that clothing will become damp or wet. Again, wetness or dampness plays a critical role in the development of hypothermia. To prevent chilling, athletes should wear warm-up suits before exercising, during activity breaks or rest periods, and at the termination of exercise. A hat should also be worn to limit heat loss from the head. Activity in cold, wet, and windy weather poses some problems because such weather reduces the insulating value of clothing; consequently, the individual may be unable to achieve energy levels equal to the subsequent body heat losses. Runners

> **Dress in thin layers of clothing that can be added and removed.**

Temperature (°F)

Wind (mph)	40	35	30	25	20	15	10	5	0	−5	−10	−15	−20	−25	−30	−35	−40	−45
Calm																		
5	36	31	25	19	13	7	1	−5	−11	−16	−22	−28	−34	−40	−46	−52	−57	−63
10	34	27	21	15	9	3	−4	−10	−16	−22	−28	−35	−41	−47	−53	−59	−66	−72
15	32	25	19	13	6	0	−7	−13	−19	−26	−32	−39	−45	−51	−58	−64	−71	−77
20	30	24	17	11	4	−2	−9	−15	−22	−29	−35	−42	−48	−55	−61	−68	−74	−81
25	29	23	16	9	3	−4	−11	−17	−24	−31	−37	−44	−51	−58	−64	−71	−78	−84
30	28	22	15	8	1	−5	−12	−19	−26	−33	−39	−46	−53	−60	−67	−73	−80	−87
35	28	21	14	7	0	−7	−14	−21	−27	−34	−41	−48	−55	−62	−69	−76	−82	−89
40	27	20	13	6	−1	−8	−15	−22	−29	−36	−43	−50	−57	−64	−71	−78	−84	−91
45	26	19	12	5	−2	−9	−16	−23	−30	−37	−44	−51	−58	−65	−72	−79	−86	−93
50	26	19	12	4	−3	−10	−17	−24	−31	−38	−45	−52	−60	−67	−74	−81	−88	−95
55	25	18	11	4	−3	−11	−18	−25	−32	−39	−46	−54	−61	−68	−75	−82	−89	−97
60	25	17	10	3	−4	−11	−19	−26	−33	−40	−48	−55	−62	−69	−76	−84	−91	−98

Frostbite times: ▢ 30 minutes ▢ 10 minutes ▢ 5 minutes

FIGURE 6–4 Low temperatures can pose serious problems for the athlete, but wind chill can be a critical factor.

who wish to continue outdoor work in cold weather should use lightweight insulating clothing and, if breathing cold air seems distressful, should use ski goggles and a ski face mask or should cover the mouth and nose with a free-hanging cloth.[4]

Inadequate clothing, improper warm-up, and a high chill factor form a triad that can lead to musculoskeletal injury, chilblains, frostbite, or the minor respiratory disorders associated with lower tissue temperatures. For work or sports in temperatures below 32°F (0°C), it is advisable to add a layer of protective clothing for every 5 mph of wind.[65]

As is true in a hot environment, athletes exercising in a cold environment need to replace fluids. Dehydration causes reduced blood volume, which means less fluid is available for warming the tissues.[55,57] Athletes performing in a cold environment should be weighed before and after practice, especially in the first 2 weeks of the season.[23] Severe overexposure to a cold climate occurs less often than hyperthermia does in a warm climate; however, it is still a major risk of winter sports, long-distance running in cold weather, and swimming in cold water.[4]

Common Cold Injuries

Local cooling of the body can result in tissue damage ranging from superficial to deep. Exposure to a damp, freezing cold can cause frost nip. In contrast, exposure to dry temperatures well below freezing more commonly produces a deep, freezing type of frostbite.[23]

Cold injuries in sports:
• Frost nip
• Frostbite

Below-freezing temperatures may cause ice crystals to form between or within the cells and may eventually destroy the cells. Local capillaries can be injured, blood clots may form, and blood may be shunted away from the injury site to ensure the survival of the nonaffected tissue.[45]

Frost Nip Frost nip affects the ears, nose, cheeks, chin, fingers, and toes. It commonly occurs when there is a high wind, severe cold, or both. The skin initially appears very firm, with cold, painless areas that may peel or blister in 24 to 72 hours. Affected areas can be treated early by firm, sustained pressure of the hand (without rubbing), by blowing hot breath on the spot, or if the injury is to the fingertips, by placing them in the armpits.

Frostbite *Chilblains* result from prolonged and constant exposure to cold for many hours. In time, there is skin redness, swelling, tingling, and pain in the toes and fingers. This adverse response is caused by problems of peripheral circulation and can be avoided by preventing further cold exposure.

Superficial frostbite involves only the skin and subcutaneous tissue. The skin appears pale, hard, cold, and waxy. Palpating the injured area will reveal a sense of hardness but with yielding of the underlying deeper tissue structures. When rewarming, by immersing the area in warm water (100°F to 110°F), the superficial frostbite will at first feel numb, then will sting and burn. Do not rub the affected area. Later the area may produce blisters and be painful for a number of weeks (Figure 6–5A).[45]

Deep frostbite is a serious injury, indicating tissues that are frozen. This medical emergency requires immediate hospitalization. As with frost nip and superficial frostbite, the tissue is initially cold, hard, pale or white, and numb. Gradual rewarming is required, including hot drinks, heating pads, or hot water bottles that are 100°F to 110°F (38°C to 43°C).[41] During rewarming, the tissue becomes blotchy red, swollen, and extremely painful. Later the injury may become gangrenous, causing a loss of tissue (Figure 6–5B). A link to the NATA position statement "Environmental cold injuries" (http://www.nata.org/sites/default/files/EnvironmentalColdInjuries.pdf) can be found at www.mhhe.com/prentice15e.

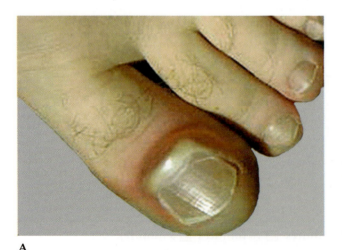
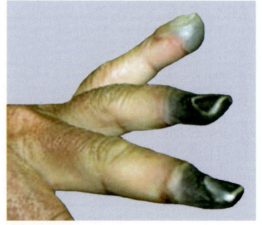

A   **B**

FIGURE 6–5   (A) Superficial frostbite on great toe. (B) Deep frostbite on tips of fingers.

ALTITUDE SICKNESS

Most athletic events are not conducted at extreme altitudes. For example, Mexico City's elevation, which is 7,600 feet (2,316 m), is considered moderate, yet at this height there is a 7 percent to 8 percent decrease in maximum oxygen uptake.[41] This

> **Most athletic events are not conducted at high altitudes.**

loss in maximum oxygen uptake represents a 4 percent to 8 percent deterioration in an athlete's performance in endurance events, depending on the duration of effort and lack of wind resistance.[50] Often, the athlete's body compensates for this decrease in maximum oxygen uptake with corresponding tachycardia.[41] When the body is suddenly without its usual oxygen supply, hyperventilation can occur. Many of these responses result from the athlete having fewer red blood cells than necessary to adequately capture the available oxygen in the air.[41]

Adaptation to Altitude

A major factor in altitude adaptation is the problem of oxygen deficiency. With a reduction in barometric pressure, the partial pressure of oxygen in inspired air is also low. Under these circumstances, the existing circulating red blood cells become less saturated, depriving tissue of needed oxygen.[50]

An individual's adaptation to high altitude depends on whether he or she is a native, resident, or visitor to the area. Natives of areas with high altitudes (e.g., the Andes and Nepal) have a larger chest capacity, more alveoli, more capillaries that transport blood to tissue, and a higher red blood cell level. In contrast, the resident or the individual who stays at a high altitude for months or years makes a partial adaptation. His or her later adaptation includes the conservation of glucose, an increased number of mitochondria (the sources of energy in a cell), and increased formation of hemoglobin. In the visitor or the person who is in an early stage of adaptation to high altitude, a number of responses represent a physiological struggle. The responses include increased breathing, increased heart action, increased hemoglobin in circulating blood, increased blood alkalinity, and increased myoglobin, as well as changes in the distribution of blood flow and cell enzyme activity. Dehydration has also been linked to altitude sickness.[50]

There are many uncertainties about when to have an athlete go to an area of high altitude to train and compete.[55] Some experts believe that having the athlete arrive 2 to 3 weeks before competition provides the best adjustment period, whereas others believe that, for psychological as well as physiological reasons, 3 days before competition is enough time.[41] This shorter adjustment period allows for the recovery of the acid-base balance in the blood but does not provide enough time for the athlete to achieve a significant adjustment in blood volume and maximum cardiac output.[50]

Altitude Illnesses

Athletic trainers must understand that some of their athletes may become ill when suddenly subjected to high altitudes.[34] These illnesses include acute mountain sickness, high altitude pulmonary edema (HAPE), high altitude cerebral edema (HACE), and an adverse reaction to the sickle-cell trait.

Acute Mountain Sickness One out of three individuals who go from a low to a moderate altitude of 7,000 to 8,000 feet (2,133 to 2,438 m) experience mild to moderate symptoms of acute mountain sickness.[9] Symptoms include headache, nausea, vomiting, sleep disturbance, and dyspnea, which may last up to 3 days.[34] These symptoms have been attributed to a tissue disruption in the brain that affects the sodium and potassium balance. This imbalance can cause excess fluid retention within the cells and the subsequent occurrence of abnormal pressure.[34]

High Altitude Pulmonary Edema (HAPE) At an altitude of 9,000 to 10,000 feet (2,743 to 3,048 m), high altitude pulmonary edema (HAPE) may occur. Characteristically, lungs at this altitude will accumulate a small amount of fluid within the alveolar walls.[50] In most individuals, this fluid is absorbed in a few days, but in some it continues to collect and forms pulmonary edema. Symptoms of high altitude pulmonary edema are dyspnea, cough, headache, weakness, and unconsciousness.[50] The treatment of choice is to move the athlete to a lower altitude as soon as possible and give oxygen. The condition rapidly resolves once the athlete is at a lower altitude.[34]

High Altitude Cerebral Edema (HACE) High altitude cerebral edema (HACE), usually in conjunction with HAPE, is a life-threatening condition that can lead to coma or death. It occurs in about 1 percent of people adjusting to altitudes above 9,000 feet (2,743 m). HACE is likely the result of increased cerebral edema caused by increased cerebral blood flow due to the increased permeability of cerebral endothelium when exposed to hypoxia. Increased cerebral blood flow results in increased intracranial pressure, which is responsible for many of the clinical manifestations of HACE. Symptoms consist of a severe headache that may precede mental dysfunction (hallucinations, bizarre behavior, and coma) and neurological abnormalities (loss of coordination, paralysis, and cerebellar signs). Descent to lower altitudes may save those afflicted with HACE.[9]

Sickle-Cell Trait Reaction Approximately 8 percent to 10 percent of African Americans (approximately 2 million persons) have the sickle-cell trait. In most, the trait is benign. It relates to an abnormality of the structure of the red blood cells and their hemoglobin content.[50] When the abnormal hemoglobin molecules become deoxygenated as a result of exercise at a high altitude, the cells tend to clump together. This process causes an abnormal sickle shape in the red blood cell, which can be destroyed easily. This condition can cause an enlarged spleen, which has been known to rupture at high altitudes (see Chapter 29).[50]

OVEREXPOSURE TO SUN

Athletes, along with coaches, athletic trainers, and other support staff, frequently spend a great deal of time outdoors in direct sunlight. Precautions to protect these individuals from overexposure to ultraviolet light by applying sunscreens are often totally ignored.

Long-Term Effects on Skin

The most serious effects of long-term exposure to ultraviolet light are premature aging of the skin and skin cancer.[30] Lightly pigmented individuals are more susceptible to these maladies. Premature aging of the skin is characterized by dryness, cracking, and a decrease in the elasticity of the skin. Skin cancer is the most common malignant tumor found in humans and has been epidemiologically and clinically associated with exposure to ultraviolet radiation. Damage to DNA is suspected as the cause of skin cancer, but the exact cause is unknown. The major types of skin cancer are basal cell carcinoma, squamous cell carcinoma, and malignant melanoma. Fortunately, the rate of cure exceeds 95 percent with early detection and treatment.[30,75]

Sunscreens

Sunscreens applied to the skin can help prevent many of the damaging effects of ultraviolet radiation. A sunscreen's effectiveness in absorbing the sunburn-inducing radiation is expressed as the sun protection factor (**SPF**). An SPF of 6 indicates that an athlete can be exposed to ultraviolet light six times longer than without a sunscreen before the skin begins to turn red. Higher numbers provide longer periods of protection. However, athletes who have a family or personal history of skin cancer may experience significant damage to the skin even when wearing an SPF-15 sunscreen. Therefore, these individuals should wear an SPF-30 sunscreen.

SPF Sun protection factor.

Sunscreen should be worn regularly by athletes, coaches, and athletic trainers who spend time outside, particularly if they have a fair complexion, light hair, blue eyes, or skin that burns easily.[29] People with dark complexions should also wear sunscreens to prevent sun damage.[30]

Sun exposure causes a premature aging of the skin (wrinkling, freckling, prominent blood vessels, coarsening of skin texture), induces the formation of precancerous growths, and increases the risk of developing basal and squamous cell skin cancers. Because 60 to 80 percent of lifetime sun exposure is often obtained by age 20, everyone over 6 months of age should use sunscreens.

Sunscreens are needed most between the months of March and November but should be used year-round. They are needed most between the hours of 10 A.M. and 4 P.M. and should be applied 15 to 30 minutes before sun exposure. Although clothing and hats provide some protection from the sun, they are not a substitute for sunscreens (a typical white cotton T-shirt provides an SPF of only 5). Reflected sunlight from water, sand, and snow may effectively increase sun exposure and the risk of burning.

LIGHTNING SAFETY

Research indicates that lightning is the number two cause of death by weather phenomena, accounting for 110 deaths per year.[51,81] As a result of the danger associated with electrical storms to athletes and staff who practice and compete outdoors, the NATA has established a position statement with guidelines for athletic trainers.[79] Each institution should develop a specific emergency action plan to be implemented in case of a lightning storm, which includes establishing

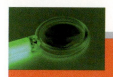

Lightning safety[79]

The following checklist includes basic guidelines that should be followed during an electrical storm.

- In situations in which thunder or lightning may be present and you feel your hair stand on end and skin tingle, immediately assume a crouched position—drop to your knees, place your hands and arms on your legs, and lower your head. Do not lie flat.
- If thunder and/or lightning can be heard or seen, and if the flash-to-bang count reaches 30, stop activity and seek protective shelter immediately. An indoor facility is recommended as the safest protective shelter. However, if an indoor facility is not available, an automobile is a relatively safe alternative. If neither of these options is available, you should avoid standing under large trees and telephone poles. If the only alternative is a tree, choose a small tree in a wooded area that is not on a hill. As a last alternative, find a ravine or valley. In all instances outdoors, assume the aforementioned crouched position.
- Avoid standing water and metal objects at all times (e.g., metal bleachers, metal cleats, umbrellas).
- Allow 30 minutes to pass after the last sound of thunder or lightning strike before resuming play.

a chain of command to determine who should monitor both the weather forecast and changing weather of a threatening nature and to determine who makes the decision to remove from, and ultimately to return a team to, the practice field, based on pre-established criteria.[10,80] If you hear thunder or see lightning, you are in immediate danger and should seek a protective shelter in an indoor facility at once. An indoor facility is recommended as the safest protective shelter. However, if an indoor facility is not available, an automobile is a relatively safe alternative. If neither of these is available, the following guidelines are recommended. Avoid standing near large trees, flagpoles, or light poles. Choose an area that is not on a hill. As a last alternative, find a ditch, ravine, or valley. At times, the only natural forewarning of a strike is feeling your hair stand on end and your skin tingle. At this point, you are in imminent danger of being struck by lightning and should drop to the ground, assuming a crouched position immediately. Do not lie flat. Should a ground strike occur near you, lying flat increases the body's surface area that is exposed to the current traveling through the ground.[81] Avoid standing water (pools),

6–6 Clinical Application Exercise

A lacrosse team is practicing on a remote field with no indoor facility in close proximity. The weather is rapidly worsening, with the sky becoming dark and the wind blowing harder. Twenty minutes are left in the practice session, and the coach is hoping to finish practice before it begins to rain. Suddenly, there is a bolt of lightning and an immediate burst of thunder.

? How should the athletic trainer manage this extremely dangerous situation?

showers, telephones, and metal objects at all times (metal bleachers, umbrellas).[79]

The most dangerous storms give little or no warning; thunder and lightning are not heard or seen.[10] Lightning is always accompanied by thunder, although 20 to 40 percent of thunder cannot be heard

> **The most dangerous storms give little or no warning.**

because of atmospheric disturbances. The **flash-to-bang** method provides an estimation of how far away lightning is occurring.[79] From the time lightning is sighted, count the number of seconds until the bang occurs and divide by 5 to calculate the number of miles away the lightning is occurring.[64] When the flash-to-bang count is at or less

> **flash-to-bang** Number of seconds from lightning flash until the sound of thunder divided by 5 to determine the distance from the lightning strike.

than 30 there is danger, and conditions should be closely monitored. When the count reaches 30, everyone should have left the field for safe shelter.[64]

Both the NATA and the National Severe Storms Service recommend that 30 minutes should pass after the last sound of thunder is heard or lightning strike is seen before resuming play.[80] This is enough time to allow the storm to pass and move out of lightning strike range. The perilous misconception that it is possible to see lightning coming and have time to act before it strikes could prove to be fatal. In reality, the lightning that we see flashing is actually the return stroke flashing upward from the ground to the cloud, not downward. When you see the lightning strike, it has already hit.[81]

Focus Box 6–7: "Lightning safety" identifies guidelines that should be followed during an

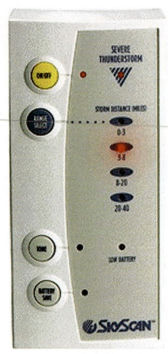

FIGURE 6–6   Portable handheld lightning detector.
(Courtesy Novalynx Corp., Grass Valley, CA)

electrical storm. A link to the NATA position statement "lightning safety for athletics and recreation" (http://www.nata.org/sites/default/files/LightningSafety4AthleticsRec.pdf) can be found at www.mhhe.com/prentice15e.

Lightning Detectors

A lightning detector is a handheld instrument with an electronic system to detect the presence and the distance of lightning/thunderstorm activity occurring within a 40-mile distance (Figure 6–6). It allows you to know the level of activity of the storm, and it determines whether the storm is moving toward, away from, or parallel to your position. When the lightning detector detects a lightning strike, it emits an audible warning tone and lights the range indicator, allowing you to see the distance to the last, closest detected lightning strike. If the lightning detector flashes in the 3–8 range, this is generally considered to be a threatening environmental condition, and all activity should immediately be moved indoors. Lightning detectors are under $200 and are thus an inexpensive alternative to contracting with a weather service to provide information on potentially dangerous weather conditions over a pager system.

AIR POLLUTION

Air pollution is a significant problem everywhere in the United States but particularly in urban areas with large industries and heavy automobile traffic.

Because athletes are outside for long periods of time during training or competition, they may be more susceptible to the effects of air pollution than is a sedentary individual who remains indoors.[58] There are two types of pollution: photochemical haze and smog. Photochemical haze consists of nitrogen dioxide and stagnant air that are acted on by sunlight to produce ozone.[66] Smog is produced by the combination of carbon monoxide, sulfur dioxide, and particulate matter that emanates from the combustion of a fossil fuel, such as coal.

> Air pollution is a major problem in urban areas with large industries and heavy automobile traffic.

Ozone

Ozone is formed by the action of sunlight on carbon-based chemicals known as hydrocarbons, acting in combination with nitrogen dioxide.[31] It is the main component of the air pollution referred to as smog. Hydrocarbons are emitted by motor vehicles, oil and chemical storage facilities, and industrial sources, such as gas stations, dry cleaners, and degreasing operations. Ozone is at its highest level when higher temperatures and the increased amount of sunlight during the summer combine with stagnant atmospheric conditions.

When individuals are engaged in physical tasks requiring minimal effort, an increase in ozone in the air does not usually reduce functional capacity in normal work output. However, when individuals increase their work output (e.g., during exercise), their work capacity is decreased. The athlete may experience shortness of breath, coughing, chest tightness, pain during deep breathing, nausea, eye irritation, fatigue, lung irritation, and a lowered resistance to lung infections. Over a period of time, individuals may to some degree become desensitized to ozone. Asthmatics are at greater risk when ozone levels increase.

Nitrogen Dioxide

Nitrogen dioxide is produced from combustive processes, such as in automobiles, power plants, home heaters, and gas stoves. Nitrogen dioxide is a light brown gas that is a component of urban haze. It plays an important role in the atmospheric reactions that generate ozone and acid rain.[2] Nitrogen dioxide can irritate the lungs and lower resistance to respiratory infections, such as influenza, and may cause increased incidences of acute respiratory disease in children.[66]

Sulfur Dioxide

Sulfur dioxide (SO_2) is a colorless gas that is a component of burning coal or petroleum. As an air contaminant, it causes an increased resistance to air

TABLE 6–4 Air Quality Guide for Ozone*

Air Quality	Air Quality Index	Protect Your Health
Good	0–50	No health impacts are expected when air quality is in this range.
Moderate	51–100	Unusually sensitive people should consider limiting prolonged outdoor exertion.
Unhealthy for sensitive groups	101–150	Active children and adults and people with respiratory disease, such as asthma, should limit prolonged outdoor exertion.
Unhealthy	151–200	Active children and adults and people with respiratory disease, such as asthma, should avoid prolonged outdoor exertion; everyone else, especially children, should limit prolonged outdoor exertion.
Very unhealthy (alert)	201–300	Active children and adults and people with respiratory disease, such as asthma, should avoid all outdoor exertion; everyone else, especially children, should limit outdoor exertion.

*Modified from United States Environmental Protection Agency, Air and Radiation, EPA-456/F-99-002, Washington, DC, 20460, 1999.

movement into and out of the lungs, a decreased ability of the lungs to rid themselves of foreign matter, shortness of breath, coughing, fatigue, and increased susceptibility to lung diseases. Sulfur dioxide causes an adverse effect mostly on asthmatics and other sensitive individuals. Nose breathing lessens the effects of sulfur dioxide because the nasal mucosa acts as a sulfur dioxide scrubber.[58]

Carbon Monoxide

Carbon monoxide (CO) is a colorless, odorless gas. In general, it reduces hemoglobin's ability to transport oxygen and restricts the release of oxygen to the tissue. Besides interfering with performance during exercise, carbon monoxide exposure interferes with various psychomotor, behavioral, and attention-related activities.[58]

> Carbon monoxide (CO) reduces hemoglobin's ability to transport and release oxygen in the body.

Particulate Matter

Particulate matter is a type of air pollution that consists of solids in the atmosphere, such as dirt, soil dust, pollens, molds, ashes, soot, and aerosols, that have been found to present a serious danger to health. Particulate pollution comes from such diverse sources as factory smokestacks, vehicle exhaust, wood burning, mining, construction, and agriculture. Fine particles, less than 2.5 microns in diameter, are easily inhaled into the lungs, where they can be absorbed into the bloodstream or remain embedded for long periods of time.[2] Exposure to particulate air pollution can trigger asthma attacks and cause wheezing, coughing, and respiratory irritation in individuals who have chronic obstructive pulmonary disease (COPD), including emphysema and bronchitis.[66]

Prevention

To avoid problems created by air pollution, the athlete must stop or significantly decrease physical activity during periods of high pollution. If activity is conducted, it should be performed when commuter traffic has lessened and when ambient temperature has lowered. Ozone levels rise during dawn, peak at midday, and are much reduced after the late-afternoon rush hour. Running should be avoided on roads containing a concentration of auto emissions and carbon monoxide.[58] Table 6–4 provides guidelines for activity based on the air quality index for ozone.

CIRCADIAN DYSRHYTHMIA (JET LAG)

Jet power makes it possible to travel thousands of miles in just a few hours. Athletes and athletic teams are quickly transported from one end of the country to the other and to foreign lands. For some athletes, such travel induces a particular physiological stress, resulting in a syndrome that is identified as *circadian dysrhythmia* and that reflects a desynchronization of the athlete's biological and biophysical time clock.[82]

> **Circadian Dysrhythmia (Jet Lag)** Disruption of biological and biophysical time clock.

The term *circadian* (from the Latin *circa dies,* "about a day") implies a period of time of approximately 24 hours. The body maintains many

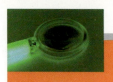

FOCUS 6–8 Focus on Injury/Illness Prevention and Wellness Protection

Minimizing the effects of jet lag

- Depart for a trip well rested.
- Preadjust circadian rhythms by getting up and going to bed 1 hour later for each time zone crossed when traveling west and 1 hour earlier for each time zone crossed when traveling east.
- When traveling west, eat light meals early and heavy meals late in the day. When traveling east, eat a heavy meal earlier in the day.[68]
- Drink plenty of fluids to avoid dehydration, which occurs because of dry, high-altitude, low-humidity cabin air.
- Consume caffeine in coffee, tea, or soda when traveling west. Avoid caffeine when traveling east.[68]

(Caffeine is only a mild diuretic and causes no greater increase in urine output than drinking water.[38])
- Exercise or training should be done later in the day if traveling west and earlier in the day if traveling east.
- Reset watches according to the new time zone after boarding the plane.
- If traveling west, get as much sunlight as possible on arrival.
- On arrival, immediately adopt the local time schedule for training, eating, and sleeping. Forget about what time it is where you came from.
- Avoid using alcohol before, during, and after travel.

6–7 Clinical Application Exercise

A college tennis team from the West Coast must travel to the East Coast to play a scheduled match. The coach has done a lot of traveling and knows that traveling from west to east seems to be more difficult than traveling east to west. This match is important, and the tennis coach asks the athletic trainer for advice to help the athletes minimize the effects of jet lag.

? What can the athletic trainer recommend to help the athletes adjust to the new time zone in as short a time as possible?

cyclical mechanisms (circadian rhythms) that follow a pattern (e.g., the daily rise and fall of body temperature or the tidal ebb and flow of the cortical steroid secretion, which produces other effects on the metabolic system that are in themselves cyclical). Body mechanisms adapt at varying rates to time changes. Some adjust immediately (e.g., protein metabolism), whereas others take time (e.g., the rise and fall of body temperature, which takes approximately 8 days to adjust). Other body mechanisms, such as the adrenal hormones, which regulate metabolism and other body functions, may take as long as 3 weeks to adjust. Even intellectual proficiency, or the ability to think clearly, is cyclical.

The term *jet lag* refers to the physical and mental effects caused by traveling rapidly across several time zones.[82] It results from the disruption of both circadian rhythms and the sleep-wake cycle. As the length of travel increases over several time zones, the effects of jet lag become more profound.[43]

Disruption of circadian rhythms has been shown to cause fatigue, headache, problems with the digestive system, and changes in blood pressure, heart rate, hormonal release, endocrine secretions, and bowel habits.[38] Any of these changes may have a negative effect on athletic performance and may predispose the athlete to injury.[82]

Younger individuals adjust more rapidly to time zone changes than do older people, although the differences are not great. The stress induced in jet travel occurs only when flying either east or west at high speed. Travel north or south has no effect on the body unless several time zones are crossed in an east or west progression. There is 30 to 50 percent faster adaptation in individuals flying westward than in individuals flying eastward.[38] In fact, flying from the west to the east has been demonstrated to decrease performance.[68] The changes in time zones, illumination, and environment prove somewhat disruptive to the human physiological mechanisms, particularly when a person flies through five or more time zones, as occurs in some international travel.[38] Some people are more susceptible to the syndrome than are others, but the symptoms can be sufficiently disruptive to interfere with an athlete's ability to perform maximally in a competitive event.[82] In some cases, an athlete becomes ill for a short period of time, with severe headache, blurred vision, dizziness, insomnia, or extreme fatigue. The negative effects of jet lag can be reduced by paying attention to the guidelines in *Focus Box 6–8:* "Minimizing the effects of jet lag."

SYNTHETIC TURF

Synthetic turf was first used in the Houston Astrodome in 1966 and was first marketed under the trade name AstroTurf. The artificial surface was said to be more durable, offer greater consistency, require less maintenance, be more "playable" during inclement weather, and offer greater performance characteristics, such as increased speed and resiliency. Since the late 1960s, a number of companies have manufactured synthetic surfaces that are variations of AstroTurf. Today synthetic surfaces have a relatively new option in "resilient infill turf," which its manufacturers claim is more similar to natural grass and considerably less expensive than other types of synthetic turf.[85] It is made of polyethylene and polypropylene yarns that sit on a base of sand, crumbled rubber pellets, or a combination of both. The consumer can choose from a number of artificial turf products, including AstroTurf, Nexturf, FieldTurf, AstroPlay, Omniturf, EasyTurf, SyntheticTurf, Sof-Step 200, SprlnTurf, and Avery SportsTurf.[70]

6–8 Clinical Application Exercise

A collegiate athletic director is trying to make a decision about replacing a natural grass playing field with a new synthetic playing surface. He asks the athletic trainer to provide him with recommendations relative to the incidence of injury on natural grass versus synthetic turf.

? What can the athletic trainer tell him?

There has been an ongoing debate over the advantages and disadvantages of synthetic surfaces compared with natural surfaces.[84] From an injury perspective, the evidence in the literature is not conclusive to indicate that a synthetic surface is more likely to cause injury than a natural surface.[26,33,49,84,85] Empirically, most athletes, coaches, and athletic trainers agree that injuries are more likely to occur on synthetic surfaces than on natural grass, and most of these individuals would rather practice and play on natural grass. In recent years, the trend in many colleges, universities, and professional arenas has been to move away from synthetic surfaces, replacing them with natural grass. New hybrid grasses are now available that are more durable.

It has been argued that synthetic surfaces lose their inherent shock absorption capability as they age.[33] It has been demonstrated that training injuries are more likely to occur if training always occurs on artificial turf.[26] Higher speeds are said to be possible on artificial surfaces; thus, injuries involving collision can be more severe because of increased force on impact.[85] A shoe that does not "stick" to the artificial surface but still provides solid footing will significantly reduce the likelihood of injury.[85]

Two injuries that seem to occur more frequently in athletes competing on an artificial surface are abrasions and turf toe (a hyperextension of the great toe). The incidence of abrasions can be greatly reduced by wearing pads on the elbows and knees. Turf toe is less likely to occur if the shoe has a stiff, firm sole.

SUMMARY

- Environmental stress can adversely affect an athlete's performance and pose a serious health problem.
- Hyperthermia is one of sport's major concerns. In times of high temperatures and humidity, athletes should always exercise caution. The key to preventing heat-related illness is rehydration, acclimatization, and common sense. Losing 2 percent or more of body weight due to fluid loss could pose a health problem.
- Cold weather requires athletes to wear the correct apparel and to warm up properly before engaging in sports activities. The wind chill factor must always be considered when performing. As is true in a hot environment, athletes in cold conditions must ingest adequate fluids. Extreme cold exposure can cause conditions such as frost nip, chilblains, and frostbite.
- An athlete going from a low to a high altitude in a short time may encounter problems with performance and may experience some health problems. Researchers are unsure about how much time it takes for adaptation to occur and about when to take the athlete to the higher altitude, especially for an endurance event. Many athletic trainers believe that 3 days at the higher altitude provides enough time for adaptation to occur. Others believe that a much longer time period is needed. An athlete who experiences a serious illness because of his or her presence at a particular altitude must be returned to a lower altitude as soon as possible.
- Air pollution can be a major decrement to performance and can cause illness. Increased ozone levels can cause respiratory distress, nausea, eye irritation, and fatigue. Sulfur dioxide, a colorless gas, can also cause physical reactions in some athletes and can be a serious problem for asthmatics. Carbon monoxide, a colorless and odorless gas, reduces hemoglobin's ability to use oxygen and, as a result, adversely affects performance.

- Travel through time zones can place a serious physiological stress on the athlete. This stress is called circadian dysrhythmia, or jet lag. This disruption of biological rhythm can adversely affect performance and may even produce health problems. The athletic trainer must pay careful attention to helping the athlete acclimatize to time-zone shifting.

- There is inconclusive evidence that the incidence of injury on artificial surfaces is higher than on natural surfaces, although most coaches, athletes, and athletic trainers seem to prefer practicing and playing on natural grass. Two frequently seen injuries that occur on artificial turf are abrasions and turf toe.

WEB SITES

A hypothermia treatment technology Web site: www.hypothermia-ca.com

American Lung Association: http://www.lung.org/
The American Lung Association site looks at outdoor air pollution and its effects on the lungs.

FEMA: Extreme Heat Fact Sheet: http://www.fema .gov/library/viewRecord.do?id=3042
Doing too much on a hot day, spending too much time in the sun, or staying too long in an overheated place can cause heat-related illnesses.

Gatorade Sport Science Institute: www.gssiweb.com
This site provides the most up-to-date recommendations for fluid replacement and preventing heat illnesses.

National Athletic Trainers' Association: www.nata.org
This site contains detailed position papers on heat illness, fluid replacement, and lightning safety.

National Lightning Safety Institute (NLSI): www.lightningsafety.com
The National Lightning Safety Institute provides consulting, education, training, and expert witnesses relating to lightning hazard mitigation.

OA Guide to Hypothermia & Cold Weather Injuries: www.princeton.edu/–oa/safety/hypocold.shtml

OnHealth: Heat Illness (Heat Exhaustion, Heatstroke, Heat Cramps): http://firstaid.webmd.com/ understanding-heat-related-illness-basics
Prolonged or intense exposure to hot temperatures can cause heat-related illnesses, such as heat exhaustion, heat cramps, and heatstroke (also known as sunstroke).

Sports Turf Managers Association: www.stma.org

SOLUTIONS TO CLINICAL APPLICATION EXERCISES

6–1 The wrestler is experiencing heat exhaustion, which results from inadequate fluid replacement or dehydration. If conscious, the athlete should be forced to drink large quantities of water. By far the most rapid method of fluid replacement is for a physician to use an IV (fluids administered intravenously). It is desirable, but not necessary, to move the athlete to a cooler environment. The athlete should be counseled about the dangers of using diuretic medication.

6–2 The athletic trainer may suspect that the athlete is experiencing heatstroke. The course of action includes checking the athlete's vitals (airway, breathing, circulation) and activating the emergency action plan. Remove his helmet and as much excess clothing as is appropriate. The first priority is to cool the individual down as quickly as possible by immersing him in a cold-water tub. Continuously monitor his vital signs until the rescue squad arrives. The athlete's core temperature should be around 100°F before he is removed from the cold tub. If a cold tub is not available, use cold packs or cold-water spray. Move the athlete into the shade or to a cooler environment, if possible.

6–3 The athletic trainer should explain to the coach that heat-related illnesses are, for the most part, preventable. The athletes should come into preseason practice at least partially acclimatized to working in a hot, humid environment and during the first week of practice should become fully acclimatized. Temperature and humidity readings should be monitored, and practice should be modified according to conditions. Practice uniforms should maximize evaporation and minimize heat absorption to the greatest extent possible. Weight records should be maintained to identify individuals

who are becoming dehydrated. Most important, the athletes must keep themselves hydrated by constantly drinking large quantities of water both during and between practice sessions.

6–4 The safest recommendation would be for the athlete to travel to Colorado 2 to 3 weeks before the event. If this arrival time is not practical, she should be in Colorado for at least 3 days before her first event.

6–5 The sun protection factor (SPF) indicates the sunscreen's effectiveness in absorbing the sunburn-inducing radiation. An SPF of 15 indicates that an athlete can be exposed to ultraviolet light 15 times longer than without a sunscreen before the skin will begin to turn red. Therefore, the athlete needs to understand that a higher SPF does not indicate a greater degree of protection. She must simply apply the sunscreen with an SPF of 15 twice as often as would be necessary with a sunscreen with an SPF of 30.

6–6 As soon as lightning is observed, the athletic trainer should immediately end practice and get the athletes under cover. If an indoor facility is not available, automobiles are a relatively safe alternative. The athletes should avoid standing under large trees or telephone poles. As a last alternative, athletes should assume a crouched position in a ditch or ravine. If possible, athletes should avoid any standing water or metal objects around the field.

6–7 Most important, the athletes should leave for the trip well rested. The day before leaving, the athletes should go to bed and get up 3 hours earlier than normal. Athletes should reset their watches according to the new time zone once they board the plane. During the trip they should drink plenty of fluids to prevent dehydration, but they should avoid caffeine. Their largest meal should be eaten earlier in the day. On arrival, athletes should immediately adopt the local time schedule for training, eating, and sleeping, and they should get as much sunlight as possible. Training sessions should be done earlier in the day.

6–8 The athletic trainer should inform the athletic director that the trend seems to be moving toward natural grass fields.

The research data collected over the years have not clearly indicated that there is a difference in injury rates between natural grass and synthetic turf. However, it does seem that most athletes, coaches, and athletic trainers prefer natural turf. It should also be stressed that the newer synthetic surfaces are more like natural grass and may warrant additional investigation.

REVIEW QUESTIONS AND CLASS ACTIVITIES

1. How do temperature and humidity cause heat illnesses?
2. What steps should be taken to prevent heat illnesses?
3. Describe the symptoms and signs of the most common heat illnesses.
4. How is heat lost from the body to produce hypothermia?
5. What should an athlete do to prevent heat loss?
6. Identify the physiological basis for the body's susceptibility to a cold disorder.
7. Describe the symptoms and signs of the major cold disorders affecting athletes.
8. How should athletes protect themselves from the effects of ultraviolet radiation from the sun?
9. What precautions can be taken to minimize the possibility of injury during an electrical storm?
10. What concerns should an athletic trainer have when athletes are to perform an endurance sport at high altitudes?
11. What altitude illnesses might be expected among some athletes, and how should those illnesses be managed?
12. What adverse effects could high air concentrations of ozone, nitrogen dioxide, sulfur dioxide, carbon monoxide, and particulate matter have on the athlete? How should they be dealt with?
13. How can the adverse effects of circadian dysrhythmia be avoided or lessened?
14. What are two common injuries in athletes who compete on artificial turf?

REFERENCES

1. American College of Sports Medicine: Position stand on exercise and fluid replacement, *Med Sci Sports Exerc* 28(17):377–90, 1996.
2. American Lung Association, www.lungusa.org.
3. Armstrong L: Caffeine, body fluid-electrolyte balance, and exercise performance, *Int J Sport Nutr* 12(2):189, 2002.
4. Armstrong LE, Epstein Y, Greenleaf JE: Heat and cold illnesses during distance running, *Med Sci Sports Exerc* 28(12):377–90, 1996.
5. Armstrong L: The American football uniform: Uncompensable heat stress and hyperthermic exhaustion, *J Athl Train*, 45(2):117–27, 2010.
6. Armstrong L: Exertional heat illness during training and competition, *Med Sci Sport Exer*, 39(3):556–72, 2007.
7. Armstrong L: Nutritional strategies for football: Counteracting heat, cold, high altitude, and jet lag, *Journal of Sports Sciences* 24(7):723, 2006.
8. Baxter R, Moore J: Diagnosis and treatment of acute exertional rhabdomyolysis, *J Ortho Sports Phys Ther* 33(3):124, 2003.
9. Bellis F: Acute mountain sickness: An unexpected management problem, *British Journal of Sports Medicine* 36(2):147, 2002.
10. Bennett B: A model lightning safety policy for athletics, *J Athl Train* 32(3):251, 1997.
11. Bergeron MF: Averting heat cramps, *Physician Sportsmed* 30(11):14, 2002.
12. Binkley H, Beckett J, Casa D: National Athletic Trainers' Association position statement: Exertional heat illnesses, *J Athl Train* 37(3):329, 2002.
13. Brukner P: Exercise in the cold. In Brukner P, editor: *Clinical sports medicine*, ed 2, Sydney, 2002, McGraw-Hill.
14. Budd G: Wet-bulb globe temperature (WBGT)—its history and its limitations, *Journal of Science and Medicine in Sports*, 11(1):20–32, 2008.
15. Capacchione J: The relationship between exertional heat illness, exertional rhabdomyolysis, and malignant hyperthermia, *Anesthesia and Analgesia*, 109(4):1065–69, 2009.
16. Cappaert T, Stone J, Castellini J: National Athletic Trainers' Association position statement: Environmental cold injuries, *J Athl Train* 43(4):640, 2008.
17. Carlson M: Exercising in the cold, *ACSM's Health & Fitness Journal* 16(1):8–12, 2012.
18. Casa D: Cold water immersion: The gold standard for exertional heatstroke treatment, *Exer & Sport Sci Rev*, 35(3):141–49, 2007.
19. Casa D: Exercise in the heat. II. Critical concepts in rehydration, exertional heat illnesses, and maximizing athletic performance, *J Athl Train* 34(3):253, 1999.
20. Casa D: Preseason heat-acclimatization guidelines for secondary school athletes, *Journal of Athletic Training* 44(3):332–33, 2009.
21. Casa DJ, Armstrong LE, Hillman S: National Athletic Trainers' Association position statement: Fluid replacement for athletes, *J Athl Train* 35(2):212, 2000.
22. Casey E: Heat emergencies, *Athletic Therapy Today* 11(3):44, 2006.
23. Castellani J: Prevention of cold injuries during exercise, 38(11):2012–29, 2006.
24. Cleary M, Casa D: Exertional hyponatremia: Considerations for athletic trainers, *Athletic Therapy Today* 10(4):61, 2005.
25. Clements J, Casa DJ, Knight C: Ice-water immersion and cold-water immersion provide similar cooling rates in runners with exercise-induced hyperthermia, *J Athl Train* 37(2):146, 2002.
26. Conklin AR: Grass gets greener: Division 1-A football programs are gradually switching from synthetic turf to grass—and the reasons behind the shift may surprise you, *Sports Med Update* 15(1):11, 2000.
27. Coris E, Ramirez A, Van Durme D: Heat illness in athletes: The dangerous combination of heat, humidity and exercise, *Sports Med* 34(1):9, 2004.
28. Coyle E: Fluid and fuel intake during exercise, *Journal of Sports Sciences* 22(1):39, 2004.
29. Davis JL: Sun and active patients: Preventing cumulative skin damage, *Physician Sportsmed* 28(7):79, 2000.
30. Davis M: Ultraviolet therapy. In Prentice W, editor: *Therapeutic modalities in sports medicine*, St. Louis, 2003, McGraw-Hill.
31. DeFranco M: Environmental issues for team physicians, *American Journal of Sports Medicine* 36(11):26–33, 2008.
32. Dotan F: Temperature regulation and elite young athletes, *Medicine and Sport Science* 56(1):126–49, 2011.
33. Dragoo J: The effect of playing surface on injury rate: A review of the current literature, *Sports Medicine* 40(11):981–90, 2010.
34. Eichner R: Acute mountain sickness: New research on causes, coping, *Sports Med Digest* 25(11):121, 2003.
35. Eichner R: Heat cramps in sports, *Current Sports Medicine Reports* 7(4):178–79, 2008.
36. Eichner R: Toward ending fatal heat stroke in football players, *J Athl Train*. 45(2):105–106, 2010.
37. Fawcett C: Fluid-electrolyte replacement, *J Athl Train*, 41(S):59, 2006.
38. Forbes S, Vadgama D: Circadian disruption and remedial interventions: Effects and interventions for jet lag for athletic peak performance, *Sports Medicine*, Mar 1;42(3):185–208, 2012.
39. Gagnon D: Aural canal, esophageal, and rectal temperatures during exertional heat stress and the subsequent recovery period, *J Athl Train*, 45(2):157–63, 2010.
40. Gagnon D: Cold-water immersion and the treatment of hyperthermia: Using 38.6°C

as a safe rectal temperature cooling limit, *J Athl Train*. 45(5):439–44, 2010.

41. Hoffman J: Exercise at altitude. In Hoffman J, editor: *Physiological aspects of sport training and performance*, Champaign, IL, 2002, Human Kinetics.

42. Inter-association task force on exertional heat illnesses consensus statement, *NATA News* 6:24, 2003.

43. Johnson R, Tulin B: *Travel fitness*, Champaign, IL, 1995, Human Kinetics.

44. Jung A, Bishop P, Barry D: Influence of hydration and electrolyte supplementation on incidence and time to onset of exercise associated muscle cramps, *J Athl Train* 40(2):71, 2005.

45. Kanzanbach TL, Dexter WW: Cold injuries: Protecting your patients from the dangers of hypothermia and frostbite, *Post Graduate Medicine* 105(1):72, 1999.

46. Kay D, Marino FE: Fluid ingestion and exercise hyperthermia: Implications for performance, thermoregulation, metabolism, and development of fatigue, *Journal of Sports Sciences* 18(2):71, 2000.

47. Kleiner DM: A new exertional heat illness scale. *Athletic Therapy Today* 7(6):65, 2002.

48. Kozack JK, MacIntyre DL: Malignant hyperthermia, *Phys Ther* 81:945, 2001.

49. Lemack L: The artificial turf debate. *Sports-Med Update* 15(1):14, 2000.

50. Levine B, Stray-Gundersen J: Exercise at high altitudes. In Torg J, Shephard R, editors: *Current therapy in sports medicine*, St. Louis, 1995, Mosby.

51. Lightning casualties on the rise in recreational and sports settings, *Athletic Therapy Today* 6(5):33, 2001.

52. Mazerolle S: Current knowledge, attitudes, and practices of certified athletic trainers regarding recognition and treatment of exertional heat stroke, *J Athl Train* 45(2):170–80, 2010.

53. Mazerolle S: Evidence-based medicine and the recognition and treatment of exertional heat stroke, Part II: A perspective from the clinical athletic trainer, *J Athl Train* 46(5):533–42, 2011.

54. Mazerolle S: Is oral temperature an accurate measurement of deep body temperature? A systematic review, *J Athl Train* 46(5):566–73, 2011.

55. McArdle WD, Katch FI, Katch VL: *Exercise physiology*, Philadelphia, 2010, Lea & Febiger.

56. McDermott B, Casa, D: Acute whole-body cooling for exercise-induced hyperthermia: A systematic review, *J Athl Train*, 44(1): 84–93, 2009.

57. Miller T: Preparing for cold weather exercise, *NSCA's Performance Training Journal* 3(1):19, 2004.

58. Mittleman M: Air pollution, exercise, and cardiovascular risk, *New England Journal of Medicine*, 357:1147–49, 2007.

59. Montain S, Cheuvront S, Sawka M: Exercise-associated hyponatremia: Quantitative analysis to understand the aetiology, *British Journal of Sports Medicine* 40(2):98, 2006.

60. Moss RI: Another look at sudden death and exertional hyperthermia, *Athletic Therapy Today* 7(3):44, 2002.

61. Muldoon S, Deuster P, Brandom B: Is there a link between malignant hyperthermia and exertional heat illness? *Exerc Sport Sci Rev* 32(4):174, 2004.

62. Murray B: Fluid replacement: The American College of Sports Medicine position stand, *Sports Science Exchange* 9(4):1, 1996.

63. Murray R: Guidelines for fluid replacement during exercise, *Australian Journal of Nutrition and Dietetics* 53(4 suppl):S17, 1996.

64. *NCAA sports medicine handbook, 2011–2012*, Indianapolis, 2011, National Collegiate Athletic Association.

65. Nimmo M: Exercise in the cold, *Journal of Sports Sciences* 22(10):886, 2004.

66. Peden DB: Air pollutants, exercise, and risk of developing asthma in children, *Clinic J Sports Med* 13(1):62, 2003.

67. Proulx C: Effect of water temperature on cooling efficiency during hyperthermia in humans, *J App Physiol* 94(4):1317, 2003.

68. Reilly T: How can traveling athletes deal with jet lag? *Kinesiology* 41(2):128–35, 2009.

69. Rush S: Winter exercise, *ACSM's Health and Fitness Journal* 5(6):23, 2001.

70. Scholand G: Straight talk: Researching synthetic turf suppliers, *Athletic management* 17(3):59, 2005.

71. Seto C: Environmental illness in athletes, *Clinics in Sports Medicine* 24(3):695–718, 2005.

72. Sherriffs S: Hydration in sport and exercise: Water, sports drinks and other drinks, *Nutrition Bulletin* 34(4):374–79, 2009.

73. Siegel A: Hydration and its disorders: New understandings, new treatments, *AMAA Journal* 19(1):13, 2006.

74. Smith J: Cooling methods used in the treatment of exertional heat illness, *British Journal of Sports Medicine* 39(8):503, 2005.

75. Taylor K: Ultraviolet radiation: Recognizing hidden potential for injury, *Athletic Therapy and Training*, 15(3):75–80, 2010.

76. Tyler C: Cooling the neck region during exercise in the heat. *J Athl Train*, 46(1):61–68, 2011.

77. Volpe S: Estimation of prepractice hydration status of National Collegiate Athletic Association Division I Athletes, *J Athl Train*, 44(6):624–29, 2009.

78. Wallace C: Fluid replacement and dehydration. In *NFHS Sports Medicine Handbook* Indianapolis, 2011, NFHS.

79. Walsh K, Bennett B, Cooper M: National Athletic Trainers' Association position statement: Lightning safety for athletics and recreation, *J Athl Train* 35(4):471, 2000.

80. Walsh K, Cooper, M: Lightening. In Casa D, editor: *Preventing sudden death in sport and physical activity*, New York, 2011, Jones and Bartlett Publishers.

81. Walters F: Position stand on lightning and thunder: The Athletic Health Care Services of the District of Columbia Public Schools, *J Athl Train* 28(3):201, 1993.

82. Waterhouse J: Identifying some determinants of "jet lag" and its symptoms: A study of athletes and other travelers, *British Journal of Sports Medicine* 36(1):54, 2002.

83. Watson G, Casa D, Fiala K: Creatine use and exercise heat tolerance in dehydrated men, *J Athl Train* 41(1):18, 2006.

84. Williams S: A review of football injuries on third and fourth generation artificial turfs compared with natural turf, *Sports Medicine* 41(11):903–23, 2011.

85. Wright J: Playing field issues in sports medicine, *Current Sports Medicine Issues*, 9(3):129–33, 2010.

86. Yeargin S: Thermoregulatory responses and hydration practices in heat-acclimatized adolescents during preseason high school football, *J Athl Train* 45(2):136–46, 2010.

ANNOTATED BIBLIOGRAPHY

Armstrong LE: *Performing in extreme environments: Training and working in intense heat, frigid cold, under water, high altitude, air pollution*, Champaign, IL, 2000, Human Kinetics.

Looks at exercise as it is affected by a variety of environmental conditions.

Giesbrecht G, Wikerson J: *Hypothermia, frostbite and other cold injuries: Prevention, recognition and treatment*, Seattle, 2006, Mountaineers Books.

A comprehensive guide to recognizing, preventing, and treating hypothermia and other cold injuries.

Graver D, Armstrong L: *Exertional heat illness*, Champaign, IL, 2003, Human Kinetics.

Focuses on all aspects of heat illness and is a good resource for the athletic trainer.

Maughan R, Murray R: *Sports drinks: Basic science and practical aspects*, Boca Raton, FL, 2001, CRC Press.

Provides a review of current knowledge on issues relating to the formulation of sports drinks and the physiological responses to their ingestion during physical activity.

NCAA sports medicine handbook, 2005–2006, Indianapolis, 2005, National Collegiate Athletic Association.

Contains guidelines and recommendations for preventing heat illness and hypohydration, for cold, for stress, and for lightning safety.

Pollard A, Murdoch D: *High altitude medicine handbook*, Abbington, England, 2003, Radcliffe Medical Press.

A compilation of pertinent information on almost every aspect of health and illness at altitudes higher than 2,500 meters.

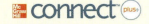

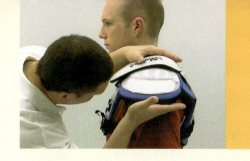

Protective Equipment

■ Objectives

When you finish this chapter you should be able to

- Fit selected protective equipment properly (e.g., football helmets, shoulder pads, and running shoes).
- Differentiate between good and bad features of selected protective devices.
- Contrast the advantages and disadvantages of customized versus off-the-shelf foot and ankle protective devices.

- Rate the protective value of various materials used in sports to make pads and orthotic devices.
- List the steps in making a customized foam pad with a thermomoldable shell.

■ Outline

■ Key Terms

pronators   supinators

■ Connect Highlights

Visit connect.mcgraw-hill.com for further exercises to apply your knowledge:

- Clinical application scenarios covering the use and application of protective equipment and the construction of pads and orthotic devices
- Click-and-drag questions covering fitting protective equipment, construction and application of protective devices
- Multiple-choice questions covering prophylactic bracing, construction of protective pads, and knowledge and application of protective equipment
- Selection questions covering anatomy of the shoe

One of the main responsibilities of the athletic trainer is to try to minimize the likelihood of injury or reinjury. A number of factors either singly or collectively can contribute to the incidence of injury. Certainly, the selection, fitting, and maintenance of protective equipment are critical not only in injury prevention but also in injury rehabilitation. Regardless of whether the athletic trainer works at the secondary-school, collegiate, or professional level or in a clinical, hospital, corporate, or industrial setting, it is essential that the athletic trainer have some knowledge about the types of protective equipment available for a particular activity and how that equipment should best be fitted and maintained to reduce the possibility of injury.[49]

This protection is particularly important in direct-collision sports, such as football, hockey, and lacrosse, but it can also be important in indirect-contact sports, such as basketball and soccer. When protective sports equipment is selected and purchased, a significant commitment is made to safeguard athletes' health and welfare.

During the rehabilitation period following injury, the athletic trainer must be knowledgeable about the types of protective rehabilitation equipment available and about how that equipment should be utilized to facilitate the recovery process.

SAFETY STANDARDS FOR SPORTS EQUIPMENT AND FACILITIES

There is serious concern about the standards for protective sports equipment, particularly material durability standards. These concerns include who should set the standards, the mass production of equipment, equipment testing methods, and requirements for wearing protective equipment. Standards are also needed for protective equipment maintenance, repair, and replacement. Too often, old, worn-out, and ill-fitting equipment is passed down from the varsity players to the younger and often less experienced players, compounding their risk of injury.[52] It is critical for those responsible for purchasing athletic equipment to be less concerned with the color, look, and style of a piece of equipment and more concerned with its ability to prevent injury.[53] Many national organizations are addressing these issues. Engineering, chemistry, biomechanics, anatomy, physiology, physics, computer science, and other related disciplines are

> Old, worn-out, poorly fitted equipment should never be passed down to younger, less experienced players because it compounds their chances for injury.

applied to solve problems inherent in safety standardization of sports equipment and facilities. *Focus Box 7–1:* "Equipment Regulatory Agencies" lists agencies that regulate protective sports equipment.

LEGAL CONCERNS IN USING PROTECTIVE EQUIPMENT

As with other aspects of sports participation, litigation related to the use of protective equipment is increasing. Both manufacturers and those who purchase sports equipment must foresee all possible uses and misuses of the equipment and must warn the user of any potential risks inherent in using or misusing that equipment.

If an injury occurs as a result of an individual using a piece of equipment that is determined to be defective or inadequate for its intended purpose, the manufacturer is considered liable. If a piece of protective equipment is modified in any way by an athlete, a coach, or an athletic trainer (e.g., removing some pads from inside a football helmet), the liability on the part of the manufacturer is voided, and the individual who modified the equipment becomes liable. *The best way for an athletic trainer to avoid litigation is to follow exactly the manufacturer's instructions for using and maintaining protective equipment.*

If an athletic trainer modifies a piece of equipment and an individual wearing that equipment is injured, it is likely that any lawsuit would involve both the athletic trainer individually and the employing institution or company. This becomes a case of tort (described in Chapter 3) in which the injured person must show that the athletic trainer was negligent in his or her decision to alter a piece of equipment and that the negligence resulted in injury. The athletic trainer would then be legally liable for that action. (See *Focus Box 7–2:* "Guidelines for selecting, purchasing, and fitting protective gear and sports equipment to help minimize liability.")

EQUIPMENT RECONDITIONING AND RECERTIFICATION

The National Operating Committee on Standards for Athletic Equipment (NOCSAE) is an organization that has established voluntary test standards to reduce head injuries by establishing minimum safety requirements for football helmets/face masks; baseball/softball batting helmets, baseballs and softballs; and lacrosse helmets/face masks.[46] These standards have been adopted by various regulatory bodies for sports, including the NCAA and the National Federation of State High School Associations (NFHS). Factors such as the type of helmet and the amount and intensity of usage determine the condition of each helmet over a period of time.

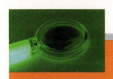
Equipment regulatory agencies

American National Standards Institute
1819 L Street NW
Washington, DC 20036
(202) 293-8020
www.ansi.org

American Society for Testing Materials
100 Barr Harbor Drive
West Conshohocken, PA 19428-2959
(610) 832-9585
www.astm.org

Athletic Equipment Manufacturers Association
Dorothy Cutting
Cornell University Athletic Department
P.O. Box 729
Ithaca, NY 14851
(607) 255-4115
www.wisc.edu/ath/aema

Hockey Equipment Certification Council
18103 Trans Canada Highway
Kirkland, QC H9J324
Canada
(514) 697-9900
www.hecc.net

National Athletic Trainers' Association
2952 Stemmons Freeway
Dallas, TX 75247-6196
(214) 637-6282
www.nata.org

National Collegiate Athletic Association
700 W. Washington Street
P.O. Box 6222
Indianapolis, IN 46206-6222
www.ncaa.org

National Association of Intercollegiate Athletics
6120 S. Yale Avenue
Suite 1450
Tulsa, OK 74136
(918) 494-8828
www.naia.org

National Federation of State High School
   Athletic Associations
P.O. Box 690
Indianapolis, IN 46200
(317) 972-6900
www.nfhs.org

National Operating Committee on Standards for
   Athletic Equipment
P.O. Box 12290
Overland, KS 66282-2290
www.nocsae.org

Sporting Goods Manufacturers Association
200 Castlewood Drive
North Palm Beach, FL 33418
(561) 842-4100
http://sgma@ix.netcom.com

U.S. Consumer Product Safety Commission
4330 East-West Highway
Bethesda, MD 20814-4408
(301) 504-0990
www.cpsc.gov

The NOCSAE helmet standard is not a warranty, but simply a statement that a particular helmet model met the requirements of performance tests when it was manufactured or reconditioned. NOCSAE does recommend that the consumer adhere to a program of periodically having used helmets reconditioned and recertified. Because of the difference in the amount and intensity of usage on each helmet, the consumer should use discretion regarding the frequency with which certain helmets are to be reconditioned and recertified. Helmets that regularly undergo the reconditioning and recertification process can meet standard performance requirements for many seasons, depending on the model and usage. *Focus Box 7–3: "Guidelines for purchasing and reconditioning helmets"* provides some guidelines.

USING OFF-THE-SHELF VERSUS CUSTOM PROTECTIVE EQUIPMENT

"Off-the-shelf" equipment is premade and packaged by the manufacturer and when taken out of the package may be used immediately without modification. Examples of off-the-shelf equipment are neoprene sleeves, sorbethane shoe inserts, and protective ankle braces. Custom equipment is

An athletic training student must acquire a basic understanding of protective sports equipment.

? What competencies relative to protective sports equipment must an athletic training student have?

7–1 Clinical Application Exercise

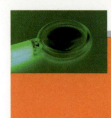

FOCUS 7-2 Focus on Injury/Illness Prevention and Wellness Protection

Guidelines for selecting, purchasing, and fitting protective gear and sports equipment to help minimize liability

- Buy sports equipment from reputable manufacturers.
- Buy the safest equipment that resources permit.
- Make sure that all equipment is assembled correctly.
- Ensure that the person who assembles equipment is competent to do so and follows the manufacturer's instructions to the letter.
- Maintain all equipment properly, according to the manufacturer's guidelines.
- Use equipment only for the purpose for which it was designed.
- If an athlete is wearing some type of immobilization device (e.g., cast, brace), make certain that this does not violate the rules of that sport.
- Warn individuals who use the equipment about all possible risks that using the equipment could entail.
- Use great caution in constructing or customizing of any piece of equipment.
- Do not use defective equipment.
- Routinely inspect all equipment for defects and render all defective equipment unusable.

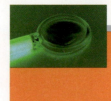

FOCUS 7-3 Focus on Injury/Illness Prevention and Wellness Protection

Guidelines for purchasing and reconditioning helmets

- Purchase only NOCSAE-approved helmets.
- Purchase helmets for the appropriate skill level. For example, do not purchase youth helmets for high-school football.
- Assign a code number to each helmet purchased, and record the date of purchase.
- Fit helmets according to manufacturer's recommendations.
- Recheck helmets for proper fit during the season.
- Review written warranty information and comply with manufacturer's requirement(s) for cleaning/reconditioning/recertification.
- Replace or repair broken or damaged helmets before returning to service.
- Develop a written accounting of player use, inspections, reconditioning, recertification, and disposal of each helmet.
- Clean helmets and other equipment according to manufacturer's recommendations on a regular schedule during the season and at the end of the season prior to off-season storage in order to avoid infections.
- Recertify/recondition each football helmet according to manufacturer's warranty.
- Recertify/recondition helmets every 2 years using a certified NOCSAE-approved vendor if no warranty exists or after the warranty expires.

constructed according to the individual characteristics of the athlete. Using off-the-shelf items may cause problems with sizing and exact fit. In contrast, a custom piece of equipment can be specifically sized and made to fit the protective and support needs of the individual. Generally, custom equipment is more expensive than off-the-shelf equipment. This increased cost may be attributed to the time that is necessary for an athletic trainer, a physical therapist, an orthotist, or an ortho tech to evaluate, construct, fit, and adjust a custom piece of equipment.

HEAD PROTECTION

Direct-collision sports, such as football and hockey, require special protective equipment, especially for the head.[19] Football and ice hockey provide frequent opportunities for body contact but hockey players generally move faster and therefore create greater impact forces. Besides direct head contact, hockey has the added injury elements of swinging sticks and fast-moving pucks. Other sports using fast-moving projectiles are baseball, with its pitched ball and swinging bat; field hockey; lacrosse; and track and field, with the javelin, discus, and shot, which can also produce serious head injuries.[19]

Football Helmets

NOCSAE has developed standards for football helmet certification.[46] An approved helmet must protect against concussive forces that may injure the brain. Collisions that cause concussions are usually with another player or the turf.[38]

> **Football helmets must be NOCSAE certified.**

Schools must provide the athlete with quality equipment, especially football helmets. All helmets must have NOCSAE[46] certification. However, a helmet that is certified is not necessarily completely fail-safe.[63] Athletes as well as their parents must be apprised of the dangers that are inherent in any sport, particularly football.[38]

> **Football helmets must withstand repeated blows that are of high mass and low velocity.**

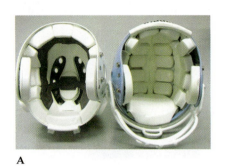
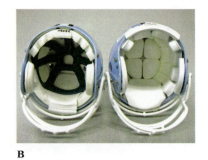
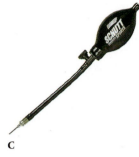

A   B   C

FIGURE 7–1 Football Helmets: **(A)** Fluid-filled helmet. **(B)** Air-filled helmet. **(C)** Pump for inflating air/helmets. (C: Courtesy Sports Authority, www.sportsauthority.com)

To make this danger especially clear, NOCSAE has adopted the following recommended warning to be placed on all football helmets:

> WARNING: Do not strike an opponent with any part of this helmet or face mask. This is a violation of football rules and may cause you to suffer severe brain or neck injury, including paralysis or death. Severe brain or neck injury may also occur accidentally while playing football. NO HELMET CAN PREVENT ALL SUCH INJURIES. USE THIS HELMET AT YOUR OWN RISK.[46]

Each player's helmet must have this visible, exterior warning label or a similar one ensuring that players have been made aware of the risks involved in the game of American football. The warning label must be attached to each helmet by both the manufacturer and the reconditioner.[46] It is important to have each player read this warning, after which it is read aloud by the equipment manager. The athlete then should sign a statement agreeing that he or she understands this warning.

A link to the NATA position statement "Head down contact and spearing in tackle football" (http://www.nata.org/sites/default/files/HeadDownContact AndSpearingInTackleFB.pdf) can be found at www.mhhe.com/prentice15e. A variety of football helmets are available on the market (Figure 7–1), although the number of companies producing these helmets has decreased significantly over the years. This decrease in the number of helmet manufacturers can be attributed primarily to the number of lawsuits and liability cases that have forced many companies out of business.

The lightweight Revolution helmet from Riddell marks the first significant structural change in football helmet design in nearly 25 years (Figure 7–2A).[44] The protective shell extends to the jaw area to provide protection to the side of the head and the jaw as well as improved front-to-back fit and stability. The distance between the helmet shell and the head has been increased. The padding inflates to provide a custom fit to every player's head shape. The face guard system is designed to isolate the attachment points of the face guard from the shell, thus reducing jarring to the player from low-level impacts to the face guard.

Another new football helmet, developed by Xenith, is lined with 18 thermoplastic airflow shock absorbers, which are embedded in a flexible cap. The helmet's design is said to adapt to the force of an impact and dissipate the energy to decrease the acceleration of the head and prevent the jarring that causes concussions (Figure 7–2B).

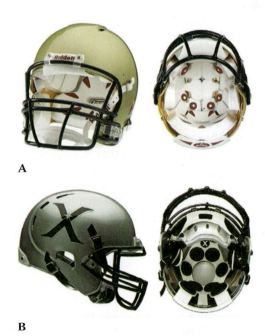

A

B

FIGURE 7–2 New helmet designs. **(A)** Revolution helmet. **(B)** Xenith helmet. (A: Courtesy Ridell; B: Courtesy Xenith)

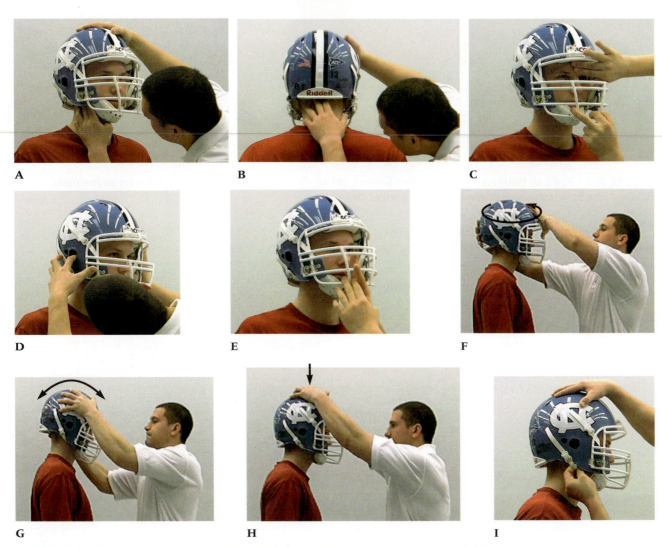

FIGURE 7–3 Properly fitting a football helmet. **(A)** Check snugness of cheek pads. **(B)** Helmet should cover base of skull. **(C)** Two finger widths above eyes. **(D)** Ear holes line up. **(E)** Three finger widths from face mask. **(F, G, H)** Helmet should not shift on head. **(I)** Check chin straps.

Fitting a Football Helmet When fitting a football helmet, closely follow the manufacturer's directions for a proper fit (Figure 7–3). (See *Focus Box 7–4: "Properly fitting the football helmet."*) The football helmet must be routinely checked for proper fit, especially in the first few days that it is worn. A check for snugness should be made by inserting a credit card between the head and the liner. Fit is proper when the credit card is resisted firmly when moved back and forth. If a team that travels to a different altitude and air pressure uses air bladder helmets, the helmet fit must be routinely rechecked.

Chin straps are also important in maintaining the proper head and helmet relationship. Three basic types of chin straps are in use today: a two-snap, a four-snap, and a six-snap strap. Many coaches prefer the four-snap chin strap because it keeps the helmet from tilting forward and backward. The chin strap should always be locked so that it cannot be released by a hard external force to the helmet.

Jaw pads are also essential to keep the helmet from rocking laterally. They should fit snugly against the player's cheekbones. Certification of a helmet's ability to withstand the forces of the game is of no avail if the helmet is not properly fitted or maintained. Loop straps should be used to fix the face mask to the helmet. These can be easily cut to remove the face mask should there be an injury that requires CPR or spinal injury.

Ice Hockey Helmets

Like football helmets, ice hockey helmets have been upgraded and standardized.[39] Blows to the head in ice hockey, in contrast to football, are

The athletic trainer explains helmet's limitations to a football team.

? Why does the football helmet have a warning label?

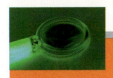

FOCUS 7–4 Focus on Injury/Illness Prevention and Wellness Protection

Properly fitting the football helmet

In general, the helmet should adhere to the following fit standards:

1. The helmet should fit snugly around all parts of the player's head (front, sides, and crown), and there should be no gaps between the cheek pads and the head or face (Figure 7–3A).
2. It should cover the base of the skull. The pads placed at the back of the neck should be snug, but not to the extent of discomfort (Figure 7–3B).
3. It should not come down over the eyes. It should set (front edge) ¾ inch (1.91 cm) above the player's eyebrows (approximately two finger widths) (Figure 7–3C).
4. The ear holes should be aligned with the external opening in the ear canal (Figure 7–3D).
5. The face mask should be attached securely to the helmet, allowing a complete field of vision and should be positioned three finger widths from the chin (Figure 7–3E).
6. It should not shift when manual pressure is applied (Figure 7–3F/G).
7. It should not recoil on impact. (Figure 7–3H)
8. The chin strap should be an equal distance from the center of the helmet. Straps must keep the helmet from moving up and down or side to side (Figure 7–3I).

usually singular rather than multiple. An ice hockey helmet must withstand not only high-velocity impacts (e.g., being hit with a stick or a puck, which produces low mass and high velocity) but also the high-mass–low-velocity forces produced by running into the boards or falling on the ice.[39] In each instance, the hockey helmet, like the football helmet, must be able to disperse the impact over a large surface area through a firm exterior shell and, at the same time, be able to decelerate forces that act on the head through a proper energy-absorbing liner. It is essential for all hockey players to wear protective helmets that carry the stamp of approval from either the Canadian Standards Association (CSA) (Figure 7–4) or the Hockey Equipment Certification Council (HECC). *Focus Box 7–5*: "Properly fitting the ice hockey helmet" offers some tips.

> Even high-quality helmets are of no use if not properly fitted and maintained.

> Ice hockey helmets must withstand the high-velocity impact from a stick or puck and the low-velocity forces from falling or hitting a board.

Baseball/Softball Batting Helmets

Like ice hockey helmets, the baseball/softball batting helmet must withstand high-velocity impacts.[19] Unlike football and ice hockey, baseball and softball have not produced a great deal of data on batting helmets. It has been suggested, however, that baseball and softball helmets do little to adequately dissipate the energy of the ball during impact (Figure 7–5). A

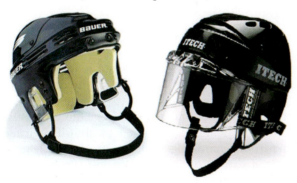

FIGURE 7–4   Ice hockey helmets. (Courtesy Sports Authority, www.sportsauthority.com)

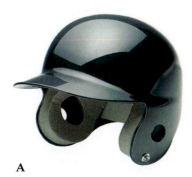

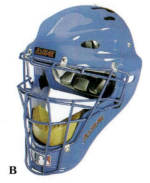

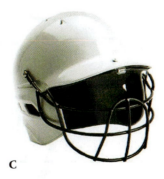

A   **B**   **C**

FIGURE 7–5   There is some question about how well baseball batting helmets protect against high-velocity impacts. **(A)** Batter's helmet. **(B)** Catcher's helmet and mask. **(C)** Batter's face mask and face shield. (Courtesy Sports Authority, www.sportsauthority.com)

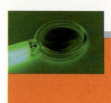

FOCUS 7–5 Focus on Injury/Illness Prevention and Wellness Protection

Properly fitting the ice hockey helmet

- The helmet should be comfortably snug at the forehead, top, back, and sides of the head.
- The helmet should not shift or wobble on the head—this will reduce protection and comfort and could also be distracting during play.
- The chin strap should be adjusted, so that it gently contacts the chin when the mouth is closed.
- The helmet should fit flat and snug on the head above the eyebrows without tilting forward or back.
- If the helmet is loose or not properly fastened, it loses its protective qualities.
- The bottom of a full cage face mask should rest gently on the chin when properly fitted.

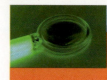

FOCUS 7–6 Focus on Injury/Illness Prevention and Wellness Protection

Guidelines for fitting a cycling helmet

- The helmet should be level on the head.
- If it is not level, adjust the fit, using the extra foam fitting pads on the inside to provide contact with the head all the way around.
- With a "one size fits all" model with a fitting ring, adjust the fit by tightening the ring if needed.
- Adjust the rear (nape) straps, then the front straps, to position the Y fitting where the straps come together just under the ear. (It may be necessary to slide the straps across the top of the helmet to get them even on both sides.)
- Next, adjust the chin strap so that it is comfortably snug.
- Next adjust the rear stabilizer if the helmet has one.
- Shake your head around violently.
- Push under the front edge and push up and back. If the helmet moves more than an inch or so from level, tighten the straps so that the helmet is level and feels solid but comfortable on the head.

possible solution is to add external padding or to improve the helmet's suspension. The use of a helmet with an ear flap can afford some additional protection to the batter. Each runner and on-deck batter is required to wear a baseball or softball helmet that carries the NOCSAE stamp, which is similar to the warning on football helmets.

Cycling Helmets

Unlike the other helmets discussed, cycling helmets are designed to protect the head during one impact. Football, hockey, and baseball helmets are more durable and can survive repeated impacts.[38] Many states require the use of cycling helmets, especially by adolescents (Figure 7–6). *Focus Box 7–6:* "Guidelines for fitting a cycling helmet" outlines fitting procedures.

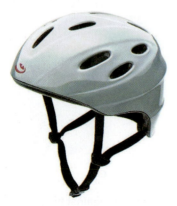

FIGURE 7–6 Cycling helmet. (Courtesy Sports Authority, www.sportsauthority.com)

Lacrosse Helmets

Helmets are required equipment for all male lacrosse players. Women's lacrosse requires only a protective eye guard. Lacrosse helmets are made of a hard plastic with a wire mesh cage, or face mask, to protect the front of the face (Figure 7–7). The face mask must have a center bar running from the top to the bottom. The helmet is designed to absorb repeated impact from a hard, high-velocity projectile. Helmets come in a variety of sizes and are usually measured in inches. Lacrosse helmets use a four-point buckling system both to ensure that they stay on and to allow for a better fit. Goalie helmets add a throat protector.[16]

Soccer Headgear

Several companies have marketed headgear for soccer players to reduce concussions and other head injuries that occur from heading a soccer ball.[11] The headgear is essentially a headband with a piece of foam in the front that is about 1½ to 2 inches (3.8 to 5 cm) wide. To date there are no studies that demonstrate that this headgear is effective in reducing the incidence of concussions or other head injuries.[57,62] It is far more likely that a soccer player will get a concussion from hitting his or her head on another player, the goalpost, or the ground than from heading a soccer ball.[57]

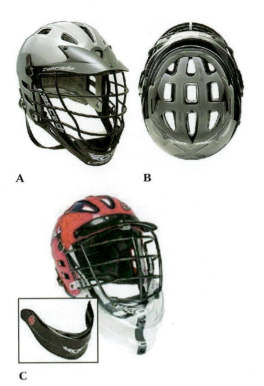

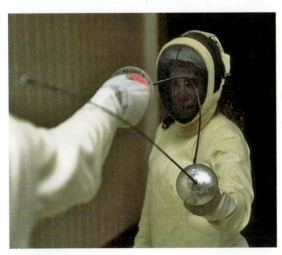

FIGURE 7–7 **(A)** Men's lacrosse helmet. **(B)** Inside padding. **(C)** Goalie helmet with throat protector. (Courtesy Sports Authority www.sportsauthority.com)

FACE PROTECTION

Devices that provide face protection fall into five categories: full face guards, throat protection, mouth guards, ear guards, and eye protection devices.

Full Face Guards

Face guards are used in a variety of sports to protect against flying or carried objects during a collision with another player (Figure 7–8).[26] Since the adoption of face guards and mouth guards for use in football, the incidence of facial injuries (e.g.,

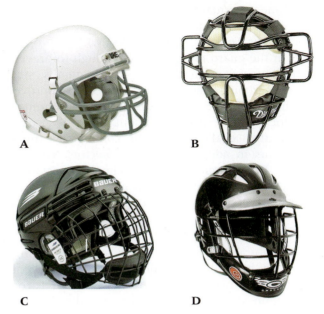

FIGURE 7–9 **(A)** Football face mask. **(B)** Baseball catcher's face mask. **(C)** Ice hockey face mask. **(D)** Lacrosse face mask.

lacerations, nose fractures, eye injuries) has dramatically decreased. However, the number of concussions and, to some extent, neck injuries has increased because the head is more often used to make initial contact. The catcher in baseball, the goalie in hockey, and the lacrosse player should all be adequately protected against facial injuries, particularly lacerations and fractures (Figure 7–9).

A variety of face masks and bars are available to the player, depending on the position played and the degree of protection needed.[26] In football, no face guard should have less than two bars. Proper mounting of the face mask and bars is imperative for maximum safety. All mountings should be made in such a way that the bar attachments are flush with the helmet. A 3-inch (7.62 cm) space should exist between the top of the face guard

Face protection
• Face guards
• Throat protection devices
• Mouth guards
• Ear guards
• Eye protection devices

and the lower edge of the helmet. No helmet should be drilled more than one time on each side, and this drilling must be done by a factory-authorized reconditioner. Attachment of a bar or face mask not specifically designed for the helmet can invalidate the manufacturer's warranty.

Ice hockey face masks have been shown to reduce the incidence of facial injuries. In high school, face masks are required not just for the goalie but for all players. Helmets should be equipped with commercial plastic-coated wire mask guards, which

FIGURE 7–8 Sports such as fencing require complete face protection.

must meet standards set by the Hockey Equipment Certification Council (HECC) and the American Society for Testing Materials (ASTM).[46] The openings in the guard must be small enough to prevent a hockey stick from entering. Plastic guards, such as polycarbonate face shields, have been approved by the HECC, the ASTM, and the CSA Committee on Hockey Protective Equipment. The rule also requires that goalkeepers wear commercial throat protectors in addition to face protectors. The National Federation of High School Associations (NFHS) rule is similar to the NCAA rule that requires players to wear face guards.

Throat (Laryngotracheal) Protection

A laryngotracheal injury, though relatively uncommon, can be fatal.[38] Baseball catchers, lacrosse goalies, and ice hockey goalies are most at risk. Throat protection should be mandatory for these sports. Throat protectors may be built into the helmet or they can be attached separately (Figure 7–10).

Mouth Guards

The majority of dental traumas can be prevented if the athlete wears a correctly fitted, customized intraoral mouth guard (Figure 7–11).[34,37,48] Although it has been argued that mouth guards reduce the likelihood of concussion, the most recent evidence suggests that they do not appear to have any effect in preventing concussions.[39] Mouth guards also minimize lacerations to the lips and cheeks and fractures to the mandible. The mouth protector should give the athlete proper and tight fit, comfort, unrestricted breathing, and unimpeded speech during competition. A loose mouth guard will soon be ejected onto the ground or left unused in the locker room.[2] The athlete's air passages should not be obstructed in any way. It is best when the mouth guard is retained on the upper jaw and projects backward only as far as the last molar, thus permitting speech. Maximum protection is afforded when the mouth guard is composed of a flexible, resilient material and is formed to fit to the teeth and upper jaw.[36]

Cutting down mouth guards to cover only the front teeth should never be permitted. This

> A properly fitted mouth guard protects the teeth, absorbs blows to the chin, and can prevent concussion.

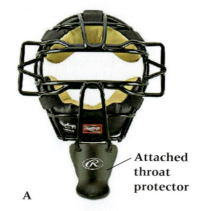
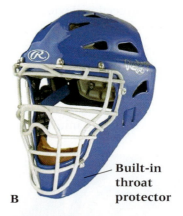

A — Attached throat protector

B — Built-in throat protector

FIGURE 7–10   A throat protector can be attached to **(A)** the catcher's face mask in baseball and softball and the **(B)** a goalie mask in lacrosse and ice hockey. (Courtesy Sports Authority, www.sportsauthority.com)

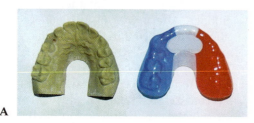
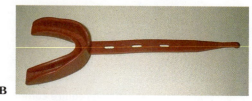

A   **B**

FIGURE 7–11   Mouth guards. **(A)** Custom-fit from a mold and **(B)** heat moldable.

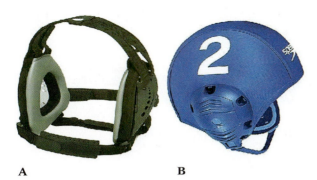

FIGURE 7–12 Ear protection.
(A) Wrestler's ear guard.(Courtesy Sports Authority, www.thesportsauthority.com)
(B) Water polo player's ear protection.
(Courtesy Speedo USA)

invalidates the manufacturer's warranty against dental injuries, and a cut-down mouth guard can become dislodged and lead to an obstructed airway.

The three types of mouth guards generally used in sports are the stock variety, the commercial mouth guard formed after submersion in boiling water, and the custom-fabricated type, which is formed over a mold made from an impression of the athlete's maxillary arch.[48,65]

Many high schools and colleges require that mouth guards be worn at all times during participation. For example, the NCAA football rules mandate that all players wear a properly manufactured mouth guard. A time-out is charged to a team if a player fails to wear the mouth guard.[29] To assist enforcement, official mouth guards are required to be in a highly visible color.

Ear Guards

With the exception of wrestling, water polo, and boxing, most contact sports do not make a special practice of protecting the ears. All these sports can cause irritation of the ears to the point that permanent deformity can ensue. To avoid this problem, ear guards should be worn routinely (Figure 7–12).

Eye Protection Devices

The National Society to Prevent Blindness estimates that the highest percentage of eye injuries are sports- or play-related. Most injuries are from blunt trauma. Protective devices must be sport specific.[31]

Glasses For the individual who must wear corrective lenses, glasses can be both a blessing and a nuisance. They may slip on sweat, get bent when hit, fog from perspiration, detract from peripheral vision, and be difficult to wear with protective headgear. Even with all these disadvantages, properly fitted and designed glasses can provide adequate protection and withstand the rigors of the sport.

Athletes should wear polycarbonate lenses, which are virtually unbreakable.[60] These are the newest type of lenses available, and they are the safest. If the athlete has glass lenses, they must be case-hardened to prevent them from splintering on impact. When a case-hardened lens breaks, it crumbles, eliminating the sharp edges that may penetrate the eye. The cost of this process is relatively low. The only disadvantages are that the glasses are heavier than average and may be scratched more easily than regular glasses.[32] Another possible sports advantage of glass-lensed glasses is that they can be created so the lenses become color-tinted when exposed to ultraviolet rays from the sun and then return to a clear state when removed from the sun's rays. These lenses are known as photochromic lenses.

Contact Lenses The individual who can wear contact lenses without discomfort can avoid many of the inconveniences of glasses. The greatest advantage to contact lenses is probably the fact that they "become a part of the eye" and move with it.

Contact lenses come mainly in two types: the corneal type, which covers just the iris of the eye, and the scleral type, which covers the entire front of the eye, including the white. Peripheral vision as well as astigmatism and corneal waviness are improved through the use of contact lenses. Unlike glasses, contact lenses do not normally cloud during temperature changes. They also can be tinted to reduce glare. For example, yellow lenses can be used against ice glare and blue ones against glare from snow. Some serious disadvantages of wearing contact lenses are the possibility of corneal irritation caused by dust getting under the lens and the possibility of a lens becoming dislodged during body contact. In addition, only certain individuals can wear contacts with comfort, and some individuals are unable to ever wear them because of certain eye idiosyncrasies. Athletes currently prefer the soft, hydrophilic lenses to the hard type. Adjustment time for the soft lenses is shorter than for the hard, they can be more easily replaced, and they are more adaptable to the sports environment. Disposable lenses and lenses that can be worn for an extended period are also available. In the last few years, the cost of contact lenses has dropped significantly.

The advent of two eye surgery procedures, radial kerotectomy (RK) and laser insitu keratomileusis (LASIK), has potentially reduced the need for individuals to wear vision-correcting glasses or contact lenses. Although relatively expensive, the LASIK procedure has proven to be a safe and effective technique for correcting faulty vision.

Eye and Glasses Guards It is essential that athletes take special precautions to protect their eyes, especially in sports that use fast-moving projectiles

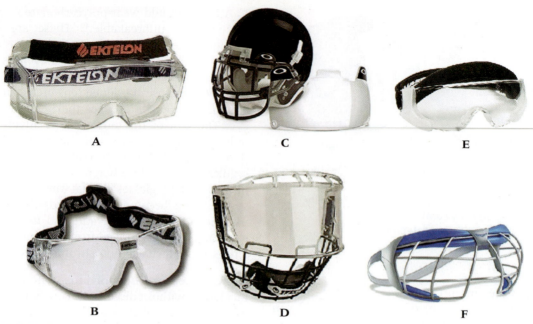

FIGURE 7–13 **(A & B)** Athletes playing sports that involve small, fast projectiles should wear closed eye guards. **(C)** Polycarbonate shield for a football helmet. **(D)** Shield for an ice hockey face mask. **(E)** Field hockey goggle. **(F)** Lacrosse goggle. (Courtesy Sports Authority, www.sportsauthority.com)

and implements, such as handball and racquetball (Figure 7–13).[32] Besides the more obvious sports of ice hockey, lacrosse, and baseball, the racquet sports can also cause serious eye injury. Athletes not wearing glasses should wear closed eye guards to protect the orbital cavity. Athletes who normally wear glasses with plastic or case-hardened lenses are to some degree already protected against eye injury from an implement or a projectile; however, greater safety is afforded by the polycarbonate frame that surrounds and fits over the athlete's glasses. The protection that the guard affords is excellent, but it hinders vision in some planes. Polycarbonate eye shields can be attached to football face masks, hockey helmets, and baseball and softball helmets.

> Eye protection must be worn by all athletes who play sports that use fast-moving projectiles.

NECK PROTECTION

Experts in cervical injuries consider the major value of commercial and customized cervical collars to be mostly a reminder to the athlete to be cautious rather than to provide a definitive restriction (see Figure 7–17C).[22]

TRUNK AND THORAX PROTECTION

Trunk and thorax protection is essential in many contact and collision sports. Sports such as football,

ice hockey, baseball, and lacrosse use extensive body protection. Areas that are most exposed to impact forces must be properly covered with some material that offers protection against soft-tissue compression. Of particular concern are the external genitalia and the exposed bony protuberances of the body that have insufficient soft tissue for protection, such as shoulders, ribs, and spine (Figure 7–14).

As discussed earlier, the problem that arises in wearing protective equipment is that, although it is armor against injury to the athlete wearing it, it can also serve as a weapon against all opponents. Standards must become more stringent in determining what equipment is absolutely necessary for body protection and at the same time is not itself a source of trauma. Proper fit and proper maintenance of equipment are essential.

Football Shoulder Pads

Two general types of shoulder pads are available: cantilevered and noncantilevered (Figure 7–15). A cantilever is a strap that extends from the front to the back of the shoulder pads that causes the shoulder pads to arch above the tip of the shoulder, thus dispersing pressure onto the pads rather than on the shoulder. The player who uses the shoulder a great deal in blocking and tackling requires the bulkier, cantilevered type, whereas a quarterback, receiver, or youth football player might prefer to use the noncantilevered pads, which don't restrict shoulder motion as much as the cantilevered pads. Over

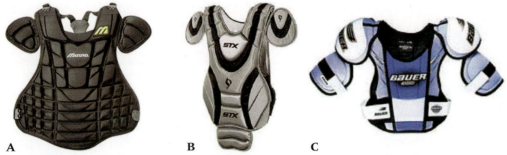

FIGURE 7–14   Chest and thorax protectors. **(A)** Baseball catcher's chest protector.
(B) Lacrosse goalie chest protector. **(C)** Ice hockey thorax protector and shoulder pads.
(Courtesy Sports Authority, www.sportsauthority.com)

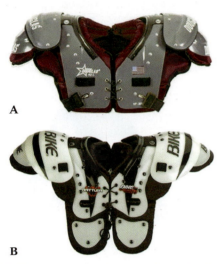

FIGURE 7–15   Shoulder pads protect both the shoulder and thorax. **(A)** Noncantilevered pads. **(B)** Cantilevered pads. (Courtesy Sports Authority, www.sportsauthority.com)

the years, the shoulder pad's front and rear panels have been extended along with the cantilever. *Focus Box 7–7:* "Rules for fitting football shoulder pads" summarizes fitting guidelines (Figure 7–16).

Some athletic trainers use a combination of football and ice hockey shoulder pads to prevent injuries high on the upper arm and shoulder. A pair of supplemental shoulder pads are placed under the football pads (Figure 7–17A&B). The deltoid cap of the hockey pad is connected to the main body of the hockey pad by an adjustable lace. The distal end of the deltoid cap is held in place by a Velcro strap. The chest pad is adjustable to ensure proper fit for any size athlete. The football shoulder pads are placed over the hockey pads. The athletic trainer should observe for a proper fit. Larger football pads may be needed. A neck collar can be attached to the shoulder pads and has been shown to be effective in minimizing neck movement (Figure 7–17C).[22]

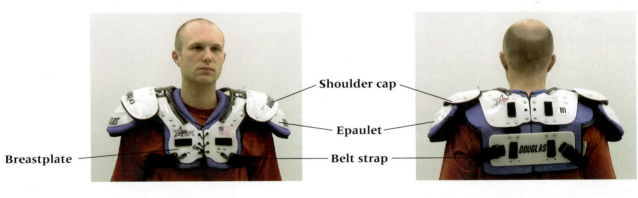

Breastplate

Shoulder cap

Epaulet

Belt strap

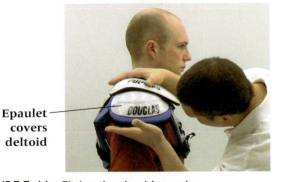

Epaulet covers deltoid

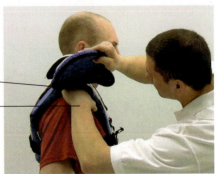

Cantilever

Hand slides under cantilever

FIGURE 7–16   Fitting the shoulder pads.

Chapter Seven ■ Protective Equipment

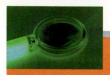
Rules for fitting football shoulder pads

- The width of the shoulder is measured to determine the proper size of pad.
- The inside shoulder pad should cover the tip of the shoulder in a direct line with the lateral aspect of the shoulder.
- The epaulets and cups should cover the deltoid muscle and allow movements required by the athlete's position.
- The neck opening must allow the athlete to raise the arm overhead, but not allow the pad to slide back and forth.

- If a split-clavicle shoulder pad is used, the channel for the top of the shoulder must be in the proper position.
- Straps underneath the arm must hold the pads firmly in place, but not so they constrict soft tissue. A collar and drop-down pads may be added to provide more protection.
- After fitting, make sure the pads don't shift when the athlete puts on the jersey.

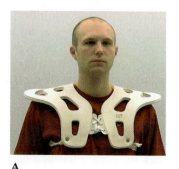
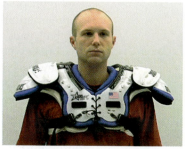
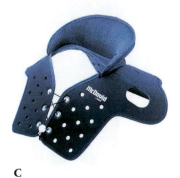

A   **B**   **C**

FIGURE 7–17   **(A & B)** Customized foam is placed on the underside of the shoulder pad to provide additional protection to the acromioclavicular joint or clavicle. **(C)** A cowboy collar can be attached to the shoulder pad.

Sports Bras

Manufacturers have made significant efforts to develop athletic support bras for women who participate in all types of physical activity. In the past, the primary concern was for breast protection against external forces that could cause bruising. Most sports bras are now designed to minimize excessive vertical and horizontal movements of the breasts that occur with running and jumping.[47]

To be effective, a bra should hold the breasts to the chest and prevent stretching of the ligaments of Cooper, which causes premature sagging (Figure 7–18). Metal parts (snaps, fasteners, underwire support) rub and abrade the skin and should be avoided.

> To be effective, a bra should hold the breasts tightly to the chest.

Shoulder straps should be at least 1 inch (2.5 cm) wide for comfort. Nonsupport bras lack sufficient padding, and seams over nipples compound the rubbing of the bra on the nipple, which can lead to irritation.[9]

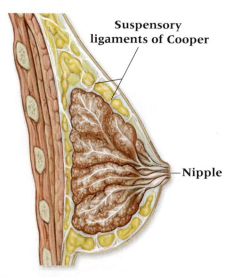

FIGURE 7–18   Stretching of ligaments of Cooper causes premature sagging.

Several styles of sports bras are now available:

1. For women with smaller breasts, it is not as critical to provide compression or support, and

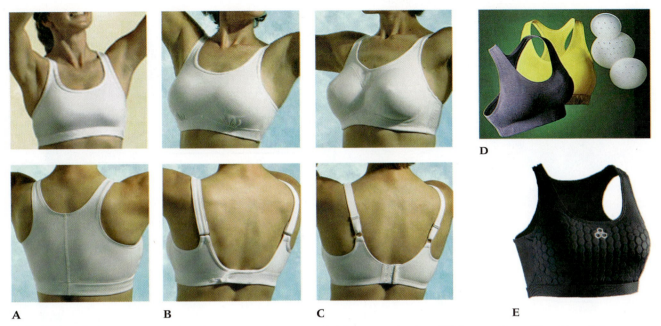

A   B   C   E

D

FIGURE 7–19   Sports bras. **(A)** Lightweight pullover bra. **(B)** Compressive bra. **(C)** Support bra with underwire. **(A–C: Courtesy Title 9 Sports, www.title9sports.com) (D)** Protective sports bra with cup inserts. (Courtesy Turtle Shells Sports Bras) **(E)** Hexpad Bra. (Courtesy McDavid)

thus a less elastic, lightweight bra is sufficient (Figure 7–19A).

2. A compressive pullover bra is perhaps the most common and is recommended for women with medium-size breasts. Compressive bras function like wide elastic bandages, binding the breasts to the chest wall (Figure 7–19B).

3. Support bras are a bit more heavy duty and provide good upward support with elastic material and an underwire. They tend to have wide bands under the breasts with elastic shoulder straps in the back. They are designed for women with larger breasts (Figure 7–19C).

In contact sports, additional padding may be placed inside the cup if needed (Figure 7–19D). Women competing in ice hockey may wear protective plastic chest pieces that attach to their shoulder pads to protect the breast tissue from contusions.

Thorax and Rib Protection

Several manufacturers provide equipment for thorax protection. Many of the thorax protectors and rib belts can be modified by replacing stock pads with customized thermomoldable plastic protective devices.[38] Many lightweight pads have been developed to protect the athlete against external forces. A jacket for the protection of a rib injury incorporates a pad composed of air-inflated, interconnected cylinders that protect against severe external forces (Figure 7–20). The same principle has been used in the development of other protective pads.

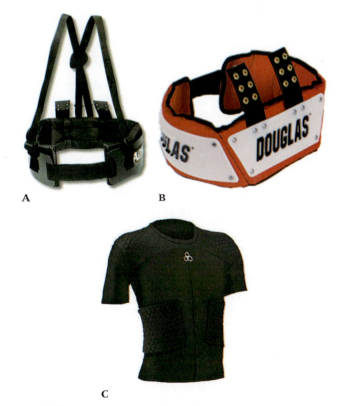

A   B

C

FIGURE 7–20   Protective rib belts. **(A)** Suspended. **(B)** Strap-on. **(C)** Hexpad shirt. (Courtesy Sports Authority, www.thesportsauthority.com)

Hip and Buttock Protection

Pads in the region of the hips and buttocks are often needed in collision and high-velocity sports, such as hockey and football. Other athletes needing

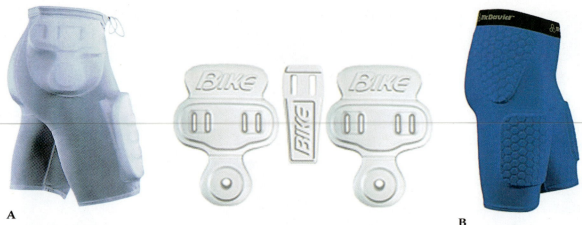

FIGURE 7–21 **(A)** Girdle-style hip and coccygeal pads. (Courtesy Sports Authority, www.thesportsauthority.com) **(B)** Hexpads. (Courtesy McDavid)

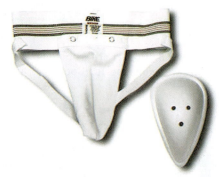

FIGURE 7–22 A cup, held in place by an athletic supporter, used for protecting the genitals against high-velocity projectiles.

protection in this region are amateur boxers, snow skiers, equestrians, jockeys, and water skiers. The most popular commercial pads are the girdle types, in which lightweight hip and coccyx pads are inserted into pockets in the girdle (Figure 7–21).

Groin and Genitalia Protection

Sports involving high-velocity projectiles (e.g., hockey, lacrosse, and baseball) require cup protection for male participants. The cup comes as an off-the-shelf item that fits into place in a jockstrap, or athletic supporter (Figure 7–22).

LOWER-EXTREMITY PROTECTIVE EQUIPMENT

Footwear

It is essential that the athletic trainer and equipment personnel make every effort to fit their athletes with proper socks and shoes.

Socks Poorly fitted socks can cause abnormal stresses on the foot. For example, socks that are too short crowd the toes, especially the fourth and fifth ones. Socks that are too long can wrinkle and cause skin irritation. All athletic socks should be clean, dry, and without holes to avoid topical fungal infections and other irritations. Manufacturers are now providing different types of socks for various sports. The composition of the sock's material also should be noted. Cotton socks can be too bulky, whereas a combination of materials such as cotton and polyester is less bulky and dries faster.

> All athletic socks should be clean and dry and without holes. Socks of the wrong size can irritate the skin.

Shoe Selection The athletic and fitness shoe manufacturing industry has become extremely sophisticated and offers a number of options when it comes to purchasing shoes for different activities.[1] Shoes are specifically manufactured and marketed for running, walking, basketball, tennis, and aerobics. If an individual participates in multiple sports, it is strongly recommended that separate shoes be purchased and worn for each sport.[30,35] It must also be stressed that shoes don't last forever. Over time, they break down, degrade, and lose shock absorption from use. For example, a running shoe is expected to last for 350 to 550 miles before it begins to develop wear patterns and break down to the point where it should no longer be used for running. Thus, for an active individual shoes must constantly be replaced.

> Running shoes tend to break down between 350 and 550 miles.

Athletes and other patients frequently ask athletic trainers about the types of shoes they should purchase or what they should look for in a shoe. Figure 7–23 shows the major parts of a shoe. The following guidelines can help in selecting the most appropriate shoe:

- *Toe box.* There should be plenty of room for the toes in the athletic shoe. A distance of ½ to

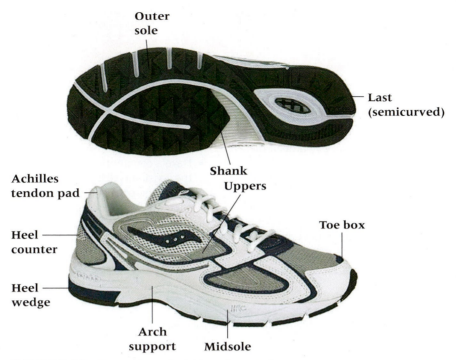

FIGURE 7–23 Parts of a well-designed sport shoe.

¾ inch (1.3 to 1.9 cm) between the longest toe and the front of the shoe is recommended. A few fitness shoes are made in varying widths. If an athlete has a very wide or narrow foot, most shoe salespersons can recommend a specific shoe for that foot. The best way to make sure the toe box offers adequate room is to have the foot measured and then try on the shoe.

- *Sole.* The sole should possess two qualities. First, it must provide shock absorption; second, it must be durable. Most shoes have three layers on the sole: a thick, spongy layer, which absorbs the force of the foot strike under the heel; a midsole, which cushions the midfoot and toes; and a hard rubber layer, which comes in contact with the ground. The average runner's feet strike the ground between 1,500 and 1,700 times per mile. Thus, it is essential that the force of the heel strike be absorbed by the spongy layer to prevent overuse injuries from occurring in the ankles and knees. Heel wedges are sometimes inserted on either the inside or the outside surface of the sole underneath the heel counter to accommodate and correct for various structural deformities of the foot that may alter normal biomechanics of the running gait. A flared heel may be appropriate for running shoes but is not recommended in aerobic or court shoes. The sole must provide good traction and must be made of tough material that is resistant to wear. Most of the better-known brands of shoes have well-designed, long-lasting soles.

- *Shank.* The shank is the part of the sole between the heel and the metatarsal heads. It is usually reinforced with material of sufficient density to support the weight of the wearer.

- *Last.* This is the form on which the shoe is built. The last may be straight, semicurved, or curved. A straight-lasted shoe is filled in on the inside/medial side of the shoe to increase stability for people who have a flat arch or run on the inside of their foot **(pronators).** A semicurved last is designed for the average or normal foot. There is a small curve on the medial side of the foot to fit a normal arch. The curved last is built with a larger curve on the medial side of the shoe and has a wider outside portion of the shoe to provide more forefoot stability. A curved last is built for people with an abnormally high arch and for runners who run on the outside of their foot **(supinators).**

> **pronators** Those who run on the inside of the foot.

> **supinators** Those who run on the outside of the foot.

- *Heel counter.* The heel counter is the portion of the shoe that prevents the foot from rolling from side to side at heel strike. The heel counter should be firm but well fitted to minimize movement of the heel up and down or side to side. A good heel counter may prevent ankle sprains and painful blisters.

- *Shoe upper.* The upper part of the shoe is made of some combination of nylon and leather. The

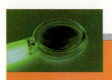
Proper running shoe design and construction[21]

To avoid injury, the running shoe should meet the following requirements.

- Have a strong heel counter that fits well around the foot and locks the shoe around the foot
- Always have good flexibility in the forefoot where toes bend
- Preferably have a fairly high heel for the individual with a tight Achilles tendon
- Have a midsole that is moderately soft but does not flatten easily

- Have a heel counter that is high enough to surround the foot but still allows room for an orthotic insert, if needed
- Have a counter that is attached to the sole to avoid the possibility of it coming loose from its attachment
- Always be of quality construction; a properly fitted shoe will bend where the foot bends

uppers should be lightweight, quick drying, and well ventilated. They should have some type of extra support in the saddle area, and there should be some extra padding in the area of the Achilles tendon just above the heel counter.

- *Arch support.* The arch support should be made of a durable yet soft supportive material and should smoothly join with the insole. The support should not have any rough seams or ridges inside the shoe, which may cause blisters.
- *Price.* Unfortunately, in many instances price is the primary consideration in buying athletic shoes. When buying athletic shoes, remember that in many activities shoes are important for performance and prevention of injury. Thus, it is worth a little extra investment to buy a quality pair of shoes.

Shoe Fitting Fitting athletic shoes can be difficult.[6] Frequently, the athlete's left foot varies in size and shape from the right foot. Therefore, measuring both feet is imperative. To fit the sports shoe properly, the athlete should approximate the conditions under which he or she will perform, such as wearing athletic socks, jumping up and down, or running. It is also desirable to fit the athlete's shoes at the end of the day to accommodate the gradual increase in foot volume that occurs during weight-bearing. The athlete must carefully consider this shoe choice because he or she will be spending countless hours in those shoes (see *Focus Box 7–8:* "Proper running shoe design and construction" for suggestions about shoe fitting).[6]

During performance conditions, the new shoe should feel snug but not too tight. The sports shoe should be long enough that all toes can be fully extended without being cramped. Its width should permit full movement of the toes, including flexion, extension, and some spreading. The wide part of the shoe should match the wide part of the foot to allow the shoe to crease evenly when the athlete is on the balls of the feet. The shoe should bend (or "break") at its widest part; when the break of the shoe and the ball joint coincide, the fit is correct. However, if the break of the shoe is in back of or in front of the normal bend of the foot (metatarsophalangeal joint), the shoe and the foot will oppose one another, causing abnormal skin and structural stresses to occur. Two measurements must be considered when fitting shoes: (1) the distance from the heel to the metatarsophalangeal joint and (2) the distance from the heel to the end of the longest toe. An individual's feet may be equal in length from the heels to the balls of the feet but different between the heels and the toes. No single type of shoe is appropriate for all athletes in a particular sport. Shoes therefore should be selected for the longer of the two measurements.[6] Other factors to consider when buying a sports shoe are the stiffness of the sole and the width of the shank, or narrowest part of the sole. A shoe with a sole that is too rigid and nonyielding places a great deal of extra strain on the foot tendons. A shoe with a shank that is too narrow also causes extra strain because it fails to adequately support the athlete's inner, longitudinal arches.[53] Lacing techniques can

> A properly fitted shoe will bend where the foot bends.

7–5 Clinical Application Exercise

A high-school basketball player asks the athletic trainer for advice on purchasing a pair of basketball shoes.

❓ What fitting factors must be taken into consideration when purchasing basketball shoes?

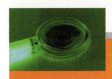
Shoe lacing techniques

A shoe that doesn't fit just right may be adjusted to provide a more secure, comfortable, and supportive fit by using specific lacing techniques to accommodate a narrow heel, a wide foot, or a low or high arch. Athletic shoes with a large number of eyelets make it easier to adjust the laces for a custom fit.

Narrow foot or heel (technique A)

If the shoe has two rows of eyelets that appear to zig-zag, use the row farthest from the tongue, tightening from the outer eyelets and pulling the body of the shoe toward the center. If there is only one row of eyelets, follow a normal lacing pattern up to the last pair of holes. At the last hole, tighten the laces and thread into the last hole, leaving a loop on each side. Cross the laces and thread each through the loop on the other side before tightening and tying.

Wide foot (technique B)

If the shoe has two rows of eyelets that appear to zig-zag, use the row closest to the tongue. If there is only a single row, thread laces through the first set of eyelets and then straight up each side without crisscrossing at all. Continue this way for two or three holes until the laces are above the forefoot and can tighten without squeezing. Then begin crisscrossing and finish lacing as normal.

Low arch (pes planus) (technique C)

Beginning at the bottom, crisscross lace shoes as normal halfway up the eyelets. Use the loop lacing technique used for a narrow heel the rest of the way.

High arch (pes cavus) (technique D)

Begin lacing as normal, crisscrossing and stopping after the first set of holes. Thread laces straight up each side, crisscrossing only before threading the last hole.

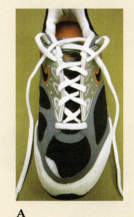

A

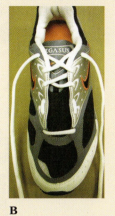

B

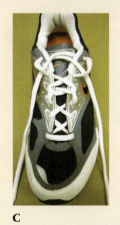

C

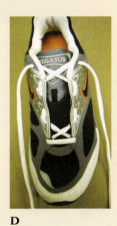

D

help adjust the width of the shoe to the foot. *Focus Box 7–9:* "Shoe lacing techniques" provides some suggestions for alternative lacing techniques. Two other shoe features to consider are insoles to reduce friction and arch supports.

Cleats can be made of polyurethane, rubber, or metal. They can be molded as part of the sole or they may be screw-ins that can be changed depending on the playing surface and weather conditions (Figure 7–24). Longer cleats are more often used on a muddy or soft field, and although they provide better traction, they are also more likely to create a lower-extremity injury because they will not slip or give away as easily as shorter cleats. Shorter cleats are most often used on synthetic or dry surfaces. (See Table 7–1 for shoe comparisons.)

Foot Orthotics An orthotic is a device for correcting biomechanical problems that exist in the foot that can potentially cause an injury.[24,55] The orthotic is a plastic, thermoplastic, rubber, sorbethane, or leather support that is placed in the shoe as a replacement for the existing insole (see Figure 7–36).[45] Ready-made orthotics can be purchased in sporting goods or shoe stores. Some athletes need orthotics that are custom made by a physician, a podiatrist, an athletic trainer, a physical therapist, or an orthotist.[18] These are more expensive but can be well worth the expense if the athlete's feet cause pain and discomfort, especially when exercising (Figure 7–25).

Heel Cups Heel cups should be used for a variety of conditions, including plantar fasciitis, a heel spur, Achilles tendinitis, and heel bursitis (Figure 7–26).

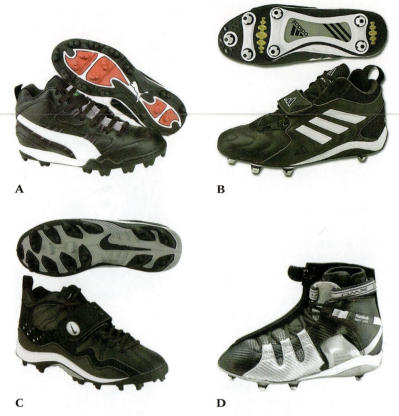

FIGURE 7–24   Variations in cleated shoes: The longer the cleat, the higher the incidence of injury. (Courtesy Sports Authority, www.sportsauthority.com)

TABLE 7–1	Shoe Comparisons		
	Tennis	**Aerobic**	**Running**
Flexibility	Firm sole, more rigid than running shoe	Sole between running and tennis shoe	Flexible ball of foot
Uppers	Leather or leather with nylon	Leather or leather with nylon	Nylon or nylon mesh
Heel Flare	None	Very little	Flared for stability
Cushioning	Less than a running shoe	Between running and tennis shoe	Heel and sole well padded
Soles (last)	Polyurethane	Rubber or polyurethane	Carbon-based material for greater durability
Tread	Flattened	Flat or pivot dot	Deep grooves for grip

The heel cup helps to compress the fat pad under the heel, providing more heel cushioning during weight-bearing activities. Heel cups may be either hard plastic or spongy rubber. They should generally be worn bilaterally.

Off-the-Shelf Foot Pads   Off-the-shelf foot pads are intended for use by the general public and are not usually designed to withstand the rigors of sports activities. Off-the-shelf pads that are suited for sports are generally not durable enough for hard, extended use. If money is no object, the ready-made off-the-shelf pad, which is replaced more often, has the advantage of saving time. Off-the-shelf pads are manufactured for almost every type of common structural foot condition, ranging from corns and bunions to fallen arches and pronated feet. Off-the-shelf foot pads are commonly used before more customized orthotic devices are made. These products offer a compromise to the custom-made foot orthotics by providing some biomechanical control.[44] Indiscriminate use of these aids, however, may intensify the pathological

> Indiscriminate use of commercial foot orthotics may give the athlete a false sense of security.

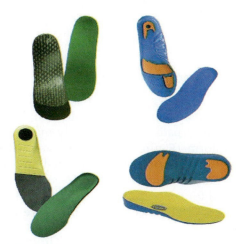

FIGURE 7–25   Commercially manufactured orthotic devices. Top view and bottom view of four different sets of orthotics. (Courtesy Sports Authority. www.sportsauthority.com)

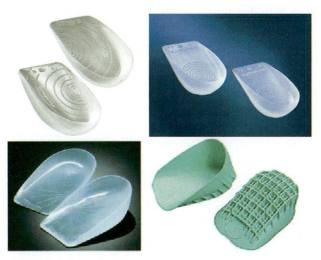

FIGURE 7–26   Different styles of heel cups.

condition or cause the athlete to delay seeing the team physician or team podiatrist for evaluation.[44]

For the most part, foot devices are fabricated and customized from a variety of materials such as foam, felt, plaster, aluminum, and spring steel (see the section "Construction of Protective and Supportive Devices" later in this chapter).

Ankle Braces

Ankle stabilizers, either alone or in combination with ankle taping, are becoming increasingly popular (Figure 7–27).[8,25,42,64] There has been significant debate regarding the efficacy of ankle supports in the prevention of ankle sprains.[23,28] Most studies indicate that bracing is effective in reducing ankle injury,[20,58] but other studies have shown no effects[7,27] or even negative effects.[7,23] Bracing probably has little or no effect on performance; any change in performance is due to the athlete's perception of support and comfort.[4] When compared with ankle taping, these devices do not loosen significantly during exercise.[54] A study that collectively analyzed the data from 19 studies of the effects of different types of ankle support on ankle motion before and after activity showed significantly greater frontal-plane ankle-motion restriction after exercise for a semirigid stirrup brace design than for taping or a lace-up-type brace.[14] Several studies have documented a beneficial effect of semirigid ankle bracing on sprain incidence, whereas others comparing the effects of taping and a lace-up brace on sprain incidence support the superiority of bracing for injury prevention.[17,23,33,61] Recent studies have focused on the proprioceptive effects and how ankle braces influence balance, postural sway, and joint position sense.[27,61,66]

7–6 Clinical Application Exercise

A basketball player with a history of ankle sprains needs support during practice.

❓ Which type of ankle support is cost efficient and most reliable: tape or commercial supports?

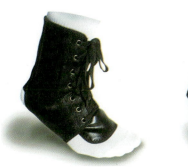
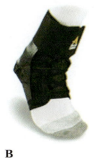
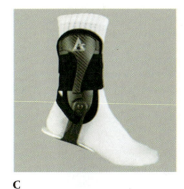
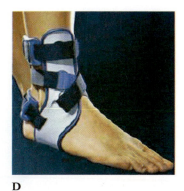

A   B   C   D

FIGURE 7–27   Commercial ankle supports for an injured ankle. **(A)** Lace-up brace. (Courtesy McDavid) **(B)** Lace-up with straps brace. (Courtesy Active Ankle) **(C)** Rigid support brace. (Courtesy Active Ankle) **(D)** Rigid support with stabilizing straps. (Courtesy Bauerfeind)

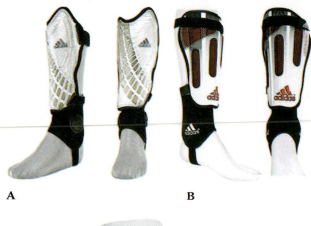

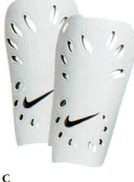

C

FIGURE 7–28 Soccer shin guards.
(A & B: Courtesy Adidas; C: Courtesy Nike)

Shin and Lower Leg

The shin and lower leg are particularly vulnerable to being kicked, especially in soccer, or hit with a stick in field hockey. The anterior surface of the tibia is exposed, lacking any soft-tissue protection. Contusion to the anterior surface of the tibia can result in swelling and significant pain. Contusion of the exposed muscle either lateral or medial to the tibia can result in compartment syndromes (see Chapter 19). Shin guards should be used to protect the anterior shin from direct blows. For maximum

protection, the shin guards should extend from just below the tibial tubercle proximally to just above the malleoli distally (Figure 7–28).

Thigh and Upper Leg

Thigh and upper-leg protection is widely used in collision sports, such as hockey, football, and soccer. Generally, pads slip into ready-made pockets in the uniform (Figure 7–29A). In some instances, customized pads should be constructed and held in place with tape or an elastic wrap. Neoprene sleeves can be used for support following strain to the hamstring, groin, or quadriceps muscles (Figure 7–29B).

Knee Supports and Protective Devices

Knee Pads Elastic knee pads or guards are extremely valuable in sports in which the athlete falls or receives a direct blow to the anterior aspect of the knee. An elastic sleeve containing a resilient pad may help dissipate an anterior striking force and reduce contusions but fails to protect the knee against lateral, medial, or twisting forces that result in stress to the ligaments.

Knee Braces Because of the high incidence of injury to the knee joint, manufacturers have designed a host of different knee braces for a variety of purposes.[10] *Protective knee braces* are used prophylactically to prevent injuries to the medial collateral ligament in contact sports such as football (Figure 7–30A).[50] Although these protective braces have been widely used in the past, the American Orthopedic Society for Sports Medicine has expressed concern about their efficacy in reducing injuries to the collateral ligaments.[43] Several studies have actually shown an increase in the incidence of injuries to the medial collateral ligament in athletes wearing these braces.[50] Others have shown a positive influence on joint position sense[3] but little or no effect on performance.[27]

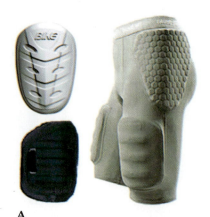

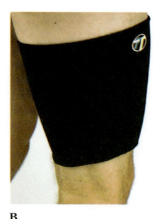

A   B

FIGURE 7–29 **(A)** Protective thigh pads (Courtesy Mueller Sports Medicine). **(B)** Neoprene thigh sleeve. (Courtesy Pro-Tech)

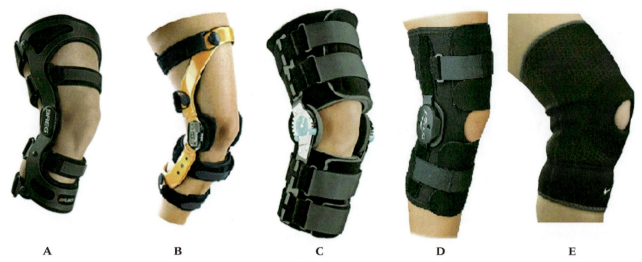

FIGURE 7–30 Knee braces. **(A)** Prophylactic knee brace. (Courtesy Breg) **(B)** Functional brace. (Courtesy DonJoy) **(C)** Rehabilitative brace. (Courtesy Breg) **(D)** Neoprene with medial support brace. (Courtesy DonJoy) **(E)** Neoprene brace. (Courtesy Nike)

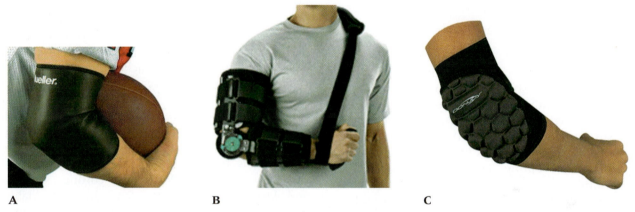

FIGURE 7–31 **(A)** Neoprene elbow sleeve. (Courtesy Mueller) **(B)** Hinged rehabilitative elbow brace. (Courtesy Breg) **(C)** Elbow pad. (Courtesy DonJoy)

Rehabilitative braces are widely used following surgical repair or reconstruction of the knee joint to allow for controlled progressive immobilization (Figure 7–30C).[4] These braces have hinges that can be easily adjusted to allow range of motion to be progressively increased.

Functional knee braces may be worn both during and following the rehabilitative period to provide support during functional activities (Figure 7–30B).[13,15,51] Functional braces can be purchased ready made or can be custom made.[59] Some physicians strongly recommend that their patients consistently[41] wear these braces during physical activity, whereas others do not feel that they are necessary.[12,63]

Neoprene braces with medial and lateral supports may be used by individuals who have sustained injury to the collateral ligaments and feel that they need extra support medially and laterally[56] (Figure 7–30D).

A variety of *neoprene sleeves* may also be used to provide some support for patellofemoral conditions (Figure 7–30E).[5]

ELBOW, WRIST, AND HAND PROTECTION

As with the lower extremity, the upper extremity requires protection from injury and prevention of further injury after trauma. Although the elbow joint is less commonly injured than the ankle, knee, or shoulder, it is still vulnerable to instability, contusion, and muscle strain. A variety of off-the-shelf protective neoprene sleeves and pads and hinged adjustable rehabilitative braces can offer protection to the elbow (Figure 7–31).

In sports medicine, injuries to the wrist, hand, and fingers are occasionally trivialized and considered insignificant. But injuries to the distal aspect of

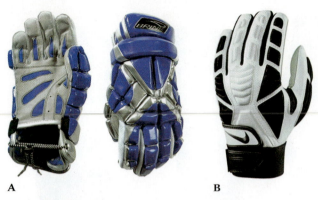

A   B

FIGURE 7–32   The hand is an often neglected area of the body in sports. **(A)** Lacrosse gloves. (Courtesy Brine) **(B)** Football lineman's glove. (Courtesy Nike)

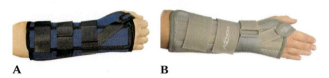

A   B

FIGURE 7–33   Wrist and hand braces and immobilizers.

the upper extremity can be functionally disabling, especially in those sports that involve throwing and catching.[21] In both contact and noncontact sport activities, the wrist, hand, and particularly the fingers are susceptible to fracture, dislocation, ligament sprains, and muscle strains.[21] Protective gloves are essential in preventing injuries in sports such as lacrosse and ice hockey (Figure 7–32). It is also common to use both off-the-shelf and custom-molded splints both for support and for immobilization of an injury (Figure 7–33).

CONSTRUCTION OF PROTECTIVE AND SUPPORTIVE DEVICES

The athletic trainer should be able to design and construct protective and supportive devices when necessary. Certainly, the athletic trainer must understand the theoretical basis for constructing protective pads and supports. However, the ability to construct an effective and appropriate protective device is more of an art than a science.

Custom Pad and Orthotic Materials

Many materials are available to the athletic trainer attempting to protect or support an injured area. In general, these materials can be divided into soft and hard materials.

Soft Materials   The primary soft-material media found in athletic training rooms are gauze padding, cotton, adhesive felt or adhesive sponge rubber felt, and an assortment of foam rubber.

Gauze padding is less versatile than other pad materials. It is assembled in varying thicknesses and can be used as an absorbent or protective pad.

Cotton is probably the cheapest and most widely used material in sports. It has the ability to absorb, to hold emollients, and to offer a mild padding effect.

Adhesive felt (moleskin) or *sponge rubber* material contains an adhesive mass on one side, thus combining a cushioning effect with the ability to be held in place by the adhesive mass. It is a versatile material that is useful on all body parts (Figure 7–34A).

Felt is a material composed of matted wool fibers pressed into varying thicknesses that range from ¼ to 1 inch (0.6 to 2.5 cm) (Figure 7–34B). Its benefit lies in its comfortable, semiresilient surface, which gives a firmer pressure than most sponge rubbers. Because felt absorbs perspiration, it clings to the skin, and it has less tendency to move than sponge rubber does. Because of its absorbent qualities, felt should be replaced daily. Currently, it is most often used as support and protection for a variety of foot conditions.

Foams are currently the materials most often used for providing injury protection in sports. They come in many different thicknesses and densities (Figure 7–34C). They are usually resilient, nonabsorbent, and able to protect the body against compressive forces. Some foams are open celled, whereas others are closed celled (Figure 7–35). The closed-cell type is preferable in sports because it rebounds to its original shape quickly. Foams can be easily worked through cutting, shaping, and faceting. Some foams are thermomoldable; when heated, they become highly pliant and easy to shape. When cooled, they retain the shape in which they were formed. A new class of foams is composed of viscoelastic polymers. Sorbothane is one example. This foam has a high energy-absorbing quality, but it also has a high density, making it heavy (Figure 7–34D). Used in inner soles in sports shoes, foam helps prevent blisters and effectively absorbs anterior/posterior and medial/lateral ground reaction forces. Foams generally range from ⅛ to ½ inch (0.3 to 1.25 cm) in thickness.

Nonyielding Materials   A number of hard, nonyielding materials are used in athletic training for making protective shells and splints.

Thermomoldable Plastics   Plastic materials are widely used in sports medicine for customized orthotics. They can brace, splint, and shield a body area. They can provide casting for a fracture; support for a foot defect; or a firm, nonyielding surface to protect a severe contusion. Plastics used for these purposes differ in their chemical composition and reaction to heat. The two categories are heat-forming plastics and heat-plastic foams.

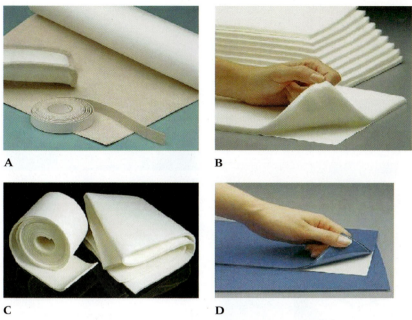

FIGURE 7–34   Soft Materials. **(A)** Adhesive moleskin. **(B)** Orthopedic felt. **(C)** Adhesive foam. **(D)** Adhesive sorbethane.

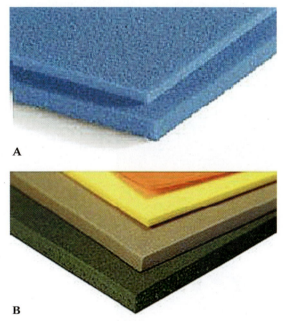

FIGURE 7–35   Foam padding. **(A)** Open-celled foam. **(B)** Closed-cell foam.

Heat-forming plastics are of the low-temperature variety and are the most popular in athletic

> **Heat-forming plastics of the low-temperature variety are the most popular in athletic training.**

training. When heated to 140°F to 180°F (60°C to 82.2°C), depending on the material, the plastic can be accurately molded to a body part. Orthoplast and X-Lite (synthetic rubber thermoplast) are popular types (Figure 7–36A&B).

Heat-plastic foams are plastics that have differences in density as a result of the addition of liquids, gas, or crystals. They are commonly used as shoe orthotic inserts and other body padding. Plastazote and Aliplast (polyethylene foams) are two commonly used products (Figure 7–36C&D).

Usually, the plastic is heated until soft and malleable. It is then molded into the desired shape and allowed to cool, thereby retaining its shape. Various pads and other materials can also be fastened in place. The rules and regulations of various sport activities may place limitations on the use of rigid thermomoldable plastics.

Casting Materials Applying plaster casts to injured body areas has long been a practice in sports medicine. The material of choice is fiberglass, which uses resin and a catalytic converter, plus water, to produce hardening. Besides casts, this material makes effective shells for splints and protective pads. Once hardened, the fiberglass is trimmed to shape with a cast saw (Figure 7–37).

Tools Used for Customizing   Many different tools are needed to work with the various materials used to customize protective equipment. These tools include adhesives, adhesive tape, heat sources, shaping tools, and fastening material.

Adhesives   A number of adhesives are used in constructing custom protective equipment. Many

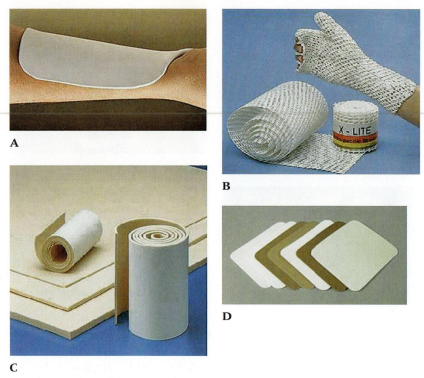

FIGURE 7–36   Thermomoldable plastics. **(A)** Orthoplast. **(B)** X-Lite.
(C) Plastazote. **(D)** Aliplast sheets.

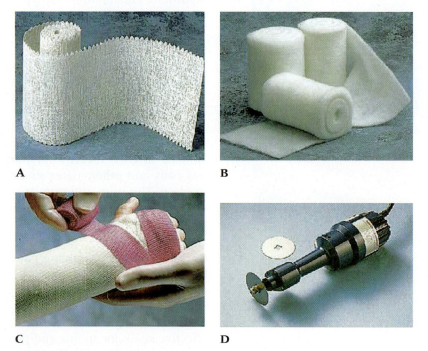

FIGURE 7–37   Casting materials and saw. **(A)** Plaster roll.
(B) Cast padding roll. **(C)** Fiberglass roll. **(D)** Cast saw.

cements and glues join plastic to plastic or join other combinations of materials.

Adhesive Tape   Adhesive tape is a major tool in holding various materials in place. Linen and elastic tape can hold pads to a rigid backing or to adhesive felt

(moleskin) and can be used to protect against sharp edges (see Chapter 8).

Heat Sources   To form thermomoldable plastics, a heat source must be available. Three sources are commonly found in training rooms: the commercial

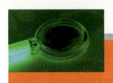

FOCUS 7–10 Focus on Injury/Illness Prevention and Wellness Protection

How to construct a hard-shell pad

1. Select proper material and tools, which might include the following:
   a. Thermomoldable plastic sheet (Orthoplast, Hexalite)
   b. Scissors
   c. Felt material
2. Palpate and mark the margins of the tender area that needs protection.
3. Cut a felt piece to fit in the area of tenderness.
4. Heat plastic until malleable.
5. Place heated plastic over felt and wrap in place with an elastic wrap.

6. When cooled, remove elastic wrap and felt pad.
7. Trim shell to desired shape; a protective shell has now been made to provide a "bubble" relief.
8. If needed, add a softer inner layer of foam to distribute and lessen force further.
   a. Cut a doughnut-type hole in softer foam material the same size as the injury site.
   b. Cut foam the same shape as the hard shell.
   c. Use tape or an adhesive to affix the foam to the shell.

---

moist heat unit, a hot air gun or hair dryer, and a convection oven with a temperature control. The usual desired temperature is 160°F (71°C) or higher.

Shaping Tools Commonly, the tools required to shape custom devices are heavy-duty scissors, sharp-blade knives, and cast saws.

Fastening Material Once formed, customized protective equipment often must be secured in place. Fastening this equipment requires the availability of a great variety of materials. For example, if something is to be held securely, Velcro can be used when a device must be continually put on and removed. Leather can be cut and riveted in place to form hinge straps with buckles attached. Various types of laces can be laced through eyelets to hold something in place. Tools that allow for this type of construction include a portable drill, a hole punch, and an ice pick.

Customized Hard-Shell Pads A hard-shell pad is often required for an athlete who has an injury, such as a painful contusion (bruise), that must be completely protected from further injury. *Focus Box 7–10:* "How to construct a hard-shell pad" provides the procedures needed to customize such a pad (Figure 7–38).

Dynamic Splints Occasionally, it is necessary to fabricate and apply a dynamic splint in treating injuries to the hand and fingers (Figure 7–39). Most often, an occupational therapist would make a dynamic splint; however, the athletic trainer is certainly capable of designing such a splint. A dynamic splint is used to provide long-duration tension on a healing structure (usually a tendon) so that it can return to normal function. Dynamic splints use a combination of thermoplastic material, Velcro, and pieces of rubber band or elastic to provide dynamic assistance.

7-7 Clinical Application Exercise

A soccer player has incurred a number of contusions to the right quadriceps muscle.

❓ How does the athletic trainer customize a hard-shell protective thigh pad for the soccer player?

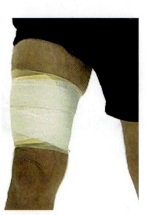

FIGURE 7–38 Hard-shell pad wrapped on the thigh.

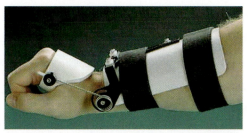

FIGURE 7–39 Dynamic splint for the hand and fingers. (Courtesy Rolyan)

SUMMARY

- The proper selection and proper fitting of protective equipment are essential in the prevention and rehabilitation of many sports injuries. Because of the number of current litigations, sports equipment standards regarding the durability of the material and the fit and wear requirements of the equipment are of serious concern. Manufacturers must foresee all possible uses and misuses of their equipment and warn the user of any potential risks.

- Athletic trainers must be concerned about head protection in many collision and contact sports. The football helmet must be used only for its intended purpose and not as a weapon. To avoid unwarranted litigation, a warning label must be placed on the outside of the helmet indicating that the helmet is not fail-safe and must be used as intended. Properly fitting the helmet is of critical importance.

- Face protection is important in sports that have fast-moving projectiles, use implements that are in close proximity to other athletes, and facilitate body collisions. Protecting teeth and eyes is of particular significance. The customized mouth guard, fitted to individual requirements, provides the best protection for the teeth and protects against concussions. Eyes must be protected against projectiles and sports implements. The safest eye guard for the athlete wearing contact lenses or glasses is the closed type that completely protects the orbital cavity.

- Many sports require protection of various parts of the athlete's body. American football players, ice hockey players, and baseball catchers are examples of players who require body protection. Commonly, the protection is for the shoulders, chest, thighs, ribs, hips, buttocks, groin, genitalia (male athletes), and breasts (female athletes).

- Footwear is essential to prevent injuries. Socks must be clean, without holes, and made of appropriate materials. Shoes must be suited to the sport and must be properly fitted. The wide part of the foot must match the wide part of the shoe. If the shoe has cleats, they must be positioned at the metatarsophalangeal joints.

- Currently, there are many off-the-shelf pieces of specialized protective equipment on the market. They may be designed to support ankles, knees, or other body parts. In addition to stock equipment, athletic trainers often construct customized equipment out of a variety of materials to pad injuries or support feet. Professionals such as athletic trainers, orthopedists, podiatrists, physical therapists, and orthotists may devise orthopedic footwear and orthotic devices to improve the biomechanics of the athlete's foot.

WEB SITES

Athletic Protective Equipment: www.rapidwear.com
Provides information on a variety of protective equipment.

Douglas Protective Equipment:
www.douglaspads.com
Manufacturer and distributor of football, hockey, and baseball protective padding.

National Operating Committee on Standards for Athletic Equipment: www.nocsae.org

Riddell: http://riddell.com
Riddell is an equipment manufacturing company, and this site gives information about the safety of the products they sell and the necessary standards for safety equipment.

The Sports Authority: www.sportsauthority.com
Provides a wide selection of protective equipment for virtually all sports.

SOLUTIONS TO CLINICAL APPLICATION EXERCISES

7–1 The athletic training student must acquire the following protective equipment competencies:
- Identify good-quality and poor-quality commercial protective equipment.
- Properly fit commercial protective equipment.
- Construct protective and supportive devices.

7–2 The athletic trainer should initiate the following steps:
1. Call a team meeting in which he or she fully explains the risks entailed in the use and fitting of the equipment.
2. Report and repair any defective pieces of equipment immediately.
3. Send out a letter to each parent or guardian, explaining equipment limitations. This letter must be signed and returned to the athletic trainer.
4. Call a meeting of parents, team members, and coaches in which he or she further explains equipment limitations.

7–3 The athletic trainer explains that the helmet cannot prevent serious neck injuries. Striking an opponent with any part of the helmet or face mask can place abnormal stress on cervical structures. Most severe neck injuries occur from striking an opponent with the top of the helmet; this action is known as axial loading.

7–4 Mouth guards serve several important purposes in preventing injury in athletics, especially contact sports, such as ice hockey. Mouth guards help prevent or minimize lacerations, fractures, and possibly reduce the incidence of cerebral concussions. For a mouth guard to work effectively, proper fit is essential and must not interfere with breathing or speech. A custom-fabricated mouth guard is produced from a mold of each athlete, causing the fit to be more precise. If the fit is improved, athletes are more likely to wear their mouth guards.

7–5 The athletic trainer provides the following advice:
- Shoes should be purchased to fit the larger foot.
- The athlete should wear athletic socks when fitting shoes.
- Shoes should be purchased at the end of the day.
- Shoes should feel snug but comfortable when the athlete jumps up and down and performs cutting motions.
- Shoe length and width should allow full toe function.
- The wide part of the foot should match the wide part of the shoe.
- The shoe should bend at its widest part.
- Each foot should be measured from the heel to the end of the largest toe.

7–6 A verified commercial ankle support provides more consistent support for a longer period of time and is more cost efficient.

7–7 To construct a hard-shell protective thigh pad, the athletic trainer follows these steps:
1. Mark the area on the athlete to be protected.
2. Cut a foam piece to cover the injury temporarily.
3. Heat thermomoldable plastic and place over the foam piece to form a bubble.
4. Cut a plastic sheet to form to the athlete's thigh.
5. Create a doughnut-shaped foam lining to surround the injury.
6. Secure the foam doughnut to the plastic piece.
7. Secure the pad in place with elastic wrap.

REVIEW QUESTIONS AND CLASS ACTIVITIES

1. What are the legal responsibilities of the athletic trainer in terms of protective equipment?
2. Invite an attorney to class to discuss product liability and its impact on the athletic trainer.
3. What are the various sports with high risk factors that require protective equipment?
4. How can the athletic trainer select and use safety equipment to decrease the possibility of sports injuries and litigation?
5. Why is continual inspection and/or replacement of used equipment important?
6. What are the standards for fitting football helmets? Are there standards for any other helmets?
7. Invite your school equipment manager to class to demonstrate all the protective equipment and how to fit it to the athlete.
8. Why are mouth guards important, and what are the advantages of custom-made mouth guards over the stock type?
9. What are the advantages and disadvantages of glasses and contact lenses in athletic competition?
10. How do you fit shoulder pads for the different-sized players and their positions?
11. Why is breast protection necessary? Which types of sports bras are available and what should the athlete look for when purchasing one?
12. How do you properly fit shoes? What type of shoes should you use for the various sports and the different floor and field surfaces?

REFERENCES

1. AAPSM Running shoes recommendations: *American Academy of Podiatric Sports Medicine Newsletter* 2, May 2006.
2. Amis T, Di Somma E, Bacha F, Wheatley J: Influence of intra-oral maxillary sports mouthguards on the airflow dynamics of oral breathing, *Med Sci Sports Exerc* 32(2): 284, 2000.
3. Baltaci G: The effect of prophylactic knee bracing on performance: Balance, proprioception, coordination, and muscular power. *Knee Surgery, Sports Traumatology Arthroscopy*, 19(10)1722–28, 2011.
4. Beynnon B, Good L, Risberg M: The effect of bracing on proprioception of knees with anterior cruciate ligament injury, *J Ortho Sports Phys Ther* 32(1):32, 2002.
5. Birmingham TB, Inglis JT, Kramer JF: Effect of a neoprene sleeve on knee joint kinesthesis: Influence of different testing procedures, *Med Sci Sports Exerc* 32(2):304, 2000.
6. Bone S: If the shoe fits …, *Athletic Therapy Today* 6(6):52, 2001.
7. Bot S: The effect of ankle bracing and taping on performance: A review of the literature *International Sports Medicine Journal I* 4(5):171, 2003.
8. Boyce S, Quigley M, Campbell S: Management of ankle sprains: A randomised controlled trial of the treatment of inversion injuries using an elastic support bandage or an Aircast ankle brace, *British Journal of Sports Medicine* 39(2):91, 2005.
9. Breast support for female athletes, *Sport Research Review/Nike Sport Research Review* 1:1, 2002.
10. Bridge M: 2008. Knee bracing in sports medicine: A review, *Techniques in Knee Surgery* 7(4):251–60.
11. Broglio S, Yan-Ying J, Broglio M: The efficacy of soccer headgear, *J Athl Train* 38(3):220–24, 2003.
12. Brownstein B: Migration and design characteristics of functional knee braces, *J Sport Rehabil* 7(1):33, 1998.
13. Campbell B, Yaggie J, Cipriani D: Temporal influences of functional knee bracing on torque production of the lower extremity, *J Sport Rehabil* 15(3):216, 2006.
14. Cardova M, Ingersoll C, LeBlane M: Influence and support on joint range of motion before and after exercise: A meta-analysis, *J Orthop Sports Phys Ther* 30(7):170, 2000.
15. Carlson L: Use of functional knee braces after ACL reconstruction, *Athletic Therapy Today* 7(3):48, 2002.
16. Caswell S, Deivert R: Lacrosse helmet designs and the effects of impact forces, *J Athl Train* 37(2):164, 2002.
17. Clanto T: Ankle sprains, ankle instability, and syndesmosis injuries. In Porter D: *Baxter's the foot and ankle in sport*, New York, 2007, Mosby.
18. Crabtree P: Design and manufacture of customized orthotics for sporting applications, *The Engineering of Sport* 1(3):309–17, 2008.
19. Daneshvar D: Helmets and mouth guards: The role of Personal Equipment in Preventing Sport-Related Concussions, *Clinics in Sports Medicine*, 30(1):145–63, 2011.
20. Dizon J: A systematic review on the effectiveness of external ankle supports in the prevention of inversion ankle sprains among elite and recreational players, *Journal of Science and Medicine in Sport*, 13(3):306–17, 2010.
21. Downing N: Orthopedic injuries to the hand and wrist. In Hutson M: *Sports Injuries,* New York, 2011, Oxford University Press.
22. Gorden J, Straub S, Swanik C: Effects of football collars on cervical hyperextension and lateral flexion, *J Athl Train* 38(3):209–15, 2003.
23. Gribble P: Bracing does not improve dynamic stability in chronic ankle instability subjects, *Physical Therapy in Sports*, 11(1): 3–7, 2010.
24. Gross MT: The impact of custom semirigid foot orthotics on pain and disability for individuals with plantar fasciitis, *J Orthop Sports Phys Ther* 32(4):149, 2002.
25. Gross M, Liu H: The role of ankle bracing for prevention of ankle sprain injuries, *J Orthop Sports Phys Ther* 33(10):572, 2003.
26. Halstead PD: Performance testing updates in head, face, and eye protection, *J Athl Train* 36(3):322, 2001.
27. Hartsell H: Effects of bracing on isokinetic torque for the chronically unstable ankle, *J Sport Rehabil* 8(2):83, 1999.

28. Hartsell H: The effects of external bracing on joint position sense awareness for the chronically unstable ankle, *J Sport Rehabil* 9(4):279, 2000.

29. Hawn K, Visser M, Sexton P: Enforcement of mouthguard use and athlete compliance in National Collegiate Athletic Association men's collegiate ice hockey competition, *J Athl Train* 37(2):204, 2002.

30. Hilgers M: Current trends in athletic shoe design, *Athletic Therapy Today* 14(6):23–26, 2009.

31. Hootman J: Use of protective eyewear among children participating in sports: National data and prevention implications (Abstract), *J Athl Train* 40(2 Suppl):S-71, 2005.

32. International Federation of Medicine: Position statement: Eye injuries and eye protection in sports, *Athletic Therapy Today* 4(5):6, 1999.

33. Kemler E: A systematic review on the treatment of acute ankle sprain: Brace versus other functional treatment types. *Sports Medicine*, 41(3):185–97, 2011.

34. Knapik J: Mouthguards in sport activities: History, physical properties and injury prevention effectiveness, *Sports Medicine* 37(2):117–44, 2007.

35. Kunde S: Relationship between running shoe fit and perceptual, biomechanical and mechanical parameters. *Footwear Science* 1(Supp.1):19–20, 2009.

36. Labella CR, Smith RW, Sigurdsson A: Effect of mouth guards on dental injuries and concussions in college basketball, *Med Sci Sports Exerc* 34(1):41, 2002.

37. Lahti H: Dental injuries in ice hockey games and training, *Med Sci Sports Exerc* 34(3):400, 2002.

38. Lord JL: Protective Athletic Equipment. In Birrer RB, O'Connor, FG, editor: *Sports medicine for the primary care physician*, ed 3, Boca Raton, FL, 2004, CRC Press.

39. McLeod TCV: Proper fit and maintenance of ice-hockey helmets, *Athletic Therapy Today* 10(6):54, 2005.

40. Mihalik J: Effectiveness of mouthguards in reducing neurocognitive deficits following sports-related cerebral concussions, *Dental Traumatology* I23(1):14–20, 2007.

41. Miller J, et al. Dynamic analysis of custom fitted functional knee braces: EMG and brace migration during physical activity, *J Sport Rehabil* 8(2):109, 1999.

42. Mogolov R: Ankle brace improvements pay off for athletes, *Training & Conditioning* 17(7):48, 2007.

43. Najibi S, Albright J: The use of knee braces, part 1: Prophylactic knee braces in contact sports, *Am J Sports Med* 33(4):602, 2005.

44. National Operating Committee on Standards for Athletic Equipment: *NOCSAE. Standard drop test method and equipment used in evaluating the performance characteristics of protective headgear/equipment*, Overland Park, KS, 2010, NOCASE.

45. New Revolution helmet being put to the test for improved safety on the field, *Sports Medicine Alert* 8(7):55, 2002.

46. Nigg BM, Nurse MA, Stefanyshyn DJ: Shoe inserts and orthotics for sport and physical activities, *Med Sci Sports Exerc* 31 (7 Suppl.):S421, 1999.

47. Page KA, Steele JR: Breast motion and sports brassiere design: Implications for future research, *Sports Med* 27(4):205, 1999.

48. Patrick D, van Noort R, Found M: Scale of protection and the various types of sports mouthguard, *British Journal of Sports Medicine* 39(5):278, 2005.

49. Peterson L, Renstrom P: Sports and protective equipment. In Peterson L, editor: *Sports injuries: Their prevention and treatment*, ed 3, Champaign, IL, 2001, Human Kinetics.

50. Pietrosimone B: A systemic review of prophylactic braces in the prevention of knee ligament injuries in college football players, *Journal of Athletic Training* 43(4):409–14, 2008.

51. Rishiraj N: Effect of functional knee brace on accellertation, agility, leg power, and speed performance in healthy athletes, *British Journal of Sports Medicine Online*, 2010, doi:10.1136/bjsm.2010.079244.

52. Rules and equipment. In *Coaching youth football*, ed 3, Champaign, IL, 2001, Human Kinetics.

53. Steinbach P: Armor for all. With player safety paramount, the purchasing of football equipment must ensure adequate supply and proper fit of helmets, shoes and everything in between, *Athletic Business* 26(8):96, 2002.

54. Stoffel K: Effect of ankle taping on knee and ankle joint biomechanics in sporting tasks, *Medicine and Science in Sport and Exercise*, 42(11):2089–97, 2010.

55. Swanik CB: Orthotics in sports medicine, *Athletic Therapy Today* 5(1):5, 2000.

56. Tiggelen D: The effects of a neoprene knee sleeve on subjects with a poor versus good joint position sense subjected to an isokinetic fatigue protocol, *Clinical Journal of Sports Medicine*, 18(3):259–65, 2008.

57. Tobianski N, Livingston S, Palmieri R: Soccer headgear increases peak acceleration of the head during purposeful heading (Abstract), *J Athl Train* 40(2 Suppl):S-82, 2005.

58. Ubell M, Boylan J, Ashton M: The effect of ankle braces on the prevention of dynamic forced ankle inversion, *Am J Sports Med* 31(6):935, 2003.

59. Vandertuin J, Grant J: The role of functional knee braces in managing ACL injuries, *Athletic Therapy Today* 9(2):58, 2004.

60. Vinger PF: A practical guide for sports eye protection, *Physician Sportsmed* 28(6):49, 2000.

61. Wilkerson GB: Biomechanical and neuromuscular effects of ankle taping and bracing, *J Athl Train* 37(4):436, 2002.

62. Withnall C, Shewchenko N, Wonnacott M: Effectiveness of headgear in football, *British Journal of Sports Medicine* 39(Suppl 1):40, 2005.

63. Wojtys EM, Huston LJ: Functional knee braces—the 25-year controversy. In Chan KM, editor: *Controversies in orthopedic sports medicine*, Champaign, IL, 2002, Human Kinetics.

64. Yaggie J, Kinzey S: A comparative analysis of selected ankle orthoses during functional tasks, *Sport Rehabil* 10(3):174, 2001.

65. Yunker C, Cameron K, Peck K: Evaluating the perceived preventative qualities associated with two different types of mouthguards (Abstract), *J Athl Train* 39 (2 Suppl):S-52, 2004.

66. Zinder S: Ankle bracing and the neuromuscular factors influencing joint stiffness, *J Athl Train*, 44(4):363–69, 2009.

ANNOTATED BIBLIOGRAPHY

Hunter S, Dolan M, Davis M: *Foot orthotics in therapy and sport*, Champaign, Ill, 1995, Human Kinetics.

  A detailed look at the fabrication of orthotic devices.

Nicholas JA, Hirshman EB, editors: *The upper extremity in sports medicine*, St. Louis, 1995, Mosby.

  Includes a chapter on protective equipment for the shoulder, elbow, wrist, and hand.

Street S, Runkle D: *Athletic protective equipment: care, selection and fitting*, Boston, 2001, McGraw-Hill.

  An overview of available athletic equipment and its usage. A resource for athletic trainers, coaches, and physical education teachers.

Werd, M: *Athletic footwear and Orthoses in sports medicine*, New York, 2010, Springer.

  A concise manual for sports medicine specialists who want to effectively prescribe footwear and orthotics for the athlete.

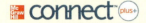

8

Wrapping and Taping

■ Objectives

When you finish this chapter you should be able to

- Discuss how the athletic trainer should approach using taping and wrapping techniques in clinical practice.
- Demonstrate the ability to apply elastic wraps to provide support, limit range of motion, or hold a protective pad in place for an injured body part.
- Identify the properties of elastic and nonelastic adhesive tape.

- Explain the process of applying and removing adhesive tape.
- Demonstrate the correct techniques for applying common taping procedures.
- Explain how Kinesio taping can be used in treating an injured patient.

■ Outline

■ Key Terms

wrap
dressing

spica

■ Connect Highlights

Visit connect.mcgraw-hill.com for further exercises to apply your knowledge:

- Clinical application scenarios covering applying and removal of adhesive tape, correct techniques for applying common taping procedures, application of protective padding, application of taping and wrapping, using taping and wrapping techniques in clinical practice
- Click-and-drag questions covering process of applying and removing adhesive tape
- Multiple-choice questions covering use and application of taping and wrapping in clinical practice, application of protective padding, properties of elastic and nonelastic adhesive tape, common taping procedures, and Kinesio taping
- Video identification of various taping techniques

Wrapping and taping techniques are used routinely by athletic trainers. They have been used to accomplish a variety of specific objectives, including the following:[5,19]

- Providing compression to minimize swelling in the initial management of injury
- Reducing the chances of injury by applying tape prophylactically before an injury occurs
- Providing additional support to an injured structure

Correctly and effectively applying a wrap or a "tape job" to a specific body part is a skill that has traditionally been left to the athletic trainer. It is true that athletic trainers have been instructed in and generally become highly proficient at applying a variety of wrapping and taping techniques to accomplish the objectives listed. Certainly, wrapping and taping skills are not difficult. They can be mastered by anyone willing to spend time practicing and learning what works best in a given situation. Of course, certain taping and wrapping techniques are more advanced and should be used only by those with some advanced experience. However, to be most effective in applying taping and wrapping techniques, the athletic trainer must have a sound background in and an understanding of anatomy and biomechanical function.

A review of the evidence-based support for using taping indicates that good research has shown the limited effectiveness of taping.[1,10] Although it is still widely used for a variety of reasons, the athletic training profession has advanced beyond simply applying a specific taping technique for every injury. In some specific instances, braces have been shown to be more effective alternatives to taping.[10,23,46]

Certainly, the taping techniques presented in this chapter are not intended to be an all-inclusive list. Applying tape to an injured body part involves more art than science. Athletic trainers utilize countless variations on basic taping techniques. Some of the techniques presented in this chapter, such as using cloth ankle wraps, triangular bandages, and open basket weave taping, have, to some extent, fallen out of favor in clinical practice in many settings. These techniques have been replaced by slings, shoulder and ankle braces, and compression wraps that some consider to be better and more effective. However, many clinicians continue to make use of these techniques because they have sound theoretical applicability and, for that reason, they are included in this chapter.

WRAPPING

A **wrap** may be used to hold a **dressing** in place over an open wound, to secure a compressive or protective pad in place over an injured area, or to provide support or limit range of motion for an injured body part. A wrap may consist of roller gauze, a cloth ankle wrap or triangular bandage, or, most commonly in athletic training, an elastic wrap.

wrap Strip of cloth or other material used to cover a wound or hold a dressing in place.

dressing Covering, protective or supportive, that is applied to an injury or wound.

Elastic Wrap Use

The *elastic wrap* is widely used by athletic trainers because of its elasticity, which allows it to conform easily to the contour of different body parts. If applied correctly it exerts consistent, even pressure.

The width and length of the elastic wrap vary according to the body part to be wrapped. The sizes most frequently used are the 2-inch (5 cm) width by 6-yard (5.5 m) length for hand, finger, toe, and head wraps; the 3-inch (7.5 cm) width or 4-inch (10 cm) width by 10-yard (9 m) length for the extremities; and the 4-inch (10 cm) or 6-inch (15 cm) width by 10-yard (9 m) length for thigh, groin, and trunk. Double-length elastic wraps are useful when wrapping large body parts or areas. For ease and convenience in the application of the elastic wrap, the strips of material are first rolled into a cylinder. When a wrap is selected, it should be a single piece that is free from wrinkles, seams, and any other imperfections that may cause skin irritation.[18]

A *cohesive elastic wrap* exerts constant, even pressure. It is lightweight and contours easily to the body part. The wrap is composed of two layers of nonwoven rayon, which are separated by strands of spandex material. The cohesive elastic wrap is coated with a substance that makes the material adhere to itself, eliminating the need for metal clips or adhesive tape to hold it in place, as is required with standard elastic wraps. Athletic trainers sometimes use cohesive elastic wraps for "speed taping" when there is not enough time to apply an appropriate taping procedure and some support is better than none.

> Wrinkles or seams in roller wraps may irritate skin.

> To apply a roller wrap, hold it in the preferred hand with the loose end extending from the bottom of the roll.

Application Application of the elastic wrap must be executed in a specific manner to maximize its effectiveness. When an elastic wrap is about to be placed on a body part, the roll should be held in the preferred hand, with the loose end extending from the bottom of the roll. The back surface of the loose end is placed on the injured area and held in position by

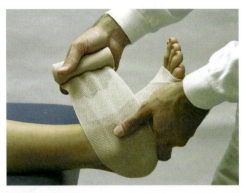

FIGURE 8–1 Elastic wraps should be applied with firm, even pressure.

8–1 Clinical Application Exercise

A freshman football player has a chronically weak ankle that he has sprained several times. He wants to have the ankle taped before games and practices but has never had it taped before.

? What can the athletic trainer do to minimize the occurrence of blisters and ensure that the tape provides support?

the other hand (Figure 8–1). The wrap cylinder is then unrolled and passed around the injured area. As the hand pulls the material from the roll, it also standardizes the wrap pressure and guides the wrap in the proper direction. To anchor and stabilize the wrap, a number of turns, one on top of the other, are made. Circling a body part requires the athletic trainer to alternate the wrap roll from one hand to the other and back again.

To provide maximum benefit, an elastic wrap should be applied uniformly and firmly but not too tightly. Excessive or unequal pressure can hinder the normal blood flow within the part. The following points should be considered when using the elastic wrap:

1. A body part should be wrapped with surrounding muscles contracted to ensure unhampered movement or circulation.
2. It is better to use a large number of turns with moderate tension than a limited number of turns applied too tightly.
3. Each turn of the wrap should be overlapped by at least one-half of the overlying wrap to prevent the separation of the material while the individual is engaged in activity. Separation of the wrap turns tends to pinch and irritate the skin and leaves a space where edema can collect.
4. When limbs are wrapped, fingers and toes should be checked often for signs of circulation impairment. Abnormally cold or blue-colored (cyanotic) phalanges are signs of excessive wrap pressure.

The usual application of elastic wraps consists of several circular wraps directly overlying each other. Whenever possible, application begins distally at the smallest circumference of a limb and is then moved proximally. Wrists and ankles are the usual sites for beginning application of wraps of the limbs. Wraps are applied to these areas in the following manner:

> **Begin application of wraps at the smallest part of the limb.**

1. The loose end of the elastic wrap is laid obliquely on the anterior aspects of the wrist or ankle and held in this position. The roll is then carried posteriorly under and completely around the limb and back to the starting point.
2. The triangular portion of the uncovered oblique end is folded over the second turn.
3. The folded triangle is covered by a third turn, which finishes a secure anchor.

After an elastic wrap has been applied, it is held in place by a locking technique. The method most often used to finish a wrap is to firmly tie or pin the wrap or place adhesive tape over several overlying turns. Anytime an athletic trainer applies an elastic wrap to the athlete, the athletic trainer must always check for decreased circulation and blueness of the extremity as well as for a blood capillary refill.

> **Check circulation after applying an elastic wrap.**

The elastic wrap can be removed either by unwrapping or by carefully cutting with scissors. Whatever method of wrap removal is used, the athletic trainer must take precautions to avoid additional injury.

Elastic Wrap Techniques

Ankle Spica The ankle and foot **spica** wrap (Figure 8–2) is primarily used for compression of acute injuries and for holding a compressive pad in place. In the ankle, a felt compressive horseshoe-shaped pad is commonly used following acute injury (see Figure 19–25).

> **spica** A figure-eight wrap with one of the two loops larger than the other.

Materials Needed Depending on the size of the ankle and foot, a 3-inch (7.5 cm) wrap is used.

Position of the Patient The patient sits with his or her ankle and foot extended over the edge of a table, with the ankle at 90 degrees.

Procedure

1. Place an anchor around the foot near the metatarsal arch.

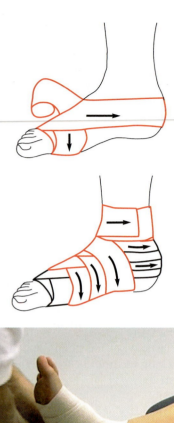

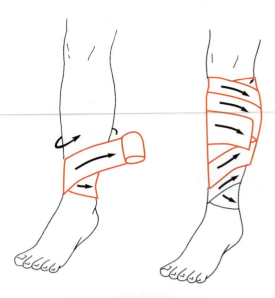

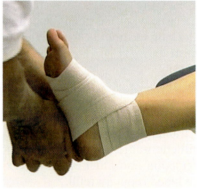

FIGURE 8–2   Ankle and foot spica.

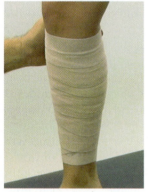

FIGURE 8–3   Spiral wrap.

2. Bring the elastic wrap across the instep and around the heel, and return to the starting point.
3. Repeat the procedure several times, with each succeeding revolution progressing upward on the foot and the ankle.
4. Overlap each spica over the preceding layer by approximately three-fourths.
5. In cases with considerable swelling, the athletic trainer may want to completely cover the heel, even though there is not typically that much swelling in that area.

Spiral Wrap   The spiral wrap (Figure 8–3) is used for covering a large area of a cylindrical part.

Materials Needed   Depending on the size of the area, a 3-inch (7.5 cm) or 4-inch (10 cm) wrap is required.

Position of the Patient   If the wrap is for the lower limb, the patient bears weight on the opposite leg.

Procedure

1. Anchor the elastic spiral wrap at the smallest distal circumference of the limb, and wrap proximally in a spiral against gravity.

2. To prevent the wrap from slipping down on a moving extremity, fold two pieces of tape lengthwise and place them on the wrap at either side of the limb, or spray tape adherent on the injured area.
3. After the wrap is anchored, carry it upward in consecutive spiral turns, each overlapping the other by at least ½ inch (1.25 cm).
4. Terminate the wrap by locking it with circular turns, and then firmly secure the wrap with tape.

Hip Spica   The following procedure is used to support a hip adductor strain (Figure 8–4).

Materials Needed   One roll of double-length 6-inch (15 cm) elastic wrap and a roll of 1½-inch (3.8 cm) adhesive tape.

Position of the Patient   The patient stands on a table and places his or her weight on the uninjured leg. The affected limb is relaxed and internally rotated.

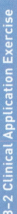

A dancer strains his right groin while performing a ballet lift

? Which elastic wrap should the athletic trainer apply when the dancer returns to dancing? Why?

8–2 Clinical Application Exercise

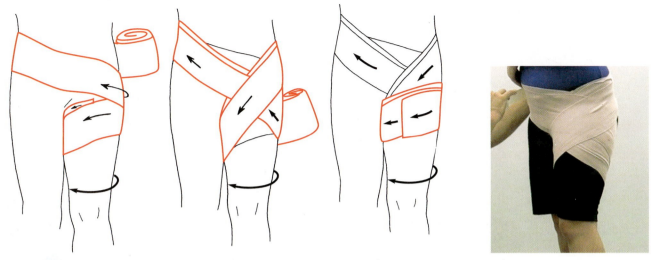

FIGURE 8–4 Hip spica using elastic wrap for hip adductor support (thigh internally rotated).

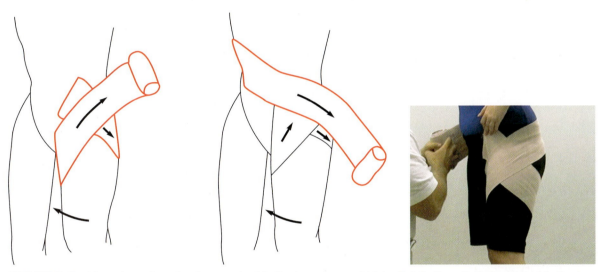

FIGURE 8–5 Hip spica using elastic wrap for hip flexion support (thigh slightly flexed). Pull up into hip flexion.

Procedure

1. Start the end of the elastic wrap at the upper part of the inner aspect of the thigh, and carry it posteriorly around the thigh. Then bring it across the lower abdomen and over the crest of the ilium on the opposite side of the body.
2. Continue the wrap around the back, repeating the same pattern and securing the wrap end with 1½-inch (3.8 cm) adhesive tape.

Variations of this method can be seen in Figure 8–5 (to support injured hip flexors) and Figure 8–6 (to support the hip extensors).

Shoulder Spica The shoulder spica (Figure 8–7) is used mainly to hold a protective pad in place or to limit shoulder flexion or abduction.

Materials Needed One roll of double-length 4-inch (10 cm) to 6-inch (15 cm) elastic wrap,

1½-inch (3.8 cm) adhesive tape, and padding for axilla.

Position of the Patient The patient stands with his or her side toward the athletic trainer.

Procedure

1. Pad the axilla well to prevent skin irritation and constriction of blood vessels.
2. Anchor the wrap by one turn around the affected upper arm.
3. After anchoring the wrap around the arm on the injured side, carry the wrap around the back under the unaffected arm and across the chest to the injured shoulder.
4. Encircle the affected arm again by the wrap, which continues around the back. Every figure-eight pattern moves progressively upward with an overlap of at least half of the previous underlying wrap.

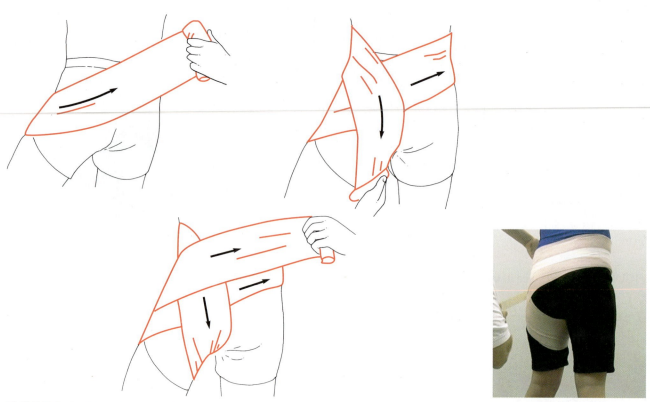

FIGURE 8–6   Hip spica using elastic wrap for hip extensor support (thigh extended and externally rotated).

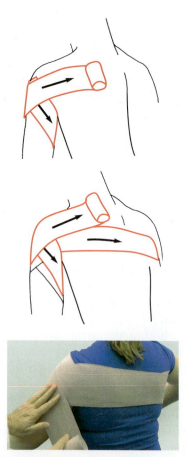

FIGURE 8–7   Shoulder spica using an elastic wrap.

Elbow Figure-Eight Wrap The elbow figure-eight wrap (Figure 8–8) can be used to secure a dressing in the antecubital fossa or to restrain full extension in hyperextension injuries. When it is reversed, it can be used on the posterior aspect of the elbow.

Materials Needed One 3-inch (7.5 cm) elastic wrap and 1½-inch (3.8 cm) adhesive tape.

Position of the Patient The patient flexes his or her elbow between 45 and 90 degrees, depending on the restriction of movement required. The fist should be clenched.

Procedure
1. Anchor the wrap by encircling the lower arm.
2. Bring the roll obliquely upward over the posterior aspect of the elbow.
3. Carry the roll obliquely upward, crossing the antecubital fossa; then pass once again completely around the upper arm and return

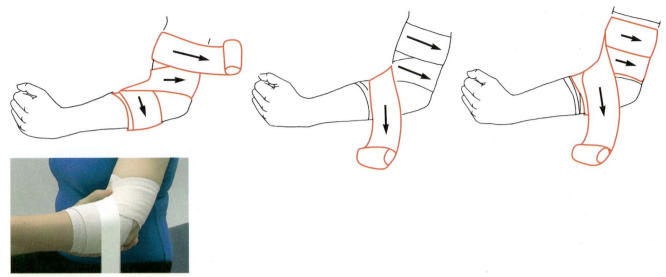

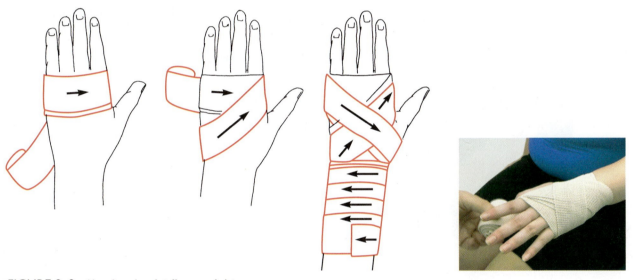

FIGURE 8–8   Elastic elbow figure-eight wrap (fist clenched).

FIGURE 8–9   Hand and wrist figure-eight wrap.

to the beginning position by again crossing the antecubital fossa.

4. Continue the procedure as described, but for every new sequence move upward toward the elbow one-half the width of the underlying wrap.

Hand and Wrist Figure-Eight Wrap   A figure-eight wrap (Figure 8–9) can be used for mild wrist and hand support and for holding dressings in place.

Materials Needed   One 2-inch (5 cm) elastic wrap and ½-inch (1.25 cm) tape.

Position of the Patient   The patient positions his or her elbow at a 45-degree angle. The fingers should be slightly spread.

Procedure

1. The anchor is executed with one or two turns of the wrap around the palm of the hand.

2. The roll is then carried obliquely across the anterior or posterior portion of the hand, depending on the position of the wound, to the wrist, which it circles once; then it is returned to the primary anchor.

3. As many figure eights as needed are applied.

Cloth Ankle Wrap

Because tape is so expensive, the ankle wrap is an inexpensive and expedient means of mildly protecting ankles (Figure 8–10). Due to an increase in the use of ankle braces and supports, the cloth ankle wrap is used infrequently in an athletic training setting.

Materials Needed   Each wrap should be 2 inches (5 cm) wide and 108 inches (270 cm) long to ensure complete coverage and protection. The purpose of this wrap is to give mild support against lateral and medial motion of the ankle. It is applied over a sock.

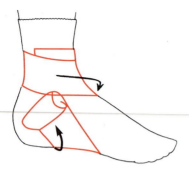

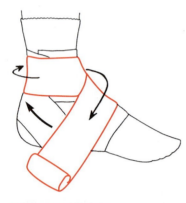

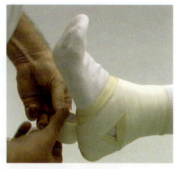

FIGURE 8–10 Ankle wrap.

Position of the Patient The patient sits on a table, extending the lower leg off the table, with the ankle flexed to 90 degrees.

Procedure

1. Anchor the wrap just above the malleoli. Circle around the ankle, moving over the top of the foot straight downward over the medial arch.
2. From the arch, move the wrap under the foot, coming up on the lateral side and then angling the wrap upward to go around the back of the ankle just above the heel.
3. Move the wrap over the top of the foot, then straight down on the lateral side toward the bottom of the foot; then go under the foot, angling upward on the medial side toward the back of the ankle just above the heel.
4. Go around the back of the ankle toward the top of the foot, thus completing one series of the wrap.
5. Complete a second and perhaps a third series with the remaining wrap.

6. For additional support apply two heel locks with 1½-inch (3.8 cm) adhesive tape over the ankle wrap.

Triangular Bandages

Triangular bandages, usually made of cotton cloth, are primarily used as first-aid devices.[18] They are valuable in emergency bandaging because they are easy and quick to apply. The principal use of the triangular bandage in athletic training is for arm slings. There are two basic kinds of slings, the cervical arm sling and the shoulder arm sling, and each has a specific purpose.

> Triangular bandages can be applied easily and quickly.

Cervical Arm Sling The cervical arm sling (Figure 8–11) is designed to support the forearm, wrist, and hand. A triangular bandage is placed around the neck and under the bent arm that is to be supported.

Materials Needed One triangular bandage.

Position of the Patient The patient stands with the affected arm bent at approximately a 70-degree angle.

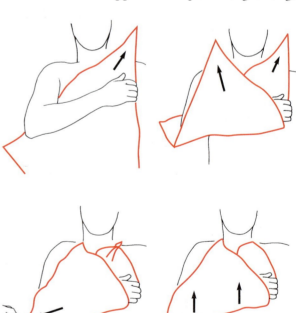

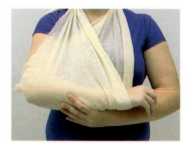

FIGURE 8–11 Cervical arm sling.

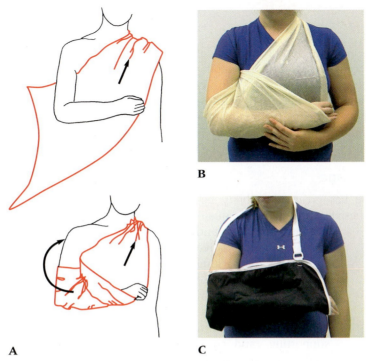

A

B

C

FIGURE 8–12 **(A)** Shoulder arm sling. **(B)** Triangular bandage. **(C)** Sling.

Procedure

1. Position the triangular bandage under the injured arm, with the apex facing the elbow.
2. Carry the end of the triangle nearest the body over the shoulder of the uninjured arm. Allow the other end to hang down loosely.
3. Pull the loose end over the shoulder of the injured side.
4. Tie the two ends of the wrap in a square knot behind the neck. For the sake of comfort, the knot should be on either side of the neck, not directly in the middle.
5. Bring the apex of the triangle around to the front of the elbow and fasten by twisting the end, then tying in a knot.

If greater arm stabilization is required than that afforded by a sling, an additional wrap can be swathed about the upper arm and body.

Shoulder Arm Sling A commercial shoulder arm sling (Figure 8–12A) is suggested for forearm support when there is an injury to the shoulder girdle or when the cervical arm sling is irritating to the patient. A triangular bandage may also be used.

Materials Needed One triangular bandage and one safety pin.

Position of the Patient The patient stands with his or her injured arm bent at approximately a 70-degree angle.

Procedure

1. Place the upper end of the shoulder sling over the uninjured shoulder side.
2. Bring the lower end of the triangle over the forearm, and draw it between the upper arm and the body, swinging it around the patient's back and then upward to meet the other end, where a square knot is tied.
3. Bring the apex end of the triangle around to the front of the elbow and fasten with a safety pin.

Sling and Swathe The sling and swathe combination is designed to stabilize the arm securely in cases of shoulder dislocation or fracture (Figure 8–13). First apply a cervical arm sling as previously described. Then stabilize the arm against the chest by wrapping a 6-inch (15.2 cm) elastic wrap completely around the torso. This is referred to as a swathe wrap. A commercial sling may also be used to create a sling and swathe.

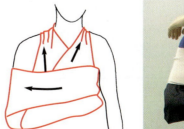
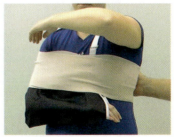

FIGURE 8–13 Sling and swathe.

NONELASTIC AND ELASTIC ADHESIVE TAPING

Historically, taping has been an important part of athletic training. In recent years, athletic taping has become decreasingly important as an adjunct to sports medicine because current research questions long-held ideas about the effectiveness of taping.[20,24,27,32,39] The psychological effect of taping is currently unknown.

Nonelastic Adhesive Tape

Nonelastic adhesive tape has great adaptability because of its uniform adhesive mass, adhering qualities, and lightness, and because of the relative strength of the backing materials.[24] All these qualities are of value in holding wound dressings in place and in supporting and protecting injured areas. This tape comes in a variety of sizes; widths of ½, 1, 1½, and 2 inches (1.25, 2.5, 3.8, and 5 cm) are commonly used in sports medicine (Figure 8–14). When linen tape is purchased, factors such as cost, grade of backing, quality of adhesive mass, and properties of unwinding should be considered.

8–4 Clinical Application Exercise

An athlete falls and sustains a dislocated right shoulder.

? How should the athlete be transported safely to the hospital?

Tape Grade Adhesive tape (usually white) is most often graded according to the number of longitudinal and vertical fibers per inch of backing material.[4] The heavier and more costly backing contains 85 or more longitudinal fibers and 65 vertical fibers per square inch. The lighter, less expensive grade has 65 or fewer longitudinal fibers and 45 vertical fibers.

> **When purchasing linen tape, consider:**
> - Grade of backing
> - Quality of adhesive mass
> - Winding tension

Adhesive Mass As a result of improvements in adhesive mass, certain essentials should be expected from tape. It should adhere readily when applied and should maintain this adherence in the presence of profuse perspiration and activity. Besides sticking well, the mass must contain as few skin irritants as possible and must be able to be removed easily without leaving a mass residue or pulling away the superficial skin.

Winding Tension The winding tension of a tape roll is important to the athletic trainer. The demands of sport activity place a unique demand on the unwinding quality of tape; if tape is to be applied for protection and support, there must be even and constant unwinding tension. In most cases, a proper wind needs little additional tension to provide sufficient tightness.

Elastic Adhesive Tape

Elastic adhesive tape is often used in combination with nonelastic adhesive tape. Because of its conforming qualities, elastic tape is used for small, angular body parts, such as the feet, wrist, hands, and fingers. It is also used when circling a soft tissue muscle group that expands with contraction or engorges with blood during activity. As with nonelastic adhesive tape, elastic tape comes in a variety of widths (1-, 2-, 3-, and 4-inch [2.5, 5, 7.5, and 10 cm]) (Figure 8–15).

Tape Storage

Tape should be stored in a cool place to avoid

> **Store tape in a cool place, and stack it flat.**

damaging the pliability of the tape fabric as well as affecting the adhesive qualities.

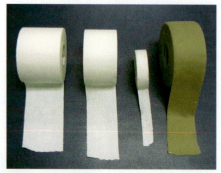

FIGURE 8–14   Nonelastic adhesive tape: 2″, 1½″, ½″ (5 cm, 3.8 cm, 1.25 cm), and Leukotape.

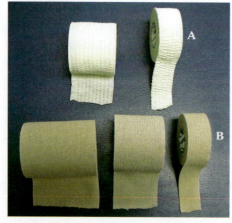

FIGURE 8–15   Elastic adhesive tape. **(A)** 2″ (5 cm) and 1″ (2.5 cm) light wrap tape. **(B)** 3″ (7.5 cm), 2″, and 1″ elastic tape.

The boxes of tape should be stacked so that the tape rests on its flat top or bottom to avoid distortion.

Using Adhesive Tape

Preparation for Taping The athletic trainer must pay special attention when applying tape directly to the skin.[31] A list of supplies needed for proper taping appears in *Focus Box 8–1:* "Taping supplies."

> Ideally, skin should be oil free and hair should be shaved before tape is applied.

Perspiration, oil, and dirt prevent tape from adhering to the skin. Whenever tape is used, ideally the skin surface should be cleaned with soap and water to remove all dirt and oil. Also, hair should be shaved to prevent additional irritation when the tape is removed (Figure 8–16A). A quick-drying tape adherent spray can be used to help the tape adhere to the skin, although it is not absolutely necessary (Figure 8–16B). Also, at certain points, such as over bony prominences, the tape can produce friction blisters. Extra foam pads (heel and lace pads) with a small amount of lubricant can help minimize the occurrence of blisters (Figure 8–16C). Taping directly on skin provides maximum immediate support. However, applying tape day after day can lead to skin irritation. A roll of foam underwrap or prewrap is thin, porous, extremely lightweight, and resilient, and it easily conforms to the contours

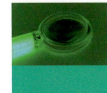

of the part to be taped and protects the skin to some degree. Underwrap should be applied only one layer thick (Figure 8–16D).[21] The underwrap should be anchored both proximally and distally (Figure 8–16E).

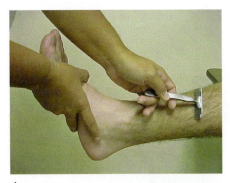

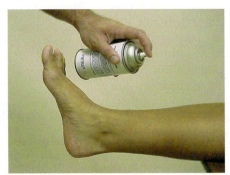

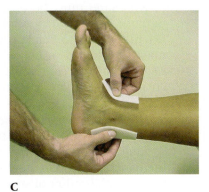

A   B   C

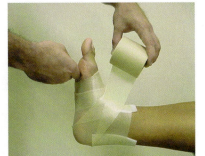

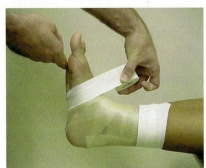

D   E

FIGURE 8–16 Taping preparation.
(A) Shaving. **(B)** Applying tape adherent. **(C)** Placing heel and lace pads. **(D)** Applying one layer of underwrap. **(E)** Applying anchor strips.

Rules for Tape Application The following are a few of the important rules to be observed in the use of adhesive tape. In practice the athletic trainer will identify others.

1. *If the part to be taped is a joint, place it in the position in which it is to be stabilized.* If the part is musculature, make the necessary allowance for contraction and expansion.
2. *Overlap the tape at least half the width of the tape below.* Unless tape is overlapped sufficiently, the active athlete will separate it, exposing the underlying skin to irritation and allowing a space in which edema can occur.
3. *Avoid continuous taping with nonelastic adhesive tape.* Tape continuously wrapped around a part may cause constriction. Make one turn at a time and tear each encirclement to overlap the starting end by approximately 1 inch (2.5 cm).
4. *Keep the tape roll in the hand whenever possible.* By learning to keep the tape roll in the hand, seldom putting it down, and by learning to tear the tape, an athletic trainer can develop taping speed and accuracy.
5. *Smooth and mold the tape as it is laid on the skin.* To save additional time, smooth and mold tape strips to the body part as they are put in place; this is done by stroking the top with the fingers, palms, and heels of both hands.
6. *Allow tape to fit the natural contour of the skin.* Each strip of tape must be placed with a particular purpose in mind. Linen-backed tape is not sufficiently elastic to bend around acute angles but must be allowed to fall as it may, fitting naturally to the body contours. Failing to allow this fit creates wrinkles and gaps that can result in skin irritations.
7. *Start taping with an anchor piece and finish by applying a lock strip.* Commence taping, if possible, by sticking the tape to an anchor piece that encircles the part. This placement affords a good medium for the stabilization of succeeding tape strips, so that they will not be affected by the movement of the part.
8. *Where maximum support is desired, tape directly over skin.* In cases of sensitive skin, prewrap may be used as a tape base. With prewrap, some movement can be expected between the skin and the base.[3]
9. *Do not apply tape if skin is hot or cold from a therapeutic treatment.*

Selecting Proper Tape Width The correct tape width depends on the area to be covered. The more acute the angles, the narrower the tape must be to fit the many contours. For example, the fingers and toes usually require ½- or 1-inch (1.25 or 2.5 cm) tape; the ankles require 1½-inch (3.8 cm) tape; and

the larger skin areas, such as thighs and back, can accommodate 2- to 3-inch (5 to 7.5 cm) tape with ease.

NOTE: Supportive tape improperly applied can aggravate an existing injury or can disrupt the mechanics of a body part, causing an initial injury to occur.

Tearing Tape Athletic trainers use various techniques to tear tape (Figure 8–17). The tearing method should permit the operator to keep the tape roll in hand most of the time.[39] The following is a suggested procedure:

> To tear tape, move hands quickly in opposite directions.

1. Hold the tape roll in the preferred hand with the middle finger hooked through the center of the tape roll and the thumb pressing its outer edge.
2. With the other hand, grasp the loose end between the thumb and index finger.
3. With both hands in place, pull both ends of the tape so that it is tight. Next, make a quick, scissorslike move to tear the tape. In tearing tape, one hand moves away from the body and the other hand moves toward the body. Remember, do not try to bend or twist the tape to tear it.

When tearing is properly executed, the torn edges of the nonelastic adhesive tape are relatively

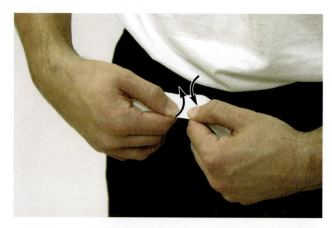

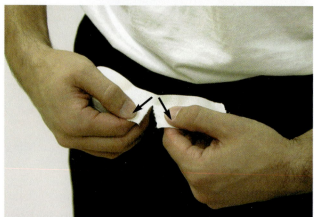

FIGURE 8–17 Technique for tearing adhesive tape.

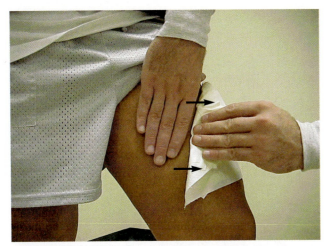

FIGURE 8–18   Removing tape by pulling in a direct line with the body.

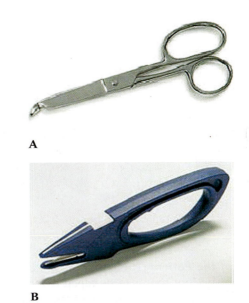

A

B

FIGURE 8–19   **(A)** Tape scissors. **(B)** Tape cutter.

straight, without curves, twists, or loose threads sticking out. Once the first thread is torn, the rest of the tape tears easily. Learning to tear tape effectively from many different positions is essential for speed and efficiency. Many tapes other than the linen-backed type cannot be torn manually but require a knife, scissors, or razor blade.

Removing Adhesive Tape Tape usually can be removed from the skin by hand, by tape scissors or tape cutters, or by chemical solvents.[1]

> Peel the skin from the tape, not the tape from the skin.

Manual Removal When pulling tape from the body, be careful not to tear or irritate the skin. Tape must not be ripped off in an outward direction from the skin but should be pulled in a direct line with the grain of the hairs (Figure 8–18). Remember to remove the skin carefully from the tape and not to peel the tape from the skin. Use one hand to gently pull the tape in one direction, and the opposite hand to gently press the skin away from the tape.

Use of Tape Scissors or Cutters The characteristic tape scissors or cutters have a blunt nose that slips underneath the tape smoothly without gouging the skin (Figure 8–19). Take care to avoid cutting the tape too near the site of the injury, so that the scissors do not aggravate the condition. Cut on the uninjured side. A general rule of thumb is to start at the superior aspect of the joint and move inferiorly.

COMMON TAPING PROCEDURES

The Arch

Arch Technique No. 1: With Arch Support Taping with an arch support strengthens weakened arches (Figure 8–20). NOTE: The longitudinal arch should be lifted. CAUTION: When applying tape around the

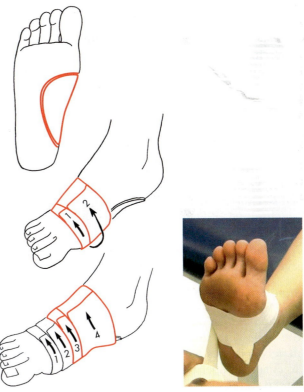

FIGURE 8–20   Arch taping technique no. 1, including an arch support and circular tape strips.

forefoot, be aware that the metatarsals must have room to spread when bearing weight.

Materials Needed One roll of 1½-inch (3.8 cm) adhesive tape, tape adherent, and a ⅛- or ¼-inch (0.3 or 0.6 cm) adhesive foam rubber pad or adhesive felt pad, cut to fit the longitudinal arch.

Site Preparation Clean foot of dirt and oil; if hairy, shave dorsum of foot. Spray area with tape adherent.

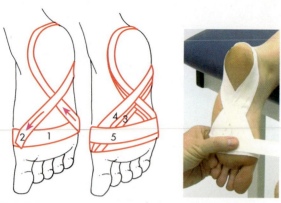

FIGURE 8–21   Arch taping technique no. 2 (X taping).

Position of the Patient The patient is seated on the table with the foot that is to be taped extending approximately 6 inches (15 cm) over the edge of the table. To ensure proper position, allow the foot to hang in a relaxed position.

Procedure

1. Place a series of strips of tape directly around the arch, pulling the arch up. If added support is required, add an arch support. The first strip should go just above the metatarsal arch (1).
2. Each successive strip overlaps the preceding piece about half the width of the tape (2 through 4).

CAUTION: Avoid putting on so many strips of tape that range of motion is limited.

Arch Technique No. 2: The X for the Longitudinal Arch

Use the figure-eight method for taping the longitudinal arch (Figure 8–21).

Materials Needed One roll of 1-inch (2.5 cm) adhesive tape and tape adherent.

Site Preparation Same as for arch technique no. 1.

Position of the Patient The patient lies face down on the table with the affected foot extending approximately 6 inches (15 cm) over the edge of the table. To ensure proper position, allow the foot to hang in a relaxed position.

Procedure

1. Lightly place an anchor strip around the ball of the foot, making certain not to restrict toe range of motion (1).
2. Start tape strip 2 from the lateral edge of the anchor. Move it upward at an acute angle, cross the center of the longitudinal arch, encircle the heel, and descend. Then cross the arch again and end at the medial aspect of the anchor (2). Repeat three or four times (3 and 4).
3. Lock the taped Xs with a single piece of tape placed around the ball of foot (5).

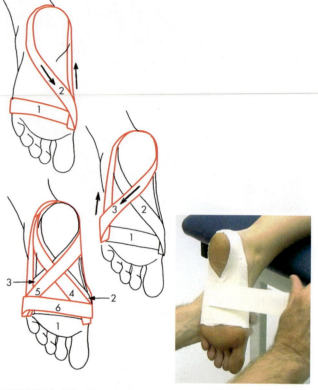

FIGURE 8–22   Teardrop arch taping technique no. 3 with double X and forefoot support.

After all the X strips are applied, an option is to cover the entire arch with 1½-inch (3.8 cm) circular adhesive tape strips.

Arch Technique No. 3: The X Teardrop Arch and Forefoot Support

As its name implies, this taping both supports the longitudinal arch and stabilizes the forefoot (Figure 8–22).

Materials Needed One roll of 1-inch (2.5 cm) adhesive tape and tape adherent.

Position of the Patient The patient lies face down on the table with the foot to be taped extending approximately 6 inches (15 cm) over the edge of the table.

Procedure

1. Place an anchor strip around the ball of the foot (1).
2. Start tape strip 2 on the side of the foot, beginning at the base of the great toe. Take the tape around the heel, crossing the arch and returning to the starting point (2).
3. The pattern of the third strip of tape is the same as the second strip except that it is started on the little toe side of the foot (3). Repeat two or three times (4 and 5).
4. Lock the series of strips by placing tape around or just proximal to the ball joint (6).

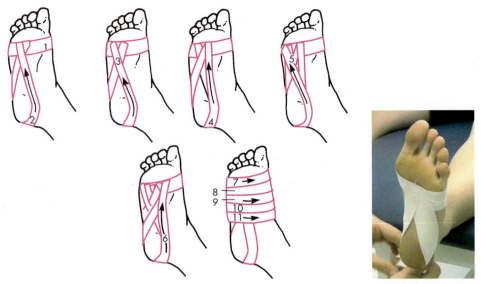

FIGURE 8–23   Fan arch taping technique.

Arch Technique No. 4: Fan Arch Support   The fan arch technique supports the entire plantar aspect of the foot (Figure 8–23).

Materials Needed   One roll of 1-inch (2.5 cm) adhesive tape, one roll of 1½-inch (3.8 cm) adhesive tape, and tape adherent.

Position of Patient   The patient is sitting on the table with the foot to be taped extending approximately 6 inches (15 cm) over the edge of the table.

Procedure

1. Using the 1-inch (2.5 cm) adhesive tape, place an anchor strip around the ball of the foot (1).
2. Starting at the third metatarsal head, take the tape around the heel from the lateral side and meet the strip where it began (2 and 3).
3. Start the next strip near the second metatarsal head and finish it on the fourth metatarsal head (4).
4. Begin the last strip on the fourth metatarsal head and finish it on the fifth metatarsal head (5). The technique, when completed, forms a fan-shaped pattern covering the metatarsal region (6).
5. Lock strips using 1½-inch (3.8 cm) adhesive tape and encircling the complete arch (7 through 11).

LowDye Technique   The LowDye technique is an excellent method for managing the fallen medial longitudinal arch, foot pronation, arch strains, and plantar fasciitis[14,17,44] (Figure 8–24).

Materials Needed   One roll of 1-inch (2.5 cm) adhesive tape, one roll of 1½-inch (3.8 cm) adhesive tape, and moleskin.

Position of the Patient   The patient sits with the foot in a neutral position with the great toe and medial aspect of the foot in plantar flexion.

Procedure

1. Grasp the forefoot with the thumb under the distal 2 to 5 metatarsal heads, pushing slightly upward, with the tips of the second and third fingers pushing downward on the first metatarsal head. Apply two or three 1-inch (2.5 cm) adhesive tape strips laterally, starting from the distal head of the fifth metatarsal bone (1 through 3). Keep these lateral strips below the outer malleolus.
2. Secure the lateral tape strips by circling the forefoot with four 1½-inch (3.8 cm) adhesive tape strips (4 through 7). Start at the lateral dorsum of the foot, circle under the plantar aspect, and finish at the medial dorsum of the foot.

The Toes

Sprained Great Toe   This procedure is used for taping a sprained great toe (Figure 8–25).

Materials Needed   One roll of 1-inch (2.5 cm) adhesive tape and tape adherent and one roll of ½-inch (1.25 cm) tape.

Site Preparation   Clean foot of dirt and oil, shave hair from toes, and spray area with tape adherent.

Position of the Patient   The patient assumes a sitting position.

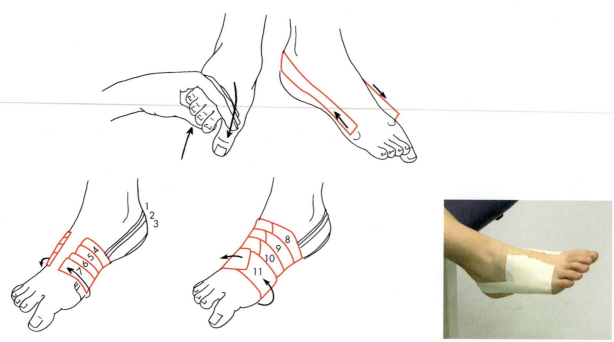

FIGURE 8–24   LowDye taping technique.

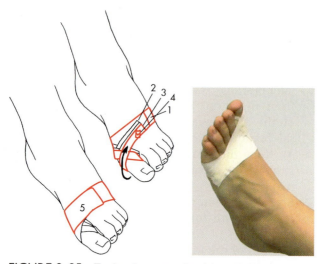

FIGURE 8–25   Taping for a sprained great toe.

Procedure

1. Use an anchor strip just proximal to metatarsal heads (1).
2. The greatest support is given to the joint by a half-figure-eight taping (2 through 4). Start the series at an acute angle on the top of the foot and swing down between the great and first toes, first encircling the great toe and then coming up, over, and across the starting point. Repeat this process, starting each series separately.
3. After the required number of half-figure-eight strips are in position, place a 1½-inch adhesive tape lock piece around the ball of the foot (5).

Hallux Valgus

Materials Needed One roll of 1-inch (2.5 cm) adhesive tape, tape adherent, and ¼-inch (0.6 cm) sponge rubber or felt (Figure 8–26).

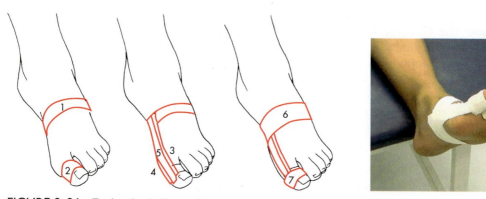

FIGURE 8–26   Taping for hallux valgus.

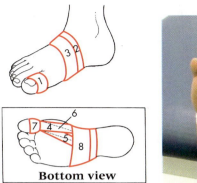
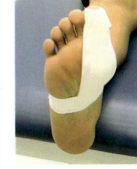

Bottom view

FIGURE 8–27   Turf toe taping.

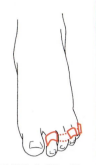
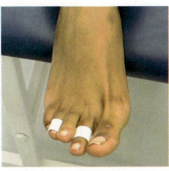

FIGURE 8–28   Hammer, or clawed, toe taping.

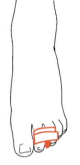
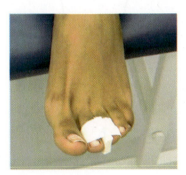

FIGURE 8–29   Fractured toe taping.

Position of the Patient The patient assumes a sitting position.

Procedure
1. Place anchor strips to encircle the midfoot and distal aspect of the great toe (1 and 2).
2. Place two or three strips on the medial aspect of the great toe to hold the toe in proper alignment (3 through 5).
3. Lock the ends of the strips with tape (6 and 7).
4. Cut a ¼-inch sponge rubber to form a wedge between the great and second toes.

Turf Toe Turf toe taping is designed to prevent excessive hyperextension of the metatarsophalangeal joint (Figure 8–27).

Materials Needed One roll of 1½-inch (3.8 cm) adhesive tape, one roll of 1-inch (2.5 cm) adhesive tape, and tape adherent.

Site Preparation Shave hair off the top of the forefoot and great toe. Spray the area with tape adherent.

Position of the Patient The great toe is in a neutral position.

Procedure
1. Apply a 1-inch (2.5 cm) adhesive tape strip around the great toe. Using 1½-inch (3.8 cm) (1) adhesive tape, apply two arch anchors to the mid-arch area (2 and 3).
2. On the middle of the great toe, attach three 1-inch (2.5 cm) adhesive tape strips to create a checkrein (4, 5, and 6).
3. Attach the checkrein to the arch anchor tapes, strip-crossing the metatarsophalangeal joint line.
4. Lock both ends of the checkrein in place (7 and 8).

Hammer, or Clawed, Toes This technique is designed to reduce the pressure of the bent toes against the shoe (Figure 8–28).[35]

Materials Needed One roll of ½- or 1-inch (1.25 or 2.5 cm) adhesive tape and tape adherent.

Position of the Patient The patient sits on the table with the affected leg extended over the edge.

Procedure
1. Tape one affected toe; then lace under the adjacent toe and over the next toe.
2. Tape can be attached to the next toe or can be continued and attached to the fifth toe.

Fractured Toes This technique splints the fractured toe with a nonfractured one (Figure 8–29).

Materials Needed One roll of ½- or 1-inch (1.25 or 2.5 cm) adhesive tape, ⅛-inch (0.3 cm) sponge rubber, and tape adherent.

Position of the Patient The patient assumes a sitting position.

Procedure
1. Cut a ⅛-inch (0.3 cm) sponge rubber wedge and place it between the affected toe and a healthy one.
2. Wrap two or three strips of tape around both toes.

The Ankle Joint

Most athletic trainers would agree that the application of adhesive tape to the ankle is the most commonly used taping technique. Both athletic trainers and patients have maintained that, if applied appropriately, taping provides comfort and support,

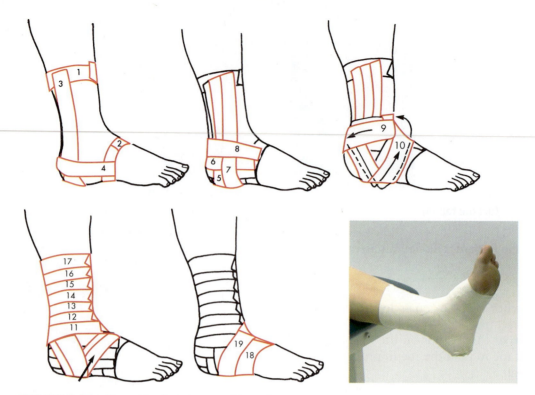

FIGURE 8–30   Closed basket weave ankle taping.

with little interference with normal ankle function. A review of the evidence-based research has questioned the effectiveness of ankle taping in reducing the incidence of ankle sprain, and a number of studies have evaluated the extent to which adhesive tape provides a mechanical restraint to excessive ankle motion.[15,25,28,33,34] Studies also describe various tape-application techniques for the ankle and explain the benefits that may be derived from ankle taping.[9,31,42,46] A few studies have indicated that ankle taping rapidly loses its initial level of resistance to motion during exercise, but a majority of studies have demonstrated that the restraining effect on extreme ankle motion is not eliminated by prolonged activity.[36,37,46] Using prewrap under adhesive tape has been shown to extend the effectiveness of tape application in controlling motion longer than if the tape is applied directly to the skin.[12,21]

As indicated in Chapter 7, a variety of ankle braces are used as alternatives to ankle taping. Some studies comparing the mechanical effects of various commercially available braces and taping have found comparable levels of postexercise motion limitation for taping and bracing.[8,10,28,46] But the majority have concluded that ankle bracing is superior to taping, based on less increase in ankle motion following exercise.[23,34,38] Despite this ongoing controversy of the relative effectiveness of taping ankles, it remains a clinical technique widely utilized by athletic trainers.

Closed Basket Weave (Gibney) Technique The closed basket weave, or Gibney, technique offers strong tape support and is primarily used in athletic training for newly sprained or chronically weak ankles (Figure 8–30).

Materials Needed One roll of 1½-inch (3.8 cm) adhesive tape, underwrap, and tape adherent.

Site Preparation Ankle taping applied directly to the athlete's skin affords the greatest support; however, when it is applied and removed daily, skin irritation will occur. To avoid this problem, apply an underwrap material. Before taping, follow these procedures:

1. Clean the foot and ankle thoroughly.
2. Shave all the hair off the foot and ankle.
3. Apply a coating of tape adherent to protect the skin and offer an adhering base.
4. Apply a gauze pad coated with friction-reducing material, such as skin lube or Vasoline over the instep and to the back of the heel.
5. If underwrap is used, apply a single layer. The tape anchors extend beyond the underwrap and adhere directly to the skin.
6. Do not apply tape if skin is cold or hot from a therapeutic treatment.

Position of the Patient The patient sits on the table with the leg extended and the foot at a 90-degree angle.

Procedure

1. Place one anchor piece around the ankle approximately 5 or 6 inches (12.5 or 15 cm) above the malleolus just below the belly of the gastrocnemius muscle. Place a second anchor around the instep directly over the styloid process of the fifth metatarsal (1 and 2).
2. Apply the first strip posteriorly to the malleolus and attach it to the ankle anchor (3). NOTE: When applying strips, pull the foot into eversion for an inversion sprain and into a neutral position for an eversion sprain.
3. Start the first Gibney directly under the malleolus and attach it to the foot anchor (4).
4. In an alternating series, place three strips and three Gibneys on the ankle, with each piece of tape overlapping at least half of the preceding strip (5 through 8).
5. After completing the conventional basket weave, apply two or three heel locks to ensure maximum stability (9 and 10). Additional support is given by a heel lock. Starting high on the instep, bring the tape along the ankle at a slight angle, hooking the heel, leading under the arch, then coming up on the opposite side, and finishing at the starting point. Tear the tape to complete half of the heel lock (9). Repeat on the opposite side of the ankle (10).
6. After applying the basket weave series, continue the Gibney strips up the ankle, thus giving circular support (11 through 17).
7. For arch support, apply two or three circular strips laterally to medially (18 and 19).

Open Basket Weave This modification of the closed basket weave, or Gibney, technique is designed to give freedom of movement in dorsiflexion and plantar flexion while providing lateral and medial support and allowing room for swelling. Taping in this pattern may be used immediately after an acute sprain in conjunction with an elastic wrap and cold applications because it allows for swelling (Figure 8–31). A U-shaped, or "horseshoe," felt pad can be used for focal compression to assist in controlling swelling (see Figure 19–25). The specific technique for controlling swelling is discussed in detail in Chapter 12.

Materials Needed One roll of 1½-inch (3.8 cm) adhesive tape and tape adherent.

Position of the Patient The patient sits on the table with the leg extended and the foot held at a 90-degree angle.

Procedure

1. Steps 1 through 4 and the first eight strips of tape applied are the same as described for the closed basket weave technique (see Figure 8–30).

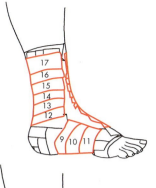
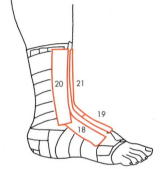
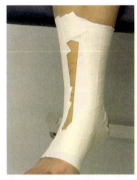

FIGURE 8–31 Open basket weave ankle taping.

2. Leave a 1- to 1½-inch (1.5 to 3.8 cm) gap between the two ends of strips 11 through 17, exposing the anterior surface of the ankle (Figure 8–31).
3. Lock the gap between the Gibney ends with either one or two pieces of tape running on either side of the instep (18 through 21). NOTE: Application of a 3- or 4-inch (7.5 or 10 cm) elastic wrap over the open basket weave affords added control of swelling. Apply the elastic wrap distal to proximal to prevent swelling from moving into the toes.

Continuous Elastic Tape Technique This technique provides a fast alternative to other taping methods for the ankle (Figure 8–32).[31]

Materials Needed One roll of 1½-inch (3.8 cm) adhesive tape, one roll of 2-inch (5 cm) elastic tape, tape adherent, and underwrap.

Position of the Patient
The patient sits on the table, with the leg extended and the foot at a 90-degree angle.

Procedure

1. Place one anchor strip around the ankle approximately 5 to 6 inches (12.5 cm to 15 cm) above the malleolus (1).
2. Apply three strips, covering the malleolli (2 through 4).

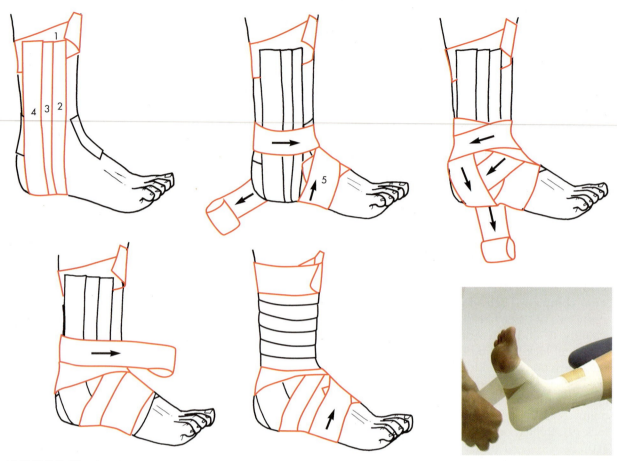

FIGURE 8–32 Continuous elastic tape technique for the ankle.

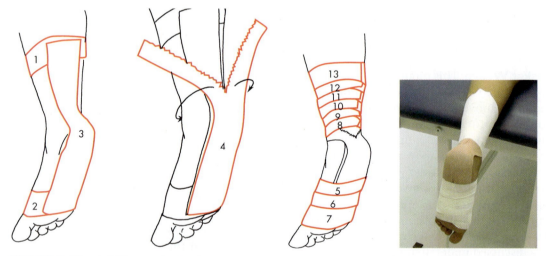

FIGURE 8–33 Achilles tendon taping.

3. Start the stretch tape in a medial-to-lateral direction above the malleoli and continue, using two heel locks, one in each direction (5).

4. After completing the heel lock, begin distally and finish proximally by closing the vertical strips.

The Lower Leg

Achilles Tendon Achilles tendon taping is designed to prevent the Achilles tendon from overstretching (Figure 8–33).

Materials Needed One roll of 3-inch (7.5 cm) elastic tape, one roll of 1½-inch (3.8 cm) adhesive tape, and tape adherent.

Site Preparation Clean and shave the area, spray with tape adherent, and apply underwrap to the lower one-third of the calf.

Position of the Patient The patient kneels or lies face down with the affected foot hanging relaxed over the edge of the table.

Procedure

1. Apply two anchors with 1½-inch (3.8 cm) adhesive tape, one circling the leg loosely approximately 7 to 9 inches (17.5 to 22.5 cm) above the malleoli, and the other encircling the ball of the foot (1 and 2).
2. Cut two strips of 3-inch (7.5 cm) elastic tape approximately 8 to 10 inches (20 to 25 cm) long. Moderately stretch the first strip from the ball of the patient's foot along its plantar aspect up to the leg anchor (3). The second elastic strip (4) follows the course of the first, but cut it and split it down the middle lengthwise. Wrap the cut ends around the lower leg to form a lock. CAUTION: Keep the wrapped ends above the level of the strain.
3. Complete the series by placing two or three lock strips of tape (5 through 7) loosely around the arch and five or six strips (8 through 13) around the patient's lower leg.

Note that locking too tightly around the lower leg and foot tends to restrict the normal action of the Achilles tendon and create more tissue irritation.

A variation on this method is to use three 2-inch (5 cm) elastic strips in place of strips 3 and 4. Apply the first strip at the plantar surface of the first metatarsal head, and end it on the lateral side of the leg anchor. Apply the second strip at the plantar surface of the fifth metatarsal head, and end it on the medial side of the leg anchor. Center the third strip between the other two strips, and end it at the posterior aspect of the calf. Lock the strips with anchors of 3-inch (7.5 cm) elastic tape around the forefoot and lower calf.[2]

The Knee

Medial Collateral Ligament Like patients with ankle instabilities, patients with unstable knees should never use tape and bracing as a replacement for proper exercise rehabilitation.[41] If properly applied, taping can help protect the knee and aid in the rehabilitation process (Figure 8–34).[41]

Materials Needed One roll of 2-inch (5 cm) adhesive tape, one roll of 3-inch (7.5 cm) elastic tape, a 1-inch (2.5 cm) heel lift, lubricant, gauze pad, tape adherent, and underwrap.

Site Preparation Clean, shave, and dry skin to be taped. Cover skin wounds. Lubricate the hamstring and popliteal areas and apply tape adherent.

Position of the Patient The patient stands on a 3-foot (90 cm) table, with the injured knee held in a moderately relaxed position by a 1-inch (2.5 cm) heel lift. Completely remove the hair from an area 6 inches (15 cm) above to 6 inches (15 cm) below the patella.

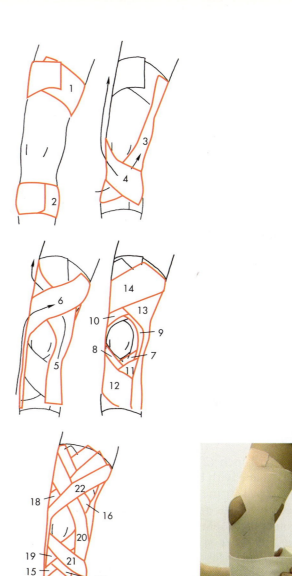

FIGURE 8–34 Collateral ligament knee taping.

Procedure

1. Lightly encircle the thigh and leg at the hairline with a 3-inch (7.5 cm) elastic tape anchor strip (1 and 2).
2. Precut 12 elastic tape strips, each approximately 9 inches (22.5 cm) long. Stretching them to their utmost, apply them to the knee as indicated in Figure 8–34 (3 through 14).
3. For additional support, a series of eight strips of 2-inch (5 cm) adhesive tape (15 through 22) may be applied in the same pattern. Some individuals find it advantageous to complete a knee taping by wrapping with an elastic wrap, thus providing an added precaution against the tape coming loose due to perspiration.

NOTE: Tape must not constrict the patella.

Rotary Taping for Instability of an Injured Knee

The rotary taping method is designed to provide the knee with support when it is unstable from injury to

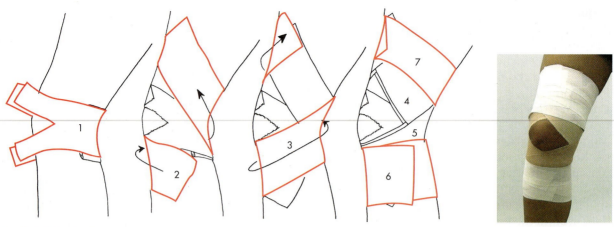

FIGURE 8–35   Rotary taping.

the medial collateral and anterior cruciate ligaments (Figure 8–35).

Materials Needed One roll of 3-inch (7.5 cm) elastic tape, tape adherent, 4-inch (10 cm) gauze pad, lubricant, scissors, and underwrap.

Position of the Patient The patient stands on the table, with the affected knee flexed 15 degrees.

Procedure

1. Cut a 10-inch (25 cm) piece of 3-inch (7.5 cm) elastic tape with both the ends snipped. Place the gauze pad in the center of the 10-inch (25 cm) piece of elastic tape, to limit skin irritation and protect the popliteal nerves and blood vessels.
2. Put the gauze with the elastic tape backing on the popliteal fossa of the athlete's knee. Stretch both ends of the tape to the fullest extent and tear them. Place the divided ends firmly around the patella and interlock them (1).
3. Starting at a midpoint on the gastrocnemius muscle, spiral a 3-inch (7.5 cm) elastic tape strip to the front of the leg, then behind, crossing the popliteal fossa, and around the thigh, finishing anteriorly (2).
4. Repeat procedure 3 on the opposite side (3).
5. Apply two or four additional spiral strips for added strength (4 and 5).
6. Once they are in place, lock the spiral strips with two strips around the thigh and two around the calf (6 and 7).

NOTE: Tracing the spiral pattern with adhesive tape yields more rigidity.

Hyperextension Hyperextension taping is designed to prevent the knee from hyperextending and may be used for a strained hamstring muscle or for slackened cruciate ligaments (Figure 8–36).

Materials Needed One roll of 2½-inch (6.25 cm) tape or 2-inch (5 cm) elastic tape, cotton or a 4-inch (10 cm) gauze pad, tape adherent, underwrap, and a 2-inch (5 cm) heel lift.

Position of the Patient Completely shave the patient's leg, including the area above midthigh and below mid-calf. The patient stands on a 3-foot (90 cm) table with the injured knee flexed by a 2-inch (5 cm) heel lift.

Procedure

1. Place four anchor strips at the hairlines, two around the thigh and two around the leg (1 through 4). The strips should be loose enough to allow for muscle expansion during exercise.
2. Place a gauze pad at the popliteal space to protect the popliteal nerves and blood vessels from constriction by the tape.
3. Start the supporting tape strips by forming an X over the popliteal space (5 and 6).
4. Cross the tape with two more strips, and place one up the middle of the leg (7 through 9).
5. Complete the technique by applying four or five locking strips around the thigh and calf (10 through 18).
6. Apply an additional series of cross-strips if the athlete is heavily muscled. Lock the additional supporting strips in place with two or three strips around the thigh and leg.

Patellofemoral Taping (McConnell Technique)

Patellofemoral orientation may be corrected to some degree by using tape.[22,40] The McConnell technique evaluates four components of patellar orientation: glide, tilt, rotation, and anteroposterior (AP) orientation.[22]

The glide component looks at side-to-side movement of the patella in the groove. The tilt component assesses the height of the lateral patellar border relative to the medial border.

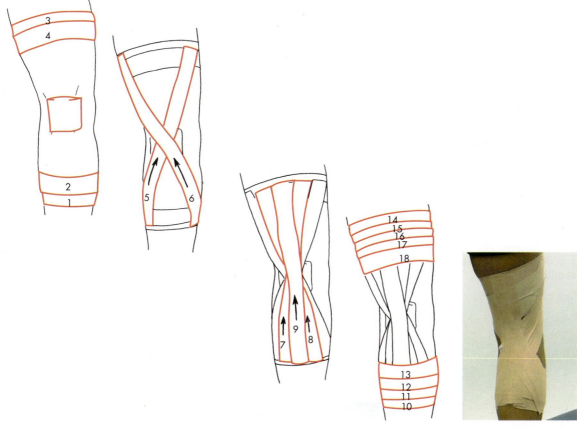

FIGURE 8–36   Hyperextension taping.

Patellar rotation is determined by looking for deviation of the long axis of the patella from the long axis of the femur. Anteroposterior alignment evaluates whether the inferior pole of the patella is tilted either anteriorly or posteriorly relative to the superior pole. Correction of patellar position and tracking is accomplished by passive taping of the patella in a more biomechanically correct position.[45,48] In addition to correcting the orientation of the patella, the tape provides a prolonged, gentle stretch to soft-tissue structure that affects patellar movement.[13,22,49]

Materials Needed Two special types of extremely sticky tape are required. Fixomull and Leuko Sportape are manufactured by Biersdorf Australia, Ltd.

Site Preparation Clean and shave, and apply tape adherent.

Position of the Patient The patient is sitting with the knee fully extended.

Procedure

1. Extend two strips of Fixomull from the lateral femoral condyle just posterior to the medial femoral condyle around the front of the knee. This tape is used as a base to which the other tape may be adhered. Leuko Sportape is used from this point on to correct patellar alignment (Figure 8–37).

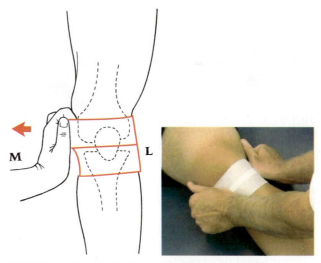

FIGURE 8–37   The McConnell patellar technique uses a base to which additional tape is adhered.

2. To correct a lateral glide, attach a short strip of tape one thumb's width from the lateral patellar border, pushing the patella medially in the frontal plane. Crease the skin between the lateral patellar border and the medial femoral condyle, and secure the tape on the medial side of the joint (Figure 8–38).

3. To correct a lateral tilt, flex the knee to 30 degrees, adhere a short strip of tape beginning at the middle of the patella, and pull medially to lift

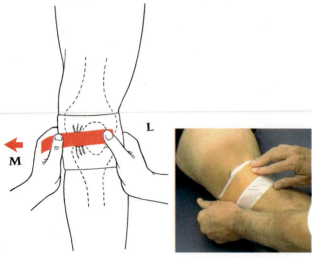

FIGURE 8–38　McConnell patellar technique to correct a lateral glide.

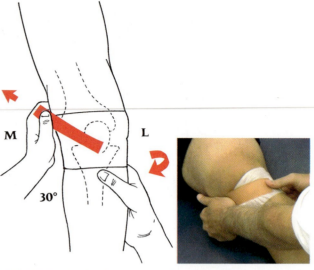

FIGURE 8–40　McConnell patellar technique to correct external rotation of the inferior pole.

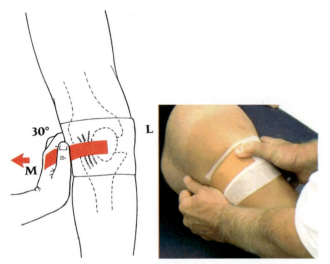

FIGURE 8–39　McConnell patellar technique to correct a lateral tilt.

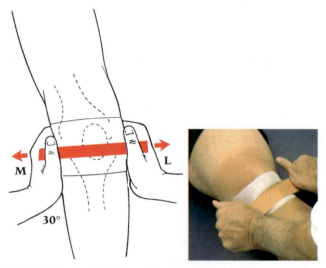

FIGURE 8–41　McConnell patellar technique to correct AP alignment with a superior tilt.

the lateral border. Again, crease the skin underneath and adhere it to the medial side of the knee (Figure 8–39).

4. To correct an external rotation of the inferior pole relative to the superior pole, adhere a strip of tape to the middle of the inferior pole, pulling upward and medially while internally rotating the patella with the free hand. The tape is attached to the medial side of the knee (Figure 8–40).

5. For correcting AP alignment in which there is a superior tilt, take a 6-inch piece of tape, place the middle of the strip over the lower one-half of the patella, and attach it equally on both sides to lift the superior pole (Figure 8–41).

6. Once patellar taping is completed, the patient should be instructed to wear the tape all day during all activities. The patient should periodically tighten the strips as they loosen.

NOTE: The McConnell technique for treating patellofemoral pain also stresses the importance of more symmetrical loading of the patella through reeducation and strengthening of the vastus medialis, although the efficacy of this technique is questionable.[7,22] Patellar taping may also enhance proprioception in the knee joint.[26]

The Elbow

Elbow Restriction Taping the elbow prevents hyperextension (Figure 8–42).[43]

Materials Needed One roll of 1½-inch (3.8 cm) adhesive tape, tape adherent, and 2-inch (5 cm) elastic tape.

Site Preparation Clean and shave area, and apply adherent.

Position of the Patient The patient has the affected elbow flexed at 90 degrees.

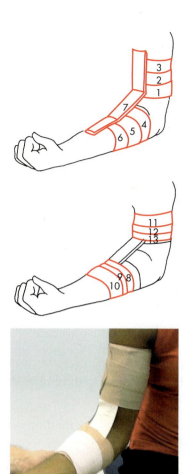

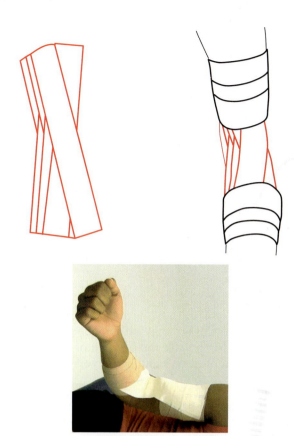

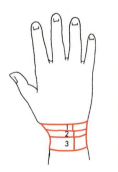

FIGURE 8–42   Elbow restriction taping.

FIGURE 8–43   Fanned checkrein technique.

Procedure

1. Apply three anchor strips loosely around the upper arm, using 2-inch (5 cm) elastic tape (1 through 3).
2. Apply three anchor strips around the upper forearm, using 2-inch (5 cm) elastic tape (4, 5, and 6).
3. Construct a checkrein by cutting a 10-inch (25 cm) and a 4-inch (10 cm) strip of tape and placing the 4-inch (10 cm) strip against the center of the 10-inch (25 cm) strip, blanking out that portion. Place the checkrein so that it spans the two anchor strips, with the blanked-out side facing downward. Leave the checkrein extended 1 to 2 inches past the anchor strips on both ends. This allows anchoring of the checkreins with circular strips to secure against slippage (7).
4. Place five additional 10-inch (25 cm) strips of tape over the basic checkrein.
5. Finish the procedure by securing the checkrein with three lock strips on each end (8 through 13). A figure-eight elastic wrap applied over the taping will prevent the tape from slipping because of perspiration.

NOTE: A variation of this method is to fan the checkreins, dispersing the force over a wider area (Figure 8–43).

FIGURE 8–44   Wrist taping technique no. 1.

The Wrist and Hand

Wrist Taping Technique No. 1 This wrist taping technique is designed for mild wrist strains and sprains (Figure 8–44).

Materials Needed One roll of 1-inch (2.5 cm) adhesive tape and tape adherent.

Position of the Patient The patient stands with the affected hand flexed toward the injured

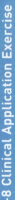

8–8 Clinical Application Exercise

A volleyball player attempts to block a ball and reports that her elbow "bent backwards."

? What taping technique can be used to prevent this incident from reoccurring?

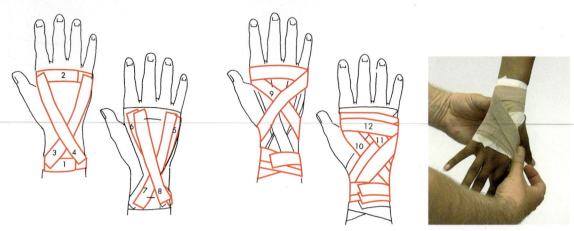

FIGURE 8–45   Wrist taping technique no. 2.

direction. The fingers may either be spread or the fist clenched to increase the breadth of the wrist for the protection of nerves and blood vessels.

Procedure

1. Starting at the base of the wrist, bring a strip of 1-inch (2.5 cm) adhesive tape around both sides of the wrist (1).
2. In the same pattern, with each strip overlapping the preceding one by at least half its width, lay two additional strips in place (2 and 3).

Wrist Taping Technique No. 2   This wrist taping technique stabilizes and protects badly injured wrists (Figure 8–45).

Materials Needed   One roll of 1-inch (2.5 cm) adhesive tape and tape adherent.

Position of the Patient   The patient stands with the affected hand flexed toward the injured side and the fingers moderately spread to increase the breadth of the wrist for the protection of nerves and blood vessels.

Procedure

1. Apply one anchor strip around the wrist approximately 3 inches (7.5 cm) from the hand (1); wrap another anchor strip around the spread hand (2).
2. With the wrist bent toward the side of the injury, run a strip of tape from the anchor strip near the little finger obliquely across the wrist joint to the wrist anchor strip. Run another strip from the anchor strip and the index finger side across the wrist joint to the wrist anchor. This forms a crisscross over the wrist joint (3 and 4). Apply a series of four or five crisscrosses, depending on the extent of splinting needed (5 through 8).
3. Apply two or three series of figure-eight tapings over the crisscross taping (9 through 11). Starting

by encircling the wrist once, carry a strip over the back of the hand obliquely upward across the back of the hand to where the figure eight started. Repeat this procedure to ensure a strong, stabilizing taping (12).

Bruised Hand   The following method is used to tape a bruised hand (Figure 8–46).

Materials Needed   One roll of 1-inch (2.5 cm) adhesive tape, one roll of ½-inch (1.25 cm) adhesive tape, ¼-inch (0.6 cm) thick sponge rubber pad, and tape adherent.

Position of the Patient   The fingers are spread moderately.

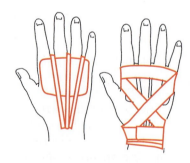

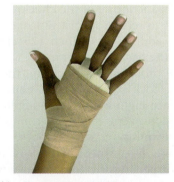

FIGURE 8–46   Bruised hand taping.

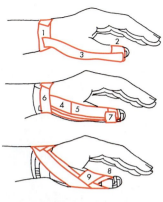

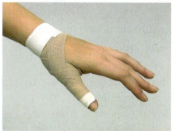

FIGURE 8–47   Sprained thumb taping.

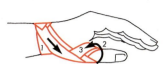
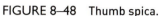

FIGURE 8–48   Thumb spica.

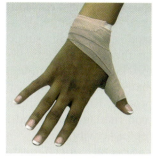

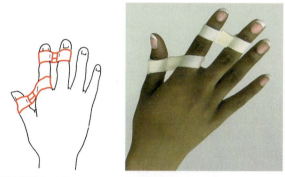

FIGURE 8–49   Finger and thumb checkreins.

Procedure

1. Lay the protective pad over the bruise and hold it in place with three strips of ½-inch (1.25 cm) tape laced through the webbing of the fingers.
2. Apply a basic figure-eight wrap made of 1-inch (2.5 cm) elastic tape.

Sprained Thumb Sprained thumb taping is designed to give protection to the joint as well as support to the thumb (Figure 8–47).[11]

Materials Needed One roll each of 1-inch (2.5 cm) adhesive tape and elastic tape and tape adherent.

Position of the Patient The patient should hold the injured thumb in a relaxed, neutral position.

Procedure

1. Place an anchor strip loosely around the wrist and another around the distal end of the thumb (1 and 2).
2. From the anchor at the tip of the thumb to the anchor around the wrist, apply four splint strips in a series on the side of greater injury (dorsal or palmar side) (3 through 5). They may be locked in place either with one lock strip around the wrist and one encircling the tip of the thumb (6 and 7) or simply with the thumb spica.
3. Add three thumb spicas. Start the first spica on the ulnar side at the wrist; carry it across the wrist; cross the strip and continue around the thumb; finish at the starting point. Each of the subsequent spica strips should overlap the preceding strip by at least ⅔-inch (1.7 cm) and adduct the thumb toward the web space (8 and 9).

The thumb spica with tape provides an excellent means of protection during recovery from an injury (Figure 8–48).

Finger and Thumb Checkreins The sprained finger or thumb may require the additional protection afforded by a restraining checkrein (Figure 8–49).[11]

Materials Needed One roll of 1-inch (2.5 cm) adhesive tape.

Position of the Patient The patient spreads the injured fingers widely but within a range that is free of pain.

Procedure

1. Bring a strip of ½-inch (1.25 cm) adhesive tape around the middle phalanx of the injured finger over to the adjacent finger and around it also. The tape left between the two fingers, which are spread apart, is called the checkrein.
2. Add strength with a lock strip around the center of the checkrein.

KINESIO TAPING

Kinesio taping is a technique developed in Japan and widely used in Europe and Asia. It has become popular in the United States despite the fact that there is little research-based evidence that supports it's effectiveness.[47] Kinesio tape differs from adhesive tape in that it is elastic and can be stretched to 140 percent of its original length before being applied to the skin, thus providing a constant tension (shear) force to the skin over which it is applied.[16] Although adhesive tape is structurally supportive, Kinesio tape is said to be therapeutic, activating neurological and circulatory systems with movement.[29] It is used both immediately following injury and during the rehabilitation process. Kinesio taping is used for edema reduction, pain management, and inhibition and facilitation of motor activity.[16]

Several mechanisms have been proposed through which Kinesio tape works, including improving circulation of blood and lymph by eliminating tissue fluid or bleeding beneath the skin; correcting muscle function by strengthening weakened muscles; decreasing pain through neurological suppression; and repositioning subluxed joints by relieving abnormal muscle tension.[29] It has also been suggested that the Kinesio tape stimulates cutaneous mechanoreceptors by applying pressure and stretching the skin, thus enhancing proprioception through increased cutaneous feedback, which signals information relative to joint movement or joint position.[30]

The basic principle of Kinesio taping is to apply the tape from one end of a muscle to the other, with very little to no stretch on the tape from origin to insertion for muscle support and from insertion to origin during rehabilitation.[15] The muscle is placed on gentle functional stretch with application of the tape at approximately 10 percent of its resting static length.[16] Because the latex-free, 100 percent cotton fabric with body heat–activated adhesive Kinesio tape is air permeable and water resistant, it can be worn continuously for 3 to 4 days before a new application is required.[29] Kinesio tape can be purchased in rolls of 1-inch (2.5 cm), 1½-inch (3.8 cm), 2-inch (5 cm), and 3-inch (7.5 cm) widths. The tape comes in a variety of colors, although there is no physical or chemical difference between the colors.

Athletic trainers are familiar and comfortable with taping techniques that provide stability and support. The therapeutic techniques of Kinesio taping are not difficult, but do require some specialized training and course work for athletic trainers who wish to use this method of taping. Figures 8–50 through 8–53 provide some common examples of Kinesio taping techniques.

Kinesio Taping Techniques

Plantar Fasciitis

Materials Needed One roll of 1-inch (2.5 cm) Kinesio tape and one roll of 3-inch (7.5 cm) Kinesio tape.

Position of the Patient The patient lies prone with the foot extending off the edge of the treatment table, with foot dorsiflexed and the toes extended (Figure 8–50).

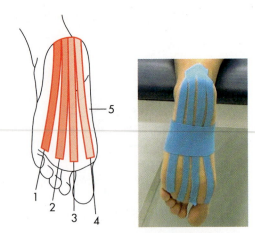

FIGURE 8–50   Kinesio taping for planter fasciitis.

Procedure

1. Place the base of 1-inch (2.5 cm) tape over heel with moderate stretch.
2. Extend four pieces of 1-inch (2.5 cm) tape over bottom of foot to the metatarsal heads while extending toes to stretch plantar fascia. Use a moderate to strong stretch (1 through 4).
3. Place one end of a 3-inch (7.5 cm) strip over the shaft of the fifth metatarsal. With the foot relaxed, extend tape over arch toward the medial side of the foot, adding moderate stretch (5).

Patellofemoral Pain

Materials Needed One roll of 2-inch (5 cm) Kinesio tape.

Position of the Patient The patient sits with the leg extended (Figure 8–51).

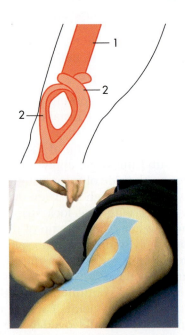

FIGURE 8–51   Kinesio taping technique for patellofemoral pain.

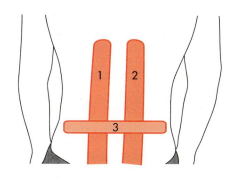

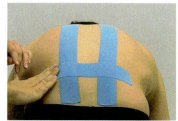

FIGURE 8–52   Kinesio taping for low back strain.

Procedure

1. Split a piece of 2-inch (5 cm) tape 10 inches (25 cm) long halfway. Position the anchor of the tape on the front of the thigh so that the Y-shape split is at the top of the patella (1).
2. Wrap tails downward around the patella, with very little or no stretch.
3. Split a piece of 2-inch (2.5 cm) tape 6 inches (15 cm) long halfway. Place the base of the second Y-shape tape slightly below the knee, and wrap tails upward around the patella, with very little or no stretch (2).

Low Back Strain

Materials Needed One roll of 3-inch (7.5 cm) Kinesio tape.

Position of the Patient The patient is standing (Figure 8–52).

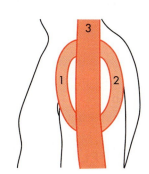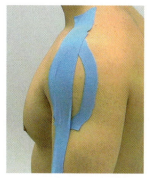

FIGURE 8–53   Kinesio taping for shoulder instability.

Procedure

1. Bend forward to stretch the back muscles. Apply two 3-inch (7.5 cm) strips beginning at the level of the waist, and extend up and along each side of the spine, adding very light stretch (1 and 2).
2. With the patient still bending forward, add light to moderate stretch and place the center of a 3-inch (7.5 cm) strip of tape over the strained area (3).

Shoulder Instability

Materials Needed One roll of 1-inch (2.5 cm) Kinesio tape and one roll of 2-inch (5 cm) Kinesio tape.

Position of the Patient The patient is standing, arm hanging at side (Figure 8–53).

Procedure

1. Using two pieces of 1-inch (2.5 cm) tape, place base of Y-shape strip below the insertion of the deltoid muscle. Extend both sides of the tape to wrap around the deltoid muscle, with no added stretch (1 and 2).
2. Abduct the shoulder to 90 degrees, and apply one strip of 2-inch (5 cm) tape over the tip of the shoulder, with little to no stretch, extending from the base of the neck to halfway down the upper arm (3).

SUMMARY

- Elastic wraps provide compression, provide support, and reduce chances of injury.
- Elastic wraps must be applied uniformly, firmly but not so tightly as to impede circulation.
- Historically, taping has been an important aspect of athletic training. However, there are limited evidence-based studies that support its use.
- For supporting and protecting musculoskeletal injuries, two types of tape are currently used—nonelastic white adhesive and elastic adhesive.
- An adherent may be applied, followed by an underwrap material, if need be, to help avoid skin irritation.

- When tape is applied, it must be done in a manner that provides the least amount of irritation and the maximum support.
- For all tape applications, the correct materials must be used, the patient must be in an appropriate position, and the proper procedures must be carefully followed.
- Kinesio taping is used for therapeutic purposes both immediately following injury and during rehabilitation.

WEB SITES

Cramer First Aider:
www.cramersportsmed.com/first_aider.jsp

Cramer Sports Medicine: www.cramersportsmed.com

Johnson & Johnson: www.jnj.com

Kinesio Taping Association: www.kinesiotaping.com

Mueller Sports Medicine—Retail Tape and Wrap:
www.muellersportsmed.com/sportcareretail.htm

Properties of Athletic Tape:
www.bloodandbones.com/tape.html

SOLUTIONS TO CLINICAL APPLICATION EXERCISES

8–1 First the ankle should be shaved. Then a tape adherent spray should be applied. Heel and lace pads with a small amount of lubricant should be applied over bony prominences. One layer of underwrap can be applied. Tape should be applied with even pressure, leaving no gaps.

8–2 The athletic trainer should apply a 6-inch (15 cm) elastic wrap as a hip adductor restraint. This technique is designed to prevent the groin from being overstretched and the hip adductors reinjured.

8–3 The athletic trainer should apply tape and a 4-inch (10 cm) double-length elastic shoulder spica to hold the doughnut in place.

8–4 The athletic trainer should apply a sling and swathe combination. This combination stabilizes the shoulder joint and upper arm.

8–5 The LowDye technique is designed to assist in the management of foot pronation and fallen medial longitudinal arch, which predisposes the patient to arch strain.

8–6 Initially, for a sprained ankle, the athletic trainer should select the open basket weave taping technique. This technique in conjunction with focal compression and cold application can also control swelling.

8–7 The McConnell taping technique can be employed to correct a lateral patellar glide.

8–8 The elbow restriction taping will help prevent elbow hyperextension.

REVIEW QUESTIONS AND CLASS ACTIVITIES

1. What are some common types of wraps used in sports medicine today?
2. Observe the athletic trainer when he or she is dressing wounds in the training clinic.
3. Demonstrate the proper use of elastic wraps.
4. What types of tape are available? What is the purpose of each type? What qualities should you look for in selecting tape?
5. How should you prepare an area to be taped?
6. How should you tear tape?
7. How should you remove tape from an area? Demonstrate the various methods and cutters that can be used to remove tape.
8. Bring the different types of tape to class. Discuss their uses and the qualities to look for in purchasing tape. Have the class practice tearing tape and preparing an area for taping.
9. Take each joint or body part and demonstrate the common taping procedures used to give support to that area. Have the students pair up and practice these tapings on each other. Discuss the advantages and disadvantages of using tape as a supportive device.
10. How is Kinesio taping different from applying regular adhesive tape?

REFERENCES

1. Abell B: *Taping and wrapping made simple*, Philadelphia, 2009, Lippincott, Williams & Wilkins.

2. Alt W, Lohrer H, Gollhofer A: Functional properties of adhesive ankle taping: Neuromuscular and mechanical effects before and after exercise, *Foot and Ankle International* 20(4):238, 1999.

3. Benefit of ankle taping is short-lived with or without prewrap, *Sports Med Digest* 19(1):130, 1997.

4. Bragg RW, Macmahon JM, Overom EK: Failure and fatigue characteristics of adhesive athletic tape, *Med Sci Sports Exerc* 34(3):403, 2002.

5. Briggs J: Bandaging, strapping and taping. In Briggs J, editor: *Sports therapy: Theoretical and practical thoughts and considerations*, Chichester, England, 2001 Corpus.

6. Callaghan M, Selfe J, Bagley P: The effects of patellar taping on knee joint proprioception, *J Athl Train* 37(1):19, 2002.

7. Camera J: The effect of patellar taping on some landing characteristics during counter movement jumps in healthy subjects, *Journal of Sport Science and Medicine* 10(1):707–11, 2011.

8. Cecchinato A, Bernier J, Cucina I: Effectiveness of ankle tape and ankle brace on joint position sense in subjects with unilateral functionally unstable ankle (Abstract), *J Athl Train* 40(2 Suppl):S-108, 2005.

9. Clay K: The impact of ankle taping upon range of movement and lower-limb balance before and after dynamic exercise. In Reilly T: *Contemporary sport, leisure and ergonomics*, 2009, Taylor and Francis.

10. Cordova M, Ingersoll C, Palmieri R: Efficacy of prophylactic ankle support: An experimental perspective, *J Athl Train* 37(4):446, 2002.

11. Deivert R: Functional thumb taping procedure, *J Athl Train* 29(4):357, 1994.

12. DesRochers DM, Cox DE: Proprioceptive benefit derived from ankle support, *Athletic Therapy Today* 7(6):44, 2002.

13. Ernst GP, Kawaguchi J, Saliba E: Effect of patellar taping on knee kinetics of patients with patellofemoral pain syndrome, *J Orthop Sports Phys Ther* 29(11):661, 1999.

14. Franettovich M: Initial neuromotor and postural effects of augmented low-dye taping do not change after continued use, *Athletic Training and Sports Healthcare* 3(1):21–28, 2011.

15. Grindstaff T: Kinesiotaping technique for patellar tendinopathy, *Athletic Training & Sports Health Care* 2(3):98–99, 2010.

16. Halseth T, McChesney J, DeBeliso M: The effects of Kinesio taping on proprioception at the ankle, *Journal of Sports Science & Medicine* 3(1):1, 2004.

17. Holmes C, Wilcox D, Fletcher J: Effect of a modified, low-dye medial longitudinal arch taping procedure on the subtalar joint neutral position before and after, light exercise, *J Orthpo Sports Phys Ther* 32(5):305–309, 2002.

18. Karren K, Limmer D, Mistovich J, Hafen B: *First aid for colleges and universities*, San Francisco, 2011, Benjamin-Cummings.

19. Knight KL: Taping, wrapping, bracing, and padding. In Knight KL, editor: *Assessing*

clinical proficiencies in athletic training: A modular approach, ed 3, Champaign, IL, 2001, Human Kinetics.

20. Magnes, S: Taping and bracing for pelvic and hip injuries. In Seidenberg P: *The hip and pelvis in sports medicine and primary care*, New York, 2010, Springer.

21. Manfroy PP, Ashton-Miller JA, Wojtys EM: The effect of exercise, prewrap, and athletic tape on the maximal active and passive ankle resistance to ankle-inversion, *Am J Sports Med* 25(2):156, 1997.

22. McConnell J: A novel approach to pain relief pre-therapeutic exercise, *Journal of Science and Medicine in Sport* 3(3):325, 2000.

23. Merrick MA: Do ankle bracing and taping work? *Athletic Therapy Today* 5(6):40, 2000.

24. Metcalfe RC, Schlabach GA, Looney MA, et al.: A comparison of moleskin tape, linen tape, and lace-up brace on joint restriction and movement performance, *J Athl Train* 32(2):136, 1997.

25. Mickel T: Prophylactic bracing versus taping for the prevention of ankle sprains in high school athletes: A prospective, randomized trial, *Journal of Foot and Ankle Surgery* 45(6):360–65, 2006.

26. Ng G: Patellar taping does not affect the onset of activities of *vastus medialis obliquus* and *vastus lateralis* before and after muscle fatigue, *American Journal of Physical Medicine and Rehabilitation* 84(2):106, 2005.

27. Olmsted L, Vela L, Denegar C: Prophylactic ankle taping and bracing: A numbers needed-to-treat and cost-benefit analysis, *J Athl Train* 39(1):95, 2004.

28. Olmsted-Kramer L, Hertel J: Preventing recurrent lateral ankle sprains: An evidence-based approach, *Athletic Therapy Today* 9(6):19, 2004.

29. Osterhues D: The use of Kinesio taping in the management of traumatic patella dislocation: A case study, *Physiotherapy Theory and Practice* 20(4):267, 2004.

30. O'Sullivan D: Utilization of kinesiotaping for fascia unloading, *Athletic Therapy and Training* 16(4):21–27, 2011.

31. Perrin DH: *Athletic taping and bracing*, Champaign, IL, 2005, Human Kinetics.

32. Purcell S: Differences in ankle range of motion before and after exercise in 2 tape conditions, *Am J Sports Med* 37(2):383–89, 2009.

33. Quackenbush K: The effects of two adhesive ankle taping methods on strength, power, and range of motion in female athletes, *North American Journal of Sorts Physical Therapy* 3(1):25–32, 2008.

34. Refshauge KM, Kilbreath SL, Raymond J: The effect of recurrent ankle inversion sprain and taping on proprioception at the ankle, *Med Sci Sports Exerc* 32(1):10, 2000.

35. Reuter B: Taping the hammer toe, *J Athl Train* 30(2):178, 1995.

36. Reuter G: Ankle spatting compared to bracing or taping during maximal effort sprint drills, *International Journal of Exercise Science* 4(1):7, 2011.

37. Ricard M, Sherwood S, Schukthies S: Effects of tape and exercise on dynamic ankle inversion, *J Athl Train* 35(1):35, 2000.

38. Riemann B, Schmitz R, Gale M: Effect of ankle taping and bracing on vertical ground reaction forces during drop landings before and after treadmill jogging, *J Orthop Sports Phys Ther* 32(5):334–38, 2002.

39. Simoneau GG, Degner RM, Kramper CA et al.: Changes in ankle joint proprioception resulting from strips of athletic tape applied over the skin, *J Athl Train* 32(2):141, 1997.

40. Somes S, et al.: Effects of patellar taping on patellar position in the open and closed kinetic chain: A preliminary study, *J Sport Rehabil* 6(4):299, 1997.

41. Stahl A: The unique benefits of therapeutic taping, *Rehab Manag* 23(6):26–29, 2010.

42. Stoffel K: Effect of ankle taping on knee and ankle joint biomechanics in sporting tasks, *Medicine and Science in Sport and Exercise* 42(11):2089–97, 2010.

43. Vicenzino B, Brooksbank J, Minto J: Initial effects of elbow taping on pain-free grip strength and pressure pain threshold, *J Orthop Sports Phys Ther* 33(7):394–96, 2003.

44. Wall K, Swanik K, Swanik C: Augmented low-dye arch taping affects on muscle activity and ground reaction forces in people with pes planus (Abstract), *J Athl Train* 40(2 Suppl):S-97, 2005.

45. Whittingham M, Palmer S, Macmillan F: Effects of taping on pain and function in patellofemoral pain syndrome: a randomized controlled trial, *J Orthop Sports Phys Ther* 34(19):504, 2004.

46. Wilkerson GB: Biomechanical and neuromuscular effects of ankle taping and bracings, *J Athl Train* 37(4):436, 2002.

47. Williams S: Kinesio taping in treatment and prevention of sports injuries: A meta-analysis of the evidence for its effectiveness, *Sports Medicine*, 42(2):153–64, 2012.

48. Wilson T, Carter N, Thomas G: A multicenter, single-masked study of medial, neutral, and lateral patellar taping in individuals with patellofemoral pain syndrome, *J Orthop Sports Phys Ther* 33(8):437–43, 2003.

49. Worrell T, et al.: Effect of patellar taping and bracing on patellar position as determined by MRI in patients with patellofemoral pain, *J Athl Train* 33(1):16, 1998.

ANNOTATED BIBLIOGRAPHY

Abell, B: Taping and wrapping made simple, Philadelphia, 2009, Lippincott, Williams & Wilkins.

Designed with the beginner or novice in mind, this text introduces essential supplies and terminology and then moves on to the basic foundations in taping and wrapping techniques.

Baxter R, Peck K: *Sports medicine taping techniques, volumes 1 and 2,* Wichita Falls, TX, 2003, Sports Medicine.

A two-volume set of CD-ROM software that presents detailed instruction on taping techniques.

Beam J: *Orthopedic taping, wrapping, bracing and padding,* Philadelphia, 2011, FA Davis.

An all-inclusive examination of taping, wrapping, bracing, and padding techniques for the prevention, treatment, and rehabilitation of common athletic injuries and conditions.

Constantinou M: *Therapeutic taping for musculoskeletal conditions,* Australia, 2010, Elsevier.

An easy-to-follow guide and instructional DVD presenting a wide range of remedial taping techniques

Hewetson T: *An illustrated guide to taping techniques,* Philadelphia, 2009, Elsevier.

This book addresses the two most essential elements of effective taping—recognition of injuries and application of techniques.

Kase K: Clinical therapeutic application of the Kinesio taping method, Albuquerque, 2003, Kinesiotaping Association.

The oringial comprehensive kinesiotaping manual available in the United States.

Keil A: Strap taping for sports and rehabilitation, Champaign, 2011, Human Kinetics.

Presents taping techniques using Leukotape for use on all body areas that help support or control joint mobility and provide greater stability.

Kumbrink B: K Taping: An Illustrated Guide—Basics, Techniques, Indications, New York, 2012, Springer.

Hands-on guidebook features a highly successful therapeutic approach using kinesiotaping to treat orthopedic, traumatological and many other conditions.

MacDonald R: *Taping techniques: principles and practice,* Philadelphia, 2009, Elsevier.

An illustrated guide to taping techniques for those involved in the treatment and rehabilitation of sports injuries and other conditions, such as muscle imbalances, unstable joints, and neural control. Chapters organized by body part give indications and instructions for taping for specific conditions.

Perrin D: *Athletic taping,* Champaign, IL, 2005, Human Kinetics.

A complete book of athletic taping for the practitioner.

Wright K, Whitehill W: *Taping technique-video series,* St. Louis, 1994, McGraw-Hill.

A series of videotapes that consists of five volumes on athletic taping techniques.

PART III

Pathology of Sports Injury

9

Mechanisms and Characteristics of Musculoskeletal and Nerve Trauma

■ Objectives

When you finish this chapter you should be able to

- Analyze the mechanical properties of tissue based on the stress–strain curve model.
- Discuss the five types of tissue loads that can produce stress and strain.
- Examine the anatomical characteristics of the musculotendinous unit, synovial joint, bone, and nerve.

- Evaluate how mechanical loads applied to the musculotendinous unit, synovial joint, bone, and nerve produce injury in these structures.
- Identify and differentiate various injuries to the musculotendinous unit, synovial joint, bone, and nerve tissue.

■ Outline

■ Key Terms

trauma	muscle guarding	diastasis
load	clonic	dislocation
stiffness	tonic	subluxation
stress	muscle soreness	osteoarthritis
strain	tendinitis	bursitis
deformation	tendon	bursae
elasticity	crepitus	osteoblasts
yield point	tendinosis	osteoclasts
plastic	tenosynovitis	closed fracture
creep	contusion	open fracture
mechanical	ecchymosis	neuropraxia
failure	myositis	neuritis
muscle strain	ossificans	referred pain
muscle cramps	synovial joints	

■ Connect Highlights   connect plus+

Visit connect.mcgraw-hill.com for further exercises to apply your knowledge:

- Clinical application scenarios covering the stress–strain curve model, anatomical characteristics, mechanical and tissue loads that produce injury, and identification of various injuries
- Click-and-drag questions covering the stress–strain curve, anatomical characteristics, mechanical and tissue loads, and various injuries sustained
- Multiple-choice questions covering the stress–strain curve, anatomical characteristics, mechanical and tissue loads, and various injuries sustained

The ability to recognize a specific injury to musculoskeletal and nerve structures and understand those mechanical factors that produce injuries or trauma is essential for the athletic trainer.[11] **Trauma** is defined as a physical injury or wound that is produced by an external or internal force.[3] This chapter provides the foundation for the identification, understanding, and management of injuries to be discussed throughout this text. It examines mechanical forces and tissue characteristics of injuries and the classification of these injuries.

| **trauma** A physical injury or wound produced by an external or internal force. |

MECHANICAL INJURY

Newtonian physics maintains that force or mechanical energy is that which changes the state of rest or uniform motion of matter. When a force applied to any part of the body results in a harmful disturbance in function and or structure, a mechanical injury is said to have been sustained.[41] Injuries are caused by external forces directed on the body that result in internal alteration in anatomical structures that are of sufficient magnitude to cause damage or destruction to that tissue.[33] How the various tissues respond to the application of an external load is determined in large part by the mechanical properties of that tissue.

Tissue Properties

Tissue properties are described according to mechanical terminology, and their relative relationships may best be illustrated by the stress–strain curve (Figure 9–1). A **load** is an external force acting on tissues that causes internal reactions within the tissues. **Stiffness** is the relative ability of a tissue to resist a particular load. The greater the stiffness, the greater the magnitude of load it can withstand. The internal resistance of the tissues to an external load is called a **stress,** and the internal **strain** placed on the tissues from that stress results in **deformation** of those tissues. However, human tissue has **elasticity,** a *property* that allows a tissue to return to normal following deformation. When tissue is deformed to the extent that it no longer reacts elastically, the **yield point** has been reached. Beyond the yield point, some deformation persists after the load is removed and this results in permanent or **plastic** changes to the tissues. **Creep** is the deformation in the shape and/or properties of a tissue that occurs with the application of a constant load over time. When the ability of the tissue to withstand stress and strain is exceeded, **mechanical failure** of the tissue ultimately occurs, manifesting itself in injury to that tissue. Depending on the amount of deformation tissues can withstand prior to mechanical failure, they can be classified as being *ductile* or *brittle*. Ductile tissues can deform

load External force or forces acting on internal tissue.

stiffness Ability of a tissue to resist a load.

stress Internal resistance to an external load.

strain Extent of deformation of tissue under loading.

deformation Change in shape of a tissue.

elasticity Property that allows a tissue to return to normal following deformation.

yield point Elastic limit of tissue.

plastic Deformation of tissues that exists after the load is removed.

creep Deformation of tissues that occurs with application of a constant load over time.

mechanical failure Exceeding the ability to withstand stress and strain, causing tissue to break down.

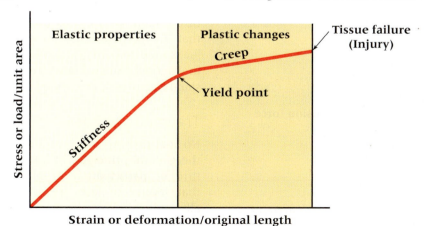

FIGURE 9–1 Stress–strain curve.

significantly before failing and consequently have a longer plastic area. Brittle tissues can deform very little before failure.[29,35]

Tissue Loading

Five types of tissue loading can produce stress and strain: compression, tension, shearing, bending, and torsion.[17]

Compression Compression is produced by external loads applied toward one another on opposite surfaces in opposite directions (Figure 9–2A).

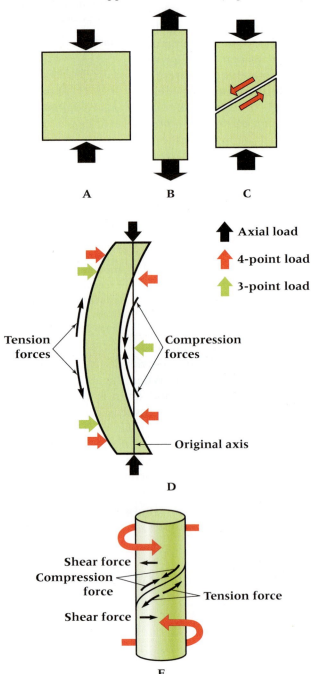

FIGURE 9–2 Types of tissue loading that can cause stress and strain. **(A)** Compression. **(B)** Tension. **(C)** Shearing. **(D)** Bending. **(E)** Torsion.

Compression shortens and widens a structure. When the force can no longer be absorbed by the tissues, injury occurs. Constant compression over a period of time can also cause injury. Arthritic changes in cartilage, fractures, and contusions are commonly caused by compression forces.

Tension Tension is the force that pulls or stretches tissue (Figure 9–2B). Tension is generated in response to equal and opposite external loads that pull a structure apart. The structure elongates and tensile stress and strain result. Muscle strains and ligament sprains both occur due to increased tension.

Shearing Shearing occurs when equal but not directly opposite loads are applied to opposing surfaces, forcing those surfaces to move in parallel directions relative to one another (Figure 9–2C). Injury occurs once shearing has exceeded the inherent strength of a tissue. Shearing stress can result in skin injuries such as blisters or abrasions or in vertebral disk injuries.

Bending Bending can occur in one of the following ways: when two force pairs act at opposite ends of a structure (4-point); when three forces cause bending (3-point); or when an already bowed structure is axially loaded (Figure 9–2D).[41] Regardless of the mechanism, the original axis is maintained while the convex side of the structure is elongated and subject to tension forces and the concave side is shortened and subject to compression forces. Shear forces also occur along the original axis. Bending of the long bones can result in fractures.

> **Tissue stresses:**
> • Compression
> • Tension
> • Shearing
> • Bending
> • Torsion

Torsion Torsion loads caused by twisting in opposite directions from the opposite ends of a structure cause shear stress over the entire cross section of that structure (Figure 9–2E). Maximal shear occurs in planes that are perpendicular and parallel to the applied loads, and maximal tension and compression occur in diagonal planes. Therefore, torsion could result in spiral fractures at an oblique angle in the long bones.

Traumatic versus Overuse Injuries

No matter how much attention is directed toward the general principles of injury prevention, the nature of participation in physical activity dictates that sooner or later injury will occur. Traditionally, injuries have been classified as either acute or chronic.[25] Some health care professionals have argued that these terms are confusing. All injuries

Injury	Classification	Load
Muscle strain	Traumatic	Tension/torsion/shearing
Muscle cramp	Overuse	Tension/compression
Muscle soreness	Overuse	Tension
Tendinitis/tendinosis	Overuse	Tension
Tenosynovitis	Overuse	Tension
Myofascial trigger point	Overuse/traumatic	Tension
Contusion	Traumatic	Compression
Ligament sprain	Traumatic	Tension/torsion/bending
Dislocation/subluxations	Traumatic	Tension/torsion/shearing
Osteoarthritis	Overuse	Compression/shearing/torsion
Bursitis	Overuse/traumatic	Compression/shearing
Capsulitis/synovitis	Overuse	Tension/compression/shearing/torsion
Bone fracture	Traumatic	Tension/compression/shearing/torsion/bending
Stress fracture	Overuse	Tension/compression/shearing/torsion/bending
Epiphyseal injury	Traumatic/overuse	Tension/compression/shearing/torsion/bending
Apophyseal injury	Traumatic/overuse	Tension/compression/shearing/torsion/bending
Neuropraxia	Traumatic	Compression/shearing
Neuritis	Overuse	Compression/tension/shearing

are acute—something initiates the injury process.[25] If the acute injury doesn't heal properly, at some point it becomes chronic. Exactly when that transition occurs is debatable. Debating how to define these terms precisely serves no useful purpose. It is perhaps less confusing to classify injuries according to the primary mechanism that causes an injury or condition. Generally, injuries are caused either by trauma or by overuse. Trauma was defined at the beginning of this chapter. Injuries that result from overuse can be either chronic, which occur with the repetitive dynamics of running, throwing, or jumping, or recurrent, which are traumatic injuries that occur multiple times.[25] Table 9–1 summarizes the general injury classifications and the types of tissue loading that produce injury for the more common injuries that the athletic trainer is likely to see.

MUSCULOTENDINOUS UNIT INJURIES

Anatomical Characteristics

The musculotendinous unit consists of the muscle, the tendon, and the fascia that surrounds the muscle. Muscles are composed of contractile cells, or fibers, that produce movement. Muscle fibers possess the ability to contract as well as the properties of irritability, conductivity, and elasticity. There are three types of muscles in the body—smooth, cardiac, and striated. Of primary concern for athletic trainers are conditions that affect striated, or skeletal, muscles. Within the muscle fiber cell is a semifluid substance called sarcoplasm (cytoplasm). Myofibrils

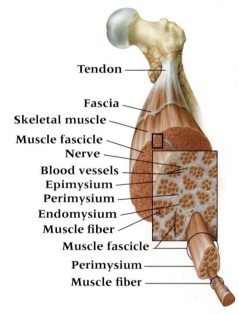

FIGURE 9–3   Connective tissue associated with skeletal muscle.

are surrounded by the endomysium, fiber bundles are surrounded by the perimysium, and the entire muscle is covered by the epimysium (Figure 9–3). The epimysium, perimysium, and endomysium may be combined with the fibrous tendon. The fibrous wrapping of a muscle may become a flat sheet of connective tissue (aponeurosis) that attaches to other muscles. Tendons and aponeuroses are extremely resilient to injuries. Occasionally, they will pull away from a bone, a bone will fracture, or a muscle will tear before tendons and aponeuroses are injured. Skeletal muscles are generally well vascularized. Arteries, veins, lymph vessels, and bundles of nerve fibers spread into the perimysium. A complex capillary network goes throughout the endomysium, coming into direct contact with the muscle fibers.[37]

Muscle Strains

The muscle is composed of separate fibers that are capable of simultaneous contraction when stimulated by the central nervous system. Each muscle is attached to bone at both ends by strong, relatively inelastic tendons that cross over joints.

If a muscle is overstretched by tension or forced to contract against too much resistance, separation or tearing of the muscle fibers occurs. This damage is referred to as a **muscle strain** (Figure 9–4).[1] Muscle strains, like ligament sprains, are subject to various classification systems. The following is a simple system of strain classification:

muscle strain A stretch, tear, or rip in the muscle or its tendon.

- *Grade 1 strain.* Some muscle fibers have been stretched or actually torn. There is some tenderness and pain on active motion. Movement is painful, but full range of motion is usually possible.
- *Grade 2 strain.* A number of muscle fibers have been torn, and active contraction of the muscle is extremely painful. Usually, a depression, or divot, can be felt somewhere in the muscle belly at the place at which the muscle fibers have been torn. Some swelling may occur because of capillary bleeding; therefore, some discoloration is possible, although it does not occur immediately. Range of motion is decreased due to pain.
- *Grade 3 strain.* A complete rupture of a muscle has occurred in the area of the muscle belly at the point

at which muscle becomes tendon or at the tendinous attachment to the bone. There is significant impairment to or perhaps total loss of movement. Initially, pain is intense but quickly diminishes because of complete nerve fiber separation.

Muscle strains can occur in any muscle and usually result from some uncoordinated activity between muscle groups.[1] Grade 3 strains are most common in the biceps tendon of the upper arm and in the Achilles heel cord in the back of the calf. When either of these tendons tears, the muscle tends to bunch toward its attachment at the bone site. Grade 3 strains involving large tendons that produce great amounts of force must be surgically repaired. Smaller musculotendinous ruptures, such as those that occur in the fingers, may heal by immobilization with a splint.

Regardless of the severity of the strain, the time required for rehabilitation is lengthy.[5] In many instances, muscle strains are incapacitating, making rehabilitation time for a muscle strain even longer than for a ligament sprain. Incapacitating muscle strains occur most frequently in the large, force-producing hamstring and quadriceps muscles of the lower extremity. The treatment of hamstring strains requires a healing period of 6 to 8 weeks and a considerable amount of patience. Trying to return to activity too soon often causes reinjury to the area of the muscle that has been strained, and the healing process must begin again.

Muscle Cramps

Muscle cramps are extremely painful involuntary muscle contractions that occur most commonly in the calf, abdomen, or hamstrings, although any muscle can be involved.[14] The occurrence of heat cramps is related to excessive loss of water and, to some extent, several electrolytes or ions (sodium, chloride, potassium, magnesium, and calcium) that are essential elements in muscle contraction (see Chapter 6).[31,39]

muscle cramps Involuntary muscle contractions.

Muscle Guarding

Following injury, the muscles that surround the injured area contract to, in effect, splint that area, thus minimizing pain by limiting movement. Quite often this "splinting" is incorrectly referred to as a muscle spasm. The terms *spasm* and *spasticity* are more correctly associated with increased tone or contractions of muscle that occur because of some upper motor neuron lesion in the brain. Thus, **muscle guarding** is a more appropriate term for the involuntary muscle contractions that occur in response to pain following musculoskeletal injury.[28]

muscle guarding Muscle contraction in response to pain.

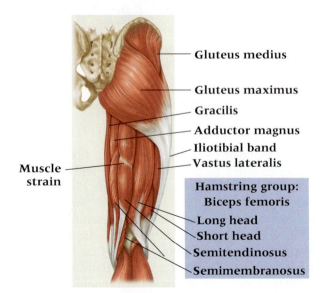

Gluteus medius
Gluteus maximus
Gracilis
Adductor magnus
Iliotibial band
Vastus lateralis
Muscle strain
Hamstring group:
Biceps femoris
Long head
Short head
Semitendinosus
Semimembranosus

FIGURE 9–4 A muscle strain results in tearing or separation of fibers.

Muscle Spasms

A spasm is a reflex reaction caused by trauma to the musculoskeletal system. The two types of spasms are the **clonic** type, with alternating involuntary muscular contraction and relaxation in quick succession, and the **tonic** type, with rigid muscle contraction that lasts a period of time. Muscle spasms may lead to a muscle strain.[10]

clonic Involuntary muscle contraction characterized by alternate contraction and relaxation in rapid succession.

tonic Type of muscle contraction characterized by constant contraction that lasts for a period of time.

Muscle Soreness

Overexertion in strenuous muscular exercise often results in muscular pain. All active people at one time or another have experienced **muscle soreness,** usually resulting from some physical activity to which they are unaccustomed. The older a person gets, the more easily muscle soreness seems to develop.

muscle soreness Pain caused by overexertion in exercise.

There are two types of muscle soreness. The first type of muscle pain is *acute-onset muscle soreness,* which accompanies fatigue. It is transient and occurs during and immediately after exercise. The second type of soreness involves delayed muscle pain that appears approximately 12 hours after injury. This *delayed-onset muscle soreness (DOMS)* becomes most intense after twenty-four to 48 hours and then gradually subsides, so that the muscle becomes symptom free after 3 or 4 days.[8] DOMS is described as a syndrome of delayed muscle pain leading to increased muscle tension, swelling, and stiffness and to resistance to stretching.[9]

DOMS has several possible causes. It may occur from very small tears in the muscle tissue, which seems to be more likely with eccentric or isometric contractions. It may also occur because of disruption of the connective tissue that holds muscle tendon fibers together.[8]

Muscle soreness may be prevented by beginning exercise at a moderate level and gradually progressing the intensity of the exercise over time. Treatment of muscle soreness usually also involves static or PNF stretching activity.

> The two major types of muscle soreness associated with severe exercise are acute- and delayed-onset muscle soreness (DOMS).

Tendon Injuries

The tendon contains wavy, parallel, collagenous fibers that are organized in bundles surrounded by a gelatinous material that decreases friction. A tendon attaches a muscle to a bone and concentrates a pulling force in a limited area. Tendons can produce and maintain a pull from 8,700 to 18,000 pounds per square inch.[40] When a tendon is loaded by tension, the wavy, collagenous fibers straighten in the direction of the load; when the tension is released, the collagen returns to its original shape. In tendons, collagen fibers will break if their physiological limits have been reached. A breaking point occurs after a 6 percent to 8 percent increase in length.[32] Because a tendon is usually double the strength of the muscle it serves, tears commonly occur at the muscle belly, musculotendinous junction, or bony attachment.[6] Clinically, however, a constant abnormal tension on tendons increases elongation by the infiltration of fibroblasts, which will cause more collagenous tissue to be produced. Repeated microtraumas can evolve into chronic muscle strain that resorbs collagen fibers and eventually weakens the tendon.[40] Collagen resorption occurs in the period of immobilization of a part. During resorption, collagenous tissues are weakened and susceptible to injury; therefore, a gradually paced conditioning program and early mobilization in the rehabilitation process are necessary.

Tendinitis/Tendinosis/Tendinopathy

Of all the overuse problems associated with activity, chronic overuse injuries involving a tendon are the most common.[42] Any term ending in the suffix *-itis* means inflammation is present. Tendinitis means inflammation of a **tendon.** During muscle activity, a tendon must move or slide on other structures around it whenever the muscle contracts. If a particular movement is performed repeatedly, the tendon becomes irritated and inflamed.[32] This inflammation is manifested by pain on movement, swelling, possibly some warmth, and usually crepitus. **Crepitus** is a crackling feeling or sound. It is usually caused by the tendon's tendency to stick to the surrounding structure while it slides back and forth. This sticking is caused primarily by the chemical products of inflammation that accumulate on the irritated tendon.

tendinitis Inflammation of a tendon.

tendon Tough band of connective tissue that attaches muscle to bone.

crepitus A crackling feel or sound.

The key to the treatment of tendinitis is rest.[40] If the repetitive motion causing irritation to the

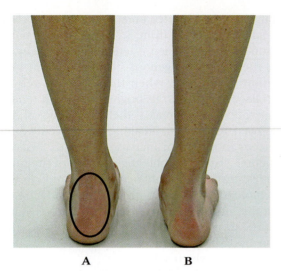

FIGURE 9–5   Tendinitis is an inflammation of the tendon. **(A)** Inflamed. **(B)** Normal.

tendon is eliminated, the inflammatory process will allow the tendon to heal. Unfortunately, athletes find it difficult to totally stop activity and rest for 2 or more weeks while the tendinitis subsides. The patient should substitute some form of activity, such as bicycling or swimming, to maintain present fitness levels while avoiding continued irritation of the inflamed tendon. In runners, tendinitis most commonly occurs in the Achilles tendon in the back of the lower leg (Figure 9–5). In swimmers, it often occurs in the muscle tendons of the shoulder joint. However, tendinitis can flare up in any activity in which overuse and repetitive movements occur.

> **The suffix *-itis* means inflammation of.**

If repetitive overuse continues and the inflamed or irritated tendon fails to heal, the tendon begins to degenerate. The primary concern shifts from tendon inflammation to tendon degeneration, a condition referred to as **tendinosis**.[32] The suffix *osis* means there is chronic degeneration without inflammation. *Most of the chronic problems that we have with tendons are correctly referred to as tendinosis.* The symptoms are somewhat similar to tendinitis. The inflammation ceases, however. The affected tendons are usually painful when moved

> **tendinosis** Breakdown of a tendon without inflammation.

or touched. The tendon sheaths may be visibly swollen with stiffness and restricted motion. Sometimes a tender lump appears. Tendinosis is more common in middle or old age as the tendons become more susceptible to injury. However, younger people who exercise vigorously as well as people who perform repetitive tasks are also susceptible. The key to treating tendinosis is engaging in exercises to strengthen the tendon and consistently stretching the tendon. *Tendinopathy* is the least often used term. The suffix *opathy* does not imply any specific type of pathology. Thus, *tendinopathy* is a more general term that refers to either tendinitis or tendinosis.

Tenosynovitis

Tenosynovitis is very similar to tendinitis in that the muscle tendons are involved in

> **tenosynovitis**
> Inflammation of a tendon and its synovial sheath.

inflammation. However, many tendons are subject to an increased amount of friction because of the tightness of the space through which they must move. In these areas of high friction, tendons are usually surrounded by synovial sheaths that reduce friction on movement. If the tendon sliding through a synovial sheath is subjected to overuse, inflammation is likely to occur. As with tendinitis, the inflammatory process produces by-products that are "sticky" and tend to cause the sliding tendon to adhere to the synovial sheath surrounding it.[4]

Tenosynovitis occurs most commonly in the long flexor tendons of the fingers as they cross over the wrist joint and in the biceps tendon around the shoulder joint. Treatment for tenosynovitis is the same as for tendinitis. Because both conditions involve inflammation, antiinflammatory drugs may be helpful in chronic cases.[4]

Myofascial Trigger Points

A *myofascial trigger point* is a discreet, hypersensitive nodule within a taut band of skeletal muscle and/or fascia.[26] Palpation of this nodule reveals an area of harder-than-normal consistency. Trigger points are classified as being latent or active, depending on their clinical characteristics. A *latent trigger point* does not cause spontaneous pain but may restrict movement or cause muscle weakness. The individual presenting with muscle restrictions or weakness may become aware of pain originating from a latent trigger point only when pressure is applied directly over the point. An *active trigger point* causes pain at rest. Firm pressure applied over the point usually elicits a "jump sign," with the patient crying out, wincing, or withdrawing from the stimulus. It is tender to palpation with a referred pain pattern that is similar to the patient's pain complaint. This referred pain is not felt at the site of the trigger point origin but rather at a remote point. The pain is often described as spreading or radiating. Referred pain is an important characteristic of a trigger point. It differentiates a trigger point from a tender point, which is associated with pain at the site of palpation only. Trigger points are palpable within muscles as cordlike bands within a sharply circumscribed area of extreme tenderness. They are found most commonly in the muscles involved in postural support.[24] Acute trauma or repetitive microtrauma may lead to the development of stress on muscle fibers and the formation of trigger points.

Contusions

A **contusion** is another word for a bruise. The mechanism that produces a contusion is familiar. A blow from some external object causes soft tissues (e.g., muscle, tendon, skin, fat) to be compressed against hard bone underneath (Figure 9–6). If the blow is hard enough, capillaries are torn, which allows bleeding into the tissues. Minor bleeding often causes **ecchymosis,** a bluish-purple discoloration of the skin that persists for several days. The contusion may be very sore to the touch, and, if damage has occurred to muscle, pain may be experienced on active movement. In most cases the pain ceases within a few days and discoloration usually disappears in a few weeks.[16]

> **contusion**
> Compression of soft tissue that results in bleeding into surrounding tissues.

> **ecchymosis** Bluish-purple discoloration of the skin.

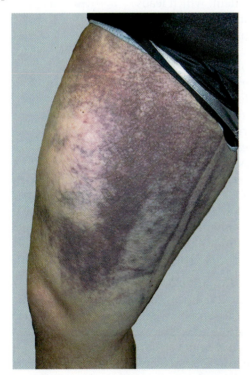

FIGURE 9–6 A contusion occurs when soft tissues are compressed between bone and some external force.

The major problem with contusions occurs in an area that is subjected to repeated blows. If the same area—or, more specifically, a muscle—is bruised over and over again, small calcium deposits may begin to accumulate in the injured area. These pieces of calcium may be found between several fibers in the muscle belly, or calcium may build up to form a spur, which projects from the underlying bone. These calcium formations may significantly impair movement and are referred to as **myositis ossificans.**[1]

> **myositis ossificans**
> Calcium deposits that result from repeated trauma.

The key to preventing the occurrence of myositis ossificans from repeated contusions is to protect the injured area with padding. If the area is properly protected after the first contusion, myositis may never develop. Protection and rest may allow the calcium to be reabsorbed, eliminating any need for surgery.

The two areas that seem to be the most vulnerable to repeated contusions during physical activity are the quadriceps muscle group on the front of the thigh and the biceps muscle on the front of the upper arm. The formation of myositis ossificans in these or any other areas may be detected by X-rays.

Atrophy and Contracture

Two complications of muscle and tendon conditions are atrophy and contracture. Muscle atrophy is the wasting away of muscle tissue. Its main causes are immobilization of a body part, inactivity, and loss of nerve innervation. A second complication is muscle contracture, an abnormal shortening of muscle tissue in which there is a great deal of resistance to passive stretch. A contracture is associated with a joint that, because of muscle injury, has developed unyielding and resisting scar tissue.

SYNOVIAL JOINT INJURIES

Anatomical Characteristics

Most of the joints in the body are **synovial joints** (Figure 9–7). All synovial joints are composed of two or more bones that articulate with one another to allow motion in one or more places.[37] The articulating surfaces of the bone are lined with a very thin, smooth, cartilaginous

> **synovial joints**
> Articulations of two bones surrounded by a joint capsule lined with synovial membrane.

A football player who plays wide receiver sustains repeated blows to his left quadriceps muscle.

? What type of injury could be sustained from repeated compressive forces to the quadriceps muscle?

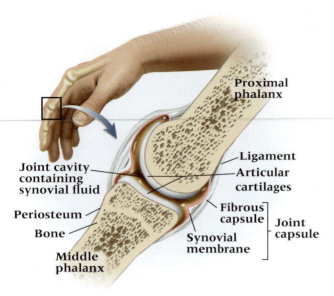

FIGURE 9–7   General anatomy of a synovial joint.

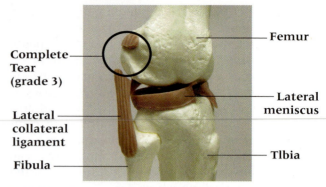

FIGURE 9–8   Grade 3 ligament sprain in the knee joint.

covering called *hyaline,* or *articular,* cartilage. All joints are entirely surrounded by a thick, ligamentous *joint capsule.* The inner surface of this joint capsule is lined by a very thin *synovial membrane* that is highly vascularized and innervated. The synovial membrane produces *synovial fluid,* which provides lubrication, shock absorption, and nutrition of the joint. The articular capsule, ligaments, outer aspects of the synovial membrane, and fat pads of the synovial joint are well supplied with nerves. The inner aspect of the synovial membrane, cartilage, and articular disks (menisci), if present, have nerves as well. These nerves, called *mechanoreceptors,* provide information about the relative position of the joint and are found in the fibrous capsule and ligaments.

Some joints contain a thick *fibrocartilage* called a meniscus. The knee joint, for example, contains two wedge-shaped *menisci* that deepen the articulation and provide shock absorption in that joint. Finally, the main structural support and joint stability are provided by the *ligaments,* which may be either thickened portions of a joint capsule or totally separate bands. Ligaments are composed of dense connective tissue arranged in parallel bundles of collagen composed of rows of fibroblasts. Although bundles are arranged in parallel, not all collagen fibers are arranged in parallel. Ligaments and tendons are very similar in structure. However, ligaments are usually more flattened than tendons, and collagen fibers in ligaments are more compact. The anatomical positioning of the ligaments determines in part what motions a joint can make.[37]

Ligament Sprains

If stress is applied to a joint that forces motion beyond its normal limits or planes of movement, injury to the ligament is likely (Figure 9–8). The severity of damage to the ligament is classified in many different ways; however, the most commonly used system involves three grades (degrees) of ligament sprain:

- *Grade 1 sprain.* There is some stretching and separation of the ligament fibers, with minimal instability of the joint. Mild to moderate pain, localized swelling, and joint stiffness should be expected.
- *Grade 2 sprain.* There is some tearing and separation of the ligament fibers, with moderate instability of the joint. Moderate to severe pain, swelling, and joint stiffness should be expected.
- *Grade 3 sprain.* There is total tearing of the ligament, which leads to instability of the joint. A grade 3 sprain can result in a subluxation. Initially, severe pain may be present, followed by little or no pain as a result of total disruption of nerve fibers. Swelling may be great, and the joint tends to become very stiff some hours after the injury. In some cases, a grade 3 sprain with marked instability requires surgical repair. Frequently, the force producing the ligament injury is so great that other ligaments or structures surrounding the joint may also be injured. Rehabilitation of grade 3 sprains involving surgery is a long-term process.

Effusion of blood and synovial fluid into the joint cavity during a sprain produces joint swelling, local temperature increase, pain or point tenderness, and skin discoloration (ecchymosis). Ligaments and capsules, like tendons, can experience forces that completely rupture or produce an avulsion fracture. Ligaments and capsules heal slowly because of a relatively poor blood supply;

however, their nerves are plentiful, often producing a great deal of pain when injured.[7]

The greatest problem in the rehabilitation of grade 1 and grade 2 sprains is restoring stability to the joint.[13] Once a ligament has been stretched or partially torn, inelastic scar tissue forms, preventing the ligament from regaining its original tension. To restore stability to the joint, the other structures surrounding that joint, primarily muscles and their tendons, must be strengthened. The increased muscle tension provided by strength training can improve stability of the injured joint.

Dislocations and Subluxations

Dislocations and subluxations both result in **diastasis,** or separation of two articulating bones.

> **diastasis** Separation of articulating bones.
>
> **dislocation** A bone is forced out of alignment and stays out until surgically or manually replaced or reduced.
>
> **subluxation** A bone is forced out of alignment but goes back into place.

A **dislocation** occurs when at least one bone in a joint (articulation) is forced completely out of its normal and proper alignment and must be manually or surgically put back into place or reduced. Dislocations most commonly occur in the shoulder joint, elbow, and fingers, but they can occur wherever two bones articulate (Figure 9–9A). A **subluxation** is like a dislocation except that a bone comes partially out of its normal articulation but then goes right back into place.[1] Subluxations most commonly occur in the shoulder joint and, in females, in the knee cap (patella) (Figure 9–9B).

In dislocations, deformity is almost always apparent; however, it may be obscured by heavy musculature, making it important for the examiner to routinely palpate, or feel, the injured site to determine the loss of normal contour. Comparison of the injured side with the uninjured side often reveals asymmetry.

Dislocations or subluxations will likely result in a rupture of the stabilizing ligaments and tendons surrounding the joint. Occasionally, an avulsion fracture occurs, in which an attached tendon or ligament pulls a small piece of bone away from the rest of the bone. In other cases, the force may separate growth plates (epiphysis) or cause a complete fracture of a long bone. These possibilities indicate the importance of administering complete and thorough medical attention to first-time dislocations. It has often been said, "Once a dislocation, always a dislocation." In most cases this statement is true because, once a joint has been either subluxated or completely dislocated, the connective tissues that bind and hold it in its correct alignment are stretched to such an extent that the joint is extremely vulnerable to subsequent dislocations.

A first-time dislocation should always be considered and treated as a possible fracture. Once it has been ascertained that the injury is a dislocation, a physician should be consulted for further evaluation. However, before the patient is taken to the physician, the injury should be properly splinted and supported to prevent any further damage. **Dislocations should not be reduced immediately, regardless of where they occur.**[1] The athlete should get an X-ray to rule out fractures or other problems before reduction. Inappropriate techniques of reduction may only exacerbate the problem. Return to activity after dislocation or subluxation is largely dependent on the degree of soft-tissue damage.

Osteoarthritis

Any mechanical system wears out with time. The joints in the body are mechanical systems, and wear and tear, even from normal activity, is inevitable.[23] The most common result of this wear and tear, a degeneration of the articular, or hyaline, cartilage, is referred to as **osteoarthritis.**[43] The cartilage may be worn away to the point of exposing, eroding, and polishing the underlying bone (Figure 9–10).

> **osteoarthritis** A wearing down of hyaline cartilage.

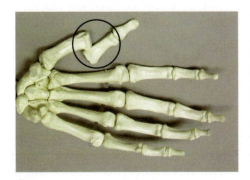
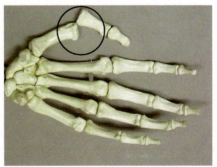

A   B

FIGURE 9–9   A joint that is forced beyond its anatomical limits can become **(A)** completely dislocated or luxated or **(B)** subluxated.

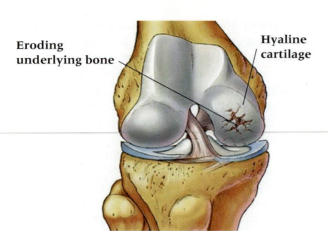

Eroding underlying bone

Hyaline cartilage

FIGURE 9–10 Osteoarthrities involves a degeneration of hyaline cartilage, exposing underlying bone.

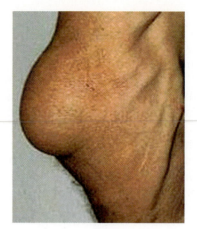

FIGURE 9–11 Elbow bursitis.

Any process that changes the mechanics of the joint eventually leads to degeneration of that joint. Degeneration is a result of repeated trauma to the joint and to the tendons, ligaments, and fasciae surrounding the joint. Such injuries may be caused by a direct blow or fall, by the pressure of carrying or lifting heavy loads, or by repeated trauma to the joint, as in running or cycling.[27]

Osteoarthritis most often affects the weight-bearing joints: the knees, hips, and lumbar spine. Also affected are the shoulders and cervical spine. Although many other joints may show pathological degenerative change, clinically the disease only occasionally produces symptoms in them. Any joint that is subjected to acute or chronic trauma may develop osteoarthritis.[42]

The symptoms of osteoarthritis are relatively local in character. Osteoarthritis may be localized to one side of the joint or may be generalized about the joint. One of the most distinctive symptoms is pain, which is brought about by friction that occurs with use and which is relieved by rest. Stiffness is a common complaint that occurs with rest and is quickly loosened with activity. This symptom is prominent upon rising in the morning. Joints may also show localized tenderness, creaking, or grating that may be heard and felt.[27] Clinical studies indicate that glucosamine sulfate is a safe and relatively effective treatment for osteoarthritis. However, no evidence to date supports or refutes a carryover effect to the athletic population and the injuries that occur in sport.[23,43]

Bursitis

Bursitis most often occurs around joints, where there is friction between tendon and bone, skin and bone, or muscle and other muscles. Without some

bursitis Inflammation of bursae at sites of bony prominences between muscle and tendon.

mechanism of protection in these high-friction areas, chronic irritation would exist (Figure 9–11).[24]

Bursae are pieces of synovial membrane that contain a small amount of fluid (synovial fluid).[37] Just as oil

bursae Pieces of synovial membrane that contain a small amount of fluid.

lubricates a hinge, these small pieces of synovium permit motion of these structures without friction.

If excessive movement or perhaps some acute trauma occurs around the bursae, they become irritated and inflamed and begin producing large amounts of synovial fluid.[30] The longer the irritation continues or the more severe the acute trauma, the more fluid is produced. As fluid continues to accumulate in the limited space available, pressure increases, causing pain in the area. Bursitis can be an extremely painful condition that may severely restrict movement, especially if it occurs around a joint. Synovial fluid continues to be produced until the movement or trauma producing the irritation is eliminated.

Occasionally, a bursa or synovial sheath completely surrounds a tendon, allowing more freedom of movement in a tight area. Irritation of this synovial sheath may restrict tendon motion. All joints are surrounded by many bursae. The three bursae that are most commonly irritated as a result of various types of physical activity are the subacromial bursa in the shoulder joint under the distal clavicle and acromion process; the olecranon bursa on the tip of the elbow; and the prepatellar bursa on the front surface of the patella. All three of these bursae produce large amounts of synovial fluid, affecting motion at their respective joints.

Capsulitis and Synovitis

After repeated joint sprains or microtraumas, a chronic inflammatory condition called capsulitis may occur.[30] Usually associated with capsulitis is synovitis. Synovitis also occurs acutely, but a chronic condition can arise with repeated joint injury or with joint injury that is improperly managed. Chronic synovitis involves active joint congestion with edema. As

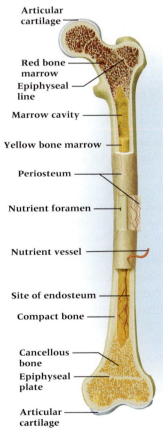

with the synovial lining of the bursa, the synovium of a joint can undergo degenerative tissue changes. The synovium becomes irregularly thickened, exudation occurs, and a fibrous underlying tissue is present. Several movements may be restricted, and there may be joint noises, such as grinding or creaking.

BONE INJURIES

Anatomical Characteristics

Bone is a specialized type of dense connective tissue consisting of bone cells (osteocytes) that are fixed in a matrix, which consists of an intercellular material. The outer surface of a bone is composed of compact tissue, and the inner aspect is composed of a more porous tissue known as *cancellous bone*, also called *trabecular* or *spongy* bone (Figure 9–12). Compact tissue is tunneled by a marrow cavity.

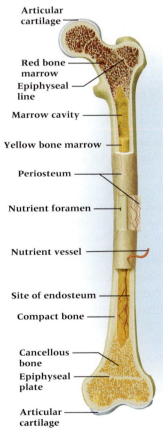

- Articular cartilage
- Red bone marrow
- Epiphyseal line
- Marrow cavity
- Yellow bone marrow
- Periosteum
- Nutrient foramen
- Nutrient vessel
- Site of endosteum
- Compact bone
- Cancellous bone
- Epiphyseal plate
- Articular cartilage

FIGURE 9–12 Anatomical characteristics of bone (longitudinal section).

Throughout the bone run countless branching canals (haversian canals), which contain blood vessels and lymphatic vessels. On the outside of a bone is a tissue covering, the *periosteum*, which contains the blood supply to the bone.[37]

Bones perform five basic functions: body support, organ protection, movement (through joints and levers), calcium storage, and formation of blood cells (hematopoiesis).

Bones are classified according to their shapes. Classifications include bones that are flat, irregular, short, and long. Flat bones are in the skull, the ribs, and the scapulae; irregular bones are in the vertebral column and the skull. Short bones are primarily in the wrist and the ankle. Long bones consist of the humerus, ulna, femur, tibia, fibula, and phalanges.

Flat, irregular, and short bones have the same inner cancellous bone with an overlying layer of compact bone. A few irregular and flat bones (e.g., the vertebrae and the sternum) have some space in the cancellous bone that is filled with red marrow and sesamoid bones.

The gross structures of bone include the diaphysis, epiphysis, articular cartilage, periosteum, medullary (marrow) cavity, and endosteum. The diaphysis is the main shaft of the long bone. It is hollow and cylindrical and is covered by compact bone. The epiphysis is located at the ends of long bones. It is bulbous in shape, providing space for the muscle attachments. The epiphysis is composed primarily of cancellous bone, giving it a spongelike appearance. As discussed previously, the ends of long bones have a layer of hyaline cartilage that covers the joint surfaces of the epiphysis. This cartilage provides protection during movement and cushions jars and blows to the joint. A dense, white, fibrous membrane, the periosteum, covers long bones except at joint surfaces. Many fibers, called Sharpey's fibers, emanate from the periosteum and penetrate the underlying bone. Interlacing with the periosteum are fibers from the muscle tendons. Throughout the periosteum on its inner layer exist countless blood vessels and osteoblasts (bone-forming cells). The blood vessels provide nutrition to the bone, and the osteoblasts provide bone growth and repair. The medullary cavity, a hollow tube in the long bone diaphysis, contains a yellow, fatty marrow in adults. Lining the medullary cavity is the endosteum.[37]

Bone Growth Bone ossification occurs from the synthesis of bone's organic matrix by osteoblasts, followed immediately by the calcification of this matrix.

The epiphyseal growth plate is a cartilaginous disk located near the end of each long bone. The growth of the long bones depends on these plates. Ossification in long bones begins in the diaphysis and in both epiphyses. It proceeds from the diaphysis toward each epiphysis and from each epiphysis toward the diaphysis. The growth plate has layers of cartilage cells in different stages of maturity, with immature cells at one end and mature ones at the other end. As the cartilage cells mature, immature osteoblasts replace them later to produce solid bone.

Epiphyseal growth plates are often less resistant to deforming forces than are ligaments of nearby joints or the outer shaft of the long bones; therefore, severe twisting or a blow to an arm or a leg can result in growth disruption. Injury can prematurely close the growth plate, causing a loss of length in the bone. Growth plate dislocation can also cause deformity of the long bone.[20]

Bone diameter may increase as a result of the combined action of **osteoblasts** and **osteoclasts.** Osteoblasts build new bone on the outside of the

osteoblasts
Bone-producing cells.

osteoclasts
Bone-remodeling cells.

bone; at the same time, osteoclasts increase the medullary cavity by breaking down bony tissue. Once a bone has reached its full size, there occurs a balance of bone formation and bone destruction, or osteogenesis and resorption, respectively. This process of balance may be disrupted by factors in sports conditioning or participation. These factors may cause greater osteogenesis than resorption. Conversely, resorption may exceed osteogenesis in situations in which the patient is out of shape but overtrains. On the other hand, women whose estrogen is decreased as a result of training may experience bone loss (see Chapter 29).[32] In general, bone loss begins to exceed bone gain by age thirty-five to forty. Gradually, bone is lost in the endosteal surfaces and then is gained on the outer surfaces. As the thickness of long bones decreases, they are less able to resist the forces of compression. This process also leads to increased bone porosity, known as osteoporosis.

Like other structures in the human body, bones are morphologically, biochemically, and biomechanically sensitive to both stress and stress deprivation. Therefore, bone's functional adaptation follows Wolff's law;[44] that is, every change in the form and function of a bone, or in its function alone, is followed by certain definite changes in its internal architecture.

Bone Fractures

Fractures generally can be classified as either closed or open. A **closed fracture** is one in which there is little or no movement or displacement of the broken bones. Conversely, in an **open fracture** (Figure 9–13) there is enough displacement of the fractured ends that the bone actually breaks

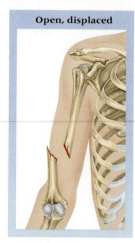

Open, displaced

FIGURE 9–13 In an open, displaced fracture, the end of the bone penetrates through the soft tissue creating an open wound.

through surrounding tissues, including the skin (Figure 9–13). An open fracture increases the possibility of infection. Both types of fracture can be serious if not managed properly.[19] Signs and symptoms of a fracture include obvious deformity, point tenderness, swelling, and pain on active and passive movement. There may also be crepitus (popping or a grating sound on movement). The only definitive technique for determining if a fracture exists is to have it X-rayed.

closed fracture
Fracture does not penetrate superficial tissue.

open fracture
Overlying skin is lacerated by protruding bone fragments.

General Fracture Classifications

Fractures can result from direct trauma; in other words, the bone breaks directly at the site where a force is applied. A fracture that occurs some distance from where force is applied is called an indirect fracture. A sudden, violent muscle contraction or repetitive abnormal stress to a bone can also cause a fracture. The most common bone fractures can be classified as follows (Figure 9–14):[18]

Greenstick fracture. Greenstick fractures are incomplete breaks in bones that have not completely ossified, such as the bones of adolescents. This injury occurs most frequently in the convex bone surface, while the concave surface remains intact. The name is derived from the similarity of the fracture to the break in a green twig taken from a tree.

Comminuted fracture. Comminuted fractures consist of three or more fragments at the fracture site. This injury could be caused by a hard blow or a fall in an awkward position. These fractures

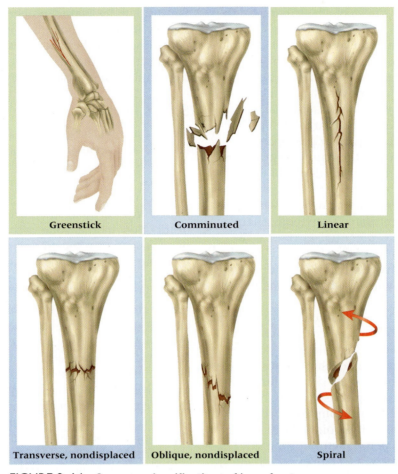

FIGURE 9–14 Common classifications of bone fractures.

9–7 Clinical Application Exercise

An alpine skier catches his right ski tip and severely twists his lower leg.

❓ What type of serious injury could be created by this mechanism?

impose a difficult healing situation because of the displacement of the bone fragments. Soft tissues are often interposed between the fragments, causing incomplete healing. Such cases may need surgical intervention.

Linear fracture. Linear fractures are those in which the bone splits along its length. They are often the result of jumping from a height and landing in such a way as to impart force or stress to the long axis.

Transverse fracture. Transverse fractures occur in a straight line, more or less at right angles to the bone shaft. A direct outside blow usually causes this injury.

Oblique fracture. Oblique fractures are similar to spiral fractures. Oblique fractures occur when one end of the bone receives sudden torsion or twisting while the other end is fixed.

Spiral fracture. Spiral fractures have an S-shaped separation. They are common in football and skiing, sports in which the foot is firmly planted when the body is suddenly rotated in an opposing direction.

Specific Fracture Types

Impacted fracture. Impacted fractures can result from a fall from a height, which causes a long bone to receive, directly on its long axis, a force of such magnitude that the osseous tissue is compressed. This stress telescopes one part of the bone on the other. Impacted fractures require immediate splinting by the athletic trainer and traction by the physician to ensure a normal length of the injured limb.

Other, less common fractures include the following:

Avulsion fracture. An avulsion fracture is the separation of a bone fragment from its cortex at an attachment of a ligament or tendon. This fracture usually occurs as a result of a sudden, powerful twist or stretch of a body part. A ligamentous avulsion can occur, for example, when a sudden eversion of the foot causes the deltoid ligament to avulse bone away from the medial malleolus. A tendinous avulsion can occur when an athlete falls forward while suddenly bending a knee, which causes a patellar fracture. The stretch of the patellar tendon pulls a portion of the inferior patellar pole apart.

Blowout fracture. Blowout fractures occur to the wall of the eye orbit as a result of a blow to the eye.

Serrated fracture. Serrated fractures, in which the two bony fragments have a sawtooth, sharp-edged fracture line, are usually caused by a direct blow. Because of the sharp and jagged bone edges, extensive internal damage, such as the severance of vital blood vessels and nerves, often occurs.

Depressed fracture. Depressed fractures occur most often in flat bones, such as those found in the skull. They are caused by falling and striking the head on a hard, immovable surface or by being hit with a hard object. Such injuries also result in gross pathology of soft areas.

Contrecoup fracture. Contrecoup fractures occur on the side opposite the point at which trauma was initiated. Fracture of the skull is, at times, a contrecoup fracture. An athlete may be hit on one side of the head with such force that the brain and internal structures compress against the opposite side of the skull, causing a fracture.

Many factors of bone structure affect its strength.[18] Anatomical strength or weakness can be affected by a bone's shape and its changes in shape or direction. Stress forces become concentrated at points at which a long bone suddenly changes shape and direction. Long bones that change shape gradually are less prone to injury than are those that change suddenly. The clavicle, for example, is prone to fracture because it changes from round to flat at the same point at which it changes direction. A hollow cylinder is one of the strongest structures for resisting both bending and torsion, stronger than a solid rod, which has much less resistance to such forces.[18] This may be why bones such as the tibia are primarily cylinders. Most spiral fractures of the tibia occur at its middle and distal third, where the bone is most solid.

Long bones can be stressed or forced to fail by compression, tension, bending, torsion, and shearing.[18] These forces, either singly or in combination, can cause a variety of fractures. For example, spiral fractures are caused by torsion, whereas oblique fractures are caused by the combined forces of axial compression, bending, and torsion. Transverse fractures occur because of bending (Figure 9–14).

Because of its elastic properties, bone will bend slightly. However, bone is generally brittle and is a poor shock absorber because of its mineral content. This brittleness increases under tension forces more than under compression forces.

Stress Fractures

Stress fractures have been variously called march, fatigue, and spontaneous fractures, although *stress fracture* is the most commonly used term. The exact cause of this fracture is not known, but there are a number of likely possibilities: an overload caused by muscle contraction, amenorrhea, an altered stress distribution in the bone accompanying muscle fatigue, a change in the ground reaction force (such as movement from a wood surface to a grass surface), or the performance of a rhythmically repetitive stress that leads up to a vibratory summation point, which appears to be the most likely cause.[36] Rhythmic muscle action performed over a period of time at a sub-threshold level causes the stress-bearing capacity of the bone to be exceeded, hence, a stress fracture. A bone may become vulnerable to fracture during the first few weeks of intense physical activity or training. Weight-bearing bones undergo bone resorption and become weaker before they become stronger. The sequence of events results from increased muscular forces plus an increased rate of remodeling that leads to bone resorption, weakening of the outer surface of the bone, and rarefaction, which progresses to produce increasingly more severe fractures.[36] The four progressively severe fractures are focal microfractures, periosteal or endosteal response (stress fractures), linear fractures (stress fractures), and displaced fractures.

Typical causes of stress fractures in sports are as follows:

1. Overtraining
2. Going back into competition too soon after an injury or illness
3. Going from one event to other without proper training in the second event
4. Starting initial training too quickly
5. Changing habits or the environment (e.g., running surfaces, the bank of a track, or shoes)

Susceptibility to fracture can also be increased by a variety of postural and foot conditions. Flatfeet, a short first metatarsal bone, or a hypermobile metatarsal region can predispose an athlete to stress fractures (see Chapter 18).

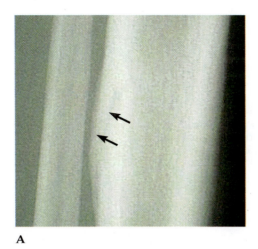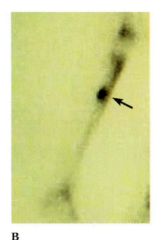

A   **B**

FIGURE 9–15 **(A)** X-ray and **(B)** bone scan of tibial stress fracture.

Early detection of the stress fracture may be difficult. Stress fractures always must be suspected in susceptible body areas that fail to respond to usual management. Until there is a reaction in the bone, which may take several weeks, X-ray examination may fail to reveal any change.[34] Although nonspecific, a bone scan can provide early indications in a given area (Figure 9–15).

The signs of a stress fracture are swelling, focal tenderness, and pain. In the early stages of the fracture, the athlete complains of pain when active but not at rest. Later, the pain is constant and becomes more intense at night. Percussion, by light tapping on the bone at a site other than the suspected fracture, will produce pain at the fracture site.[34]

The most common sites of stress fracture are the tibia, fibula, metatarsal shaft, calcaneus, femur, pars interarticularis of the lumbar vertebrae, ribs, and humerus.

The management of stress fractures varies with the individual, injury site, and extent of injury. Stress fractures that occur on the compression side of bone heal more rapidly and are managed more easily compared with those on the tension side. Stress fractures on the tension side can rapidly produce a complete fracture.[18]

Epiphyseal Conditions

Three types of epiphyseal growth site injuries can be sustained by children and adolescents performing sports activities. They are injury to the epiphyseal growth plate, physis articular epiphyseal injuries, and apophyseal injuries.[21] The most prevalent age range for these injuries is from 10 to 16 years.

Epiphyseal growth plate injuries (Figure 9–16) have been classified by Salter-Harris into five types as follows:[2,22]

- Type I—complete separation of the physis in relation to the metaphysis without fracture to the bone
- Type II—separation of the growth plate and a small portion of the metaphysis
- Type III—fracture of the physis
- Type IV—fracture of a portion of the physis and metaphysis
- Type V—no displacement of the physis, but the crushing force can cause a growth deformity

Apophyseal Injuries The young, physically immature athlete is particularly prone to apophyseal injuries.[12] The apophyses are traction epiphyses, in contrast to the pressure epiphyses of the long bones. These apophyses serve as origins, or insertions, for muscles on growing bone that provide bone shape but not length. Common apophyseal avulsion conditions found in sports are Severs disease and Osgood-Schlatter disease[12] (see Chapter 20).

Osteochondrosis

Osteochondrosis is a category of conditions of which the causes are not well understood. In general, the term refers to degenerative changes in the ossification centers of the epiphyses of bones, especially during periods of rapid growth in children.[12] Synonyms for this condition are as follows: if it is located in a point such as the knee, *osteochondritis dissecans* and, if located at a tubercle or tuberosity,

A musculoskeletal injury to a child or an adolescent should always be considered to involve a possible epiphyseal condition.

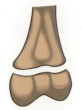 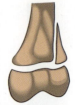 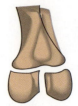

**Type I—Separation
of the physis**

**Type II—Fracture–separation
of growth plate and small
part of metaphysis**

**Type III—Fracture–part
of physis**

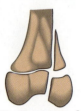 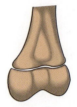

**Type IV—Fracture–physis
and metaphysis**

**Type V—Crushing of physis with
no displacement–may cause
premature closure**

FIGURE 9–16   Salter-Harris classification of long bone epiphyseal injuries in children.

apophysitis. Apophyseal conditions are discussed in the section on bone trauma in this chapter.

One suggested cause of osteochondrosis is aseptic necrosis, in which circulation to the epiphysis has been disrupted. Another suggestion is that trauma causes particles of the articular cartilage to fracture, eventually resulting in fissures that penetrate to the subchondral bone. If trauma to a joint occurs, pieces of cartilage may be dislodged, which can cause joint locking, swelling, and pain. If the condition occurs in an apophysis, there may be an avulsion fracture and fragmentation of the epiphysis along with pain, swelling, and disability.

NERVE TRAUMA

A number of abnormal nerve responses can be attributed to athletic participation or injury. The most frequent type of nerve injury is neuropraxia produced by a direct trauma. A laceration can cut nerves, causing complications in healing of the injury. Fractures and dislocation can avulse or abnormally compress nerves.

Anatomical Characteristics

Nerve tissue provides sensitivity and communication from the central nervous system (brain and spinal cord) to the muscles, sensory organs, various systems, and the periphery. The basic nerve cell is the neuron (Figure 9–17). The neuron cell body contains a large nucleus and branched extensions called dendrites, which respond to neurotransmitter substances released from other nerve cells.

From each nerve cell arises a single axon, which conducts the nerve impulses. Large axons found in peripheral nerves are enclosed in neurilemmal sheaths composed of Schwann cells and satellite cells, which are tightly wound around the axon. In the central nervous system, various types of neuroglial cells, including astrocytes, oligodendrocytes, ependymal cells, and microglia, function collectively to bind neurons together and provide a supportive framework for the nervous tissue.[35]

Nerve Injuries

Nerve injuries, as with injuries to other tissues in the body, can be traumatic or overuse. Trauma directly affecting nerves can produce a variety of sensory responses, including hypoesthesia (diminished sense of feeling), hyperesthesia (increased sense of feelings such as pain or touch), and paresthesia (numbness, prickling, or tingling, which may occur from a direct blow to or stretch of an area).[15] For example, a sudden nerve stretch or pinch can produce both a sharp or burning pain that radiates down a limb and muscle weakness. In **neuropraxia,**

neuropraxia
Interruption in conduction of an impulse down the nerve fiber.

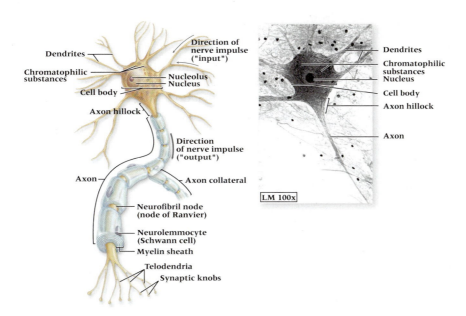

FIGURE 9–17   Basic anatomy of a neuron.

BODY MECHANICS AND INJURY SUSCEPTIBILITY

there is an interruption in conduction of the impulse down the nerve fiber. This is the mildest form of nerve injury. Neuropraxia is brought about by compression or relatively mild, blunt blows close to the nerve. It results in a temporary loss of function, which is reversible within hours to months of the injury (on average, 6 to 8 weeks). There is frequently greater involvement of motor than sensory function.[15] **Neuritis,** a chronic nerve problem,

| **neuritis** Inflammation of a nerve.

can be caused by a variety of forces that usually have been repeated or continued for a long time. Symptoms of neuritis can range from minor nerve problems to paralysis. More serious injuries involve the crushing of a nerve or complete division (severing). This type of injury may produce a lifelong physical disability, such as paraplegia or quadriplegia, and should therefore not be overlooked in any circumstance.

Specialized tissue, such as nerve cells, cannot regenerate once the nerve cell dies. In an injured peripheral nerve, however, the nerve fiber can regenerate significantly if the injury does not affect the cell body. For regeneration to occur, an optimal environment for healing must exist.

Regeneration is slow, at a rate of only 3 to 4 mm per day. Damaged nerves within the central nervous system regenerate very poorly compared with nerves in the peripheral nervous system.[15]

Pain that is felt at a point of the body other than its actual origin is known as **referred pain.** Another potential cause of referred pain is a trigger

| **referred pain** Pain that is felt at a point of the body other than its origin.

point, which occurs in the muscular system but refers pain to some other distant body part.

If one carefully studies the mechanical structure of the human body, it is amazing that humans can move so effectively in the upright posture. Not only must the body overcome constant gravitational force, but it also must be manipulated through space by a complex system of somewhat inefficient levers, fueled by a machinery that operates at an efficiency level of approximately 30 percent. The bony levers that move the body must overcome considerable resistance in the form of inertia and muscle viscosity and in most instances must work at an extremely unfavorable angle of pull. All these factors mitigate the effectiveness of lever action to the extent that most movement is achieved at an efficiency level of less than 25 percent.

When determining the mechanical reasons for injuries to the musculoskeletal system, many factors can be identified. Hereditary, congenital, or acquired defects may predispose an athlete to a specific type of injury. Anomalies in anatomical structure or in body build (somatotype) may make an individual prone to injuries. The habitually incorrect application of skill is a common cause of overuse injuries.

Microtrauma and Overuse Syndrome

Injuries as a result of abnormal and repetitive stress and microtraumas fall into a class with certain identifiable syndromes.[38] Such stress injuries frequently result in either limitation or curtailment of performance. Most of these injuries are directly related to the dynamics of running, throwing, or jumping. The injuries may result from constant and repetitive stresses placed on bones, joints, or soft tissues; from forcing a joint into an extreme range of motion; or from prolonged strenuous activity. Some of the injuries falling into this category may be relatively minor; still, they can be disabling. Among injuries classified as repetitive stress and microtrauma are Achilles tendinitis; shinsplints; stress fractures, particularly of the fibula and second and fifth metatarsal bones; Osgood-Schlatter disease; runner's and jumper's knee; patellar chondromalacia; apophyseal avulsion, especially in the lower extremities of young, growing individuals; and intertarsal neuroma.

Postural Deviations

Postural deviations are often an underlying cause of injuries.[38] Postural malalignment may be the result of unilateral muscle and soft-tissue asymmetries or bony asymmetries. As a result, the individual engages in poor mechanics of movement (pathomechanics). Many activities are unilateral, thus leading to asymmetries in body development. The resulting imbalance is manifested by a postural deviation as the body seeks to reestablish itself in relation to its center of gravity. Often, such deviations are a primary cause of injury. For example, a consistent pattern of knee injury may be related to asymmetries within the pelvis and the legs (short-leg syndrome). Unfortunately, not much in the form of remedial work is usually performed. As a result, an injury often becomes chronic—sometimes to the point that participation in activity must be halted. When possible, the athletic trainer should seek to ameliorate or eliminate faulty postural conditions through therapeutic exercise. A number of postural conditions offer genuine hazards to athletes by making them exceedingly prone to specific injuries.[21] Some of the more important are discussed in the chapters on foot and leg anomalies, spinal anomalies, and various stress syndromes.

SUMMARY

- "When a force applied to any part of the body results in a harmful disturbance in function or structure, a mechanical injury is said to have been sustained."[17] Mechanical terminology is used to describe tissue properties. Examples of this terminology are *load, stiffness, stress, strain, deformation, elastic, plastic, yield point,* and *tissue failure.*
- The five primary stresses leading to tissue trauma are compression, tension, shearing, bending, and torsion. Bending strain can produce a torque on a bone followed by injury. A torsion, or twisting, load can produce a spiral fracture along the long axis of a bone.
- Skeletal muscle trauma can involve any aspect of the musculotendinous unit. Forces that injure muscles are compression, tension, and shearing. Injuries to the musculotendinous unit include strains, cramps, muscle guarding, spasm, soreness, tendonosis/tendinitis/tendinopathy, tenosynovitis, myofacial trigger points, contusions, and atrophy.
- Injuries to the synovial joints are common. Anatomically, synovial joints have relative strengths or weaknesses based on their ligamentous or capsular type and their muscle arrangements. Forces that can injure synovial joints are tension, compression, torsion, and shearing. Sprains involve injury to ligaments or the joint capsule. A grade 3 sprain may cause ligament rupture or an avulsion fracture. Synovial joint injuries include dislocation or subluxation, osteoarthritis, bursitis, and capsulitis and synovitis. Two major chronic synovial joint conditions are osteochondrosis and traumatic arthritis.
- Because of their shape, long bones are anatomically susceptible to fractures caused by changes in direction of the force applied to them. Mechanical forces that cause injury are compression, tension, bending, torsion, and shearing. Bending and torsional forces are forms of tension. Types of fractures include avulsion, blowout, comminuted, depressed, greenstick, impacted, longitudinal, oblique, serrated, spiral, transverse, and contrecoup. Stress fractures are commonly the result of overload to a given bone area. Three major epiphyseal injuries occur to the growth plate, the articular cartilage, and the apophysis.
- Nerve trauma can be produced by overstretching or compression. The sudden stretch of a nerve can cause a burning sensation. A variety of traumas to nerves can produce acute pain or a chronic pain, such as neuritis.
- Any individual with faulty body mechanics has an increased potential for injury.

WEB SITES

American Red Cross: www.redcross.org
Cramer First Aider:
   www.cramersportsmed.com/resources/first-aider

National Institutes of Health: www.nih.gov
Wheeless' Textbook of Orthopedics:
   www.wheelessonline.com

SOLUTIONS TO CLINICAL APPLICATION EXERCISES

9–1   An external tension load causes internal strain and deformation to the ligament. When the ligament can no longer respond elastically, the yield point has been exceeded and a ligament sprain occurs.

9–2   The football player has sustained a tension force to the long head of the biceps tendon, which caused a rupture or severe strain.

9–3   The mechanism of this elbow injury is repeated tension to the extensor tendons attached to the lateral epicondyle, causing microtraumas. Stress to this area can be reduced by increasing the grip circumference and flattening the backhand stroke.

9–4   Repeated contusion of any muscle may lead to the development of myositis ossificans. The key to treating myositis ossificans is prevention. An initial contusion to any muscle should be immediately protected with padding to prevent reinjury.

9–5   In stepping on another player's foot, the basketball player produces an abnormal ankle torsion and lateral ankle tension, stretching and tearing ligaments.

9–6   The athletic trainer should suspect that the wrestler has developed bursitis from constantly kneeling on the mat. Inflammation may best be treated by rest, ice, antiinflammatory medication, and protective padding of the knee.

9–7   Catching the ski tip produces a torsional force that could cause a boot-top spiral fracture.

9–8   During the jump, a powerful stretch of the biceps femoris could cause a serious strain or an avulsion fracture in the region of the ischial tuberosity.

9–9   A stress fracture is not an actual break of the bone; it is simply an irritation of the bone. Treatment of a stress fracture requires about 2 to 4 weeks of rest. However, the athletic trainer should point out that a stress fracture can become a true fracture if it is not rested; if that happens, 4 to 6 weeks of immobilization in a cast is necessary. Thus, it is critical that this athlete rest for the required amount of time.

9–10   An epiphyseal condition, such as an epiphyseal growth plate fracture, can occur in children and adolescents and needs to be considered with any musculoskeletal injury. These injuries can impair growth and further skeletal development.

REVIEW QUESTIONS AND CLASS ACTIVITIES

1. Discuss the stress–strain curve and its associated tissue properties.
2. Differentiate among muscle strains, muscle cramps, muscle guarding, and muscle soreness.
3. How does a damaged nerve heal?
4. What are myofascial trigger points, where are they most likely to occur, and what are the signs and symptoms?
5. What is myositis ossificans and how can it be prevented?
6. How are tendinitis, tenosynovitis, and bursitis related to one another? Explain how osteoarthritis develops.
7. What structures are found at a joint? What are their functions?
8. Describe the injuries occurring to synovial joint structures.
9. Differentiate between a subluxation and a dislocation.
10. How do the three grades of ligament sprains differ?
11. Describe various types of fractures and the mechanisms that cause fractures to occur.
12. How does a stress fracture differ from a regular fracture?
13. Describe the most common epiphyseal conditions.
14. What are the relationships of postural deviations to injuries?
15. Discuss the concept of pathomechanics as it relates to microtraumas and overuse syndromes.
16. What forces injure muscle tissue?
17. Describe all types of muscle tendinous injuries.
18. What mechanical forces traumatize the musculotendinous unit and the synovial joint? How are the forces similar to one another, and how are they different?
19. What forces gradually weaken tendons and ligaments?
20. Contrast two synovial joint injuries.
21. List the structural characteristics that make a long bone susceptible to fracture.
22. What mechanical forces cause fracture of a bone?
23. How do stress fractures probably occur?

REFERENCES

1. Blavelt CT, Nelson FRT: *A manual of orthopaedic terminology,* ed 7, Philadelphia, PA, 2007, Elsevier.
2. Brinker M: *Review of orthopaedic trauma,* Philadelphia, 2001, WB Saunders.
3. Browner B: *Skeletal trauma: Basic science, management, and reconstruction,* Philadelphia, 2002, WB Saunders.
4. Brukner P, Khan K: Sports injuries. In Brukner P, editor: *Clinical sports medicine,* ed 3, Sydney, 2011, McGraw-Hill.
5. Buckwalter J: 2005. Musculoskeletal tissue healing. In Weinstein S: *Turek's Orthopedics: Principles and their application.* Baltimore, Lippincott, Williams and Wilkins.
6. Butterwick DJ: Recognition of complete muscle or tendon ruptures, *Athletic Therapy Today* 7(l):43, 2002.
7. Cailliet R: *Medical orthopedics: Conservative management of musculoskeletal injuries,* Chicago, 2004, AMA Press.
8. Cheung K: Delayed onset muscle soreness: Treatment strategies and performance factors, *Sports Medicine* 33(2):145–64, 2003.
9. Cleary M, Kimura I, Sitler M: Temporal pattern of the repeated bout effect of eccentric exercise on delayed-onset muscle soreness, *J Athl Train* 37(1):32, 2002.
10. Delee J, Drez D, Miller M: *Delee and Drez's orthopaedic sports medicine: Principles and practice,* Philadelphia, 2009, WB Saunders.
11. Delforge G: *Musculoskeletal trauma: Implications for sports injury management,* Champaign, IL, 2002, Human Kinetics.
12. DiFiori JP: Overuse injuries in young athletes: An overview, *Athletic Therapy Today* 7(6):25, 2002.
13. Drake D: Sports and performing arts medicine for traumatic injuries in sports, *Arch Phys Med Rehabil* 85(3 Suppl):S67, 2004.
14. Dumke CL: Muscle cramps are not all created equal, *Athletic Therapy Today* (3):42, 2003.
15. Feinberg J, Spielholz N: *Peripheral nerve injuries in the athlete,* Champaign, IL, 2003, Human Kinetics.
16. Gallaspie J, May D: *Signs and symptoms of athletic injuries,* St. Louis, 1996, McGraw-Hill.

17. Gomez M: *Biomechanics of soft-tissue injury,* Tuscon, AZ, 2000, Lawyers & Judges.
18. Gonza ER: Biomechanics of long bone injuries. In Gonza ER, Harrington IJ, editors: *Biomechanics of musculoskeletal injury,* Baltimore, 2007, Williams and Wilkins.
19. Hoppenfeld S, Murthy V, Taylor K: *Treatment and rehabilitation of fractures,* Philadelphia, 2000, Lippincott Williams and Wilkins.
20. Hunt T, Amato H: Epiphyseal-plate fracture in an adolescent athlete, *Athletic Therapy Today* 8(1):34, 2003.
21. Hutson M: *Sports injuries: Recognition and management,* ed 3, Oxford, England, 2001, Oxford University Press.
22. Jacobs D: Salter-Harris Type III fracture in a high school football player, *Athletic Therapy Today,* 14(6):238, 2009.
23. James C, Uhl T: A review of articular cartilage pathology and the use of glucosamine sulfate, *J Athl Train* 36(4):413, 2001.
24. Johnson J: Overuse injuries in young athletes: Cause and prevention, *Strength and Conditioning Journal* 30(2):27–31, 2008.
25. Knight K: More precise classification of orthopedic injury types and treatment will improve patient care, *J Athl Train,* 43(2):117–18, 2008.
26. Lavell E: Myofascial trigger points, *Anesthesiology Clinics* 25(4):841–51, 2007.
27. Levine D: Running and the development of osteoarthritis, part II: Human studies, *Athletic Therapy Today* 8(1):2, 2003.
28. Maehlum S: *Clinical guide to sports injuries,* Champaign, IL, 2004, Human Kinetics.
29. Martin R: *Skeletal tissue mechanics,* New York, 2010, Springer-Verlag.
30. Merrick M: Secondary injury after musculoskeletal trauma: A review and update, *J Athl Train* 37(2):209, 2002.
31. Miller K: Exercise-associated muscle cramps causes, treatment and prevention, *Sports Health,* 2(4):279–83, 2010.
32. Molina F: The physiologic basis of tendinopathy development, *Athletic Therapy and Training,* 16(6):5–8, 2011.
33. Norkin C: *Joint structure and function: A comprehensive analysis,* Philadelphia, 2011, F.A. Davis.
34. Patel D: Stress fractures: Diagnosis, treatment, and prevention, *American Family Physician,* 83(1):39–46, 2011.
35. Porth CM: *Pathophysiology: Concepts of altered health states,* ed 8, Philadelphia, 2010, Lippincott, Williams and Wilkins.
36. Romani W, Gieck J, Perrin D: Mechanisms and management of stress fractures in physically active persons, *J Athl Train* 37(3):306, 2002.
37. Saladin K: *Anatomy and physiology,* New York, 2012, McGraw-Hill.
38. Shamus E, Shamus L: *Sports injury: Prevention and rehabilitation,* New York, 2001, McGraw-Hill.
39. Stone MB: Exercise-associated muscle cramps, *Athletic Therapy Today* 8(3):30, 2003.
40. Weintraub W: *Tendon and ligament healing: A new approach to sports and overuse injury,* Herndon, VA, 2003, Paradigm.
41. Whiting W: Biomechanics of musculoskeletal injury, Champaign, IL, 2008, Human Kinetics.
42. Wilder R, Sethi S: Overuse injuries: Tendinopathies, stress fractures, compartment syndrome, and shin splints, *Clin Sports Med* 23(1):55, 2004.
43. Wilson TC: Articular-cartilage lesions of the knee and osteoarthritis in athletes: An overview, *Athletic Therapy Today* 8(1):20, 2003.
44. Wolff J: *Das geset der transformation der knockan,* Berlin, 1892, Hirschwald.

ANNOTATED BIBLIOGRAPHY

Blavelt CT, Nelson RRT: *A manual of orthopaedic terminology,* ed 6, Philadelphia, 2007, Elsevier.

A resource book for all individuals who need to identify medical words or their acronyms.

Berry, D: *Athletic and Orthopedic Injury Assessment: A Case Study Approach,* 2010 Holcomb Hathaway.

Case studies in this book use injury assessment examples to help readers link theory and clinical practice with the goal of becoming competent clinicians.

Dandy D, Edwards D: *Essential orthopaedics and trauma,* St. Louis, 2009, Elsevier.

Presents essential core information for students and emphasizes common conditions and current orthopedic practice.

Delforge G: *Musculoskeletal trauma: implications for sport injury management,* Champaign, IL, 2003, Human Kinetics.

Focuses on the therapeutic management of sport-related soft-tissue injuries, fractures, and proprioceptive/sensorimotor impairments.

Griffith HW, Pederson M: *Complete guide to sports injuries: how to treat fractures, bruises, sprains, dislocations, and head injuries,* New York, 2004, Penguin.

Tells readers how to treat, avoid, and rehabilitate nearly 200 of the most common sports injuries, including fractures, bruises, sprains, strains, dislocations, and head injuries.

Kjaer, M: *Textbook of sports medicine: basic science and clinical aspects of sports injury and physical activity,* Oxford, England, 2003, Blackwell Science.

Provides capsule summaries of the history, diagnosis, and treatment of orthopedic problems that respond to nonsurgical intervention in this primer for clinicians. Brief yet detailed entries explain the causes and treatment of impairments of the musculoskeletal system.

Maehlum S: *Clinical guide to sports injuries,* Champaign, IL, 2004, Human Kinetics.

Covers each step of the injury management process, beginning with the patient's presentation.

Norris C: *Sports injuries: diagnosis and management,* Philadelphia, 2004, Elsevier.

An overview of musculoskeletal injuries that are unique to sports and exercise.

Peacinn M, Bojanic I: *Overuse injuries of musculoskeletal system,* Boca Raton, FL, 2003, CRC Press.

A comprehensive text describing overuse injuries of the tendon, tendon sheath, bursae, muscle, muscle-tendon function, cartilage, and nerve.

Szendroi, M: 2010. *Color Atlas of Clinical Orthopedics,* New York, Springer.

This book is composed of a vast number of pictures presenting the clinical symptoms of the various orthopedic conditions. An in-depth overview of the characteristic clinical features of orthopedic conditions.

Weintraub W: *Tendon and ligament healing: a new approach to sports and overuse injury,* Herndon, VA, 2003, Paradigm.

Gives readers a clear understanding of the dynamic nature of tendons and ligaments from an excellent review of their structure, function, mechanics, injury, and healing processes.

Williams JGP: *Color atlas of injury in sport,* Chicago, 1993, Mosby.

An excellent visual guide to the area of sports injuries that covers the nature and incidence of sport injury, types of tissue damage, and regional injuries caused by a variety of sports activities.

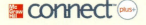

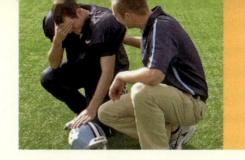

10

Tissue Response to Injury

■ Objectives

When you finish this chapter you should be able to

- Contrast the three phases of the healing process.
- Classify the physiological events that must take place during each phase of healing.
- Identify those factors that may impede the healing process.
- Discuss treatment techniques for modifying soft tissue healing, including using anti-inflammatory medications, therapeutic modalities, exercise rehabilitation, and platelet-rich plasma injections.
- Discuss the healing process relative to various soft-tissue structures, including cartilage, ligament, muscle, tendon, and nerve.

- Describe the healing process as it occurs in bone.
- Formulate a management plan for treating acute fractures.
- Define pain and discuss the various types of pain.
- Understand the neurophysiology of pain.
- Differentiate among the three mechanisms of pain control.
- Examine the various techniques for assessing pain.

■ Outline

■ Key Terms

margination
leukocytes
diapedesis
exudate
neutrophils
phagocytes
vasoconstriction
macrophages
lymphocytes
fibroblasts
fibroplasia

collagen
proteoglycans
glycosaminoglycans
microtears
macrotears
NSAIDs
prolotherapy
platelet-rich plasma (PRP)
avascular necrosis
trigger points
nociceptors

■ Connect Highlights

Visit connect.mcgraw-hill.com for further exercises to apply your knowledge:

- Clinical application scenarios covering physiological events that occur during healing, healing process in bone, and assessment of pain
- Click-and-drag questions covering tissue response to injury, inflammatory response, and soft-tissue healing
- Multiple-choice questions covering healing process, management of acute injuries, techniques and mechanisms for assessing pain, and factors that impede healing
- Selection questions covering factors that impede healing and treatment of inflammation

THE HEALING PROCESS

It is essential for the athletic trainer to possess an in-depth understanding of the healing process. The healing process consists of three phases: the inflammatory response phase, the fibroblastic repair phase, and the maturation-remodeling phase. The athletic trainer should recognize both the sequence and the time frames for these phases of healing and realize that certain physiological events must occur during each of the phases. Anything that an athletic trainer does that interferes with this healing process will likely slow the return to full activity. The healing process must have an opportunity to accomplish what it is supposed to. At best, the goal of the athletic trainer should be to try to create an environment that is conducive to the healing process. There is little that can be done to speed up the process physiologically, but there are many things that may be done during rehabilitation to impede healing. Although the phases of healing are often discussed as three separate entities, the healing process is a continuum. Phases of the healing process overlap one another and have no definitive beginning or end points (Figure 10–1).

Inflammatory Response Phase

Once a tissue is injured, the process of healing begins immediately (Figure 10–2A).[17,44] The destruction of tissue produces direct injury to the cells of the various soft tissues.[45] Cellular injury results in altered metabolism and the liberation of chemical mediators that initiate the inflammatory response (Figure 10–3). It is characterized symptomatically by redness (*rubor*), swelling (*tumor*), tenderness and pain (*dolor*), increased temperature (*calor*), and loss of function (*functio laesa*).[38] *This initial inflammatory response is critical to the entire healing process. If this response does not accomplish what it is supposed to, or if it does not subside, normal healing cannot take place.*[15]

Signs of inflammation:

- Redness (rubor)
- Swelling (tumor)
- Tenderness (dolor)
- Increased temperature (calor)
- Loss of function (functio laesa)

Chemical Mediators The events in the inflammatory response are initiated by a series of interactions involving several chemical mediators.[16] Some of these chemical mediators are derived from the invading organism, some are released by the damaged tissue, others are generated by several plasma enzyme systems, and still others are products of various white blood cells participating in the inflammatory response. Three chemical mediators, *histamine, leukotrienes,* and *cytokines,* are important in limiting the amount of exudate, and thus swelling, after injury.[3] Histamine, released from the injured mast cells, causes vasodilation and increased cell permeability, owing to a swelling of endothelial cells and then separation between the cells. Leukotrienes and prostaglandins are responsible for **margination,** in which **leukocytes** (neutrophils and macrophages) adhere along the cell walls (Figure 10–2B). They also increase cell permeability locally, thus affecting the passage of fluid, proteins, and neutrophils through cellwalls via **diapedesis** to form **exudate** in the extravascular spaces. Therefore, vasodilation and active hyperemia are important in exudate (plasma) formation and in supplying **neutrophils** to the injured area. As swelling continues and the extravascular pressure increases, the vascular flow to and the lymphatic flow from the area are decreased. The amount of swelling that occurs is directly related to the extent of vessel damage. Cytokines—in particular,

Chemical mediators:

- Histamine
- Leukotrienes
- Cytokines

margination Neutrophils and macrophages line up along the cell wall.

leukocytes Phagocytic cells.

diapedesis Movement of white blood cells out of small arterial vessels.

exudate Accumulation of fluid that penetrates through vessel walls into and joining extravascular space.

neutrophils A type of leukocyte.

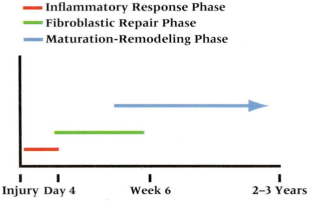

Inflammatory Response Phase
Fibroblastic Repair Phase
Maturation-Remodeling Phase

Injury · Day 4 · Week 6 · 2–3 Years

FIGURE 10–1 The three phases of the healing process fall along a continuum.

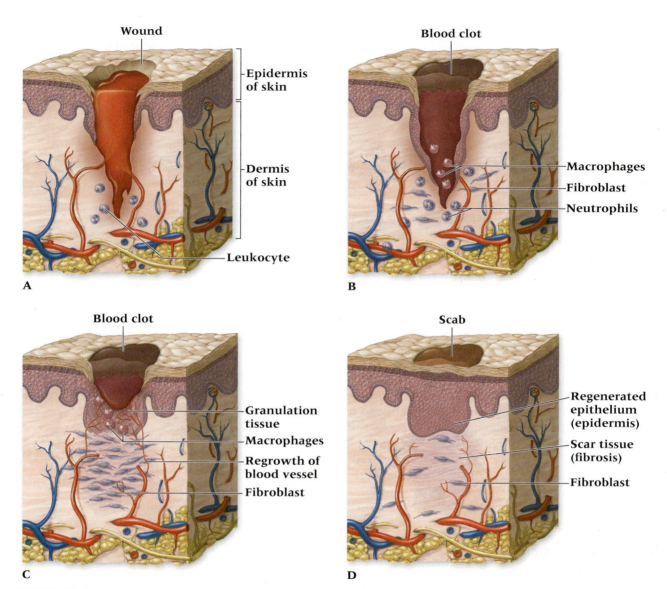

FIGURE 10–2 Initial injury and inflammatory response phase of the healing process. **(A)** Cut blood vessels bleed into the wound. **(B)** Blood clot forms, and leukocytes clean the wound. **(C)** Blood vessels regrow, and granulation tissue forms in the fibroblastic repair phase of the healing process. **(D)** Epithelium regenerates, and connective tissue fibrosis occurs in the maturation-remodeling phase of the healing process.

chemokines and interleukin, are the primary regulators of leukocyte traffic and help attract **phagocytes** to the site of inflammation.[16]

phagocytes Neutrophils, macrophages, and leukocytes that ingest microorganisms, other cells, and foreign particles.

Responding to the presence of chemokines, macrophages and leukocytes migrate to the site of inflammation within a few hours.

Vascular Reaction The vascular reaction is controlled by chemical mediators and involves vascular spasm, the formation of a platelet plug, blood coagulation, and the growth of fibrous tissue.[22] The immediate vascular response to tissue damage is **vasoconstriction** of the vascular walls in the vessels leading away from the site of injury that lasts for approximately 5 to 10 minutes. This vasoconstriction presses the opposing endothelial wall linings together to produce a local anemia that is rapidly replaced by hyperemia of the area due to vasodilation. This increase in blood flow is transitory and gives way to slowing of the flow in the dilated vessels, thus enabling the leukocytes to slow down and adhere to the vascular endothelium. Eventually, there is stagnation and stasis.[23] The initial effusion of blood and plasma lasts for 24 to 36 hours.

vasoconstriction Decrease in diameter of a blood vessel.

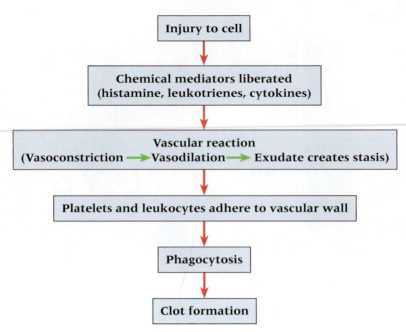

FIGURE 10–3 Inflammatory response sequence.

Function of Platelets Platelets do not normally adhere to the vascular wall. However, injury to a vessel disrupts the endothelium and exposes the collagen fibers. Platelets adhere to the collagen fibers to create a sticky matrix on the vascular wall, to which additional platelets and leukocytes adhere, eventually forming a plug. These plugs obstruct local lymphatic fluid drainage and thus localize the injury response.[15]

Formation of a Clot The initial event that precipitates clot formation is the conversion of *fibrinogen* to *fibrin*. This transformation occurs because of a cascading effect beginning with the release of a protein molecule called *thromboplastin* from the damaged cell. Thromboplastin causes *prothrombin* to be changed into *thrombin* which in turn causes the conversion of fibrinogen into a very sticky fibrin clot that shuts off blood supply to the injured area.[52] Clot formation begins around 12 hours after injury and is completed within 48 hours.

As a result of a combination of these factors, the injured area becomes walled off during the inflammatory stage of healing. The leukocytes phagocytize most of the foreign debris toward the end of the inflammatory phase, setting the stage for the fibroblastic phase. This initial inflammatory

Blood coagulation:
Thromboplastin
↓
Prothrombin
↓
Thrombin
↓
Fibrinogen
↓
Insoluble fibrin clot

response lasts for approximately 2 to 4 days after initial injury.

Chronic Inflammation A distinction must be made between the acute inflammatory response as previously described and chronic inflammation.[47] Chronic inflammation occurs when the acute inflammatory response does not respond sufficiently to eliminate the injuring agent and restore tissue to its normal physiological state. Thus, only low concentrations of the chemical mediators are present. The neutrophils that are normally present during acute inflammation are replaced by **macrophages, lymphocytes, fibroblasts,** and plasma cells.[47] As this low-grade inflammation persists, damage occurs to connective tissue, resulting in tissue necrosis and fibrosis, prolonging the healing and repair process. Chronic inflammation involves the production of granulation tissue and fibrous connective tissue. These cells accumulate in a highly vascularized and innervated loose connective tissue matrix in the area of injury.[47] The specific mechanisms that cause an insufficient acute inflammatory response are unknown, but they appear to be related to situations that involve overuse or overload with cumulative microtrauma to a particular structure.[15,23] There is

> Chronic inflammation occurs from repeated acute microtraumas and overuse.

macrophages Phagocytic cells of the immune system.

lymphocytes Cells that are the primary means of providing the body with immune capabilities.

fibroblasts Cells that produce collagen and elastin.

no specific time frame in which the acute inflammation transitions to chronic inflammation. It does appear that chronic inflammation is resistant to both physical and pharmacological treatments.[18]

Fibroblastic Repair Phase

During the fibroblastic repair phase of healing, proliferative and regenerative activity leading to scar formation and repair of the injured tissue follows the vascular and exudative phenomena of inflammation (see Figure 10–2C).[22] The period of scar formation, referred to as **fibroplasia**, begins within the first few days after injury and may last for as long as 4 to 6 weeks. During this period, many of the signs and symptoms associated with the inflammatory response subside. The patient may still indicate some tenderness to touch and will usually complain of pain when particular movements stress the injured structure. As scar formation progresses, complaints of tenderness or pain gradually disappear.[44]

During this phase, the growth of endothelial capillary buds into the wound is stimulated by a lack of oxygen, after which the wound is capable of healing aerobically. Along with increased oxygen delivery comes an increase in blood flow, which delivers nutrients essential for tissue regeneration in the area.[3]

The formation of a delicate connective tissue called *granulation tissue* occurs with the breakdown of the fibrin clot. Granulation tissue consists of fibroblasts, **collagen,** and capillaries. It appears as a reddish, granular mass of connective tissue that fills in the gaps during the healing process.

As the capillaries continue to grow into the area, fibroblasts accumulate at the wound site, arranging themselves parallel to the capillaries. Fibroblastic cells begin to synthesize an *extracellular matrix* that contains protein fibers of *collagen* and *elastin,* a *ground substance* that consists of nonfibrous proteins called **proteoglycans, glycosaminoglycans,** and fluid. On about the sixth or seventh day, fibroblasts also begin producing collagen fibers that are deposited in a random fashion throughout the forming scar. There are at least 16 types of collagen, but 80 to 90 percent of the collagen in the body consists of Types I, II, and III. Type I collagen is found in skin, fasciae, tendon, bone, ligaments, cartilage, and interstitial tissues; Type II can be found in hyaline cartilage and vertebral disks; and Type III is found in skin, smooth muscle, nerves, and blood vessels. Type III collagen has less tensile strength than does Type I and tends to be found more in the fibroblastic repair phase.[37] As the collagen continues to proliferate, the tensile strength of the wound rapidly increases in proportion to the rate of collagen synthesis. As the tensile strength increases, the number of fibroblasts diminishes to signal the beginning of the maturation phase.

This normal sequence of events in the repair phase leads to the formation of minimal scar tissue. Occasionally, a persistent inflammatory response and continued release of inflammatory products promotes extended fibroplasia and excessive fibrogenesis that can lead to irreversible tissue damage.[12] Fibrosis can occur in synovial structures, as with adhesive capsulitis in the shoulder; in extraarticular tissues, such as tendons and ligaments; in bursae; or in muscle.

Maturation-Remodeling Phase

The maturation-remodeling phase of healing is a long-term process (Figure 10–2D). This phase features a realignment or remodeling of the collagen fibers that make up scar tissue according to the tensile forces to which that scar is subjected. It involves a decrease in Type III collagen fibers and an increase in Type I fibers.[12] Ongoing breakdown and synthesis of collagen occur with a steady increase in the tensile strength of the scar matrix as well as a decrease in capillaries in that scar. With increased stress and strain, the collagen fibers realign in a position of maximum efficiency parallel to the lines of tension. The tissue gradually assumes normal appearance and function, although a scar is rarely as strong as the normal uninjured tissue. Usually, by the end of approximately 3 weeks, a firm, strong, contracted, nonvascular scar exists. The maturation phase of healing may require several years to be complete.

---

fibroplasia Period of scar formation.

collagen A strong, fibrous protein found in connective tissue.

Granulation tissue:
- Fibroblasts
- Collagen
- Capillaries

Extracellular matrix:
- Collagen
- Elastin
- Ground substance
- Proteoglycans
- Glycosaminoglycans

proteoglycans Molecules made of protein and carbohydrate.

glycosaminoglycans Carbohydrates that partially compose proteoglycans.

10–2 Clinical Application Exercise

A football player sustains a grade 2 medial collateral ligament sprain in his left knee. The athlete expresses concern with prolonged immobilization because he does not want to lose strength.

? What methods can be used to prevent atrophy from occurring but still allow healing to take place?

The Role of Progressive Controlled Mobility during the Healing Process Wolff's law states that bone and soft tissue will respond to the physical demands placed on them, causing them to remodel or realign along lines of tensile force.[37] Therefore, it is critical that injured structures be exposed to progressively increasing loads throughout the rehabilitative process.[25]

Controlled mobilization is superior to immobilization for scar formation, revascularization, muscle regeneration, and reorientation of muscle fibers and tensile properties in animal models.[29] However, a brief period of immobilization of the injured tissue during the inflammatory response phase is recommended and will likely facilitate the process of healing by controlling inflammation, thus reducing clinical symptoms. As healing progresses to the repair phase, controlled activity directed toward return to normal flexibility and strength should be combined with protective support or bracing.[17] Generally, clinical signs and symptoms disappear at the end of this phase.

As the remodeling phase begins, aggressive active range of motion and strengthening exercises should be incorporated to facilitate tissue remodeling and realignment.[48] To a great extent, pain dictates the rate of progression. With initial injury, pain is intense and tends to decrease and eventually subside altogether as healing progresses. Any exacerbation of pain, swelling, or other clinical symptoms during or after a particular exercise or activity indicates that the load is too great for the level of tissue repair or remodeling. The athletic trainer must be aware of the time required for the healing process and realize that being overly aggressive can interfere with that process.

Factors That Impede Healing

Extent of Injury The nature or amount of the inflammatory response is determined by the extent of the tissue injury. **Microtears** of soft tissue involve only minor damage and are most often associated with overuse. **Macrotears** involve significantly greater destruction of soft tissue and result in clinical symptoms and functional alterations. Macrotears are generally caused by acute trauma.[16]

microtears Overuse.

macrotears Acute trauma.

Edema The increased pressure caused by swelling retards the healing process, causes separation of tissues, inhibits neuromuscular control, produces reflexive neurological changes, and impedes nutrition in the injured part. Edema is best controlled and managed during the initial first-aid management period, as described previously.[32]

Hemorrhage Bleeding occurs with even the smallest amount of damage to the capillaries. Bleeding produces the same negative effects on healing as does the accumulation of edema, and its presence produces additional tissue damage and thus exacerbation of the injury.[52]

Poor Vascular Supply Injuries to tissues with a poor vascular supply heal poorly and slowly. This response is likely related to a failure in the initial delivery of phagocytic cells and fibroblasts necessary for scar formation.[52]

Separation of Tissue Mechanical separation of tissue can significantly affect the course of healing. A wound that has smooth edges that are in good apposition will tend to heal by *primary intention* with minimal scarring. Conversely, a wound that has jagged, separated edges must heal by *secondary intention,* with granulation tissue filling the defect and excessive scarring.[9,52]

Muscle Spasm Muscle spasm causes traction on the torn tissue, separates the two ends, and prevents approximation. Local and generalized ischemia may result from spasm.

Atrophy Wasting away of muscle tissue begins immediately with injury. Strengthening and early mobilization of the injured structure retard atrophy.[9]

Corticosteroids The use of corticosteroids in the treatment of inflammation is controversial. Steroid use in the early stages of healing has been demonstrated to inhibit fibroplasia, capillary proliferation, collagen synthesis, and increases in tensile strength of the healing scar. Their use in the later stages of healing and with chronic inflammation is debatable.[16]

Keloids and Hypertrophic Scars Keloids occur when the rate of collagen production exceeds the rate of collagen breakdown during the maturation phase of healing. This process leads to hypertrophy of scar tissue, particularly around the periphery of the wound.

Infection The presence of bacteria in the wound can delay healing and cause excessive granulation tissue, and frequently causes large, deformed scars.[16]

Humidity, Climate, and Oxygen Tension Humidity significantly influences the process of epithelization. Occlusive dressings stimulate the epithelium to migrate twice as fast without crust or scab formation. The formation of a scab occurs with dehydration of the wound and traps wound drainage, which promotes infection. Keeping the wound moist allows the necrotic debris to more easily go to the surface and be shed.

Oxygen tension relates to the neovascularization of the wound, which translates into optimal saturation and maximal tensile strength development. Circulation to the wound can be affected by ischemia, venous stasis, hematomas, and vessel trauma.

Health, Age, and Nutrition The elastic qualities of the skin decrease with aging. Degenerative diseases, such as diabetes and arteriosclerosis, also become a concern for older patients and may affect wound healing.[43] Nutrition is important for wound healing. In particular, vitamins C (collagen synthesis and immune system), K (clotting), and A (immune system); zinc for the enzyme systems; and amino acids play critical roles in the healing process.[28] Meeting the Dietary Recommended Intake (DRI) for vitamins is sufficient for wound healing.

SOFT-TISSUE HEALING
Cell Structure and Function

All organisms, from the simplest to the most complex, are composed of cells (Figure 10–4). The properties of a specific soft tissue of the body are derived from the structure and function of the cells. Individual cells contain a *nucleus* surrounded by *cytoplasm* and are enclosed by a *cell membrane* that selectively allows substances to enter and leave the cell. The nucleus contains *chromosomes,* which consist of DNA and protein. The functional and structural elements within the cell are called *organelles* and include *mitochondria, ribosomes, endoplasmic reticulum, centrioles, Golgi apparatusus,* and *microtubules.*[37]

All the tissues of the body can be defined as soft tissue except for bone. The human body has four types of soft tissue: epithelial tissue, which consists of the skin and the lining of vessels and many organs; connective tissue, which consists of tendons, ligaments, cartilage, fat, and blood vessels; muscle, which can be skeletal (striated), cardiac, or smooth; and nervous tissue, which consists of the brain, spinal cord, and nerves.[37]

Soft tissue can undergo adaptations as a result of healing and of the rehabilitative process following injury.[13] Soft-tissue adaptations include the following:

- Metaplasia—coversion of one kind of tissue into a form that is not normal for that tissue.
- Dysplasia—abnormal development of tissue
- Hyperplasia—excessive proliferation of normal cells in the normal tissue arrangement.
- Atrophy—a decrease in the size of tissue due to cell death and resorption or decreased cell proliferation.
- Hypertrophy—an increase in the size of a tissue without necessarily increasing the number of cells.

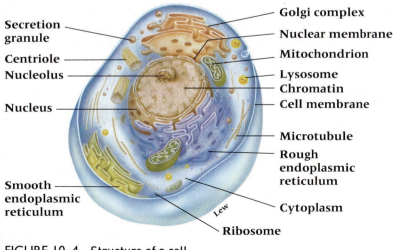

Golgi complex
Nuclear membrane
Mitochondrion
Lysosome
Chromatin
Cell membrane
Microtubule
Rough endoplasmic reticulum
Cytoplasm
Ribosome
Secretion granule
Centriole
Nucleolus
Nucleus
Smooth endoplasmic reticulum

FIGURE 10–4   Structure of a cell.

Cartilage Healing

Cartilage has a relatively limited healing capacity.[30] When chondrocytes are destroyed and the matrix is disrupted, the course of healing is variable, depending on whether damage is to cartilage alone or also to subchondral bone.[46] Injuries to articular cartilage alone fail to elicit clot formation or a cellular response. For the most part, the chondrocytes adjacent to the injury are the only cells that show any signs of proliferation and synthesis of matrix. Thus, the defect fails to heal, although the extent of the damage tends to remain the same.[19]

If subchondral bone is also affected, inflammatory cells enter the damaged area and formulate granulation tissue. In this case, the healing process proceeds normally, with differentiation of granulation tissue cells into chondrocytes occurring in about 2 weeks.[19] By approximately 2 months, normal collagen has been formed.[8]

Ligament Healing

The healing process in the sprained ligament follows a course of repair similar to that of other vascular tissues.[41] Immediately after injury and for approximately 72 hours, there is a loss of blood from damaged vessels and an attraction of inflammatory cells into the injured area. If a ligament is sprained outside of a joint capsule (extraarticular ligament), bleeding occurs in a subcutaneous space. If an intraarticular ligament is injured, bleeding occurs inside the joint capsule until either clotting occurs or the pressure becomes so great that bleeding ceases.[10]

During the next 6 weeks, vascular proliferation with new capillary growth begins to occur, along with fibroblastic activity, resulting in the formation of a fibrin clot.[27] It is essential that the torn ends of the ligament be reconnected by bridging of this clot. A synthesis of collagen and a ground substance of proteoglycan in an intracellular matrix contributes to the proliferation of the scar that bridges the torn ends of the ligament. Initially, this scar is soft and viscous, but eventually it becomes more elastic. Collagen fibers are arranged in a random woven pattern with little organization. Gradually, there is a decrease in fibroblastic activity, a decrease in vascularity, and a maximum increase in the collagen density of the scar.[41] Failure to produce enough scar and failure to reconnect the ligament to the appropriate location on a bone are the two reasons ligaments are likely to fail.

Over the next several months, the scar continues to mature, with the realignment of collagen occurring in response to progressive stresses and strains.[27] The maturation of the scar may require as long as 12 months to complete.[3] The exact length of time required for maturation depends on mechanical factors, such as apposition of torn ends and length of immobilization.[51]

Factors Affecting Ligament Healing Surgically repaired extraarticular ligaments have healed with decreased scar formation and are generally stronger than unrepaired ligaments initially, although this strength advantage may not be maintained as time progresses.[10] Nonrepaired ligaments heal by fibrous scarring, effectively lengthening the ligament and producing some degree of joint instability. With intraarticular ligament tears, the presence of synovial fluid dilutes the hematoma, thus preventing the formation of a fibrin clot and spontaneous healing.[51]

Several studies have shown that actively exercised ligaments are stronger than those that are immobilized. Ligaments that are immobilized for several weeks after injury tend to decrease in tensile strength and exhibit weakening of the insertion of the ligament to bone.[41] Thus, it is important to minimize periods of immobilization and progressively stress the injured ligaments while exercising caution relative to biomechanical considerations for specific ligaments.[21]

It is not likely that the inherent stability of the joint provided by the ligament before injury will be regained. Thus, to restore stability to the joint, the structures that surround that joint, primarily muscles and their tendons, must be strengthened. The increased muscle tension provided by strength training can improve the stability of the injured joint.[25]

Muscle Healing

Injuries to muscle tissue involve processes of healing and repair similar to those of other tissues. Initially, there will be hemorrhage and edema followed almost immediately by phagocytosis to clear debris. Within a few days, there is a proliferation of ground substance, and fibroblasts begin producing a gel-type matrix that surrounds the connective tissue, leading to fibrosis and scarring. At the same time, myoblastic cells (satellite cells) form in the area of injury, which eventually leads to the regeneration of new myofibrils. Thus, the regeneration of both connective tissue and muscle tissue has begun.[25]

Collagen fibers undergo maturation and orient themselves along lines of tensile force according to Wolff's law. Active contraction of the muscle is critical in regaining normal tensile strength.[25,50]

Regardless of the severity of the strain, the time required for rehabilitation is fairly lengthy. In many instances, rehabilitation time for a muscle strain is longer than for a ligament sprain. These incapacitating muscle strains occur most often in the large, force-producing hamstring and quadriceps muscles of the lower extremity. The treatment of hamstring strains requires a healing period of at least 6 to 8 weeks and a considerable amount of patience. Trying to return to activity too soon often causes reinjury to the area of the musculotendinous unit that has been strained, and the healing process must begin again.

Tendon Healing

Unlike most soft-tissue healing, tendon injuries pose a problem.[4,17] The injured tendon requires dense fibrous union of the separated ends and both extensibility and flexibility at the site of attachment.[33] Thus, an abundance of collagen is required to achieve good tensile strength. Unfortunately, collagen synthesis can become excessive, resulting in fibrosis, in which adhesions form in surrounding tissues and interfere with the gliding that is essential for smooth motion.[36] Fortunately, over a period of time the scar tissue of the surrounding tissues becomes elongated in its structure because of a breakdown in the cross-links between fibrin units and thus allows the necessary gliding motion. A tendon injury that occurs where the tendon is surrounded by a synovial sheath can be potentially devastating.[49]

A typical time frame for tendon healing would be that during the second week the healing tendon adheres to the surrounding tissue to form a single mass.[29] During the third week, the tendon separates to varying degrees from the surrounding tissues. However, the tensile strength is not sufficient to permit a strong pull on the tendon for at least 4 to 5 weeks, the danger being that a strong contraction can pull the tendon ends apart.[24,35,42]

Nerve Healing

Specialized tissue, such as nerve cells, cannot regenerate once the nerve cell dies. In an injured peripheral nerve, however, the nerve fiber can regenerate significantly if the injury does not affect the cell body.[37] The proximity of the axonal injury to the cell body can significantly affect the time required for healing. The closer an injury is to the cell body, the more difficult the regenerative process. In the case of a severed nerve, surgical intervention can markedly enhance regeneration.

For regeneration to occur, an optimal environment for healing must exist.[5] When a nerve is cut, several degenerative changes occur that interfere with the neural pathways (Figure 10–5). Within the first 3 to 5 days, the portion of the axon distal to the cut begins to degenerate and breaks into irregular segments. There is also a concomitant increase in metabolism and protein production by the nerve cell body to facilitate the regenerative process. The neuron in the cell body contains the genetic material and produces the chemicals necessary to maintain the axon. These substances cannot be transmitted to the distal part of the axon, and eventually there will be complete degeneration.[37]

In addition, the myelin portion of the Schwann cells around the degenerating axon also degenerates,

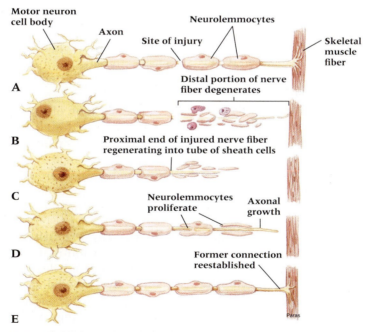

FIGURE 10–5   Neuron regeneration.
(A) If a neuron is severed through a myelinated axon, the proximal portion may survive, but **(B)** the distal portion will degenerate through phagocytosis. **(C & D)** The myelin layer provides a pathway for regeneration of the axon. **(E)** Innervation is restored.

and the myelin is phagocytized. The Schwann cells divide, forming a column of cells in place of the axon. If the cut ends of the axon contact this column of Schwann cells, the chances are good that an axon will eventually reinnervate distal structures. If the proximal end of the axon does not make contact with the column of Schwann cells, reinnervation will not occur.[37]

The axon proximal to the cut has minimal degeneration initially and then begins the regenerative process with growth from the proximal axon. Bulbous enlargements and several axon sprouts form at the end of the proximal axon. Within about two weeks, these sprouts grow across the scar that has developed in the area of the cut and enter the column of Schwann cells. Only one of these sprouts will form the new axon, while the others will degenerate. Once the axon grows through the Schwann cell columns, remaining Schwann cells proliferate along the length of the degenerating fiber and the neurolemmocytes form new myelin around the growing axon, which will eventually reinnervate distal structures.[20]

Regeneration is slow, at a rate of only 3 to 4 millimeters per day. Axon regeneration can be obstructed by scar formation due to excessive fibroplasia. Damaged nerves within the central nervous system regenerate very poorly compared with nerves in the peripheral nervous system. Central nervous system axons lack connective tissue sheaths, and the myelin-producing Schwann cells fail to proliferate.[7]

Modifying Soft-Tissue Healing

The healing process is unique in each patient. In addition, different tissues vary in their ability to regenerate. For example, cartilage regenerates to some degree from the perichondrium, striated muscle is limited in its regeneration, and peripheral nerve fibers can regenerate only if their damaged ends are opposed. Usually, connective tissue will readily regenerate, but, as is true of all tissue, this possibility is dependent on the availability of nutrients.

Age and general nutrition can play a role in healing. Older patients may be more delayed in healing than are younger patients. In a patient with a poor nutritional status, injuries may heal more slowly than normal. Patients with certain organic disorders may heal slowly. For example, blood conditions such as anemia and diabetes often inhibit the healing process because of markedly impaired collagen deposition. Many of the current treatment approaches are designed to enhance the healing process. Current treatments are anti-inflammatory medications, therapeutic modalities, exercise rehabilitation, and prolotherapy.

Methods to modify soft-tissue healing:
• Anti-inflammatory medications
• Therapeutic modalities
• Exercise rehabilitation

Anti-inflammatory Medications It is a common practice for a physician to routinely prescribe nonsteroidal anti-inflammatory drugs **(NSAIDs)** for patients who have sustained an injury.[18] These medications are certainly effective in minimizing the pain and swelling associated with inflammation and may enhance a return to full activity. However, there are some concerns that the use of NSAIDs acutely following injury may actually interfere with inflammation, thus delaying the healing process. The use of NSAIDs is further discussed in Chapter 17.

NSAIDs Nonsteroidal anti-inflammatory drugs.

Therapeutic Modalities Both cold and heat are used for different conditions. In general, heat facilitates an acute inflammatory response and cold slows the inflammatory response.[32]

A number of electrical modalities are used for the treatment of inflammation stemming from sports injuries. These procedures involve penetrating heat devices, such as shortwave and ultrasound therapy, and electrical stimulation, including transcutaneous electrical nerve stimulation (TENS) and electrical muscle stimulation (EMS)[32] (see Chapter 15).

Exercise Rehabilitation A major aim of soft-tissue rehabilitation through exercise is pain-free movement, full-strength power, and full extensibility of associated muscles. The ligamentous tissue, if related to the injury, should become pain free and have full tensile strength and full range of motion. The dynamic joint stabilizers should regain full strength and power.[18]

Immobilization of a part after injury or surgery is not always good for all injuries. When a part is immobilized over an extended period of time, adverse biochemical changes occur in collagenous tissue. Early mobilization used in exercise rehabilitation that is highly controlled may enhance the healing process[19] (see Chapter 16).

Prolotherapy Prolotherapy is a technique that involves injection of an irritant, nonpharmacological solution (e.g., dextrose, phenol, glycerine, lidocaine) into soft tissue for the purpose of increasing the inflammatory response, thus enhancing the healing process.[39] It is also referred to in the literature as proliferation therapy, proliferative injection therapy, and regenerative injection

Prolotherapy Injecting an irritant solution into a tendon or ligament to facilitate healing.

therapy. Prolotherapy has been used primarily to facilitate strengthening of weakened connective tissue (i.e., tendons and ligaments) and to reduce pain although it has also been used in treating a variety of other musculoskeletal conditions.[39] Injections are typically repeated every 3 to 6 weeks until no longer necessary. There is currently limited evidence in the literature to support the use of prolotherapy, although a number of randomized clinical trials are looking at this technique. Consequently, third-party payers are reluctant to reimburse for this therapeutic treatment.

Platelet-Rich Plasma (PRP) Injections **Platelet-rich plasma (PRP)** injections are a type of prolotherapy that uses the patient's own platelets to promote the natural healing of a variety of musculoskeletal conditions such as tendinosis, tendinitis, ligament sprains, muscle strains, injuries to fibrocartilage, osteoarthritis, and wound healing.[6,31] To prepare a PRP injection, a small amount of the patient's own blood is drawn into a vial. The blood is then spun in a centrifuge to separate the blood into its various components: plasma, platelets and white blood cells, and red blood cells. The red blood cells are drained away, and the concentrated platelets, white cells, and some plasma are centrifuged again to separate the platelet-rich plasma from the platelet-poor plasma; then an anticoagulant is added to prevent early platelet clotting. The PRP is then injected into and around the injured tissues.[34] The concentrated platelets release bioactive proteins that include growth factors and signaling proteins that stimulate wound healing and tissue repair. Growth factors are peptides secreted by many different tissues (including platelets) that activate intracellular pathways

> **Platelet-rich plasma (PRP)** Using blood plasma that has been enriched with platelets to stimulate healing of bone and soft tissue.

responsible for growth, differentiation, and development of cells. Specific growth factors are responsible for healing in musculoskeletal tissues.[6] The concentrated platelets can increase the growth factors by as much as eightfold.[31] The signaling proteins attract stem cells that multiply and function to repair and rebuild damaged tissue. Following an injection, there is usually an increase in pain for 5 to 10 days. The number of injections that are necessary depends upon the type of condition, severity, and the age of the patient.[34] Because this is a relatively new technique for treating musculoskeletal injuries, there are comparatively few randomized controlled trial studies that offer strong evidence supporting its effectiveness. Also, it is currently an expensive treatment, costing about $1,000 per injection.

BONE HEALING

Healing of injured bone tissue is similar to soft-tissue healing in that all phases of the healing process may be identified, although bone regeneration capabilities are somewhat limited. However, the functional elements of healing differ significantly from those of soft tissue. The tensile strength of the scar is the single most critical factor in soft-tissue healing, whereas bone has to contend with a number of additional forces, including torsion, bending, and compression.[26] Trauma to bone may vary from contusions of the periosteum to closed, nondisplaced fractures to severely displaced open fractures that also involve significant soft-tissue damage. When a fracture occurs, blood vessels in the bone and the periosteum are damaged, resulting in bleeding and subsequent clot formation (Figure 10–6). Hemorrhaging from the marrow is contained by the periosteum and the surrounding soft tissue in the region of the fracture. In about

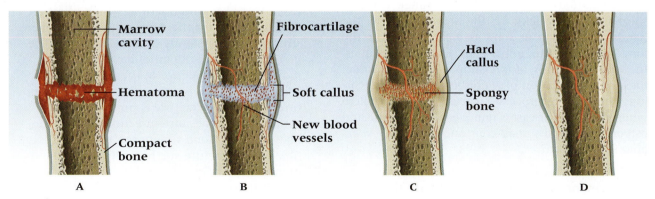

FIGURE 10–6 The healing of a fracture.
(A) Blood vessels are broken at the fracture line; the blood clots and forms a fracture hematoma. **(B)** Blood vessels grow into the fracture and a fibrocartilage soft callus forms. **(C)** The fibrocartilage becomes ossified and forms a bony callus made of spongy bone. **(D)** Osteoclasts remove excess tissue from the bony callus and the bone eventually resembles its original appearance.

one week, fibroblasts have begun laying down a fibrous collagen network. The fibrin strands within the clot serve as the framework for proliferating vessels. *Chondroblast* cells begin producing fibrocartilage, creating a *callus* between the broken bones. At first, the callus is soft and firm because it is composed primarily of collagenous fibrin. The callus becomes firm and more rubbery as cartilage begins to predominate. Bone-producing cells called osteoblasts begin to proliferate and enter the callus, forming cancellous bone trabeculae, which eventually replace the cartilage. Finally, the callus crystallizes into bone, at which point remodeling of the bone begins. The callus can be divided into two portions, the external callus located around the periosteum on the outside of the fracture and the internal callus found between the bone fragments. The size of the callus is proportional both to the damage and to the amount of irritation to the fracture site during the healing process. Also during this time, osteoclasts begin to appear in the area to resorb bone fragments and clean up debris.[26,37]

The remodeling process is similar to the growth process of bone in that the fibrous cartilage is gradually replaced by fibrous bone and then by more structurally efficient lamellar bone. Remodeling involves an ongoing process during which osteoblasts lay down new bone and osteoclasts remove and break down bone according to the forces placed on the healing bone.[26] Wolff's law maintains that a bone will adapt to mechanical stresses and strains by changing size, shape, and structure. Therefore, once the cast is removed, the bone must be subjected to normal stresses and strains, so that tensile strength may be regained before the healing process is complete.[2]

The time required for bone healing is variable and based on a number of factors, such as the severity of the fracture, site of the fracture, extensiveness of the trauma, and age of the patient.[2] Normal periods of immobilization range from as short as three weeks for the small bones in the hands and feet to as long as eight weeks for the long bones of the upper and lower extremities. In some instances—for example, the four small toes—immobilization may not be required for healing. The healing process is certainly not complete when the splint or cast is removed. Osteoblastic and osteoclastic activity may continue for 2 to 3 years after severe fractures.

Management of Acute Fractures In the treatment of acute fractures, the bones commonly must be immobilized completely until X-ray studies reveal that the hard callus has been formed. It is up to the physician to know the various types of fractures and the best form of immobilization for each

fracture.[26] Fractures can keep a patient from activity for several weeks or months, depending on the nature, extent, and site of the fracture. During this period, certain conditions can seriously interfere with the healing process:[2,26,37]

- If there is *a poor blood supply to the fractured area* and one of the parts of the fractured bone is not properly supplied by the blood, that part will die and union or healing of the fracture will not take place. This condition is known as **avascular necrosis** and often occurs in the head of the femur, the navicular bone in the wrist, the talus in the ankle, and isolated bone fragments. The condition is relatively rare among vital, healthy, young patients except in the navicular bone of the wrist.

- *Poor immobilization of the fracture site*, resulting from poor casting by the physician and permitting motion between the bone parts, may not only prevent proper union but also, in the event that union does transpire, cause deformity to develop.

- *Infection* can materially interfere with the normal healing process, particularly in the case of a compound fracture, which offers an ideal situation for the development of a severe streptococcal or staphylococcal infection. The increased use of antibiotics has considerably reduced the prevalence of these infections coincidental with or immediately after a fracture. The closed fracture is not immune to contamination because infections within the body or poor blood supply can render it susceptible. If the fracture site becomes and remains infected, the infection can interfere with the proper union of the bone.

- Soft tissues that become positioned between the severed ends of the bone—such as muscle, connective tissue, or other soft tissue immediately adjacent to the fracture—can prevent proper bone union, often necessitating surgical intervention.

10–6 Clinical Application Exercise

A field hockey player falls and sustains an acute fracture of the left humerus.

? What are the healing events typical of this acute bone fracture?

Conditions that interfere with fracture healing:

- Poor blood supply
- Poor immobilization
- Infection
- Soft tissues between severed ends of bone.

avascular necrosis
A portion of the bone degenerates due to a poor blood supply.

Healing of Stress Fractures

As discussed in Chapter 9, stress fractures may be created by cyclic forces that adversely load a bone at a susceptible site. Fractures may be the result of axial compression or tension created by the pull of muscles. Stress on ligamentous and bony tissue can be either positive and increase relative strength or negative and lead to tissue weakness. Bone produces an electrical potential in response to the stress of tension and compression. As a bone bends, tension is created on its convex side along with a positive electrical charge; conversely, on the concave or compressional side, a negative electrical charge is created. Torsional forces produce tension circumferentially. Constant tension caused by axial compression or stress by muscular activity can result in an increase in bone resorption and, subsequently, a microfracture. In other words, if the osteoclastic activity is greater than the osteoblastic activity, the bone becomes increasingly susceptible to stress fractures.[14]

Like the healing of acute fractures, the healing of stress fractures involves restoring a balance of osteoclastic and osteoblastic activity. Achieving this balance requires recognition of the situation as early as possible. Stress fractures that go unhealed will eventually develop into complete cortical fractures that may, over a period of time, become displaced. A decrease in activity and the elimination of other factors in training that cause stress will allow the bone to remodel and to develop the ability to withstand stress.[14]

PAIN

Pain can be defined as "an unpleasant sensory and emotional experience associated with actual or potential tissue damage, or described in terms of such damage."[1] Pain is a subjective sensation with more than one dimension and an abundance of descriptors of its qualities and characteristics. Pain is composed of a variety of human discomforts, rather than being a single entity. The perception of pain can be subjectively modified by past experiences and expectations. Much of what is done to treat patients' pain is to change their perceptions of pain. Certainly, reducing pain is an essential part of treatment. The athletic trainer's goal is to control acute pain by encouraging the body to heal through exercise designed to progressively increase functional capacity and to return the patient to full activity as swiftly and safely as possible.

Types of Pain

Pain can be described according to a number of categories, such as pain sources, acute versus chronic pain, and referred pain.[12]

Pain Sources Pain sources are cutaneous, deep somatic, visceral, and psychogenic.[11] Cutaneous pain is usually sharp, bright, and burning and can have a fast or slow onset. Deep somatic pain stems from structures such as tendons, muscles, joints, periosteum, and blood vessels. Visceral pain originates from internal organs. Visceral pain is diffused at first and later may be localized, as in appendicitis. In psychogenic pain, the individual feels pain but the cause is emotional rather than physical.[12]

Acute versus Chronic Pain Acute pain lasts less than 6 months. Tissue damage occurs and serves as a warning to the patient. Chronic pain, on the other hand, has a duration longer than 6 months. The International Association for the Study of Pain describes chronic pain as that which continues beyond the usual normal healing time.[8]

Referred Pain Referred pain occurs away from the actual site of irritation. This pain has been called an error in perception. Each referred pain site must also be considered unique to each individual. Symptoms and signs vary according to the nerve fibers affected. Response may be motor, sensory, or both. Four types of referred pain are myofascial, sclerotomic, myotomic, and dermatomic pain.

Myofascial Pain As discussed in Chapter 9, **trigger points** are small, hyperirritable areas within a muscle in which nerve impulses bombard the central nervous system and are expressed as a referred pain.

> **trigger points** Small, hyperirritable areas within a muscle.

Acute and chronic musculoskeletal pain can be caused by myofascial trigger points.[12] Such pain sites have variously been described as fibrositis, myositis, myalgia, myofasciitis, and muscular strain.

An active trigger point is hyperirritable and causes an obvious complaint. Pain radiating from an active trigger point does not follow a usual area of distribution, such as sclerotomes, dermatomes, or peripheral nerves. The trigger point pain area is called the reference zone, which can be close to the point of irritation or a considerable distance from it.[12]

Sclerotomic, Myotomic, and Dermatomic Pain Deep pain may originate from sclerotomic, myotomic, or dermatomic nerve irritation or injury.[11] A sclerotome is an area of bone or fascia that is supplied by a single nerve root. Myotomes are muscles supplied by a single nerve root. Dermatomes also are in an area of skin supplied by a single nerve root.

Sclerotomic pain is deep, aching, and poorly localized pain. Sclerotomic pain impulses can be projected to regions in the brain such as the hypothalamus, limbic system, and reticular formation and can cause depression, anxiety, fear, or anger. Autonomic changes, such as changes in vasomotor tone, blood pressure, and sweating, may also occur.

Dermatomic pain, in contrast to sclerotomic pain, is sharp and well localized. Unlike sclerotomic pain, dermatomic pain projects mainly to the thalamus and is relayed directly to the cortex, skipping autonomic and affective responses.

Nociceptors and Neural Transmission

Pain receptors known as **nociceptors,** or free nerve endings, are sensitive to mechanical, thermal, and chemical energy.[11] They are commonly found in skin, periosteum surrounding bone, teeth, meninges, and some organs.

nociceptors Pain receptors.

Afferent nerve fibers transmit impulses from the nociceptors toward the spinal cord, while *efferent* nerve fibers, such as motor neurons, transmit impulses from the spinal cord toward the periphery. First-order, or primary, afferents transmit impulses from a nociceptor to the dorsal horn of the spinal cord. There are four types of first-order neurons: Aα, Aβ, Aδ, and C. Aα and Aβ fibers are characterized as large-diameter afferents and Aδ and C fibers as small-diameter afferents. Aδ and C fibers transmit sensations of pain and temperature. Aδ neurons originate from nociceptors located in skin and transmit "fast pain," while C neurons originate from both superficial tissue (skin) and deeper tissue (ligaments and muscle) and transmit "slow pain."[12]

Second-order afferent fibers carry sensory messages from the dorsal horn to the brain and are categorized as nociceptive specific. Second-order afferents receive input from Aβ, Aδ, and C fibers. Second-order afferents serve relatively large, overlapping receptor fields. Nociceptive-specific second-order afferents respond exclusively to noxious stimulation and receive input only from Aδ and C fibers. All of these neurons synapse with third-order neurons, which carry information via ascending spinal tracts to various brain centers, where the input is integrated, interpreted, and acted upon.[12]

Facilitators and Inhibitors of Synaptic Transmission

For information to pass between neurons, a transmitter substance must be released from one neuron terminal, enter the synaptic cleft, and attach to a receptor site on the next neuron. This occurs primarily due to chemicals called *neurotransmitters.* However, it has been shown that several compounds that are not true neurotransmitters can facilitate or inhibit synaptic activity. These include *serotonin,* which is active in descending pathways; *norepinephrine,* which inhibits pain transmission between first- and second-order neurons; *substance P,* which is active in small-diameter primary afferent neurons; *enkephalins,* found in descending pathways; and *β-endorphin,* found in the central nervous system.[40]

Neurotransmitters:
• Serotonin
• Norepinephrine
• Substance P
• Enkephalins
• β-endorphin

Mechanisms of Pain Control

The neurophysiological mechanisms of pain control have not been fully explained. To date, three models of pain control have been proposed: the gate control theory, descending pathway pain control, and the release of β-endorphin. It is likely that some as-yet-unexplained combination of these three models is responsible for pain modulation.[1]

Gate Control Theory Sensory information coming from cutaneous receptors in the skin enters the ascending Aβ afferents and is carried to the substantia gelatinosa in the dorsal horn of the spinal cord (Figure 10–7). Likewise, pain messages from the nociceptors are carried along the Aδ and C afferent fibers and enter the dorsal horn. Sensory information coming from Aβ fibers overrides or inhibits the "pain information" carried along Aδ and C fibers, thus inhibiting, or effectively "closing the gate" to, the transmission of pain information to second-order neurons. Consequently, pain information is not transmitted and never reaches sensory centers in the brain. The gate control theory of pain control occurs at the spinal cord level.[12]

Descending Pathway Pain Control Stimulation of descending pathways in the spinal cord may also inhibit pain impulses carried along the Aδ and C afferent fibers (Figure 10–8). It is theorized that previous experiences, emotional influences, sensory

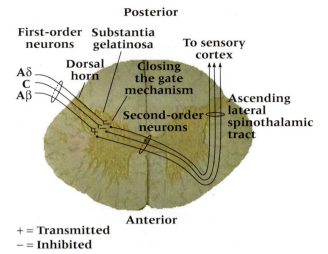

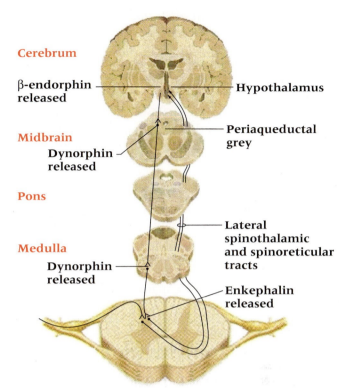

FIGURE 10–7 Gate control theory. Sensory information carried on Aβ fibers "closes the gate" to pain information carried on Aδ and C fibers in the substantia gelatinosa, preventing the transmission of pain to sensory centers in the cortex.

+ = Transmitted
− = Inhibited

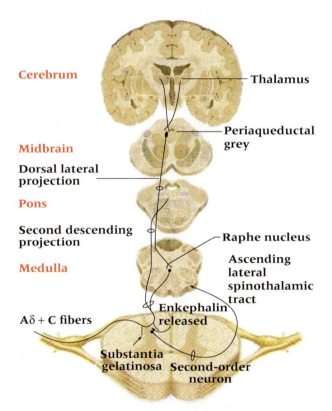

FIGURE 10–8 Descending pathway pain control. Influence from the thalamus stimulates the periaqueductal grey, the raphe nucleus, and the pons to inhibit the transmission of pain impulses through the ascending tracts.

FIGURE 10–9 β-endorphin released from the hypothalamus and dynorphin released from the periaqueductal grey and the medulla.

perception, and other factors influence the transmission of pain messages and thus the perception of pain. The information coming from higher centers in the brain along efferent descending pathways in the spinal cord causes a release of two neurotransmitter-like substances, enkephalin and norepinephrine, into the dorsal horn, which together block or inhibit the synaptic transmission of impulses from the Aδ and C afferent fibers to second-order afferent neurons.[12]

Release of β-Endorphin It has been shown that noxious (painful) stimulation of nociceptors resulting in the transmission of pain information along Aδ and C afferents can stimulate the release of an opiate-like chemical called β-endorphin from the hypothalamus and anterior pituitary (Figure 10–9). β-endorphin is endogenous to the central nervous system and is known to have strong analgesic effects. The exact mechanisms by which β-endorphin produces these potent analgesic effects are unclear. Acupuncture, acupressure, and point stimulation using electrical currents are all techniques that may stimulate the release of β-endorphin.[12]

Pain Assessment

Pain is a complex phenomenon that is difficult to evaluate and quantify because it is subjective. Thus, obtaining an accurate and standardized assessment of pain is problematic. A number of validated assessment tools are available that allow the athletic trainer to develop a pain profile by identifying the type of pain a patient is experiencing, quantifying the intensity of pain, evaluating the effect of the pain experience on a patient's level of functioning, and assessing the psychosocial impact of pain.

Pain measurement tools include simple *unidimensional scales* or *multidimensional questionnaires.* Pain measurement should include both the time frame and the clinical context of the pain. With unidimensional scales, individuals with acute pain are usually asked to describe their pain "right now" and may be asked about the average intensity over a fixed period to provide information on the course of the pain. Examples of commonly used unidimensional scales are verbal rating scales, the numeric rating scale, and the visual analog scale. Multidimensional pain assessment tools are more comprehensive pain assessments that require the determination of the quality of the pain and its effect on mood and function. They are used mainly to quantify these aspects of pain, and they take longer to administer than the unidimensional scales. The McGill Pain Questionnaire is an example of a multidimensional pain assessment tool.

Visual Analog Scales Visual analog scales are quick and simple tests that consist of a line, usually 2½ inches (10 cm) in length, the extremes of which are taken to represent the limits of the pain experience. The patient simply places a mark on that line based on the perceived level of pain. Scales can be completed daily or more often (Figure 10–10).

Pain Charts Pain charts are used to establish spatial properties of pain. They involve a two-dimensional graphic chart on which the patient assesses the location of pain and a number of subjective components. The patient colors the chart in areas that correspond to pain (Figure 10–11).

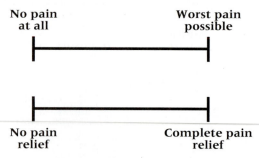

FIGURE 10–10 Visual analog scales.

McGill Pain Questionnaire The McGill Pain Questionnaire lists 78 words that describe pain, which are grouped into 20 sets and divided into four categories representing dimensions of the pain experience. It may take up to 20 minutes to complete, and the questionnaire is administered every 2 to 4 weeks (Figure 10–12).

Activity Pain Indicators Profile The Activity Pain Indicators Profile is a 64-question self-report tool used to assess functional impairment associated with pain. It measures the frequency of certain behaviors, such as housework, recreation, and social activities, that produce pain.

Numeric Rating Scale The numeric rating scale is the most common acute pain profile used in sports medicine. The patient is asked to verbally rate pain on a scale from 1 to 10, with 10 representing the worst pain he or she has experienced or can imagine. Usually, the scale is administered verbally before

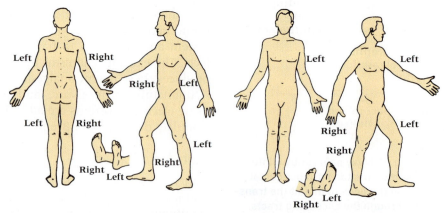

FIGURE 10–11 Pain chart. Use the following instructions: "Please use all of the figures to show me exactly where all your pains are, and where they radiate to. Shade or draw with *blue marker.* Only the athlete is to fill out this sheet. Please be as precise and detailed as possible. Use *yellow marker* for numbness and tingling. Use *red marker* for burning or hot areas, and *green marker* for cramping. Please remember: blue = pain, yellow = numbness and tingling, red = burning or hot areas, green = cramping." Used with permission from Melzack R: *Pain measurement and assessment,* New York, 1983, Raven Press.

McGill Pain Questionnaire

Patient's Name _____ Date _____ Time _____ am/pm

PRI S _____ A _____ E _____ M _____ PRI (T) _____ PPI _____
    (1–10)   (11–15)   (16)   (17–20)   (1–20)

1 Flickering / Quivering / Pulsing / Throbbing / Beating / Pounding	11 Tiring / Exhausting
2 Jumping / Flashing / Shooting	12 Sickening / Suffocating
3 Pricking / Boring / Drilling / Stabbing / Lancinating	13 Fearful / Frightful / Terrifying
4 Sharp / Cutting / Lacerating	14 Punishing / Gruelling / Cruel / Vicious / Killing
5 Pinching / Pressing / Gnawing / Cramping / Crushing	15 Wretched / Blinding
6 Tugging / Pulling / Wrenching	16 Annoying / Troublesome / Miserable / Intense / Unbearable
7 Hot / Burning / Scalding / Searing	17 Spreading / Radiating / Penetrating / Piercing
8 Tingling / Itchy / Smarting / Stinging	18 Tight / Numb / Drawing / Squeezing / Tearing
9 Dull / Sore / Hurting / Aching / Heavy	19 Cool / Cold / Freezing
10 Tender / Taut / Rasping / Splitting	20 Nagging / Nauseating / Agonizing / Dreadful / Torturing

Brief / Momentary / Transient	Rhythmic / Periodic / Intermittent	Continuous / Steady / Constant

E = External
I = Internal

PPI
0 No pain
1 Mild
2 Discomforting
3 Distressing
4 Horrible
5 Excruciating

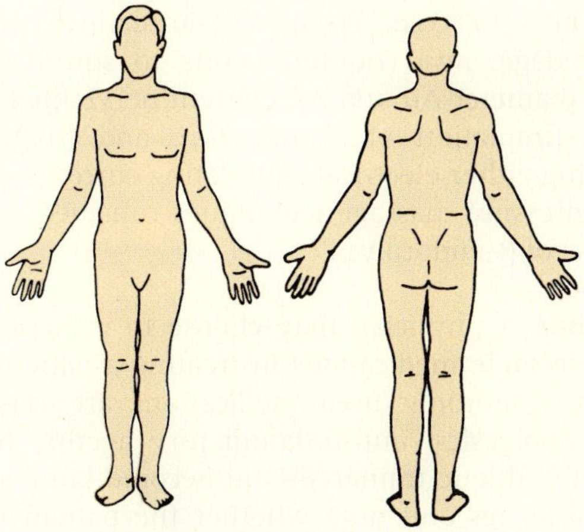

COMMENTS

FIGURE 10–12   McGill Pain Questionnaire. The descriptors fall into four groups: sensory, 1 to 10; affective, 11 to 15; evaluative, 16; and miscellaneous, 17 to 20. The rank value for each descriptor is based on its position in the word set. The sum of the rank values is the pain rating index (PRI). The present pain intensity (PPI) is based on a scale of 0 to 5.
Used with permission from Melzack R: *Pain measurement and assessment*, New York, 1983, Raven Press.

and after treatment. When treatments provide pain relief, questions are asked about the extent and duration of the relief.

Treating Pain

An athletic trainer can approach pain management using a variety of treatment options, including therapeutic modalities and medications.

Therapeutic Modalities Many therapeutic modalities can provide pain relief.[32] There is not one best therapeutic agent for pain control. The athletic trainer must select the therapeutic agent that is most appropriate for each athlete, based on the athletic trainer's knowledge of the modalities and professional judgment (see Chapter 15). In no situation should the athletic trainer apply a therapeutic agent without first developing a clear rationale for the treatment. The therapeutic modalities used to control pain do little to promote tissue healing. They should be used to relieve acute pain following injury or surgery or to control pain and other symptoms, such as swelling, to promote progressive exercise. The athletic trainer should not lose sight of the effects of the modalities or the importance of progressive exercise in restoring the athlete's functional ability.

The athletic trainer can make use of the gate control mechanism of pain control by using superficial heat or cold, electrical stimulating currents, massage, and counterirritants to stimulate the large-diameter Aα and Aβ efferent nerve fibers. Noxious stimulation of acupuncture and trigger points using either electrical stimulating currents or deep acupressure massage techniques can mediate the release of β-endorphin.[12]

Medications A physician may choose to prescribe oral or injectable medications in treating a patient. The most commonly used medications are classified as analgesics, anti-inflammatory agents, or both.[10] The athletic trainer should become familiar with these drugs and note whether the patient is taking any medications (see Chapter 17). It is also important to work with the referring physician or a pharmacist to make sure that the patient takes the medications appropriately.

Psychological Aspect of Pain

Pain, especially chronic pain, is a subjective psychological phenomenon.[40] When painful injuries are treated, the total patient must be considered, not just the pain or condition. Even in the most well-adjusted person, pain creates emotional changes. Constant pain often causes self-centeredness and an increased sense of dependency. Chapter 11 discusses in great detail the psychosocial aspects of dealing with injury and managing pain.

Patients vary in their pain thresholds (Figure 10–13). Some can tolerate enormous pain, whereas others find mild pain almost unbearable. Pain is perceived as being worse at night because persons are alone, more aware of themselves, and

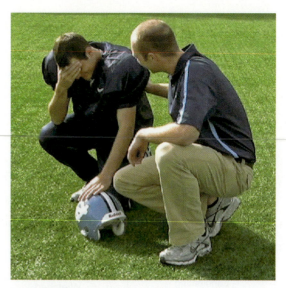

FIGURE 10–13 Coping with pain in sports is as much psychological as it is physical.

devoid of external diversions. Personality differences can also cause differences in pain toleration. For example, patients who are anxious, dependent, and immature have less tolerance for pain than those who are relaxed and emotionally in control.

A number of theories about how pain is produced and perceived by the brain have been advanced. Only in the last few decades has science demonstrated that pain is both a psychological and a physiological phenomenon and is therefore unique to each individual.[4,40] Sports activities demonstrate this fact clearly. Through conditioning, an athlete learns to endure the pain of rigorous activity and to block the sensations of a minor injury. It is perhaps most critical for the athletic trainer to recognize that all pain is very real to the patient.

SUMMARY

- The three phases of the healing process are the inflammatory response phase, the fibroblastic repair phase, and the maturation-remodeling phase, which occur in sequence but overlap one another in a continuum.
- During the inflammatory response phase, debris is phagocytized (cleaned up). The fibroblastic repair phase involves the deposition of collagen fibers to form a firm scar. During the maturation-remodeling phase, collagen is realigned along lines of tensile force and the tissue gradually assumes normal appearance and function.
- Factors that may impede the healing process include the extent of the injury, edema,

hemorrhage, poor vascular supply, separation of tissue, muscle spasm, atrophy, corticosteroids, keloids and hypertrophic scars, infection, climate and oxygen tension, health, age, and nutrition.

- Treatment techniques that can be used to modify soft-tissue healing include anti-inflammatory medications, therapeutic modalities, exercise rehabilitation, and platelet-rich plasma injections.
- The healing of soft tissues, including cartilage, ligament, muscle, and nerve, follows a similar course. Unlike the other tissues, nerve has the capability of regenerating.
- Bone healing following fracture involves increased activity of osteoblastic cells and osteoclastic cells.

- Pain is a response to a noxious stimulus that is subjectively modified by past experiences and expectations.
- Pain is classified as either acute or chronic and can exhibit many different patterns.
- Three models of pain control are the gate control theory, descending pathway pain control, and the release of β-endorphin from higher centers of the brain.
- Pain perception may be influenced by a variety of cognitive processes mediated by the higher brain centers.

WEB SITES

American Academy of Pain Management: www.aapainmanage.org

American Pain Society: www.ampainsoc.org

World Union of Wound Healing Societies: www.wuwhs.org

SOLUTIONS TO CLINICAL APPLICATION EXERCISES

10–1 Little can be done to speed up the healing process physiologically. This athlete must realize that certain physiological events must occur during each phase of the healing process. Any interference with this healing process during a rehabilitation program will likely slow return to full activity. The healing process must have an opportunity to accomplish what it is supposed to.

10–2 Immobilization during the inflammatory process may be beneficial; however, controlled mobilization helps the tissue decrease atrophy and enhance the healing process. Controlled mobilization allows the athlete to perform progressive strengthening exercises in a timely manner.

10–3 Initially, a transitory vasoconstriction with the start of blood coagulation of the broken blood vessels occurs. Dilation of the vessels in the region of injury follows, along with the activation of chemical mediators via key cells.

10–4 A grade 2 lateral ankle sprain implies that the joint capsule and ligaments are partially torn. At 3 weeks, the injury has been cleaned of debris and is undergoing the process of

secondary healing. Granulation tissue fills the torn areas, and fibroblasts are beginning to form scar tissue.

10–5 In its acute phase, the injury was not allowed to heal properly. As a result, the injury became chronic, with a proliferation of scar tissue, lymphocytes, plasma cells, and macrophages.

10–6 Uncomplicated acute bone healing goes through five stages: hematoma formation, cellular proliferation, callus formation, ossification, and remodeling.

10–7 Because it is shorter, the left leg has the greater stress during running. This stress creates increased tension on the tibia's concave side, causing an increase in osteoclastic activity.

10–8 The pain is considered to be chronic, deep somatic pain stemming from the low back muscles. It is conducted primarily by the C-type nerve fibers.

10–9 The purpose is to stimulate the large, rapidly conducting nerve fibers to inhibit the smaller and slower nerves that carry pain impulses.

REVIEW QUESTIONS AND CLASS ACTIVITIES

1. What are the three phases of healing, and what are the approximate time frames for each of these three phases?
2. What are the physiological events associated with the inflammatory response phase of the healing process?
3. How can you differentiate between acute and chronic inflammation?
4. How is collagen laid down in the area of injury during the fibroblastic repair phase of healing?
5. Explain Wolff's law and the importance of controlled mobility during the maturation-remodeling phase of healing.
6. What are some of the factors that can have a negative impact on the healing process?
7. Discuss treatment techniques for modifying soft-tissue healing, including anti-inflammatory medications, therapeutic modalities, exercise rehabilitation, and platelet-rich plasma injections.

8. Compare and contrast the course of healing in cartilage, ligaments, muscle, and nerve.
9. What is a basic definition of pain?
10. What are the different types of pain?
11. What are the characteristics of the various sensory receptors?
12. How does the nervous system relay information about painful stimuli?
13. Describe how the gate control mechanism of pain modulation may be used to modulate pain.
14. How does descending pathway pain control modulate pain?
15. What are the opiate-like substances, and how do they modulate pain?
16. What are the assessment scales available to help the athletic trainer determine the extent of pain perception?
17. How can pain perception be modified by cognitive factors?

Chapter Ten ■ Tissue Response to Injury

REFERENCES

1. Aronson PA: Pain theories: A review for application in athletic training and therapy, *Athletic Therapy Today* 7(4):8, 2002.
2. Bailon-Plaza A: Beneficial effects of moderate, early loading and adverse effects of delayed or excessive loading on bone healing, *Journal of Biomechanics* 36(8):1069, 2003.
3. Barrientos S: Growth factors and cytokines in wound healing, *Wound Repair and Regeneration*, 16(5):585–602, 2008.
4. Battery L: Inflammation in overuse tendon injuries, *Sports Medicine and Arthroscopy Reviews*, 19(3):213–17, 2011.
5. Black KP: Perpheral afferent nerve regeneration. In Lephart S, Fu F, editors: *Proprioception and neuromuscular control in joint stability*, Champaign, IL, 2000, Human Kinetics.
6. Borrione P: Platelet-rich plasma in muscle healing, *American Journal of Physical Medicine and Rehabilitation*, 89(1):854, 2010.
7. Campbell W: Evaluation on management of peripheral nerve injury, *Clinical Neurophysiology*, 119(9):1951–65, 2008.
8. Casey C: Transition from acute to chronic pain and disability: A model including cognitive, affective and trauma factors, *Pain*, 134(2):69–79, 2008.
9. Clark B: In vivo alterations in skeletal muscle form and function after disuse atrophy, *Medicine and Science in Sport and Exercise*, 2009.
10. Creighton A, Spang J, Dahners L: Basic science of ligament healing: Medial collateral ligament healing with and without treatment, *Sports Med Arthroscopy Review* 13(3):145, 2005.
11. Deleo J: Basic science of pain, *Bone Joint Surg* 88(s):58, 2006.
12. Denegar CR, Prentice W: Managing pain with therapeutic modalities. In Prentice WE, editor: *Therapeutic modalities in sports medicine and athletic training*, ed 6, San Francisco, 2010, McGraw-Hill.
13. Diegelmann R: Wound healing: An overview of acute, fibrotic, and delayed healing, *Frontiers in Bioscience*, (2):283–89, 2004.
14. Ferrry A: Stress fractures in athletes, *Physician and Sports Medicine*, 38(2):109–18, 2010.
15. Gallin J, Snyderman R, Haynes B: *Inflammation: Basic principles and clinical correlates*, Baltimore, 1999, Lippincott Williams and Wilkins.
16. Hildebrand KA, Behm C, Kydd A: The basics of soft tissue healing and general factors that influence such healing, *Sports Med Arthroscopy Review* 13(3):136, 2005.
17. Hill C: Rehabilitation of soft tissue and musculoskeletal injury. In O'Young B: *Physical medicine and rehabilitation secrets*, Philadelphia, 2007, Hanley-Belfus.
18. Hubbel S, Buschbacher R: Tissue injury and healing: Using medications, modalities, and exercise to maximize recovery. In Bushbacher R, Branddom R, editors: *Sports medicine and rehabilitation: A sport specific approach*, Philadelphia, 2008, Elsevier Health Services.
19. Irrgang JJ, Pezzullo D: Rehabilitation following surgical procedures to address articular cartilage lesions in the knee, *J Orthop Sports Phys Ther* 28(4):232, 1998.
20. Isaacs J: Treatmnt of acute peripheral nerve injuries: Current concepts, *Journal of Hand Surgery*, 35(3):491–97, 2010.
21. Kocher MS: Ligament healing and augmentation. In *Proceedings, National Athletic Trainers' Association, 10th annual meeting and clinical symposia*, Champaign, IL, 1999, Human Kinetics.
22. Ley K: *Physiology of inflammation*, Bethesda, MD, 2001, American Physiological Society.
23. Li J: Pathophysiology of acute wound healing, *Clinics in Dermatology*, 25(1):9–18, 1997.
24. Maffulli N: Basic science of tendons, *Sports Med Arthroscopy Review* 8(1):1, 2000.
25. Malone T, Garrett W, Zachewski J: Muscle: Deformation, injury and repair. In Zachazewski J, Magee D, Quillen W, editors: *Athletic injuries and rehabilitation*, Philadelphia, 1996, WB Saunders.
26. Marsell R: The biology of fracture healing, *Injury*, 42(6):551–55, 2011.
27. Molloy T: The roles of growth factors in tendon and ligament healing, *Sports Med* 33(5):381, 2003.
28. Murdoch S: Managing the inflammatory response through nutritional supplements, *Athletic Therapy Today* 6(5):46, 2001.
29. Murrell GAC, Jang D, Lily E, Best T: The effects of immobilization and exercise on tendon healing, *Journal of Science and Medicine in Sport* 2(1 Supplement):40, 1999.
30. Musahl V: Cartilage injuries. In Ranawat A: *Musculoskeletal examination of the hip and knee*, Thorofare, NJ, 2011, Slack.
31. Paoloni J: Platelet-rich plasma treatment for ligament and tendon injuries, *Clinical Journal of Sports Medicine*, 21(1):37–45, 2011.
32. Prentice WE: *Therapeutic modalities in rehabilitation*, ed 4, New York, 2011, McGraw-Hill.
33. Rees J: Management of tendinopathy, *American Journal of Sports Medicine*, 37(9):1855–67, 2009.
34. Redler L: Platelet-rich plasma therapy: An systematic literature review and evidence for clinical use, *Physician and SportsMedicine* 39(1):42–51, 2011.
35. Sandrey M: Acute and chronic tendon injuries: Factors affecting the healing response and treatment, *J Sport Rehabil* 12(1):70, 2003.
36. Sandrey MA: Effects of acute and chronic pathomechanics on the normal histology and biomechanics of tendons: A review, *J Sport Rehabil* 9(4):339, 2000.
37. Seeley R, Stephens T, Tate P: *Seeley's anatomy and physiology*, St. Louis, 2010, McGraw-Hill.
38. Serhan C: *Fundamentals of inflammation*, Cambridge, UK, 2010, Cambridge University Press.
39. Shah R: Utilization of prolotherapy for facilitation of ligament and tendon healing, *Athletic Therapy Today*, 15(6):25, 2010.
40. Shelemay K: *Pain and its transformations: The interface of biology and culture*, Boston, 2007, Harvard University Press.
41. Steiner D: Pathophysiology of ligament injuries. In Comfort P: *Sports rehabilitation and injury prevention*, New York, 2010, John Wiley & Sons.
42. Taylor M: Treating chronic tendon injuries, *Athletic Therapy Today* 5(6):50, 2000.
43. Thompson L: Skeletal muscle adaptations with age, inactivity, and therapeutic exercise, *J Orthop Sports Phys Ther* 32(2):2002.
44. Velnar T: The wound healing process: An overview of the cellular and molecular mechanisms, *Journal of International Medical Research*, 37(5):1528–42, 2009.
45. Volgas D: *A manual of soft tissue management in orthopedic trauma*, New York, 2011, Thieme.
46. Walker JM: Pathomechanics and classification of cartilage lesions, facilitation of repair, *J Orthop Sports Phys Ther* 28(4):216, 1998.
47. Ward P: Acute inflammation and chronic inflammation. In Serhan C: *Fundamentals of inflammation*, Cambridge, UK, 2010, Cambridge University Press.
48. Warren G, Ingalls C, Lowe D: What mechanisms contribute to the strength loss that occurs during and in the recovery from skeletal muscle injury? *J Orthop Sports Phys Ther* 32(2):2002.
49. Weintraub W: *Tendon and ligament healing: A new approach to sports and overuse injury*, Brookline , MA, 2005, Paradigm.
50. Westerblad H: Skeletal muscle: Energy metabolism, fiber types fatigue and adaptability, *Experimental Cell Research*, 316(18):3093–99, 2010.
51. Woo S, Moon D, Miura K: Basic science of ligament healing: anterior cruciate ligament graft biomechanics and knee kinematics, *Sports Med Arthroscopy Review* 13(3):161, 2005.
52. Young, A: The physiology of wound healing, *Surgery*, 29(10):475–79, 2011.

ANNOTATED BIBLIOGRAPHY

Damjanov I, editor: *Anderson's pathology*, ed 10, Philadelphia, 1996, Elsevier Science.

A major pathology text that discusses inflammation and healing in depth.

Kloth L, McCulloch J: *Wound healing: alternatives in management*, Philadelphia, 2001, Davis.

An excellent discussion of factors influencing wound healing, evaluation, and methods of treatment.

Melzack R, Wall P: *Handbook of pain management*, Philadelphia, 2003, Elsevier.

A summary of current knowledge of pain states and their management for all health care professionals involved in the diagnosis and treatment of patients with a wide variety of acute and chronic pain problems.

Porth CM: *Pathophysiology: Concepts of altered health states*, ed 8, Philadelphia, 2010, Lippincott, Williams and Wilkins.

An in-depth text on the physiology of altered health; contains an excellent discussion on inflammation, healing, and pain.

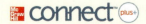

PART IV

Management Skills

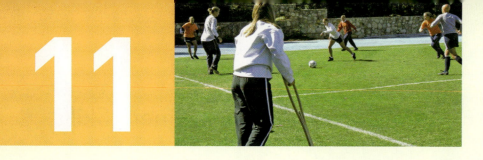

11

Psychosocial Intervention for Sports Injuries and Illnesses

■ Objectives

When you finish this chapter you should be able to

- Analyze the patient's psychological response to injury.
- Recognize the importance of social support for the injured athlete.
- Explain the relationship of stress and overtraining to the risk of injury.
- Describe the role of the athletic trainer as a counselor to the injured athlete.
- Identify the psychological factors important to rehabilitating the injured athlete.
- Compare and contrast the mental training techniques that are used to manage the psychological aspects of injury.
- Recognize the different mental disorders and the appropriate referral and treatment techniques.

■ Outline

■ Key Terms

stressor
anxiety

catecholamine

■ Connect Highlights

Visit connect.mcgraw-hill.com for further exercises to apply your knowledge:

- Clinical application scenarios covering psychological response to injury, social support, relationship of stress and overtraining, athletic trainer as a counselor, psychological factors in rehabilitation, mental training techniques, and mental disorders
- Click-and-drag questions covering psychological response to injury, and the athletic trainer as a counselor
- Multiple-choice questions covering social support, relationship of stress and overtraining, psychological factors important in rehabilitation, mental training techniques, and mental disorders

Certainly, the injured or ill patient experiences physical disability. But for many individuals, the psychological and sociological consequences of injury can be as debilitating as the physical injuries.[47] These psychological and sociological reactions, combined with the physical injury itself, can have an adverse impact on the injured athlete's successful return to competition. All of those involved with the health care of an injured patient must understand how the psyche, especially feelings and emotions, enters into that individual's reactions to injury or illness and ultimately how it affects the rehabilitation process (Figure 11–1).[17,35] The athletic trainer must also be aware of the cultural factors of an injured patient that may come into play during the rehabilitative process, and must be sensitive to those concerns on the part of the patient.[14]

Each individual reacts to injury and illness in a very personal way and makes unique adaptations to these challenges.[7] Some individuals view an injury or illness as devastating; others take such a setback in stride.[25] Some have problems with emotional control after sustaining an injury or illness. The athletic trainer must be aware that returning an injured patient to full, all-out competition requires that individual to be completely ready psychologically as well as physically.[14] Success in sports performance requires fundamental skills, such as speed, attention, concentration, stress management, and the ability to perform cognitive strategies.

Some individuals have a tendency to sustain injuries, whereas others under similar circumstances can stay injury free.[28] Countless physical and psychosocial factors can interact to predispose a person to injury as well as influence the effectiveness of the rehabilitation process.[61] No one personality type can be associated with accident-proneness. However, individuals who are risk takers seem to be more prone to injury. These individuals have a higher competition anxiety, demonstrate sensation-seeking behaviors, and have a high motivation for success, but they lack the appropriate coping skills to address these stressors.[28]

THE PSYCHOLOGICAL RESPONSE TO INJURY

Not all patients deal with injury in the same manner.[7] One person may view an injury as disastrous; another may view it as an opportunity to show courage; a third may embrace the injury to avoid embarrassment over poor performance, to provide an escape from a losing team, or to discourage a domineering parent.[25]

Some factors are common among patients who are adjusting to injury and rehabilitation. The severity of the injury usually determines the length of rehabilitation.[25] Generally, injuries are classified as short-term (less than 4 weeks),

> **Reactive phases:**
> - Reaction to injury
> - Reaction to rehabilitation
> - Reaction to return

long-term (more than 4 weeks), chronic (recurring), or terminating (career-ending). Regardless of the severity of the injury and the corresponding length of time required for rehabilitation, the injured athlete has to deal with a variety of emotions that may occur during three reactive phases of the injury and rehabilitation process (Figure 11–2). These reactive phases are reaction to injury, reaction to rehabilitation, and reaction to return to competition or career termination.[25] Not all individuals have all of these reactions, nor do all reactions fall precisely into the suggested sequence. Some psychologists have applied five stages of psychological reaction to injury. Based on Kübler-Ross's classic model of reactions to death and dying, which includes *denial, anger, bargaining, depression,* and *acceptance* (Figure 11–3).[33] Although this model is commonly considered to be applicable to terminal illnesses or death, it is generally not considered to be applicable to less significant injuries such as those that occur in sport. An alternative cognitive appraisal model has been proposed that focuses more on injured athletes' personal and situational factors and how these influence their cognitive appraisal of the injury situation.[61] It focuses on their interpretation of the injury rather than on the actual severity of the injury. Cognitive appraisal is what determines the athlete's emotional response (e.g., anger, depression, tension) and behavioral response (i.e., adherence to rehabilitation). These cognitive, emotional, and behavioral responses are interdependent and collectively influence recovery outcome. Other factors that can influence reactions to injury

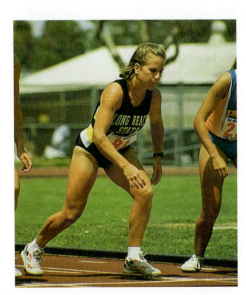

FIGURE 11–1 Sports participation can cause the athlete to experience either negative or positive stress.

Length of rehabilitation	Reaction to injury	Reaction to rehabilitation	Reaction to return
Short (<4 weeks)	Shock Relief	Impatience Optimism	Eagerness Anticipation
Long (>4 weeks)	Fear Anger	Loss of vigor Irrational thoughts Alienation	Acknowledgment
Chronic (recurring)	Anger Frustration	Dependence or independence Apprehension	Confidence or skepticism
Terminating (career-ending)	Isolation Grief process	Loss of athletic identity	Closure and renewal

FIGURE 11–2 Progressive reactions of athletes based on severity of injury and length of rehabilitation.

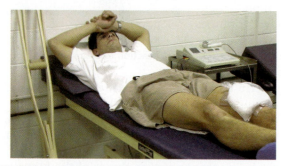

FIGURE 11–3 A sports injury can create psychological reactions characteristic of a sudden loss.

and rehabilitation are the athlete's coping skills, history of injury, social support, and personality traits.[31]

With any type of injury, but particularly with those that require a lengthy period of rehabilitation, athletes whose whole life tends to revolve around a sport may have to make major adjustments in how they perceive themselves and may have to come to terms with how they are perceived by others.[50] Therefore, many athletes have difficulty controlling their emotions when they sustain an injury (see *Focus Box 11-1:* "Psychological barriers to rehabilitation").

Injury might mean major changes in the way an athlete behaves socially.

THE ATHLETE AND THE SOCIOLOGICAL RESPONSE TO INJURY

Following injury, particularly one that requires long-term rehabilitation, all patients and especially athletes may have problems adjusting socially and may feel alienated from the rest of the team.[23] Athletes with an injury that requires weeks or months of rehabilitation before they can return to competition often feel that the coaches have ceased to care, that teammates have no time to spend with them, that friends are no longer around, and that their social life consists of time put into rehabilitation. Some athletes feel that they have received little support from coaches and teammates.[25,62]

Injured athletes may understand that the coach cares but has no expertise in injury management and must be concerned with getting the team ready without them. The athletic trainer has no expertise in coaching but is primarily interested in rehabilitating injuries. Injured athletes may feel unable to maintain or regain normal relationships with teammates.[57] The injured athlete is a reminder that injury can happen, and teammates may pull away from that constant reminder. Friendships based on athletic identification are now compromised because the athletic identification is gone; friends and team members may relate to injured athletes only in terms of what they did yesterday or as injured teammates, not as individuals. Injured athletes no longer feel the team camaraderie that provided a sense of belonging or importance. Athletes who can remain involved with the team,

11-1 Clinical Application Exercise

Patients who are injured must deal with both the physiological and the psychological aspects of injury.

? What stages of psychological reaction does the patient typically go through following injury?

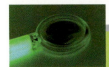

FOCUS 11–1 Focus on Treatment and Rehabilitation

Psychological barriers to rehabilitation

- Depression or grief
- Anxiety
- Anger, agitation, or aggression
- Denial
- Sleep disturbance
- Psychosocial isolation
- Substance abuse

From NATA brochure, *Psychological hints for rehabilitation success,* Dallas, TX.

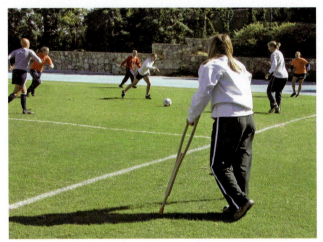

FIGURE 11–4 It is important to make sure that injured athletes still feel that they are part of the team.

however, feel less isolated and less guilty about not being able to help the team (Figure 11–4).[25]

The Athlete's Need for Social Support

The loss of social support can be lessened by the organization of support groups or similar injury groups or by mentoring by athletes who have completed rehabilitation successfully.[18] After injury, athletes need the support of teammates to prevent feelings of negative self-worth and loss of identity. Support groups need to stress the importance of the athlete as a person as well as a team member.[30]

A supporting relationship between the athlete and the athletic trainer is critical to successful rehabilitation.[55] Establishing this relationship may be difficult. Injured athletes often question many aspects of the rehabilitation procedure. They question the doctor's diagnosis; they question the athletic trainer for working them too much and the coach

for not paying attention to them. They wonder whether they are thought of as malingerers. They doubt that the athletic trainer, coach, or teammates know how important competition is to them.[25]

Toward the end of rehabilitation, the athlete should begin sport-specific drills during practice time with his or her athletic team. The athlete then begins to reenter the team culture and is not isolated from the team environment.[64] Thus, the athlete puts more effort into functional, sport-specific situations that are generally less boring. In so doing, the athlete gains a more realistic appreciation of the skills needed to attain preinjury performance levels. Athletes can more easily tolerate the rehabilitation routine if they can see some carryover to their sport.[25]

The Athletic Trainer's Role in Providing Social Support

The athletic trainer is often the first person an athlete interacts with after injury. When an athlete is injured and becomes a patient, he or she should get the perception that the athletic trainer cares for him or her as a person and not just as a part of the team.[29] His or her perception of the athletic trainer makes a difference in terms of recovery time and effort.[41] First the patient has to respect the athletic trainer as a person before he or she can trust the athletic trainer in the rehabilitative setting. Successful communication between the athletic trainer and the patient is essential for effective rehabilitation.[5] Taking an interest in athletes before injuries occur enables the athletic trainer to know their personalities and work with them to help build their confidence.[25]

Be a Good Listener Active listening is one of the athletic trainer's most important skills. The athletic trainer must learn to listen to the patient beyond the complaining and listen for fear, anger, depression, or anxiety. With *fear,* the patient may be wondering what the pain means in terms of function and if he or she will be accepted by peers. *Anger* is often a feeling of being victimized by the injury and the unfairness of it. In *depression,* the patient may have an overwhelming feeling of hopelessness or loneliness. With *anxiety,* the patient may wonder how he or she can survive the injury and what will happen if he or she cannot return to full competition.[45]

Find Out What the Problem Is During an injury evaluation, the athletic trainer should allow the patient to provide as much input about the injury as possible. Paraphrasing or restating the information to the patient will be invaluable to the athletic trainer who is unsure of the mechanism of injury or its results. Statements such as "I see" or "Go ahead" or simply silence allow patients to fully express themselves. One of the most important bits of information can be the question the athletic trainer poses at the end of gathering subjective information— "What else have I not asked you?" or "What else do I need to know about this injury?" Then the athletic trainer should give the patient input in the decision of how the rehabilitation will proceed.

Be Aware of Body Language Body language is important. The athletic trainer who continues to work on paperwork while talking to the patient is sending a message that he or she does not care. The athletic trainer needs to be concerned and should make eye contact with the patient and show a genuine interest in his or her problems. This will go a long way toward gaining the patient's confidence and respect.[25]

Project a Caring Image It is important for the athletic trainer to consider the patient as an individual instead of as an injury. If the injury is the only consideration, the athletic trainer is caring for the patient superficially, and the patient's attitude will project this.

The relationship between the athletic trainer and the patient should be a personal one. When the athletic trainer treats the patient as an equal, the relationship improves, and it helps the patient accept responsibility for his or her own rehabilitation. With injury, athletes lose control over their physical efforts. They have gone from practicing or competing 3 to 4 hours a day to no activity. They experience a temporary lifestyle change, and their feelings will affect the success or failure of the rehabilitation process. The athletic trainer must establish rapport and show a sense of genuine concern and caring for the patient.

Neglecting injured patients or giving them the perception that they are outcasts can also contribute to injury and reinjury. Athletic trainers who foster this attitude are communicating to patients that they have no self-worth if they are injured. Some athletic trainers go so far as to prevent injured patients from having contact with the team until they are ready to return, or they belittle the patient in front of his or her peers, believing that this will make the patient want to get back to competition quicker. This tactic may work with some patients who have minor injuries, but it may cause major adjustment difficulties for patients who suffer severe injuries.[25]

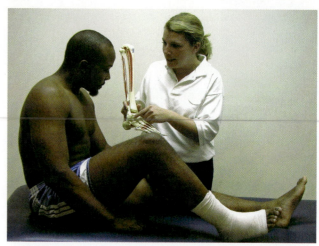

FIGURE 11–5 Educating the athlete about his or her injury is a major goal in the rehabilitation process.

Explain the Injury to the Patient The athletic trainer is often the person who effectively explains the injury to the patient (Figure 11–5). The athletic trainer should take care to explain the situation to the patient in understandable terms, avoiding the use of excessive medical terminology. The athletic trainer should avoid making false promises to make the patient feel better. In most cases, providing the patient with the simplest explanation acceptable is best. Athletes must be satisfied with the explanation of their injury. Disseminating injury information that is appropriate to a patient's emotional and intellectual level can be a challenge. The rate and degree of acceptance is not the same in all patients. The severity of the injury is important, but the patient's perception of that severity is what matters in the rehabilitation process.[25] Thus, the physiological must be interrelated with the psychological.

Manage the Stress of Injury The amount of stress associated with playing a sport and the meaning the sport has to the injured patient can impact the patient's compliance with rehabilitation.[22] The patient will have a more successful rehabilitation when he or she is fully engaged in it, much as an athlete will have a more successful sports career when he or she is interested and involved in the sport. Stress can be a deterrent to engaging in rehabilitation. Several techniques the athletic trainer can use, such as relaxation, imagery, cognitive restructuring, and thought stopping (discussed later in this chapter), may lessen a patient's stressful reaction to injury. Often a change in a patient's perception of his or her injury and rehabilitation can affect their outcome.[25]

Help the Athlete Return to Competition Returning to competition is another area in which the athletic trainer can help the injured patient. Often, the patient's perception is that he or she is ready to return and is not being allowed to or that he or she is being forced to return before being ready. The athletic trainer can help the patient make a decision based on facts, not clouded by emotions.

The athletic trainer can be of great help when an injured patient is unable or unwilling to continue to participate in his or her sport. Frequently, the athlete's identity is intertwined with the sport.[30] The transition into a completely different culture can be a stressful, frustrating, and traumatic experience for an injured patient.[25]

PREDICTORS OF INJURY

The Injury-Prone Athlete

Some athletes seem to have a pattern of injury, whereas others in exactly the same position with the same physical makeup are injury free.[33] It has been suggested that some psychological traits may predispose an athlete to repeated injury. No single personality type has been recognized as injury prone. However,

> Many injury-prone athletes are risk takers.

the person who likes to take risks often seems injury prone.[30] Other types of athletes who may be predisposed to injury are reserved, detached, or tender-minded players[19] and apprehensive, overprotective, or easily distracted players.[10] These individuals usually also lack the ability to cope with the stress associated with the risks and their consequences. Some other factors may also contribute to the likelihood of injury, such as trying to reduce anxiety by being more aggressive or continuing to play while injured because of fear of failure or guilt over unobtainable or unrealistic goals.[1,30]

11–3 Clinical Application Exercise

Some athletes seem to get injured more often than others.

? What factors should the athletic trainer look for that might make the possibility of injury more likely in certain athletes?

stressor The positive and negative forces that can disrupt the body's equilibrium.

Stress and the Risk of Injury

A **Stressor** is not something that an athlete can do to his or her body, but it is something that the brain tells the athlete is happening.[48] When change occurs, the brain interprets that change and tells the body how to react to it. Stress does not always imply a morbid change—it could also be associated with intense pleasure.[48] Stress is caused or triggered by stressors that

may be physical, social, or psychological and that may be negative or positive in nature. Positive beneficial stress is referred to as *eustress*, whereas the term *distress* describes detrimental responses or negative stressors. Often, there is a fine line between eustress and distress. Sometimes the difference between eustress and distress is only a matter of interpretation; a stressor can be interpreted as either a threat or a challenge.

A number of studies on adverse stress have shown a relationship between life events or personal losses and physical injury among athletes who engage in high-intensity sports.[19] Negative stress tends to decrease the athlete's attentional focus and create muscle tension, which may lead to a reduction in flexibility, problems in coordination, and an overall decrease in movement efficiency. A loss of attentional focus can cause the athlete to miss important cues.[58]

All living organisms are endowed with the ability to cope effectively with stressful situations. Without stress, there would be very little constructive activity or positive change.[22]

> Sports participation is both a physical and an emotional stressor.

Negative stress can contribute to poor health, whereas positive stress can enhance growth and development. A healthy life must have a balance of stress; too little stress causes a "rusting out," and too much can cause burnout.[33]

Every day athletes place their bodies in stressful situations. Their bodies undergo numerous "flight-or-fight" reactions to avoid injury or other physically and emotionally threatening situations.

Physical Response to Stress Many stress responses are apparent when athletes adjust to a physical injury and/or undergo a program of rehabilitation.[15]

Stress is a psychosomatic phenomenon. Injury can be a major stressor. Hormonal responses are reflected by an increase in the secretion of cortisol. Negative stress can produce fear and anxiety. Initially, in an acute reaction to a negative stress situation, secretions from the adrenal gland sharply increase, creating the well-known flight-or-fight response. With adrenaline in the bloodstream, pupils dilate, hearing becomes more acute, muscles

11–4 Clinical Application Exercise

Most athletic trainers do not have academic training as counselors or psychologists.

? If an injured patient is not responding psychologically to the efforts of the athletic trainer to rehabilitate and return that individual to full activity, what options does the athletic trainer have for referring this patient for additional help?

become more responsive, and blood pressure increases to facilitate the absorption of oxygen. In addition to these responses, respiration and heart rate increase to further prepare the body for action.

In general, stress can be acute and chronic. During acute stress, the threat is immediate and the response is instantaneous. Physiologically, the primary reaction in the acute stage is produced by the release of epinephrine and norepinephrine from the adrenal medulla. Chronic stress persists over time and leads to an increase of blood corticoids from the adrenal cortex.

An athlete who is taken out of a sport because of an injury or illness reacts in a personal way. The athlete who has trained diligently, has looked forward to a successful season, and is suddenly thwarted in that goal by an injury or illness can be emotionally devastated.

At the time of injury or illness, the patient may normally fear the experience of pain or possible disability. The patient may feel a sense of anxiety about suddenly becoming disabled and being unable to continue sport participation.[48] An injury or illness is a stressor that results from an external or internal sensory stimulus. Coping with the stressor depends on the patient's cognitive appraisal.

Emotional Response to Stress Sports are stressors to the athlete. An athlete often walks a fine line between reaching and maintaining peak performance and overtraining. Besides performance concerns, many peripheral stressors can be imposed on the athlete, such as unreasonable expectations by the athlete, the coaches, or the parents. Worries that stem from school, work, and family can also be major causes of emotional stress.

The coach is often the first person to notice that an athlete is stressed emotionally. The athlete whose performance is declining and whose personality is changing may need a training program that is less demanding. Conferring with the athlete might reveal emotional and physical problems that need to be dealt with by a counselor, psychologist, or physician.

Injury prevention is both psychological and physiological. The athlete who enters a contest while angry, frustrated, or discouraged or while experiencing some other disturbing emotional state is more prone to injury than is the one who is better adjusted emotionally. The angry player, for example, wants to vent that anger in some way and therefore often loses perspective on desirable and approved conduct. In the grip of emotion, skill and coordination are sacrificed, resulting in an injury that otherwise would have been avoided.

Although athletic trainers are typically not educated as professional counselors or psychologists, they must nevertheless be concerned about the feelings of the athletes they work with.[51] No one can work closely with human beings without becoming involved with their emotions and, at times, their personal problems. The athletic trainer is usually a car-

> The athletic trainer must have some counseling skills.

ing person and, as such, is placed in numerous daily situations in which close interpersonal relationships are important. The athletic trainer must have appropriate counseling skills to confront an athlete's fears, frustrations, and daily crises and to refer individuals with serious emotional problems to the proper professionals. Athletic trainers should be prepared to handle these situations by seeking formal education in counseling.[49]

The team physician, like the coach and the athletic trainer, plays an integral part in helping the athlete who is overly stressed. Many psychophysiological responses thought to be emotional are, in fact, caused by some undetected physical dysfunction. Therefore, referral to a physician, sport psychologist, clinical psychologist, or psychiatrist should be routine. (See *Focus Box 11–10:* "Keys to referral.")

Overtraining

Overtraining occurs because of an imbalance between a physical load placed on an athlete and his or her coping capacity.[2,32] Both physiological and psychological factors underlie overtraining. Overtraining can lead to staleness and eventual burnout.

Staleness There are countless reasons some athletes become "stale." The athlete could be training too hard and long without proper rest. Seasons can be long and practices can become repetitious and boring. Staleness is often attributed to emotional problems stemming from daily worries, fears, and anxieties. **Anxiety** is one of the most common mental and emotional stress producers. It is a vague fear, a sense of apprehension, and restlessness.[9] Typically, the anxious athlete is unable to describe the problem. The athlete feels inadequate

> **anxiety** A feeling of uncertainty or apprehension.

in a certain situation but is unable to say why. Heart palpitations, shortness of breath, sweaty palms, a constricted throat, and headaches may accompany anxiety. Children who are pushed too hard by parents may acquire a number of psychological problems. They may even fail purposely in their sport just to rid themselves of the painful stress of achieving. A coach who acts as a drill sergeant—one who continually gives negative reinforcements—will likely cause athletes to develop symptoms of overstress. Athletes are more prone to staleness if the rewards of their efforts are minimal. A losing season commonly causes many athletes to become stale.

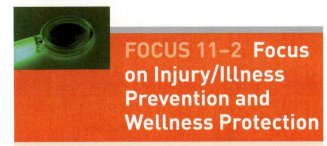

Recognizing signs and symptoms of staleness in athletes

An athlete who is becoming stale will often display some or most of the following signs:

- A decrease in performance level
- Difficulty falling asleep
- Awakening from sleep for no apparent reason
- A loss of appetite and a loss of weight; conversely, the athlete may overeat because of chronic worry
- Indigestion
- Difficulty concentrating
- Difficulty enjoying sex
- Nausea for no apparent reason
- Head colds or allergic reactions
- Behavioral signs of restlessness, irritability, anxiety, or depression
- An elevated resting heart rate and elevated blood pressure
- Psychosomatic episodes of perceiving bodily pains, such as sore muscles, especially before competing
- Arriving late to practice and/or rehabilitation sessions

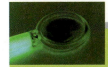

Sudden exercise abstinence syndrome[60]

Symptoms include the following:

- Heart palpitations
- Irregular heartbeat
- Chest pain
- Disturbed appetite and digestion
- Sleep disorders
- Increased sweating
- Depression
- Emotional instability

Symptoms of Staleness Staleness is evidenced by a wide variety of symptoms: a deterioration in the usual standard of performance, chronic fatigue, apathy, loss of appetite, indigestion, weight loss, and an inability to sleep or rest properly.[19] Many athletes will exhibit higher blood pressure or an increased pulse rate, both at rest and during activity, as well as increased **catecholamine** release. All these signs indicate adrenal exhaustion. Stale athletes become irritable and restless, have to force themselves to practice, and exhibit signs of boredom and lassitude about everything connected with the activity (see *Focus Box 11–2:* "Recognizing signs and symptoms of staleness in athletes").[26]

catecholamine Active amines, epinephrine, and norepinephrine, which affect the nervous and cardiovascular systems.

Athletes who show signs of staleness also increase their potential for both acute and overuse injuries and infections.[30] Stress fractures and tendinitis are typical injuries that can occur with overtraining.

Overtraining must be recognized early and dealt with immediately.[60] The athlete should take a short break from training or decrease the workload by performing less work but with the same intensity.[60] When the athlete shows signs of a full recovery, a gradual return to the same workload can be initiated. Competition must be stopped. An abrupt cessation of training, however, can produce a serious physiological and psychological condition known as sudden exercise abstinence syndrome (see *Focus Box 11–3:* "Sudden exercise abstinence syndrome").

Burnout Burnout is a syndrome related to physical and emotional exhaustion that leads to a negative self-concept, negative job or sport attitudes, and loss of concern for the feelings of others.[12] Burnout stems from overwork and can affect both the athlete and the athletic trainer. Athletes are often pulled in many directions trying to satisfy the demands of school, friends, family, and maybe a job in addition to their sport.

Burnout can be detrimental to an athlete's general health.[12] Symptoms include frequent headaches, gastrointestinal disturbances, sleeplessness, and chronic fatigue. Athletes suffering from burnout may also experience feelings of depersonalization, increased emotional exhaustion, a reduced sense of accomplishment, cynicism, and a depressed mood.[61]

REACTING TO ATHLETES WITH INJURIES

Even though athletic trainers need to be proficient in counseling in the areas of injury prevention, injury rehabilitation, and nutrition, they are not usually academically trained for other areas.[37] To meet other counseling needs of the athlete, the athletic trainer needs additional academic preparation or should refer the athlete to a sport psychologist.[11,46]

No matter what reaction the injured athlete displays, the athletic trainer should respond to the

TABLE 11–1 Emotional First Aid

Type of Emotional Reaction	Outward Signs	Athletic Trainer's Reactions	
		Yes	**No**
Normal	Weakness, trembling	Be calm and reassuring	Avoid pity
	Nausea, vomiting		
	Perspiration		
	Diarrhea		
	Fear, anxiety		
	Heart pounding		
Overreaction	Excessive talking	Allow athlete to vent emotions	Avoid telling athlete he or she is acting abnormally
	Argumentativeness		
	Inappropriate joke telling		
	Hyperactivity		
Underreaction	Depression; sitting or standing numbly	Be empathetic; encourage talking to express feelings	Avoid being abrupt; avoid pity
	Little or no talking		
	Lack of emotion		
	Confusion		
	Failure to respond to questions		

patient as a person, not as an injury. An injured patient can be difficult to be around, especially in the early stages of a serious injury. The injury may suddenly force the patient to be dependent and helpless.[26] The patient may regress to childlike behavior, crying or displacing anger toward the person administering first aid. Table 11–1 provides some suggestions on rendering emotional first aid. During this time, comfort, care, and communication should be given freely.[40]

Those involved with health care for the injured patient must be honest, supportive, and respectful of the patient during the time of disability. They need to understand the patient at a deeper level and how he or she is coping with this stressful event.[63] A number of questions should be answered. Does the doctor-patient relationship contain confidence, trust, and optimism?[30] Does the patient fear that a pending surgery will be more painful or will make him or her unable to continue in the sport?[40] How long is the recovery? What is the possibility of reinjury?[40] Is forced retirement possible? If so, how well will the patient adjust? What are the athlete's attitudes toward rehabilitation?

The Catastrophic Injury

A permanent functional disability is a catastrophic injury. Intervention must be directed toward the psychological impact of the trauma and the patient's ability to cope during medical treatment.[43] A catastrophic injury profoundly affects all aspects of a person's functioning. The athletic trainer must arrange for counseling from a psychologist or a psychiatrist to make certain that the patient is receiving the best possible care.[56] The athletic trainer should also be cognizant of the effects of such an injury on other team members.

The Psychological Effects of Injury on the Athletic Trainer

The relationships that an athletic trainer develops with a particular athlete or group of athletes are often very special. Athletic trainers tend to be very caring individuals and when one of those athletes is injured it is likely that the athletic trainer will be psychologically and emotionally affected by that injury as well. It is essential that the athletic trainer make decisions regarding care and management of that injury based on professional training and knowledge of the most appropriate course of action, given the circumstances and severity of the injury. The athletic trainer needs to make sure that emotional attachment to the injured athlete does not cloud or otherwise influence his or her decisions. The athletic trainer must be prepared to deal with significant injuries, to people he or she cares about, that may be psychologically disturbing or catastrophic. An athletic trainer must deal with the injured athlete and situation at hand and worry about how the injury has affected him or her personally at a later time. While the athletic trainer must be strong and confident in managing the initial injury, he or she may need to seek counseling to deal with the impact of that injury on his or her own emotional and psychological state.

PSYCHOLOGICAL FACTORS IN THE REHABILITATION PROCESS

A successful program of rehabilitation takes the patient's psyche into consideration. Successful treatment that involves therapeutic modalities and exercise rehabilitation depends on rapport, cooperation, and education.[26]

> **The psychology of sports rehabilitation must include establishing**
> - Rapport
> - Cooperation
> - Education

Rapport is a relationship of mutual trust and understanding. Patients must thoroughly trust their athletic trainers or therapists to achieve maximum rehabilitation, and they must believe that their best interests are being considered at all times.[26]

A highly motivated athlete begrudges every moment spent out of action and can become somewhat difficult to handle if the rehabilitative process moves slowly.[8] Often, the patient blames the physician or the athletic trainer for not doing all that he or she can. To avoid this situation, the patient must learn early in the rehabilitative process that healing is a cooperative undertaking with the patient, physician, and athletic trainer acting as a team, working toward the same end—the return to full function as soon as physically and physiologically possible. To create this atmosphere, the patient must feel free to vent frustrations, to ask questions, and to expect clear answers about any aspect of the rehabilitative process. The patient must feel a major responsibility to come into the athletic training clinic on time and not skip appointments. He or she must be motivated to perform all exercises correctly and all home exercises regularly.[6]

Many injured athletes lack patience. Nevertheless, patience and desire are necessary adjuncts in securing a reasonable rate of recovery.[23]

To ensure maximum positive responses from the patient in all aspects of rehabilitation, he or she must receive continual education. All education must be provided in layman's language and at a level appropriate for the patient's background and education. *Focus Box 11–4:* "Educating the injured patient about the rehabilitation process" is a list of educational matters that athletic trainers and therapists must address carefully.

Psychological Approaches during the Phases of Rehabilitation

The rehabilitation process incorporates both therapeutic modalities and exercise rehabilitation. During each phase of rehabilitation, the athletic trainer or therapist must address the patient's specific psychological issues.[65]

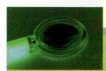

Educating the injured patient about the rehabilitation process

1. Describe the injury clearly, using anatomy charts or other visual aids. The athlete must fully understand the nature of his or her injury and its prognosis (expected outcome), based on similar cases. A false hope for a fast comeback should not be engendered if a full recovery is doubtful.
2. Explain how the healing process occurs and estimate the time needed for such healing.
3. Describe in detail the consequences of not following proper procedures.
4. Describe an overall rehabilitative plan, including progressive steps or phases within the plan.
5. Explain each physical modality or exercise, how it works, and its purpose.
6. Make the athlete aware that recovery depends as much on his or her attitude toward the rehabilitative process as on what therapy is being given. A positive attitude leads to a conscientious and persistent effort to speed recovery.
7. Realize that the athlete needs to see immediate results.[14]
8. Plan rehabilitation around the athlete's schedule.[14]
9. Ensure that the rehabilitation facility is convenient to the athlete.
10. Monitor the athlete regularly.

Immediate Postinjury Period The immediate postinjury period is a time of fear and denial for the patient, who often has severe pain and disability. Emotional first aid must be administered.[67] The physician must give an accurate diagnosis and a full explanation of that diagnosis to the patient and family members. As much as possible, the patient needs to know the course of treatment, the prognosis, and the planned goals. The patient must know from the beginning that he or she is an integral part of rehabilitation.

> A patient has been rehabilitating a surgically repaired knee for 6 months. Physically, she is capable of returning to activity but seems very hesitant to engage in an activity where there is potential contact.
>
> **?** Should the athletic trainer push her back into activity despite her apprehension?
>
> **11–5 Clinical Application Exercise**

Early Postoperative Period When surgery is performed, the injured athlete becomes a disabled patient. Each phase of the healing process and the purpose of each treatment procedure should be explained to the patient. The patient should be encouraged to maintain aerobic conditioning by exercising the noninjured body parts.

Advanced Postoperative, or Rehabilitation, Period

While the patient rehabilitates the injured body part, he or she should continue to condition unaffected body regions both aerobically and anaerobically. The patient must feel that he or she is in control and can make choices. The patient's confidence is increased by small successes. Milestones must be kept realistic, and positive verbal reinforcement must be given by the coach, peers, and sports medicine team.[67]

This period places greater emphasis on movement patterns that mimic a specific sport. Injured athletes need reassurance that they will be able to return to their sport and once again achieve success. Their fear of failure and anxiety should be dealt with by positive reinforcement.[63]

Return to Full Activity Many patients return to participation physically ready but psychologically ill prepared.[43] Although few patients will admit it, they return to participation feeling anxious about getting hurt again. This feeling may, in some ways, be a self-fulfilling prophecy. In other words, anxiety can lead to muscle tension, which in turn can lead to disruption of normal coordination, thus producing conditions that are favorable for reinjury or for injury to another body part.[43] The following are suggestions for helping an athlete regain competitive confidence:

1. The athletic trainer allows the patient to regain full performance by progressing in small increments.[24] Return might include, first, performing all the necessary skills away from the team. This action may be followed by engaging in a highly controlled small-group practice and then attempting participation in full-team noncontact practice. The patient should be encouraged to express freely any anxiety that he or she may feel and to engage in full contact only when anxiety is at a minimum.
2. The athletic trainer can teach the patient the technique of systematic desensitization. The patient first learns to relax consciously as much as possible through the Jacobson progressive relaxation method (described later in this chapter).[27] When the athlete can achieve relaxation at will, he or she, with the help of the athletic trainer, develops a fear hierarchy related to returning to the sport and playing all out.[4] The patient imagines each fear-related step while fully relaxed. If the athlete experiences fear or anxiety at a specific step, the thought processes are halted while

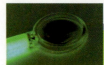

the athlete restores and holds total relaxation until the anxiety has passed. The patient then continues to the next, more anxiety-producing step and repeats the relaxation process until he or she feels no anxiety. The patient who completes the entire list of steps without anxiety and who has completed the proper physical rehabilitation is ready for competition. The use of scales developed specifically for the purpose of assessing the athlete's readiness to return to competitive activity can be helpful to both the athletic trainer, the physician, and the coach who must make that decision.[16]

Goal Setting as a Motivator for Compliance during Rehabilitation

Goal setting has been shown to be an effective motivator for compliance to the rehabilitation of an athletic injury, as well as for reaching goals in a general sport setting.[59] Athletes have set goals since their first competition, usually starting at an early age. They have set goals to run faster, jump higher, shoot straighter, throw longer, hit harder, and so on. These goals have all had one thing in common: They were not achieved with one burst of effort but resulted from meeting many short-term goals before achieving the long-term goal. See *Focus Box 11–5:* "Nine factors to incorporate into goal setting for the athlete."[59]

> **Establishing progressive, attainable goals is essential in rehabilitation.**

In any rehabilitation setting, patients need to know exactly what the goal is and have a sense that they can meet it.[59] For example, telling a patient that, by a certain day, he or she should be bearing partial weight with crutches is neither specific nor measurable. It is more effective to say that, by achieving a certain range of motion and strength level, the foot can be placed on the ground with weight bearing and that the measurement of success is that the partial weight bearing is without pain. The goal must be a challenge but one that the patient can reach with reasonable rehabilitation effort.[2] Goals that are easily reached have no reward in success. Goals must be personal and internally satisfying, not goals imposed on the patient by the athletic trainer. Setting goals needs to be a joint venture between the patient and the athletic trainer to be successful.[14] **The injured patient has to take responsibility for the progress of the injury and be responsible for doing the necessary rehabilitation.[7]**

Goal setting incorporates a multitude of other motivating factors that intuitively appear to increase the odds of compliance by reducing the stress associated with injury rehabilitation. These buffers incorporated within the goal-setting paradigm include positive reinforcement when goals are met, time management for incorporating goals into a lifestyle, a feeling of social support when goals are set with the athletic trainer, and feelings of increased self-efficacy when goals are achieved. Goals are easily understood by athletes, are concrete concepts, are active events, and are a natural part of their sport.[59] Goals can be set daily for a sense of accomplishment, weekly for a sense of progress, and monthly or yearly for long-term achievement.

In general, athletes are highly motivated individuals.

? What can the athletic trainer do to motivate an injured patient to be compliant with the rehabilitation program?

11–6 Clinical Application Exercise

MENTAL TRAINING TECHNIQUES

Mental training techniques have long been used to enhance sports skills.[39] Many of these techniques are appropriate for injured athletes in the process of healing and rehabilitating a serious injury or illness.[39]

Athletic trainers can help injured athletes to respond positively to their injuries via specific mental training techniques.[66] It should be noted that serious emotional instabilities must be referred to a professional psychologist.[52] Some techniques that are available are quieting the anxious mind, mental and emotional assessment, pain control, and healing approaches.

Techniques for Reducing Tension and Anxiety

Fear and anxiety are always present to some degree in a serious sports injury or illness. Fear of pain, loss of control, and unknown consequences of disability can create physical and emotional tensions. Two techniques that the athlete can learn to deal with anxiety and tension are meditation and progressive relaxation.

An athlete who has experienced several different injuries throughout the season is anxious about performing at his usual level.

? What can the athletic trainer recommend to help the patient relax before a game?

11–7 Clinical Application Exercise

Meditation Meditators focus on a constant mental stimulus, such as a phrase, a sound, or a single word repeated silently or audibly, or they gaze steadily at some object. The passive attitude of meditation takes a "don't work at it" approach. As thoughts come into the consciousness, they are quietly turned away, and the individual returns to the focus of attention. The meditator takes a comfortable position and relaxes the various major body areas. To effectively conduct a meditation session, a quiet environment is essential. Normally, the eyes are closed unless the meditator is focusing on some external object (see *Focus Box 11–6:* "The meditation technique").

Progressive Relaxation Progressive muscle relaxation is probably the most extensively used technique for relaxation.[27] It can be considered intense training in the awareness of tension and tension's release. Progressive relaxation may be practiced in a reclining position or while seated in a chair. Each muscle group is tensed from 5 to 7 seconds, then relaxed for 20 to 30 seconds. In most cases, one repetition of the procedure is sufficient; however, if tension remains in the area, repeated contraction and relaxation is permitted. The sequence of tensing and releasing is systematically applied to the following body areas: the dominant hand and forearm; dominant upper

An athlete has a chronic back injury.

? How can the athletic trainer help the athlete deal with the chronic pain?

11–8 Clinical Application Exercise

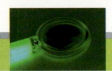
The meditation technique

Quieting the body

The person sits comfortably in a position that maintains a straight back; the head is erect and the hands are placed loosely on each leg or on the arm of a chair, with both feet firmly planted on the floor. To ensure a relaxed state, the meditator should mentally relax each body part, starting at the feet. If a great deal of tension is present, Jacobson's relaxation exercise (see Focus Box 11–7) might be appropriate, or several deep breaths are taken in and exhaled slowly and completely, allowing the body to settle more and more into a relaxed state after each emptying of the lungs.

The meditative technique

Once the person is in a quiet environment and fully physically relaxed, the meditative process can begin. With each exhalation, the person emits a repetitive self-talk of a short word, such as *one* or *peace*. The word is repeated for 10 to 20 minutes. Such words as *peace* and *relaxed* are excellent relaxers; however, Benson[3] has suggested that the word *one* produces the same physiological responses as any other word. If extraneous thoughts occur, the person just returns to the meditation process.

After meditating

After repeating the special word, the person comes back to physical reality slowly and gently. As awareness increases, physical activity should also increase. Moving too quickly or standing up suddenly might produce lightheadedness or dizziness.

---

arm; nondominant hand and forearm; nondominant upper arm; forehead; eyes and nose; cheeks and mouth; neck and throat; chest; back; respiratory muscles; abdomen; dominant upper leg, calf, and foot; and nondominant upper leg, calf, and foot. Throughout the session, a number of expressions for relaxing may be used: "Let the tension dissolve. Let go of the tension. I am bringing my muscles to zero. Let the tension flow out of my body."

After the individual has become aware of the tension in the body, the contraction is gradually decreased until little remains. At this point, the individual focuses on one area and mentally wills the tension to decrease to zero, or complete relaxation.

Jacobson's progressive relaxation normally takes longer than the time allowed in a typical session or than the individual would want to spend.[27] A short form can be developed that, although not as satisfactory, helps the individual become better aware of the body (see *Focus Box 11–7:* "Jacobson's progressive relaxation"). The essence of Jacobson's method is to recognize and consciously release muscular tension.

11–9 Clinical Application Exercise

A collegiate gymnast suffers a season-ending shoulder injury. She expresses concern about gaining weight due to the lack of exercise.

❓ How should the athletic trainer deal with this situation? What tools should he or she use?

Techniques for Cognitive Restructuring

Some injured athletes practice irrational thinking and negative self-talk. This habit can hinder the treatment progress. An important approach to negative thoughts is cognitive restructuring.[22] Two successful methods to thought restructuring are refuting irrational thoughts and thought stopping.[26]

Refuting Irrational Thoughts This method is designed to deal with a person's internal dialogue. Psychologist Albert Ellis developed a system to change irrational ideas and beliefs.[26] His system is called rational emotive therapy. The basic premise is that actual events do not create emotions; rather, it is the self-talk after the event that does. In other words, irrational self-talk causes anxiety, anger, and depression.

Individuals who are under severe stress should explore their self-talk. Following are two examples:

1. *Facts and events:* A tennis player, after surgical repair of her shoulder, is impatient about the speed of recovery. Emotions of anger and depression are present.
   Negative self-talk:
   "I was stupid to get hurt."
   "Why me? Why did I have to get hurt?"
   "I have never been laid up before. It's not fair!"
   Positive self-talk:
   "I was hurt and now I am doing my best to get well."
   "Every day I am getting better."
   "The athletic trainers are doing their best for me."

2. *Facts and events:* A football player blows a knee out and requires surgery. Emotions of anger and denial are present.
   Negative self-talk:
   "I was blindsided and no penalty was called."
   "I could have avoided such a serious injury if the coaches coached better."

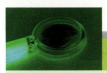

Jacobson's progressive relaxation[27]

Beginning instructions

1. Get into a position that is relaxed and comfortable.
2. Breathe in and out easily and allow yourself to relax as much as possible.
3. Make yourself aware of your total body and the tensions that your muscles might have within them.

The arms

1. Clench your right fist. Increase the grip more and more until you feel the tension created in your hand and forearm.
2. Slowly open your fist and allow the tension to flow out slowly until there is no tension left in your hand and forearm.
3. Feel how soft and relaxed the hand and forearm are, and contrast this feeling with the left hand.
4. Repeat this procedure with the left hand, gripping hard and bringing the tension into the fist and forearm.
5. Bend your right elbow and bring tension into the right biceps, tensing it as hard as you possibly can and observing the tightness of the muscle.
6. Relax and straighten the arm, allowing the tension to flow out.
7. Repeat the tension and relaxation technique with the left biceps.

The head

1. Wrinkle your forehead as hard as you can and hold that tension for 5 seconds or longer.
2. Relax and allow the forehead and face to smooth out completely.
3. Frown and feel the tension that comes in between the eyes and eyebrows.
4. Let go to a completely blank expression. Feel the tension flow out of your face.
5. Squint your eyes tighter and tighter, feeling the tension creep into the eyes.
6. Relax and gently allow your eyes to be closed without tension.
7. Clench your jaw, bite down hard, then harder. Notice the tension in your jaw.
8. Relax. When you are relaxed, allow your lips to be slightly parted and your face to be completely without expression, without wrinkles or tension.
9. Stick your tongue up against the roof of your mouth as hard as possible, feeling the tension in the tongue and the mouth. Hold that tension.
10. Relax, allowing the face and the mouth to be completely relaxed. Allow the tongue to be suspended lightly in the mouth. Relax.
11. Form an O with your lips. Purse the lips hard together, so that you feel the tension around the lips only.
12. Relax, allowing the tension to leave around the lips. Allow your lips to be slightly parted, and allow tension to be completely gone from the face.

The neck and shoulders

1. Press your head back against the mat or chair and feel the tension come into the neck region. Hold that tension. Be aware of it; sense it.
2. Slowly allow the tension to leave, decreasing the amount of pressure applied until the tension has completely gone and you are as relaxed as possible.
3. Bring your head forward, so that your chin is pressing against your chest and tension is brought into your throat and back of your neck. Hold that tension.
4. Slowly return to the beginning position and feel the tension leave your neck. Relax completely.
5. Shrug your shoulders upward, raising your shoulders as far as you can toward your ears, hunching your head between your shoulders. Feel the tension creep into your shoulders. Hold that tension.
6. Slowly let the tension leave by returning your shoulders to their original position. Allow the tension to completely leave the neck and shoulder region. Have a sense of bringing the muscles to zero, where they are completely at ease and without strain.

Respiration and the trunk

1. When the body is completely relaxed and you have a sense of heaviness, allow tension to move to your respiration. Fill the lungs completely and hold your breath for 5 seconds, feeling the tension go into the chest and upper back muscles.
2. Exhale slowly, allowing the air to go out slowly as you feel the tension being released slowly.
3. While your breath is coming slowly and easily, sense the contrast of the breath holding to the breath that is coming freely and gently.
4. Tighten the abdominal muscles by pressing downward on your stomach. Note the tension that comes into your abdominal region, respiratory center, and back region.
5. Relax your abdominal area and feel the tension leave your trunk region.
6. Slightly arch your back against the mat or back of the chair. This should be done without hyperextending or straining. Feel the tension that creeps into and along your spine. Hold that tension.

(continued)

7. Gradually allow your body to sink back into its original position. Feel the tension leave the long muscles of your back.
8. Flatten your lower back by rolling your hips forward. Feel the tension come into your lower back by rolling your hips forward. Hold that tension. Try to isolate that tension from all the other parts of your body.
9. Gradually return to the original position, and feel the tension leave your body. Be aware of any tension that might have crept into body regions that you have already relaxed. Allow your mind to scan your body; go back over the areas that you have released from tension and become aware of whether any tension has returned.

The buttocks and thighs

1. Tense your buttocks for 5 seconds. Try to isolate just the contraction of the buttocks region.
2. Slowly allow the buttocks to return to their normal state, relaxing completely.
3. Contract your thighs by straightening your knees. Hold that contraction, feeling the tension; isolate the tension just to that region, focusing just on the thighs.
4. Slowly allow the tension to leave the region, bringing your entire body to a relaxed state, especially the thighs.
5. To bring the tension to the back of your thighs, press your heels as hard as you can against the floor or mat, slightly bending your knees; bring the tension to the hamstring region and the back

of your thighs. Hold this tension; study it; concentrate on it. Try to isolate the tension from other tensions that might have crept into your body.
6. Relax. Allow the tension to flow out. Return your legs to the original position, and let go of all the tensions of the body.

The lower legs and feet

1. With the legs fully extended, point your feet downward as hard as possible, bringing tension into both calves. Hold that tension. Hold it as hard as you can without cramping.
2. Slowly allow one foot to return to a neutral position, and allow relaxation to occur within the calf muscle. Bring it to zero, if possible—no tension.
3. Curl the toes of the feet downward as hard as you can without pointing the feet downward, isolating the tension just in the bottoms of the feet and toes. Hold that tension. Isolate the tension, if possible, from the calves. Hold it, feeling the tension on the bottoms of your feet.
4. Slowly relax and allow the tension to release from your feet as your toes straighten out.
5. Curl your toes backward toward your kneecaps and bring your feet back into dorsiflexion, so that you feel the tension in the tops of your toes, the tops of your feet, and your shins. Hold that tension. Be aware of it; study the tension.
6. After 5 seconds or longer, return to a neutral state, where your feet are completely relaxed and your toes have returned to their normal position. Feel the tension leave your body.

Positive self-talk:

"I am hurt, but because of my good fitness level I will recover quickly."

"I plan to do everything I am told to recover quickly."

Thought Stopping Thought stopping is an excellent cognitive technique for helping the athlete overcome worries and doubts. The anxious athlete, especially one who is hurt, will often repeat negative, unproductive, and unrealistic statements during self-talk, such as "I am no good to anyone now that I am hurt" or "Everyone on the team is going to pass me by while I am recovering." Thought stopping consists of focusing on the undesired thoughts and stopping them with the command "stop" or a loud noise. After the thought interruption, a positive statement is inserted, such as "My shoulder is healing and I'll play as well as or maybe better than before"[23] (see *Focus Box 11–8:* "Thought stopping").

Imagery

Imagery is the use of the senses to create or re-create an experience in the mind.[13] Visual images used in the rehabilitation process include visual rehearsal,

emotive imagery rehearsal, and body rehearsal.[36] Visual rehearsal uses both coping and mastery rehearsal. In coping rehearsal, athletes visually rehearse problems they feel may stand in the way of their return to competition. They then rehearse how they will overcome these problems.[36] Mastery rehearsal aids in gaining the confidence and motivational skills necessary. Athletes visualize their successful return to competition, beginning with early practice drills and continuing on to the game situation.

Emotive rehearsal aids the injured athlete in gaining confidence and security by visualizing scenes relating to the positive feelings of enthusiasm, confidence, and pride—in other words, the emotional rewards of praise and success from participating well in competition.[10] Body rehearsal empirically helps patients in the healing process. It is suggested that patients visualize their bodies healing internally both during the rehabilitation procedures and throughout their daily activities.[50] To do this, patients have to have a good understanding of the injury and of the type of healing occurring during the rehabilitation process.[38]

Care should be taken to explain the healing and rehabilitative process clearly but not overwhelm

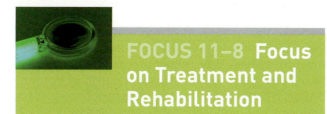

FOCUS 11–8 Focus on Treatment and Rehabilitation

Thought stopping

1. Thoughts immediately precede actions.
2. Patient experiences negative thoughts.
3. Patient recognizes negative thoughts.
4. Patient subconsciously says, "Stop."
5. Patient substitutes a positive statement for a negative thought.

From NATA brochure, *Psychological hints for rehabilitation success*, Dallas, TX.

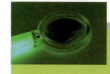

FOCUS 11–9 Focus on Treatment and Rehabilitation

Healing images

Treatment modalities

- Ultrasound increases circulation, bringing healthy new tissue to the area.
- Cold application inhibits pain.

Exercise rehabilitation

- Muscle fibers increase in size and become stronger.
- Joint range of motion increases, so joints become fully functional.

Medications

- Antiinflammatories decrease inflammation and swelling.
- Pain medication inhibits pain.

patients with so much information that they become intimidated and fearful.[53] Educate patients only to the amount of knowledge they require (see *Focus Box 11–9:* "Healing images").

Techniques for Coping with Pain

The injured patient can be taught relatively simple techniques to inhibit pain.[1] At no time should pain be completely inhibited because pain is a protective mechanism. The patient can reduce pain in three ways: reducing muscle tension, diverting attention away from the pain, and changing the pain sensation to another sensation.

Reducing Muscle Tension The pain response can be associated with general muscular tension stemming from anxiety or from the pain-spasm-pain cycle of the injury. In both of these situations, muscle tension increases the sensation of pain. Conversely, relaxation methods that reduce muscle tension can also decrease the awareness of pain. Both the Benson[4] and the Jacobson[27] techniques of stress reduction can be advantageous in pain reduction.

Diverting Attention A positive method for decreasing pain perception is to divert attention from the injury.[28] The athletic trainer should engage the patient in mental problem solving, such as adding or subtracting a column of numbers or counting spots on the floor. The patient can also divert pain by fantasizing about pleasant activities, such as sunbathing at the beach, sailing, or skiing.

Altering the Pain Sensation Imagination is one of the most powerful forces available to human beings. Negative imagination can be a major cause of illness, stress, and muscular tension, whereas positive imagination can produce wellness and counteract stress.

Through imagination, the patient can alter pain sensation to another sensation.[28] For example, immersing a body part in ice-cold water can change the pain to a sensation of cold dampness. The patient can visualize that the injured part is relaxed and comfortable instead of painful. Imagining a peaceful scene at a pleasant spot, such as the beach or mountains, can both relax the athlete and divert attention from the pain.

MENTAL DISORDERS

A mental illness is any disorder that affects the mind or behavior. Mental disorders are common in our society, and it is not uncommon for an athletic trainer to deal with an athlete who has a mental illness.[44] Although the typical athletic trainer has little or no training to deal with this type of illness, he or she must be able to recognize when an individual is having a problem and make a referral to a psychiatrist, psychologist, counselor, or social worker[44,52] (see *Focus Box 11–10:* "Keys to referral"). In the past, mental disorders were generally classified as being either *neuroses* or *psychoses*.[20] A neurosis was thought to be an unpleasant mental symptom in a person who has intact reality testing. Symptoms

An athlete goes to the athletic trainer concerned about her recent changes in mood. She says she feels positive and upbeat one minute but the next minute feels sad and apprehensive.

? What mood disorder might the athlete have, and how should this condition be managed?

11–10 Clinical Application Exercise

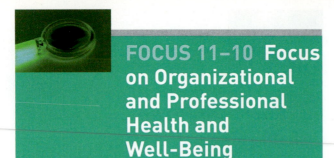

of neurotic behavior included anxiousness, depression, or obsession with a solid base in reality. A psychosis was described as a disturbance in which there was a disintegration in personality and loss of contact with reality, characterized by delusions and hallucinations.[54] Mental illnesses are no longer classified as neuroses or psychoses. Instead, some 300 different mental problems have been identified.[20]

Mood Disorders

Mood swings ranging from happiness to sadness are normal. However, a mood swing is pathological when it disrupts normal behavior, is prolonged, and is accompanied by physical symptoms (such as sleep disturbances or appetite disturbances).

Mood disorders:

- Depression
- Seasonal affective disorder

Depression *Depression* (unipolar) is a disease in which an individual experiences helplessness and misery, loss of energy, excessive guilt, diminished ability to think, changes in eating and sleeping habits, and recurrent thoughts of hurting themselves, suicide, or death.[3] One in five people suffer from some form of depression. In *bipolar depression* (formerly called manic depression), an individual goes from exaggerated feelings of happiness and great energy to extreme states of depression.[42] Treatment must be individualized and might include psychotherapy and antidepressant medication.

Seasonal Affective Disorder Seasonal affective disorder (SAD) is characterized by mental depression related to a certain season of the year.[42] SAD is most likely to occur during the winter months due to a decrease in the amount of sunlight. The symptoms include fatigue, diminished concentration, and daytime drowsiness.[32] It usually occurs in adults and is four times more common in women than in men. SAD is commonly treated with light therapy, stress management, antidepressants, and exercise.

Anxiety Disorders

Anxiety disorders contribute to about 20 percent of all medical conditions among Americans seeking medical care.[20] Everyone occasionally experiences anxiety. Anxiety can cause a number of physiological responses, including sweating, increased heart rate, increased blood pressure, stomach discomfort, chills, dry mouth, difficulty concentrating, irritability, and sleep disturbances. Anxiety is abnormal when it begins to interfere with emotional well-being or normal daily functioning. *General anxiety* consists of persistent or unrealistic worrying that lasts for 6 months or longer.

Panic Attacks A *panic attack* is an unexpected and unprovoked emotionally intense experience of terror and fear. The physiological responses are similar to those of someone who fears he or she is in a life-threatening situation. Panic

Anxiety disorders:

- Panic attacks
- Phobias

attacks occur in about 30 percent of young adults, are most likely to occur at night, and tend to run in families. Behavioral modification and medications that suppress fear are helpful in controlling panic attacks.[42]

Phobias A *phobia* is a persistent and irrational fear of a specific situation, activity, or object that creates an intense desire to avoid the feared stimulus.[42] Some common phobias are fear of social situations, fear of height, fear of closed spaces, and fear of flying. Symptoms include increased heart rate, difficulty breathing, sweating, and dizziness. Treatments include behavioral modification, antidepressant or antianxiety medications, and systematic desensitization, a therapeutic technique in which the patient gradually confronts the source of the fear.

Personality Disorders

All of us have individual personality traits that make us who we are. A personality disorder is a pathological disturbance in cognition, affect, interpersonal functioning, or impulse control.[20] Usually, the personality disorder is of long duration and can be traced to some event or

Personality disorders:

- Paranoia
- Obsessive-compulsive disorder
- Posttraumatic stress disorder

circumstance occurring in adolescence. Treatment may involve psychotherapy and the use of psychopharmacological drugs.

Paranoia *Paranoia* is having unrealistic and unfounded suspicions about specific people or things.[54] Paranoid individuals are constantly on guard and cannot be convinced that their suspicions are not correct. Over time, resentment and anger develop toward a specific person or object. Paranoid individuals are often forced to seek medical care.

Obsessive-Compulsive Disorder *Obsessive-compulsive disorder* is characterized by a combination of emotional and behavioral symptoms. The symptoms of obsessive behavior are recurrent, inappropriate thoughts, feelings, impulses, or images arising from within that a person cannot eliminate by ignoring or neutralizing through other actions, even though they realize that they are wrong.[42] Compulsive behavior involves engaging in unreasonable repetitive acts, such as washing hands or counting in response to obsessive thoughts. This behavior interferes with normal daily functioning. Behavioral psychotherapy that attempts to restructure the environment to minimize the tendency to act compulsively, in addition to appropriate medication, is helpful.[1]

Posttraumatic Stress Disorder Individuals who suffer a psychologically traumatic event, such as a personal assault or abuse, a sexual assault or harassment, or a plane crash, may reexperience this event through nightmares or an exaggerated startle response.[20] They may experience a numbing of general responsiveness, insomnia, and increased aggression. This disorder may persist for decades. Group therapy with others who have had similar experiences seems to be beneficial.

11–11 Clinical Application Exercise

A patient was in a car accident in which a close friend was seriously injured. He has had difficulty sleeping and is beginning to have nightmares, which further compound his insomnia.

? What might the athletic trainer suspect is affecting this individual?

SUMMARY

- The injured or ill patient experiences not only physical disability but also major psychological reactions. Sport can be a major psychophysiological stressor.
- The athlete who sustains a serious injury may experience psychological characteristics of sudden loss, including denial, anger, bargaining, depression, and acceptance. Injury can cause the athlete to have physical, emotional, social, and self-concept reactions.
- Some athletes, because of personality factors, experience an inordinate number of injuries and illnesses. Anxiety, low self-esteem, and poor discipline may cause an athlete to be accident-prone.
- Overtraining and staleness result in a physical load being placed on the athlete's ability to cope. Athletes who are pushed or who push themselves too hard may experience burnout. These conditions generate a higher incidence of overuse injuries.
- At all times, the injured or ill athlete must be treated as a person, not as an injury. Health care providers should offer comfort, care, and good communication.
- The rehabilitation process requires mutual trust, understanding, and cooperation. Rehabilitation must be an educational process. Education is carried out through each phase of rehabilitation. Health care personnel may encounter athletes who overcomply or comply poorly.
- Many mental training aids can help the injured athlete through the rehabilitation process to reenter competition. Some of these aids are systematic desensitization, mental and emotional assessment, refuting irrational thoughts, and thought stopping.
- A mental illness is any disorder that affects the mind or behavior. The athletic trainer should recognize when a potential problem exists and refer the patient to an appropriate psychiatrist, psychologist, or counselor.

WEB SITES

Exercise and Sport Psychology: www.apadivisions
.org/division-47/index.aspx
This site belongs to the sports and exercise division of the American Psychological Association.

Mind Games: Applied Sport Psychology for Every Athlete: www.drrelax.com
This is a new, Web-based system of individualized psychological training.

North American Society for Psychology of Sport and Physical Activity: www.naspspa.org

Sport Psychology for Athletes: www.drrelax.com/
baseball.htm
Discuss the use of psychological training and preparation.

SOLUTIONS TO CLINICAL APPLICATION EXERCISES

11–1 The athletic trainer can be a good listener, find out what the problem is, be aware of his or her body language, project a caring image, explain the injury to the patient, help manage the stress of injury, and prepare the athlete physically and psychologically to return to competition.

11–2 Many patients experience five stages of psychological reaction, beginning with denial that they are injured, followed by anger, bargaining, depression, and finally acceptance.

11–3 The athletic trainer should look for athletes who have personality characteristics that make them more prone to injury, athletes who are under stress, and athletes who are overtraining and exhibiting signs of staleness and/or burnout.

11–4 If the athletic trainer needs help with the psychological aspects of a rehabilitation program, the patient can be referred to a physician, a sport psychologist, a clinical psychologist, a psychiatrist, a school guidance counselor, or a social worker.

11–5 The athletic trainer must appreciate that, even though she is physically ready to return, she is not psychologically prepared and has not yet realized that she can compete physically. The athletic trainer should have her engage in

practice activities that will progressively expose her to more chance of physical risk until she is totally confident that she is ready to return.

11–6 Athletes tend to be goal-oriented individuals. They are used to having goals set for them and striving to meet them. The athletic trainer can motivate the athlete by setting an ultimate goal and devising a series of short-term goals that should be met sequentially to achieve the long-term goal.

11–7 The athletic trainer should recommend and lead the athlete through meditation and/or progressive relaxation techniques in a quiet environment that will allow the athlete to relax mentally and focus on his abilities to perform at a high level.

11–8 The patient can be taught to inhibit pain by reducing tension and stress using the Benson and Jacobson techniques; by diverting attention from the chronic pain by engaging in problem solving; or by imagining or visualizing pleasant thoughts.

11–9 It is likely that the emotional distress caused by the accident is triggering posttraumatic stress disorder. Group therapy with others who have had similar experiences may be helpful.

REVIEW QUESTIONS AND CLASS ACTIVITIES

1. What is the importance of psychology to sports injuries?
2. How does stress relate to athlete injuries and illnesses?
3. Discuss the psychology of loss in sports injuries.
4. Describe the physical, emotional, social, and self-concept factors in sports injuries.
5. As an athletic trainer, how would you psychologically assist the athlete who is about to undergo major knee surgery?
6. Discuss overtraining, staleness, and overuse injuries.
7. What actions would you take with an athlete who is stale?
8. Psychologically, how should an athletic trainer react to serious injury immediately after injury and during the disability?
9. Psychologically, what makes for a successful rehabilitation climate?
10. Discuss psychological problems common to the rehabilitation process and possible ways of intervening.
11. What mental training techniques might be employed to assist the athlete who is fearful and anxious?
12. Practice teaching mental training techniques.

REFERENCES

1. Albinson C, Petrie T: Cognitive appraisals, stress, and coping: Preinjury and postinjury factors influencing psychological adjustment to sport injury, *J Sport Rehabil* 12(4):306, 2003.
2. Armstrong N: The elite young athlete. *Med Sport Sci.* 56(1):97–105, 2011.
3. Baum A: Suicide in athletes: A review and commentary, *Clinics in Sports Medicine*, 24(4):853–69, 2005.
4. Benson HH: *Beyond the relaxation response,* New York, 1984, Times.
5. Bone J, Fry M: The influence of injured athletes' perceptions of social support from ATCs on their beliefs about rehabilitation, *J Sport Rehabil* 15(2):156, 2006.
6. Brewer B: Adherence to sport injury rehabilitation. In Andersen M: *Routledge handbook of applied sport psychology* New York, 2010, Taylor & Francis.
7. Brewer B: Developmental differences in psychological aspects of sport-injury rehabilitation, *J Athl Train* 38(2):152, 2003.
8. Brinkman R: The motivational climate in the rehabilitation setting, *Athletic Therapy Today,* 15(2):44–46, 2010.
9. Cassidy C: Understanding sport-injury anxiety, *Athletic Therapy Today* 11(4):57, 2006.
10. Coote D, Tenenbaum G: Can emotive imagery aid in tolerating exertion efficiently? *J Sports Med Phys Fitness* 38(4):344, 1998.
11. Cramer-Roh JL, Perna FM: Psychology/counseling: A universal competency in athletic training, *J Athl Train* 35(4):458, 2000.
12. Cresswell S, Eklund R: The athlete burnout syndrome: Possible early signs, *Journal of Science and Medicine in Sport* 7(4):481, 2004.
13. Driediger M: Imagery use by injured athletes: A qualitative analysis, *Journal of Sport Sciences,* 24(3):261–72, 2007.
14. Fisher L, Wrisberg C: What athletic training students want to know about sport psychology, *Athletic Therapy Today* 11(3):32, 2006.
15. Ford I, Gordon S: Guidelines for using sport psychology in rehabilitation, *Athletic Therapy Today* 3(2):41, 1998.
16. Glazer D: Development and preliminary validation of the injury-psychological readiness to return to sport (I-PRRS) scale, *J Athl Train,* 44(2):185–89, 2009.
17. Gourlay L: Recognizing psychological disorders, part 1: Overview, *Athletic Therapy and Training,* 15(6):15–18, 2010.
18. Granquist M: Development of a measure of rehabilitation adherence for athletic training, *Journal of Sport Rehabilitation,* 19:249–67, 2010.
19. Gunnoe A, Horodyski ML, Tennant K: The effect of life events on incidence of injury in high school football players, *J Athl Train* 36(2):150, 2001.
20. Hales D: *An invitation to health,* Stamford, CT, 2000, Brooks/Cole.
21. Hamson-Utley J: Athletic trainers' and physical therapists' perceptions of the effectiveness of psychological skills within sport injury rehabilitation programs, *J Athl Train,* 43(3):258–64, 2008.
22. Hanley C: Stress-management interventions for female athletes: Relaxation and cognitive restructuring, *International Journal of Sport Psychology* 35(2):109, 2004.
23. Harris L: Development of the injured collegiate athlete, *J Athl Train* 38(1):75, 2003.
24. Hayden L: The role of athletic trainers in helping coaches to facilitate return to play, *Athletic Therapy and Training,* 16(1):24–26, 2011.
25. Hedgpeth EB, Gieck JJ: Considerations for rehabilitation of the injured athlete. In Prentice WE, editor: *Rehabilitation techniques in sports medicine and athletic training,* ed 5, San Francisco, 2010, McGraw-Hill.
26. Horn TS: *Advances in sport psychology,* ed 3, Champaign, IL, 2008, Human Kinetics.
27. Jacobson E: *Progressive relaxation: A physiological & clinical investigation of muscular states & their significance in psychology and medical practice,* Chicago, 1974, University of Chicago Press.
28. Johnson U: Athletes experiences of psychosocial risk factors preceding injury, *Qualitative Research in Sport, Exercise, Health,* 3(1):99–115, 2011.

29. Johnston L, Carroll D: Coping, social support, and injury changes over time and the effects of pain and exercise involvement, *J Sport Rehabil* 9(4):291, 2000.

30. Johnston L, Carroll D: The provision of social support to injured athletes: A qualitative analysis, *J Sport Rehabil* 7(4):267, 1998.

31. Kolt GS: Doing sport psychology with injured athletes. In Andersen MB, editor: *Sport Psychology in Practice,* Champaign, IL, 2005, Human Kinetics.

32. Koutedakis Y, Sharp NC: Seasonal variations of injury and overtraining in elite athletes, *Cl J Sports Med* 8(1):18, 1998.

33. Kübler-Ross E: *On death and dying.* London, 1969, Tavistock.

34. Marra J: Assessment of certified athletic trainers' levels of cultural competence in the delivery of health care, *J Athl Train,* 45(4):380–85, 2010.

35. Mihalik J: Recognition of psychological conditions in adolescent athletes, *Athletic Therapy Today* 9(3):54, 2004.

36. Milne M, Hall C, Forwell L: Self-efficacy, imagery use, and adherence to rehabilitation by injured athletes, *J Sport Rehabil* 14(2):150, 2005.

37. Misasi S, Redmond C, Kemler D: Counseling skills and the athletic therapist, *Athletic Therapy Today* 3(1):35, 1998.

38. Monsma E: Keeping your head in the game: Sport-specific imagery and anxiety among injured athletes, *J Athl Train,* 44(4):410–17, 2009.

39. Naylor A: The role of mental training in injury prevention, *Athletic Therapy Today,* 14(2):27–29, 2009.

40. Newcomer R, Perna F: Features of post-traumatic distress among adolescent athletes, *J Athl Train* 38(2):163, 2003.

41. Newsom J, Knight P, Balnave R: Use of mental imagery to limit strength loss after immobilization, *J Sport Rehabil* 12(3):249, 2003.

42. Payne W, Hahn D: *Understanding your health,* New York, 2010, McGraw-Hill.

43. Podlog L, Eklund R: Return to sport after serious injury: A retrospective examination of motivation and psychological outcomes, *J Sport Rehabil* 14(1):20, 2005.

44. Reardon C: Sport psychiatry: A systematic review of diagnosis and medical treatment of mental illness in athletes, *Sports Medicine,* 40(11):961–80, 2010.

45. Robbins JE, Rosenfeld LB: Athletes' perceptions of social support provided by their head coach, assistant coach, and athletic trainer, pre-injury and during rehabilitation, *Journal of Sport Behavior* 24(3):277, 2001.

46. Rock JA, Jones MV: A preliminary investigation into the use of counseling skills in support of rehabilitation from sport injury, *J Sport Rehabil* 11(4):284, 2002.

47. Schwenz SJ: Psychology of injury and rehabilitation, *Athletic Therapy Today* 6(1):44, 2001.

48. Selye H: *Stress without distress,* New York, 1974, Lippincott.

49. Sharon P, et al.: Academic preparation of athletic trainers as counselors, *J Athl Train* 31(1):39–43, 1996.

50. Shell D, Ferrante AP: Recognition of adjustment disorders in college athletes: A case study, *Cl J Sports Med* 6(1):60–62, 1996.

51. Shelley G, Trowbridge C, Detling N: Practical counseling skills for athletic therapists, *Athletic Therapy Today* 8(2):57, 2003.

52. Smith R: Recognition, management, and referral of the injured athlete with psychological problems, *Athletic Therapy Today* 3(1):14, 1998.

53. Sordoni C, Hall C, Forwell L: The use of imagery by athletes during injury rehabilitation, *J Sport Rehabil* 9(4):329, 2000.

54. *Taber's cyclopedic medical dictionary,* Philadelphia, 2011, F.A. Davis.

55. Udry E: Staying connected: Optimizing social support for injured athletes, *Athletic Therapy Today* 7(3):42, 2002.

56. Van Raalte J: Referring clients to other professionals. In Andersen M: *Routledge handbook of applied sport psychology,* New York, 2010, Taylor & Francis.

57. Vela L: Transient disablement in the physically active with musculoskeletal injuries, part I: A descriptive model, *J Athl Train,* 45(6):615–29, 2010.

58. Walsh, A: The relaxation response: A strategy to address stress, *Athletic Therapy and Training,* 16(2):20–23, 2011.

59. Wayda V, Armenth-Brothers F, Boyce B: Goal setting: A key to injury rehabilitation, *Athletic Therapy Today* 3(1):21, 1998.

60. Weinberg R, Gould D; Burnout and overtraining. In Gould D, editor: *Foundations of sport and exercise psychology,* ed 5, Champaign, IL, 2010, Human Kinetics.

61. Weiss-Bjornstal M: An integrated model of response to sport injury: Psychological and sociological dynamics, *Journal of applied Sports Psychology* 10:46–69, 1998.

62. Wiese-Bjornstal D: Psychology and socioculture affect injury risk, response, and recovery in high-intensity athletes: A consensus statement, *Scandinavian Journal of Medicine and Science in Sports,* 20(2):103–11, 2010.

63. Williams A: Social support and sport injury, *Athletic Therapy Today,* 15(4):46, 2010.

64. Wrisberg C: Recommendations for successfully integrating sport psychology into athletic therapy, *Athletic Therapy Today* 11(2):60, 2006.

65. Wrisberg C, Fisher L: Mental rehearsal during rehabilitation, *Athletic Therapy Today* 10(6):58, 2005.

66. Wrisberg C, Fisher L: Staying connected to teammates during rehabilitation, *Athletic Therapy Today* 10(2):62, 2005.

67. Yang, J: Social support patterns of collegiate athletes before and after injury, *J Athl Train,* 45(4):372–79, 2010.

ANNOTATED BIBLIOGRAPHY

Gould D, Weinberg R: *Foundations of sport and exercise psychology,* Champaign, IL, 2010, Human Kinetics.

Discusses the techniques that a coach should use for contributing to the success of an athlete.

Heil J, editor: *Psychology of sport injury,* Champaign, IL, 1995, Human Kinetics.

An in-depth look at the psychology of sport injury for sport psychologists.

Kreider RB et al.: *Overtraining in sport,* Champaign, IL, 1998, Human Kinetics.

An excellent secondary reference covering the psychological, immunological, nutritional, and psychological considerations of overtraining in sport.

Pargman, D: *Psychological Bases of Sports Injuries,* Morgantown, WV, 2007, Fitness Information Technologies.

Provides a thorough examination of the psychological aspects of prevention, treatment, and rehabilitation of sport injuries.

Selye H: *Stress without distress,* New York, 1974, Lippincott.

A practical guide to understanding the role of stress in life.

Singer RN, Hausenblas HA, Janelle CM: *Handbook of sport psychology,* ed 2, New York, 2001, Wiley.

A good resource for sport psychologists, coaches, and athletes searching for new and effective approaches to pain management, exercise psychology, and building self-confidence. It combines theoretical explanations and practical applications and emphasizes the value of basic and applied research to practice.

Taylor J, Taylor S: *Psychological approaches to sports injury rehabilitation,* Gaithersburg, MD, 2004, Aspen.

Provides practical techniques and strategies for sports rehabilitation.

Van Raalte JL, editor: *Exploring sport and exercise psychology,* ed 2, Washington, DC, 2002, American Psychological Association.

An overview of the field of sport and exercise psychology, connecting theory and practice and discussing practical issues.

Williams JM: *Applied sport psychology: personal growth to peak performance,* San Francisco, 2009, McGraw-Hill.

Leading sports psychologists presenting both the "whys" and "how tos" of the intervention techniques in sport psychology.

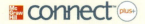

12

On-the-Field Acute Care and Emergency Procedures

■ Objectives

When you finish this chapter you should be able to

- Establish a plan for handling emergency situations.
- Explain the importance of knowing cardiopulmonary resuscitation and how to manage an obstructed airway.
- Describe the types of hemorrhage and their management.

- Assess the types of shock and their management.
- Describe the emergency management of musculoskeletal injuries.
- Describe techniques for moving and transporting the injured patient.

■ Outline

■ Key Terms

primary survey
secondary survey
systolic blood pressure
diastolic blood pressure
mm Hg

■ Connect Highlights

Visit connect.mcgraw-hill.com for further exercises to apply your knowledge:

- Clinical application scenarios covering handling emergency situations, shock, and emergency management of musculoskeletal injuries
- Click-and-drag questions covering emergency action plans, emergency managements, and cardiopulmonary resuscitation
- Multiple-choice questions covering emergency management of musculoskeletal injuries, transporting an injured patient, emergency action plans, and management of hemorrhage
- Selection questions covering musculoskeletal injuries and vital signs

Most sports injuries do not result in life-or-death emergency situations, but when such situations do arise, prompt care is essential.[11] An emergency is an unexpected serious occurrence that may cause injuries that require immediate medical attention. It has been suggested that the first hour following injury—the so-called Golden Hour—is most critical in treating injury. Although research evidence has shown that the Golden Hour is simply an arbitrary myth, it is certainly true that providing correct immediate care is important.[60] Time is the critical factor, and assistance to the injured person must be based on knowledge of what to do and how to do it—on how to perform effective first aid immediately.[23] There is no room for uncertainty, indecision, or error. A mistake in the initial management of an injury can prolong the length of time required for rehabilitation and can create a life-threatening situation for the athlete.[12]

> Time is critical in an emergency situation.

THE EMERGENCY ACTION PLAN

The prime concern of emergency aid is to maintain cardiovascular function and, indirectly, central nervous system function.[14] Failure of either of these systems may lead to death. Regardless of the setting, whether on an athletic field or in a clinic, hospital, or fitness center, emergency action should be developed for every situation in which an athletic trainer works.[26] The key to emergency aid is the initial evaluation of the injured patient. Time is of the essence, so this evaluation must be done rapidly and accurately, so that proper first aid can be rendered without delay.[9] In some instances, these first steps not only will be lifesaving but also will determine the degree and extent of permanent disability.

As discussed in Chapters 1 and 3, any individual who provides emergency care—the athletic trainer, the team physician, the coach—must act reasonably and prudently at all times.[46] This behavior is especially important during emergencies.

All health care programs must have a prearranged emergency action plan (EAP) that can be implemented immediately when necessary.[27,31,65] The following issues must be addressed when developing the emergency action for athletic settings:

> All sports programs must have an emergency action plan.

1. Develop separate emergency action plans for each sport's field, courts, or gymnasiums (see *Focus Box 12–1:* "Sample emergency action plan").

   a. Determine the personnel who will be on the field during practices and competitions (e.g., athletic trainers, athletic training students, physicians, emergency medical technicians, rescue squad). Each person should understand exactly what his or her role and responsibilities are if an emergency occurs. It is also recommended that the sports medicine team practice the use and operation of emergency equipment, such as stretchers and automatic external defibrillators.[23]

   b. Decide what emergency equipment should be available for each sport. The emergency equipment needs for football will likely be different from those of the cross-country team.

2. Establish specific procedures and policies regarding the removal of protective equipment, particularly the helmet and shoulder pads. These procedures are discussed later in this chapter.[31,37]

3. Make sure phones are readily accessible. Cell or digital phones are recommended. However, a land line should also be readily available in case cell phone service is not available. If cell phones are not available, the athletic training students, coaches, all staff personnel, and athletes should know the location of the telephone; phones should be clearly marked. Use 911 if available, but realize that in some areas not all service is accessible by cell phones and thus land lines should be used to access the emergency medical system.

4. All staff should be familiar with the community-based emergency health care delivery plan, including existing communication and transportation policies.[44] It is also critical for the athletic trainer to be familiar with emergency care facility admission and treatment policies, particularly when rendering emergency care to a minor. The athletic trainer should designate someone to make an emergency phone call. Most emergency medical systems can be accessed by dialing 911, which connects the caller to a dispatcher who has access to rescue squad, police, and fire personnel. The person making the emergency phone call must provide the following information:

   a. Type of emergency situation
   b. Type of suspected injury
   c. Present condition of the athlete
   d. Current assistance being given (e.g., cardiopulmonary resuscitation)
   e. Location of telephone being used
   f. Exact location of emergency (give names of streets and cross-streets) and how to enter facility
   g. Any limitations in the building (such as no elevator to the third floor)

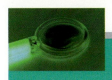
Sample emergency action plan

Emergency action plan for women's ice hockey

Emergency Personnel:
Certified athletic trainer and athletic training students on-site for practice and competition; additional sports medicine staff accessible from main athletic training facility (across street from arena)

Emergency Communication:
Fixed telephone line in ice hockey satellite athletic training room (_____-_____)

Emergency Equipment:
Supplies (AED, trauma kit, splint kit, spine board) maintained in ice hockey satellite athletic training room; additional emergency equipment accessible from athletic training facility across street from arena (_____-_____)

Roles of First Responders:
Immediate care of the injured or ill student-athlete
Emergency equipment retrieval

Activation of Emergency Medical System (EMS):
911 call (provide name, title or position, address, telephone number, number of individuals injured, condition of injured, first, aid treatment, specific directions, other information as requested)
Direct EMS to scene
 Open appropriate doors
 Designate individual to "flag down" EMS and direct to scene
Scene control: Limit scene to first-aid providers and move bystanders away from area

Venue Directions:
Ice hockey arena is located on corner of _____ Street and _____ Street adjacent to _____. Two gates provide access to the arena:_____ Street: drive leads to arena as well as rear door of complex (locker room, athletic training room)

Sports Medicine Staff and Phone Numbers:
Athletic Trainer in Charge 929-0000 (cell)
Head Athletic Trainer 929-0001 (office)
Team Physician 929-0002 (office)

From *NCAA Sports Medicine Handbook 2011–2012.*[38]

---

5. Make sure keys to gates or padlocks are easily accessible. The athletic trainer, staff members, and the coach should have the appropriate keys. Make sure an elevator in a building can accommodate a gurney or spine board.

6. Inform all coaches, athletic directors, school nurses, staff, and maintenance personnel of the emergency plan at a meeting held annually before the beginning of the school year. Each individual must know his or her responsibilities, should an emergency occur. This plan should be reviewed, revised, and rehearsed at least once a year.

7. Assign someone to accompany the injured athlete to the hospital.

8. Carry contact information for all athletes, coaches, and other personnel at all times, particularly when traveling (see Figure 3–1). For minors, consent forms should also be available when traveling.

9. In certain situations in both secondary schools and colleges, the athletic trainer may be called upon to provide emergency services not only to athletes but also to coaches, referees, and in some cases parents and other spectators who develop an emergent condition during an athletic event. The emergency action plan should include plans for managing these situations with the help of emergency medical services and other local health care providers.

An athletic trainer working in a clinic, hospital, corporate, or industrial setting should also develop an emergency action plan to make certain that appropriate procedures will be followed, should an emergency occur. If the athletic trainer is working in a hospital, he or she should become familiar with the hospital's pre-established emergency action plan for dealing with in-house emergencies and should follow it. For emergent situations that occur in a clinic, corporate, or industrial setting, similar procedures and considerations should be followed as described for managing injuries in an athletic setting.

In 2002, the NATA released a position statement relative to an emergency action plan.[4] The objective was to provide guidelines for athletic trainers in the development of emergency plans and to advocate the documentation of emergency planning. A link to the NATA position statement "Emergency planning in athletics (http://www.nata.org/sites/default/files/EmergencyPlanningInAthletics.pdf) can be found at www.mhhe.com/prentice15e.

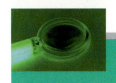

FOCUS 12–2 Focus on Organizational and Professional Health and Well-Being

Consent form for medical treatment of a minor

By this signature, I hereby consent to allow the physician(s) and other health care provider(s) selected by me or the school to perform a preparticipation examination on my child and to provide treatment for any injury or condition resulting from participating in athletics and activities for his or her school during the school year covered by this form. I further consent to allow said physician(s) or health care provider(s) to share appropriate information concerning my child that is relevant to participation in athletics and activities with coaches and other school personnel as deemed necessary.

_____
Parent or Guardian

_____
Date

Subsequently in 2007, representatives from the NATA worked on an interassociation task force official statement *Recommendations on emergency preparedness and management of sudden cardiac arrest in high school and college athletic programs* (http://www.nata.org/sites/default/files/sudden-cardiac-arrest-consensus-statement.pdf). A link to this official statement can be found at www.mhhe.com/prentice15e.

Cooperation between Emergency Care Providers

Individuals providing emergency care to injured athletes must cooperate and act professionally. The athletic trainer should make every effort to nurture the relationship with the emergency medical technicians (EMTs) and, if possible, incorporate them into the development and implementation of the emergency action plan. Occasionally, disagreements arise between rescue squad personnel, the physician, and the athletic trainer over exactly how the injured athlete should be handled and transported. The athletic trainer is usually the first to deal with the emergency situation. The athletic trainer has generally had more training and experience in moving and transporting an injured athlete than the physician has. If an athletic trainer or a physician is not available, the coach should not hesitate to call 911 to let the rescue squad handle an emergency situation. If the rescue squad is called and responds, the EMTs should have the final say on how that patient is to be transported while the athletic trainer assumes an assistive role.

To alleviate potential conflicts, the athletic trainer should establish procedures and guidelines and should arrange practice sessions at least once a year that include everyone responsible for handling an injured athlete.[19] Rescue squad personnel may not be experienced in dealing with someone who is wearing a football, lacrosse, or hockey helmet or other protective equipment; thus, athletic trainer should make sure before an incident occurs that the EMTs understand the correct management of athletes wearing various types of athletic equipment.

> Emergency practice sessions for athletic trainers and EMTs should be held at least once a year.

Parental Notification

If the injured patient is a minor, the athletic trainer should try to obtain consent from the parent before it becomes necessary to treat the patient during an emergency.[4] *Focus Box 12–2:* "Consent form for medical treatment of a minor" provides an example of a consent form that may be signed by the parents or guardians of a minor. Consent may be given in writing either before or during an emergency. This consent is notification that the parent has been informed about what the athletic trainer thinks is wrong and what the athletic trainer intends to do, and parental permission is granted to give treatment for a specific incident. If the patient's parents cannot be contacted, the predetermined wishes of the parent given at the beginning of a season or school year can be enacted. The athletic trainer should have these consent forms available when traveling in case the need for medical care arises. If no informed consent exists, the patient's implied consent to save his or her life takes precedence.

PRINCIPLES OF ON-THE-FIELD INJURY ASSESSMENT

The athletic trainer cannot deliver appropriate acute medical care to the injured patient until a systematic assessment of the situation has been made on the playing field or court where the injury occurs.[52] This *on-the-field assessment* helps determine the nature of the injury and provides direction in the decision-making process concerning the emergency care that must be rendered (Figure 12–1).[16] The on-the-field assessment may be subdivided into a primary survey and a secondary survey.

The **primary survey**, which is done initially, determines the existence of potentially life-threatening situations, including problems with level of consciousness, airway, breathing, circulation, severe bleeding, and shock.

primary survey
Assesses life-threatening injuries.

The primary survey takes precedence over all other aspects of victim assessment and should be used to correct life-threatening situations.[40] Any patient who has a life-threatening situation should be transported to an emergency care facility as soon as possible.

Once the primary survey has ruled out the existence of a life-threatening injury or illness, the **secondary survey** takes a closer look at the injury. The secondary survey gathers specific information about the injury from the patient, systematically assesses vital signs and symptoms, and allows for a more detailed evaluation of the injury. The secondary survey is done to uncover problems that do not pose an immediate threat to life but that may do so if they remain uncorrected.[40]

secondary survey
Performed after life-threatening injuries have been ruled out.

An injured patient who is conscious and stable does not require a primary survey. However, an unconscious patient must be monitored for life-threatening problems throughout the assessment process.

THE PRIMARY SURVEY

Treatment of Life-Threatening Injuries

Life-threatening injuries take precedence over all other injuries. Situations that are considered life-threatening include those that require cardiopulmonary resuscitation (i.e., obstruction of the airway, no breathing, no circulation), profuse bleeding, and shock.[21,23] In the primary survey, it is first necessary to assess the level of consciousness.

Life-threatening conditions:

- Airway obstruction
- No breathing
- No circulation
- Profuse bleeding
- Shock

Dealing with the Unconscious Patient

The state of unconsciousness provides one of the greatest dilemmas for the athletic trainer. Whether to move the injured athlete and allow the game to resume or to await the arrival of a physician is a decision that too often is resolved hastily and without much forethought. Unconsciousness is a state of insensibility in which the athlete exhibits a lack of conscious awareness. This condition can be brought about by a blow to either the head or the solar plexus; it may result from general shock, or it may result from fainting (syncope) due to inadequate blood flow to the brain. It is often difficult to determine the exact cause of unconsciousness (Table 12–1).

With an unconscious victim, the athletic trainer should call 911 immediately.

The unconscious patient always must be considered to have a life-threatening injury, which requires that the athletic trainer call 911

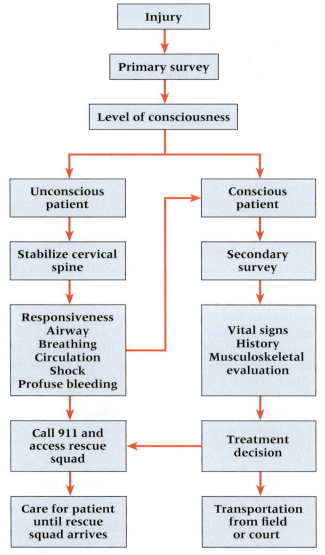

FIGURE 12–1   Flowchart showing the appropriate emergency procedures for the injured patient.

TABLE 12-1 Evaluating the Unconscious Athlete

Functional Signs	Selected Conditions						
	Fainting	Concussion	Grand Mal Epilepsy	Brain Compression and Injury	Heatstroke	Diabetic Coma	Shock
Onset	Usually sudden	Usually sudden	Sudden	Usually gradual	Gradual or sudden	Gradual	Gradual
Level of consciousness	Complete unconsciousness	Confusion or unconsciousness	Unconsciousness	Unconsciousness, gradually deepening	Delirium or unconsciousness	Drowsiness, later unconsciousness	Listlessness, later unconsciousness
Pulse	Fast and weak	Weak and irregular	Fast	Gradually slower	Fast and weak	Fast and weak	Fast and weak
Respiration	Quick and shallow	Shallow and irregular	Noisy, later deep and slow	Slow and noisy	Difficult	Deep and sighing	Rapid and shallow, with occasional deep sighs
Skin	Pale, cold, and clammy	Pale and cold	Livid, later pale	Hot and flushed	Hot and limited sweating	Livid, later pale	Pale, cold, and clammy
Pupils	Equal and dilated	Equal	Equal and dilated	Unequal	Equal	Equal	Equal and dilated
Paralysis	None	None	None	May be present in leg, arm, or both	None	None	None
Convulsions	None	None	None	Present in some cases	Present in some cases	None	None
Breath	N/A	N/A	N/A	N/A	N/A	Acetone smell	N/A
Special features	Giddiness and sway before collapse	Signs of head injury, vomiting during recovery	Bites tongue, voids urine and feces, may injure self while falling	Signs of head injury, delayed onset of symptoms	Vomiting in some cases	In early stages, headache, restlessness, and nausea	May vomit; early stages shivering, thirst, defective vision, and ear noises

immediately. The following guidelines should be used when working with the unconscious:

12–1 Clinical Application Exercise

A football defensive back is making a tackle and drops his head on contact with the ball-carrier. He hits the ground and does not move. When the athletic trainer gets to him, the patient is lying prone, is unconscious, but is breathing.

? How should the athletic trainer manage this situation?

1. The athletic trainer should immediately note the body position and determine the level of consciousness and responsiveness.
2. Circulation, airway, and breathing should be established immediately.
3. Injury to the neck and cervical spine should always be considered a possibility in the unconscious patient.[53]
4. If an athlete is wearing a helmet, it should never be removed until neck and spine injuries have been unequivocally ruled out. However, the face mask must be cut away and removed to allow for cardiopulmonary resuscitation (CPR).[66]
5. An airway, breathing, and circulation (ABC) should be established immediately if the patient is not breathing.
6. If the patient is supine and breathing, monitor closely until he or she regains consciousness.
7. If the patient is prone and not breathing, he or she should be logrolled carefully to the supine position, and CPR should begin immediately.
8. If the patient is prone and breathing, monitor closely until he or she regains consciousness; then the patient should be carefully logrolled onto a spine board because CPR could be necessary at any time.
9. Life support for the unconscious patient should be maintained and monitored until emergency medical personnel arrive.
10. Once the patient is stabilized (no longer exhibits a life-threatening condition), the athletic trainer should begin a secondary survey.

Overview of Emergency Cardiopulmonary Resuscitation

A careful evaluation of the injured person must be made to determine whether CPR should be conducted. This overview of adult and child CPR is not intended to be used by persons who are not certified in CPR. Because of the serious nature of CPR, athletic trainers should routinely be recertified in *CPR/AED for the Professional Rescuer* through the American Red Cross or the American Heart Association.[1,2,40]

In 2008, the American Heart Association, proposed changes that simplify CPR techniques for those people

who have not been certified in CPR. This technique, referred to as "hands-only CPR," only requires a rescuer to call 911, then to perform uninterrupted chest compressions—100 a minute—until paramedics take over or an automated external defibrillator is available to restore a normal heart rhythm.[1] This action should be taken only for adults who unexpectedly collapse, stop breathing, and are unresponsive. In 2010, the American Heart Association changed its acronym of ABC to CAB—circulation, airway, breathing—to help individuals who are certified in CPR remember the order of the procedures.[1] This change emphasized the importance of chest compressions in creating circulation. *Focus Box 12–3: "CPR summary"* summarizes the basics of performing CPR for the adult, child, and infant.

Equipment Considerations Protective equipment worn by an athlete may complicate lifesaving CPR procedures. The presence of a football, ice hockey, or lacrosse helmet as well as a face mask and various types of shoulder pads will obviously make CPR more difficult if not impossible. Over the years, significant debate has raged in the sports medicine community about removing the helmet of an athlete with suspected cervical spine injury, and a number of differing opinions have been expressed.[30,32,37,38,41,53,56,66,67,68] It has been proposed that removing the face mask should be the first step.[10] The face mask does not hinder the evaluation of the airway, but it may hinder treatment.[30] Thus, the face mask should be removed immediately when a decision is made to transport the patient to a medical care facility, regardless of the current respiratory status.[10,54,55,57,58]

The face mask is attached to the football helmet, usually by four fasteners. There are different types of fasteners, including loop strap fasteners, shock-blaster fasteners, stabilizer fasteners, and revolution fasteners (Figure 12–2).[12] It is recommended that the face mask be removed completely by cutting all of the fasteners, rather than simply cutting the bottom two fasteners, and retracting the face guard.[12] Using an electric screwdriver has been shown to be faster and produce less torque on the helmet than using tools that cut through the fasteners, as long as the screws are not rusted.[14,28,30] Three cutting devices—the Anvil Pruner, the Trainer's Angel, and the FM Extractor—have been recommended for their effectiveness in quickly cutting the plastic fasteners (Figure 12–3).[55] Most recently, the recommendation has been to use a combination of an electric screwdriver and one of the three cutting devices.[24] It also has been suggested that the athletic trainer should be proficient in removing the face mask within 30 seconds.[56] Studies comparing the efficacy of using these various devices suggest that the Anvil Pruner seems to be easier to use than the Trainer's Angel.[32] Other studies have shown

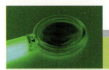

CPR summary

Instructions for individuals certified in CPR

For an adult

- Establish unresponsiveness, then call 911.
- If an AED is available, deliver 1 shock if instructed by the device and begin CPR.
- Restore blood circulation, using chest compressions at a rate of 100 per minute.
- Perform 30 compressions.
- Use two hands for compression.
- Compress chest at least 2 inches (5 mm).
- Perform mouth-to-mouth breathing after opening the airway.
- Give two breaths (1 second per ventilation).
- Breathe until the chest rises.
- Resume chest compressions.
- After five cycles or 2 minutes with no response, use an automatic external defibrillator (AED) (Figure 12–6).
- Administer one shock if instructed by the device, then continue CPR
- Continue CPR 30 compressions: 2 breaths until the person begins to breathe or EMS takes over.

For a child (ages 1–12)

- Establish unresponsiveness, then call 911.
- Restore blood circulation, using chest compressions at a rate of 100 per minute.
- Perform 30 compressions.
- Use two hands for compressions.
- Compress chest about 2 inches (5 mm).
- Perform mouth-to-mouth breathing after opening the airway.
- Give two breaths (1 second per ventilation).

- Breathe until the chest rises.
- Resume chest compressions.
- After five cycles or 2 minutes with no response, use an automatic external defibrillator (AED).
- Use pediatric pads if available.
- Administer 1 shock if instructed by the device, then continue CPR.
- Continue CPR 30 compressions: 2 breaths until the child begins to breathe or EMS takes over.

For an infant (< 1 year)

- Establish unresponsiveness, then call 911.
- Make sure airway is clear.
- Restore blood circulation with chest compressions at a rate of 100 per minute.
- Perform 30 compressions.
- Use only two fingers on sternum just below nipple line for compressions.
- Perform mouth-to-mouth/nose breathing after opening the airway.
- Give two breaths.
- Breathe more gently than for an adult.
- Resume chest compressions.
- After five cycles or 2 minutes with no response, reassess.
- Continue CPR until the child begins to breathe or EMS takes over.

Instructions for individuals who are not certified in CPR

- Perform chest compressions only at a rate of 100 per minute continuously until EMS arrives.

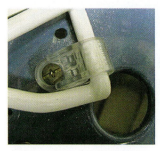
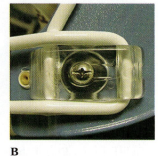

A   B

FIGURE 12–2 Football helmet face mask fasteners. **(A)** Loop strap. **(B)** Revolution.

that the Anvil Pruner and the FM Extractor are faster in removing the face mask than the Trainer's Angel.[12] Furthermore, using a Trainer's Angel seems to cause more motion in the cervical spine than using either a manual or powered screwdriver.[14] Various other tools have been recommended to remove the face mask, including wire

cutters, bolt cutters, PVC pipe cutters, tape scissors, and scalpels, none of which work very well. Thus, using any of these tools as a primary means of removing a face mask is not recommended.

In 1992, the Occupational Safety and Health Administration (OSHA) mandated the use of a barrier device or pocket mask to protect the athletic trainer from the transmission of bloodborne pathogens during CPR (see Figure 12–14B).[49] Sometimes it is possible to slip the pocket mask under the face mask, attach the one-way mouthpiece or valve through the bars of the face mask, and begin CPR within 5 to 10 seconds, without removing the face mask.[56] Also, the use of a pocket mask appears to cause less extraneous motion in the cervical spine than does the use of either screwdrivers or the Trainer's Angel to remove the face mask.[48] It also has been shown that using a pocket mask is quicker for initiating rescue breathing than rotation of the face mask using screwdriver removal.[48] It has been shown that removing a lacrosse

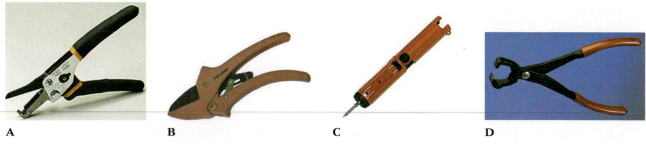

A B C D

FIGURE 12–3   A variety of tools can be used to cut or remove the plastic grommets that hold the face mask. (A) FM Extractor. (B) Anvil Pruner. (C) Electric cordless screwdriver. (D) Trainer's Angel.

helmet instead of the face mask is a faster and safer way to gain access to the airway.[15]

As mentioned earlier, controversy has existed for some time as to whether the helmet and shoulder pads should be left in place or removed.[41] The current recommendation is to leave the helmet and shoulder pads in place.[37,38,39] The football helmet and chin strap should be removed only if (1) the helmet and chin strap do not hold the head securely and immobilizing the helmet does not immobilize the head; (2) the design of the helmet and chin strap is such that, even after removal of the face mask, the airway cannot be controlled or ventilation provided; (3) the face mask cannot be removed after a reasonable period of time; or (4) the helmet prevents the athlete from being immobilized appropriately for transportation.[39] If the helmet must be removed, spinal immobilization must be maintained during removal. In most circumstances, it may be helpful to remove cheek padding and/or deflate air padding prior to removing the helmet.

The athletic trainer must either remove both the helmet and shoulder pads or leave them both in place. Removing one or the other independently will force the cervical spine into either flexion or extension. If they are left in place, the face mask should be dealt with as recommended previously, and the jersey and shoulder pad strings or straps should be cut, spreading the shoulder pads apart, so that the chest may be compressed according to CPR guidelines. Although some individuals recommend removal of the helmet and shoulder pads, it seems that, no matter how much care is taken, removal creates unnecessary movement of the cervical spine and delays the initiation of CPR, neither of which is best for the injured patient.[33,63] If cervical neck injury is suspected, yet the patient is conscious and breathing and does not require CPR, the patient should be transported with the helmet, chin strap, and shoulder pads in place. The face mask should be removed in case CPR becomes necessary.

Establishing Unresponsiveness   Initially, the athletic trainer should check for any life-threatening conditions (i.e., no breathing, no pulse, severe bleeding). The athletic trainer should, first, assess the situation to make sure there is no chance of additional injury. The next step is to establish the responsiveness of the victim by asking "Are you okay?" and then tapping the shoulder or using a painful pinch of the distal extremity (Figure 12–4). Note that shaking should be avoided if there is a possible neck injury. Quickly check for signs of breathing and pulse. If the victim does not respond to any stimuli, the emergency medical system (EMS) should be activated immediately by directing a specific person to dial 911. That person should also be directed to get an automatic external defibrillator (AED) if available. A victim who is lying prone or on his or her side and is breathing should be placed on his or her left side in the recovery position (Figure 12–5). This position can be maintained for as long as 30 minutes. If the victim is not breathing, he or she should be carefully placed in the supine position. If the victim is in a position other than supine, he or she must be carefully rolled over as a unit, avoiding any twisting of the body, because CPR can be administered only with the victim lying flat on the back with knees straight

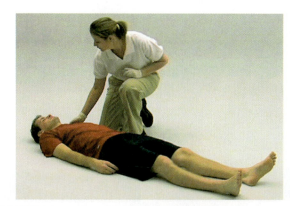

FIGURE 12–4   Establish responsiveness by gently tapping the victim's shoulder and asking "Are you okay?"

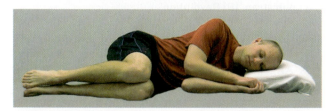

FIGURE 12–5   Victims who are breathing should be placed on their left side in the recovery position.

or slightly flexed. In cases of suspected cervical spine injury, cervical movement must be minimized during logrolling. Then CPR should be performed.[40] If an Automated External Defibrillator (AED) is available it should be used immediately after it has been determined that the victim is unresponsive. If not it should be used as soon as it becomes available.

Using an Automated External Defibrillator An automated external defibrillator (AED) is a device that evaluates the heart rhythm of a victim of sudden cardiac arrest.[49] It is capable of delivering an electrical charge to the heart and does not require the expertise of a medical professional.[51] To prevent human error, all machines have computers that evaluate heart rhythm and decide if deployment is appropriate. AEDs have become an essential tool in the treatment of out-of-hospital cardiac arrest.[20] The American Heart Association estimates that 100,000 deaths could be prevented each year with rapid defibrillation. Over the years, the devices have become safer, more reliable, and more maintenance free. The new technologies used in these devices make them suitable for use by anyone who has had basic training.[51]

AEDs are extremely easy to use; anyone trained to use cardiopulmonary resuscitation (CPR) can be trained to use an AED. Most AEDs are designed to be used by people without medical backgrounds, such as police, firefighters, flight attendants, security guards, and lay rescuers, as long as the procedure is coordinated with existing EMS systems and the person administering the procedure has received proper training. Public places where AEDs might be located include police cars, theaters, sports arenas, public buildings, business offices, and airports. An increasing number of commercial airplanes are now equipped with AEDs and enhanced medical kits. Formal training programs, such as those offered by the American Heart Association's Heartsaver AED course, can be taught in as little as 4 hours. However, operating an AED is so simple that it can be done successfully even without formal training. Training is recommended for as many people as possible. Local and state regulations determine the training requirements for public access defibrillator (PAD) programs.[51]

The legal requirements that allow the lay public to use AEDs are determined on a state-by-state basis. In some states, there is true public access defibrillation, meaning that anyone with knowledge of an AED can use one any time it is available. For example, a traveler in an airport may retrieve and use an AED mounted in a public location. In other states, use of AEDs is more restricted. Some states require a formal training program or the direct involvement of an authorizing doctor, or the AED rescuer must be part of a formal in-house response team. In most states, any individual using an AED in a good-faith attempt to save the life of a cardiac arrest victim will be covered by some form of a "good Samaritan" statute.[40]

Anyone can be certified to use an AED in most states and can learn to use an AED in about an hour.[62] AED users also need yearly training, not only on the use of the device but also in CPR. Athletic trainers must be certified in both CPR and AED use. Maintenance is minimal on AEDs. The devices are equipped with long-life batteries and have features that notify the users when the batteries need replacement. To date, most professional teams and many college teams have AEDs readily available.

To use an AED, the rescuer simply applies the two electrodes to the right apex and the left base of the chest (Figure 12–6). To operate most devices, push the "on" button and listen for a voice on the machine to direct you whether to push the defibrillator button. If the pulse does not resume after one shock, perform CPR for two minutes; then deliver another shock from the AED. If the pulse resumes, place the victim into the recovery position on his or her left side (see Figure 12–6) until the rescue squad arrives. If the pulse does not resume, continue external compressions at a 30 (compressions) to two (breaths) ratio. The victim should not be on a metal stretcher, the ground should not be wet, and the chest should be dry (not sweaty). It is best to shave chest hair if quickly possible. NATA's official statement on using AEDs appears in *Focus Box 12–4:* "Official statement—automated external defibrillators."

Establishing Circulation

1. In the adult and child victim, feel for a pulse at the carotid artery. Place two fingers on the Adam's apple and slide them toward you into the groove on the side of the neck (Figure 12–7). Monitor for 5 to 10 seconds.

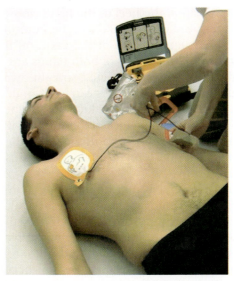

FIGURE 12–6 An automatic external defibrillator (AED) can be used if the victim has no heartbeat.

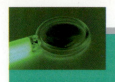

FOCUS 12–4 Focus on Organizational and Professional Health and Well-Being

Official statement—automated external defibrillators

The National Athletic Trainers' Association (NATA), as a leader in health care for the physically active, strongly believes that the treatment of sudden cardiac arrest is a priority. An AED program should be part of an athletic trainer's emergency action plan. NATA strongly encourages athletic trainers, in every work setting, to have access to an AED. Athletic trainers are encouraged to make an AED part of their standard emergency equipment. In addition, in conjunction and coordination with local EMS, athletic trainers should take a primary role in implementing a comprehensive AED program within their work setting.

From NATA official statement "Automated external defibrillators" http://www.nata.org/sites/default/files/AutomatedExternalDefibrillators.pdf

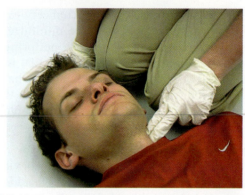

FIGURE 12–7   Checking for a pulse at the carotid artery.

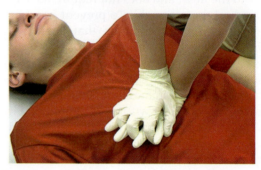

FIGURE 12–8   Chest compressions should be performed with pressure from both hands over the sternum and between the nipples.

2. If an AED is available, use it as soon as possible (see the section on AED). Deliver one shock followed immediately by chest compressions.

3. If no AED is available and there are no evident signs of circulation (i.e., breathing, coughing, or movement), begin chest compressions immediately after giving two rescue breaths.

4. Maintain an open airway. Position yourself close to the side of the victim's chest.

5. Next, position the heel of the hand closest to the victim's head on the middle of the sternum. Place the other hand on top of the hand on the sternum, so that the heels of both hands are parallel and the fingers are directed straight away from you (Figure 12–8). Fingers can be extended or interlaced, but they must be kept off the chest wall.

6. Keep elbows in a locked position, with arms straight and shoulders positioned over the hands, bending at the hips to enable the thrust to be straight down.

7. In a normal-sized adult, apply enough force to depress the sternum at least 2 inches (5 cm). (In the child, the sternum should be compressed up to 2 inches [5 cm].) After compression, completely release the sternum to allow the heart to refill. The time of release should equal the time of compression. For one rescuer, compression must be given at the rate of 100 times per minute, maintaining a ratio of 30 chest compressions to two full breaths (30:2) for all victims, from infants to adults.[2]

8. After about 2 minutes or five cycles of 30 compressions and two breaths (30:2), recheck the pulse at the carotid artery for 5 seconds while maintaining the head tilt. If no pulse is found, continue the 30:2 cycle, beginning with chest compressions.[2]

NOTE: In 2008, the American Heart Association, proposed changes that simplify CPR techniques for those people who have not been certified in CPR. This technique, referred to as "hands-only CPR," only requires a rescuer to call 911, then to perform uninterrupted chest compressions—100 a minute—until paramedics take over or an automated external defibrillator is available to restore a normal heartrhythm.[1] This action should be taken only for adults who unexpectedly collapse, stop breathing, and are unresponsive.

Opening the Airway There are several techniques that the athletic trainer can use to open the airway. [64] The most common method is to open the airway by using the head-tilt/chin-lift method (Figure 12–9A).[2] Lift under the chin with one hand while pushing down on the victim's forehead with the other, avoiding the use of excessive force. The tongue is the most common cause of airway obstruction; the forward lift of the jaw raises the tongue away from the back of the throat, thus clearing the airway.

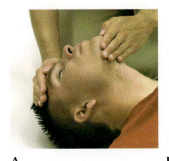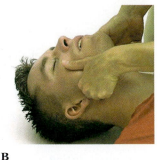

A   **B**

FIGURE 12–9 Opening the airway. **(A)** Head-tilt/ chin-lift method. **(B)** Modified jaw thrust technique.

In the modified jaw thrust technique, grasp each side of the mandible at the angles and pull upward to open the airway. Studies have shown that this technique (Figure 12–9B) does not consistently open the airway effectively, and even professional rescuers move the cervical spine when using it. Therefore, this technique is not recommended for the lay rescuer. The athletic trainer should use the head-tilt/ chin-lift method to open the airway of a person with no suspected cervical injury. If there is a suspected cervical injury, the modified jaw thrust technique should be used. If the jaw thrust maneuver fails to open the airway, use the head-tilt/chin-lift method.

Airway Adjunct Devices A suction device can be used if there is some substance (e.g., blood, fluids, vomitus) in the mouth or throat that appears to be obstructing the airway and that cannot be cleared by using a finger sweep.[36] Suction units can be portable manual units (hand-suctioning), portable mechanical units, or wall-mounted mechanical units. (Figure 12–10). Each of these works by creating a negative pressure that suctions fluid and small particles into a collecting chamber. Suctioning helps to reduce the risk of aspiration into the lungs and should be done as quickly as possible so that normal ventilation procedures can be reimplemented. The suction tube should reach only to the base of the tongue, suctioning only what can be visualized. The length of the tube inserted into the throat can be estimated by measuring the distance from the corner of the mouth to the same side earlobe. Suctioning should move from back to front, using a small circular motion with the tip of the tube.

Oropharyngeal (OPA) airways, nasopharyngeal (NPA) airways, and supraglottic (SGA) airways are types of airway adjunct devices that are used to make it easier to maintain an open airway once it has been established. Their purpose is essentially to prevent the tongue from obstructing the airway. These devices may be used by certified first responders, EMTs, paramedics, and athletic trainers who have been properly trained in their use.[8]

An oropharyngeal airways is essentially a curved, J-shaped plastic tube, designed to fit the natural contour of the mouth and throat, that is inserted into the mouth and through the posterior pharynx. (Figure 12–11). It should only be used in unconscious (unresponsive) patients with no gag reflex. If a victim gags, it should be removed

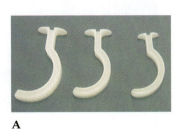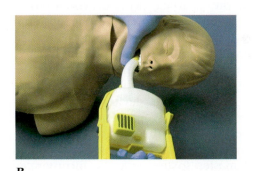

A   **B**

FIGURE 12–10 Using a suction device. **(A)** Rotate the head to the side or log roll the patient onto their side and perform a finger sweep. **(B)** Insert the suction tip into the throat and suction from the back of the throat outward using a circular movement. Always visualize the tip.

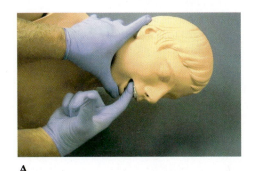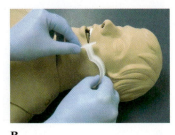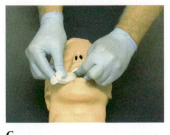

A   **B**   **C**

FIGURE 12–11 Establishing an oropharyngeal airway. **(A)** OPAs come in different sizes. **(B)** Measure from the corner of the mouth to the same side earlobe to select the correct size. **(C)** Insert the airway into the pharynx.

immediately. OPA's come in different sizes from large adult to infant. It is critical to select the correct size to avoid displacing the tongue into the posterior pharynx, causing additional airway obstruction. The size of the OPA can be estimated by measuring the distance from the corner of the mouth to the same side earlobe. If there is difficulty ventilating the patient after the airway is inserted, it should be removed and reinserted. Once correctly inserted, the flange should lie on the patient's lips. The OPA can facilitate the delivery of adequate ventilation with a bag/valvemask by preventing the tongue from occluding the airway.[36]

A nasopharyngeal airway is a soft rubber tube that is passed through the right side of the nose into the posterior pharynx. (Figure 12–12). It is used on a responsive, semiconscious patient and does not cause a gag reflex unless it is too long. Insertion of the NPA requires a water-soluble lubricating agent to avoid injuring the nasal mucosa. The tubes come in different sizes based on the diameter of the opening, which ranges from 6.5 to 8.5 mm. The length of the tube inserted into the nose can be estimated by measuring the distance from the nostril to the same side earlobe. When correctly inserted, the flared end of the tube should rest just outside of the nasal passage and a bag/valve mask should fit easily over the airway. An NPA should not be used in any patient who has head trauma.[8]

A supraglottic airway is used with patients who are unresponsive with no gag reflex. The airway is inserted into the pharynx, without visualization, and is designed to create a seal in the posterior pharynx above the glottis (vocal chords), obstructing the esophagus and forcing air into the trachea. Currently, only EMTs and paramedics may use SGAs outside of a hospital.[36]

Using the airway adjunct devices has not traditionally been within the scope of practice for the athletic trainer. However, these skills are now considered a competency that athletic trainers should practice and master so they may be incorporated into clinical practice.[8]

See *Focus Box 12–5* "Procedures for using airway adjunct devices" for a more detailed description of specific techniques.

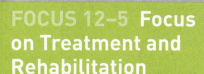

FOCUS 12–5 Focus on Treatment and Rehabilitation

Procedures for using airway adjunct devices

Manual suction

- If there is no cervical injury, logroll patient onto his or her side.
- Open patient's mouth and perform a finger sweep to remove large foreign bodies.
- Measure distance from corner of the mouth to the earlobe.
- Use this as a guide when inserting tube into the mouth. (Don't suction below base of tongue.)
- Suction from back to front in a circular pattern, moving quickly, for no more than 15 sec.
- If there is gag reflex, remove the suction tip.

Oropharyngeal (OPA) airway

- Choose the correct size by measuring from the corner of the mouth to the earlobe.
- Open the patient's mouth and lift the lower jaw and tongue up.
- Insert OPA with curved end up, then rotate tip down as it reaches the back of the throat.
- Slide it down the back of the throat behind the tongue.
- Flared end should rest on the patient's lips.

Nasopharyngeal (NPA) airway

- Choose the correct size by measuring from the nostril to the earlobe.
- Apply lubricant to tube.
- Insert tube in right nostril with gentle pressure (do not force), moving along the nasal floor.
- Flared end should rest on the patient's nostril.

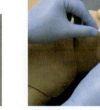
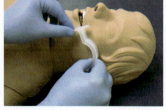
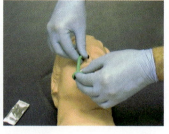

A **B** **C**

FIGURE 12–12 Establishing a nasopharyngeal airway. **(A)** NPAs come in different sizes. **(B)** Measure from the nostril to the same side earlobe to select the correct size. **(C)** Lubricate and insert the airway into the right nostril.

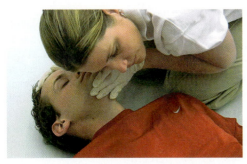

FIGURE 12–13 Once the airway is established, look, listen, and feel for breathing.

Establishing Breathing

1. To determine whether the victim is breathing, maintain the open airway; place your ear over the victim's mouth; observe the chest; and look, listen, and feel for breath sounds for 5 to 10 seconds. If the victim is prone, look for the back to rise and fall with breathing (Figure 12–13).
2. If the victim is not breathing, using the hand on the victim's forehead, pinch the nose shut, keeping the heel of the hand in place to hold the head back (if there is no neck injury). OSHA has mandated the use of barrier shields (and disposable gloves, if available) by athletic trainers to minimize the risk of transmitting bloodborne pathogens (Figure 12–14A and C).[2] These shields have a plastic or silicone sheet that spreads over the face and separates the athletic trainer from the victim. Some models have a tubelike mouthpiece, which may help in situations in which the athlete is wearing a face mask. Take a normal breath, place your mouth over the barrier mask to provide an airtight seal, and give two slow, full breaths at a rate of one breath per second. Observe the chest rise and fall. Remove your mouth, and listen for the air to escape through passive exhalation. If the airway is obstructed, reposition the victim's head and try again to ventilate. If the airway is still obstructed, give thirty chest compressions; then look for an object in the mouth. If the object is visible, perform a finger sweep with the index finger to clear visible objects from the mouth.[25] Be careful not to push an object further into the throat. Continue to repeat this sequence until ventilation occurs. If the victim is breathing but there is no pulse, give one ventilation every

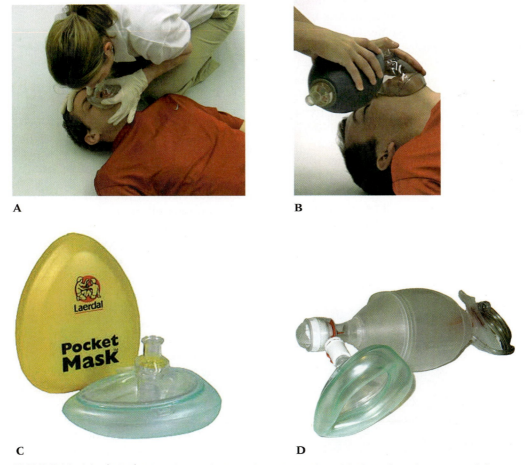

A

B

C

D

FIGURE 12–14 **(A&C)** A barrier pocket mask protects the athletic trainer from potential exposure to bloodborne pathogens. **(B&D)** A bag/valve mask can be used for respiration.

5 seconds in an adult and one breath every 3 seconds for a child or infant. Recheck for breathing and pulse every 2 minutes.

If available, use a bag/valve mask for artificial respiration. Although the bag/valve mask is easy to use, some instruction and practice in its use is recommended (Figure 12–14B and D).

NOTE: Asthma is a chronic inflammatory condition that involves spontaneous spasm and narrowing of the bronchial airways and excessive production of mucus. The patient experiencing an asthma attack exhibits respiratory distress in breathing and wheezing. However, this condition does not require basic life support intervention and is effectively managed using medication delivered via an inhaler. Asthma is discussed in detail in Chapter 29, and the use of an inhaler is discussed in Chapter 17.

Administering Supplemental Oxygen Serious and life-threatening medical emergencies often cause oxygen to be depleted in the body, leaving the victim at risk for cardiac arrest or brain damage. Supplemental oxygen may prove to be a critical step in treating a severe or life-threatening illness or injury. An athletic trainer who has been specifically trained in supplemental oxygen administration should routinely give oxygen to a victim who is having trouble breathing. Administering supplemental oxygen requires using a bag/valve mask and a pressurized cylinder or canister containing oxygen (Figure 12–15).

The air that a person normally breathes contains about 21 percent oxygen. During rescue breathing, the victim receives only about 16 percent oxygen, but a bag/valve mask provides about 21 percent oxygen. Giving supplemental oxygen can provide the victim with a significantly higher oxygen concentration.[2]

All oxygen cylinders are easily identified because they are green with a yellow diamond that clearly says "oxygen." During administration, a face mask with an attached oxygen reservoir bag

and a one-way valve between the mask and the bag are attached to the oxygen cylinder. As the athlete breathes, the concentrated oxygen is inhaled from the bag, and exhaled air freely escapes from the side of the mask. As much as 90 percent oxygen can be delivered to the victim.[2] The oxygen should be delivered at a rate of 10 to 15 liters per minute as indicated by a flow rate meter.

In some states it is illegal to administer oxygen without a physician's prescription.

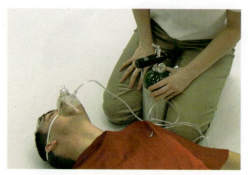

FIGURE 12–15 Administering supplemental oxygen to facilitate breathing.

A football player is injured while making a tackle. The athletic trainer quickly realizes that the victim is not breathing and immediately begins CPR. After only a few seconds, the victim begins breathing spontaneously and regains consciousness.

? What might the athletic trainer choose to do while waiting for the rescue squad to arrive to facilitate the victim's recovery from this life-threatening incident?

12–2 Clinical Application Exercise

Obstructed Airway Management Choking is a possibility in many sports activities; for example, an athlete may choke on a mouth guard, a broken piece of dental work, tongue rings, chewing gum, or even a chew of tobacco. When such emergencies arise, early recognition and prompt, knowledgeable action are necessary to avert a tragedy. An unconscious victim can have

All athletic trainers must have current CPR/AED.

an obstructed airway when the tongue falls back in the throat, thus blocking the upper airway.[42] Blood clots resulting from head, facial, or dental injuries may impede normal breathing, as may vomiting. When complete airway obstruction occurs, the individual is unable to speak, cough, or breathe.

Conscious Victim If the victim is conscious, there is a tremendous effort made to breeath, the head is forced back, and the face initially is flushed and then becomes cyanotic as oxygen deprivation occurs. If partial airway obstruction is causing the choking, some air passage can be detected, but during a complete obstruction no air movement is discernible. If the victim is coughing, he or she should be encouraged to continue coughing.[2]

First, if the victim cannot cough, speak, or breathe, have someone call 911. Obtain consent from the victim before proceeding. Lean the victim forward, supporting the chest with one hand and with the other hand deliver five back blows between the scapulae (Figure 12–16A). Then, stand behind and to one side of the victim. Place both arms around the waist just above the belt line, and permit the victim's head, arms, and upper trunk to hang forward (Figure 12–16B). Grasp one of your

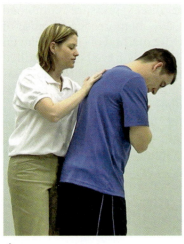
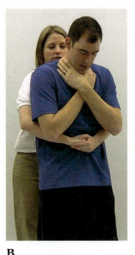

A   **B**

FIGURE 12–16   In attempting to clear an obstructed airway for a conscious victim. **(A)** deliver five back blows followed by **(B)** five abdominal thrusts.

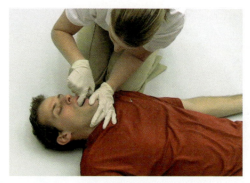

FIGURE 12–17   A finger sweep of the mouth is essential in attempting to remove a foreign object from a choking victim. The finger sweep should be performed only if the object is visible.

fists with the other, placing the thumb side of the grasped fist immediately below the xiphoid process of the sternum, clear of the rib cage. Now sharply and forcefully thrust the fists into the abdomen, inward, and upward, five times. This thrust pushes up on the diaphragm, compressing the air in the lungs, creating forceful pressure against the blockage, and thus usually causing the obstruction to be promptly expelled. Repeat the maneuver until the victim is relieved or becomes unconscious.

Unconscious Victim If a conscious victim with an obstructed airway eventually loses consciousness, help the victim get to the ground without falling. The victim must be on his or her back. If the victim loses consciousness, open the airway[1] and try to ventilate. Give two rescue breaths. If the chest does not rise, reposition the head and give two additional rescue breaths. If the chest does not rise, move to the side of the victim and give 30 chest compressions, as previously described. After 30 compressions, look for an object in the mouth. If there is a visible object, remove it by performing a finger sweep (Figure 12–17). Then try again to ventilate. Repeat this sequence as long as necessary. Victims who begin breathing on their own should be placed on their left side in the recovery position (see Figure 12–5).[1,2] Care must be taken to avoid applying extreme force over the rib cage because fractures of the ribs and damage to the organs can result.

Finger sweeping If a foreign object, such as a mouth guard, is lodged in the mouth or the throat and is visible, it may be possible to remove or release it with the fingers.[1] Care must be taken that the probing does not drive the object deeper into the throat. It is usually impossible to open the mouth of a conscious victim who is in distress, so the abdominal thrust technique should be used immediately. In the unconscious athlete, turn the head either to the side or face up, open the mouth by grasping the tongue and the lower jaw, hold them firmly between the thumb and fingers, and lift—an action that pulls the tongue away from the back of the throat and from the impediment. If this action is difficult to do, the crossed finger method can usually be used effectively. The index finger of the free hand (or, if both hands are used, an assistant can probe) should be inserted into one side of the mouth along the cheek deeply into the throat; using a hooking maneuver, attempt to free the impediment, moving it into a position from which it can be removed (Figure 12–17). Once the object is removed, if the victim is not already breathing, attempt to ventilate.[1]

Control of Hemorrhage

An abnormal discharge of blood is called a hemorrhage. The hemorrhage may be venous, capillary, or arterial and may be external or internal. Venous blood is characteristically dark red with a continuous flow; capillary bleeding exudes from tissue and is a reddish color; and arterial bleeding flows in spurts and is bright red.

NOTE: The athletic trainer must be concerned with exposure to bloodborne pathogens and other diseases when coming into contact with blood or other body fluids. It is essential to take universal precautions to minimize this risk. The athletic trainer should use disposable latex gloves whenever he or she comes in contact with blood or other body fluids. This topic is discussed in detail in Chapter 14.

12–3 Clinical Application Exercise

A patient is being treated in a sports medicine clinic. She is chewing gum while doing her exercises and suddenly begins to choke and is having difficulty breathing.

? What should the athletic trainer do for her?

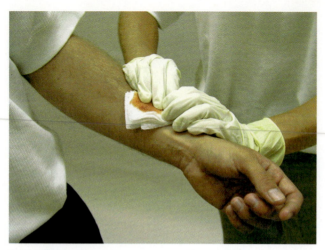

FIGURE 12–18 Direct pressure for the control of bleeding is applied with the hand over a sterile gauze pad.

External Bleeding
External bleeding stems from open skin wounds, such as abrasions, incisions, lacerations, punctures, and avulsions (see Chapter 28 for further discussion). It can also occur from an open fracture. The control of external bleeding includes the use of direct pressure, elevation, and pressure points.[40]

Direct Pressure
Pressure is directly applied with the hand over a sterile gauze pad. The pressure is applied firmly against the resistance of a bone (Figure 12–18).

> External bleeding can usually be managed through direct pressure, elevation, or pressure points.

Elevation
Elevation in combination with direct pressure provides an additional means for reducing external hemorrhaging. Elevating a hemorrhaging part against gravity reduces hydrostatic blood pressure and facilitates venous and lymphatic drainage, which slows bleeding.

Pressure Points
When direct pressure combined with elevation fails to slow hemorrhage, the use of pressure points may be the method of choice. Eleven points on each side of the body have been identified for controlling external bleeding, including the dosalis pedis, popliteal, femoral (anterior thigh), femoral (femoral triangle), radial and ulnar, brachial, axillary, subclavian, carotid, facial, and temporal pressure points. The two most commonly used are the brachial artery in the upper limb and the femoral artery in the lower limb. The brachial artery is compressed against the medial aspect of the humerus, and the femoral artery is compressed as it is detected within the femoral triangle (Figure 12–19).[7]

Internal Hemorrhaging
Internal hemorrhage is invisible to the eye unless manifested through some body opening or identified through X-ray studies or other diagnostic techniques. Its danger lies in the difficulty of diagnosis. When internal hemorrhaging occurs—subcutaneously, such as in a bruise or contusion; intramuscularly; or in joints—the patient may be moved without danger in most instances. However, the detection of bleeding within a body cavity, such as the skull, thorax, or abdomen, is a life-and-death situation. Because the symptoms are obscure, internal hemorrhage is difficult to diagnose properly. If an internal hemorrhage is suspected, blood pressure should be closely monitored.[29] As a result, patients with internal injuries require hospitalization under complete and constant observation by a medical staff to determine the nature and extent of the injuries. All severe hemorrhaging will eventually result in shock and should therefore be treated on this premise. Even if the patient shows no outward indication of shock, he or she should be kept quiet and body heat should be maintained at a constant and suitable temperature.[40] (See the following section for the preferred body position.)

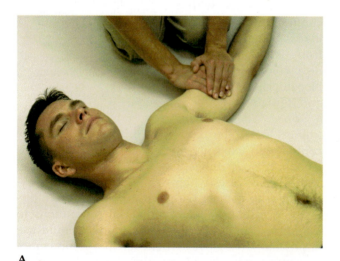

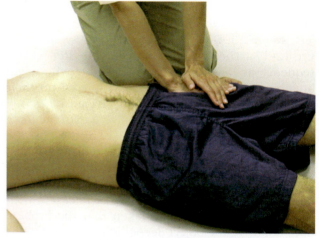

A   B

FIGURE 12–19 The two most common sites for direct pressure. **(A)** The brachial artery. **(B)** The femoral artery.

Shock

With any injury, shock is a possibility.[60] However, when severe bleeding, fractures, or internal injuries are present, the development of shock is more likely. Shock occurs when a diminished amount of blood is available to the circulatory system—that is, when the vascular system loses its capacity to hold the fluid portion of the blood because of dilation of the blood vessels.[60] When shock occurs, a quantity of plasma moves from the blood vessels into the tissue spaces of the body, leaving the blood cells within the vessels, causing stagnation and slowing the blood flow. As a result, not enough oxygen-carrying blood cells are available to the tissues, particularly those of the nervous system. With this general collapse of the vascular system comes widespread tissue death, which will eventually cause the death of the individual unless treatment is given.

Certain conditions, such as extreme fatigue, extreme exposure to heat or cold, extreme dehydration of fluids and mineral loss, or illness, predispose a patient to shock. In a situation in which there is a potential shock condition, there are other signs by which the athletic trainer should assess the possibility of the patient's lapsing into a state of shock as an aftermath of the injury. The most important clue to potential shock is the recognition of a severe injury. It may happen that none of the usual signs of shock are present.[40]

The main types of shock are hypovolemic, respiratory, neurogenic, psychogenic, cardiogenic, septic, anaphylactic, and metabolic shock.[29]

Hypovolemic shock stems from trauma in which there is blood loss. Decreased blood volume causes a decrease in blood pressure. Without enough blood in the circulatory system, the organs are not properly supplied with oxygen.

Respiratory shock occurs when the lungs are unable to supply enough oxygen to the circulating blood. Trauma that produces a pneumothorax or an injury to the breathing control mechanism can produce respiratory shock.

Neurogenic shock is caused by the general dilation of blood vessels within the cardiovascular system. When it occurs, the typical 6 liters of blood can no longer fill the system. As a result, the cardiovascular system can no longer supply oxygen to the body.

Psychogenic shock is commonly known as fainting (syncope). It is caused by a temporary dilation of blood vessels that reduces the normal amount of blood in the brain.

Cardiogenic shock is the inability of the heart to pump enough blood to the body.

Septic shock occurs from a severe, usually bacterial, infection. Toxins liberated from the bacteria cause small blood vessels in the body to dilate.

Anaphylactic shock is the result of a severe allergic reaction caused by foods, insect stings, or drugs or by inhaling dusts, pollens, or other substances. Management of anaphylaxis, using an EpiPen (see Figure 17–2) is discussed in Chapter 17.

Metabolic shock happens when a severe illness, such as diabetes, goes untreated. Another cause is an extreme loss of body fluid (e.g., through urination, vomiting, or diarrhea).

Symptoms and Signs The major signs of shock are moist, pale, cool, clammy skin; weak and rapid pulse; increased and shallow respiratory rate; decreased blood pressure; and, in severe situations, urinary retention and fecal incontinence.[29,40] If conscious, the patient may display a disinterest in his or her surroundings, irritability, restlessness, or excitement. He or she may also exhibit extreme thirst.

> **Signs of shock:**
> - Blood pressure is low.
> - Systolic pressure is usually below 90 mm Hg.
> - Pulse is rapid and weak.
> - Patient may be drowsy and appear sluggish.
> - Respiration is shallow and extremely rapid.
> - Skin is pale, cool, and clammy.

Management Depending on the cause of the shock, the following emergency care should be given:

1. Maintain body temperature as close to normal as possible.
2. Elevate the feet and legs 8 to 12 inches (20 to 30 cm) for most situations. However, shock positioning varies according to the type of injury.[29] For a neck injury, for example, the athlete should be immobilized as found; for a head injury, the head and shoulders should be elevated; for a leg fracture, the legs should be kept level and should be raised after splinting.

Shock can also be compounded or even initially produced by the patient's psychological reaction to an injury situation. Fear or the sudden realization that a serious situation has occurred can result in shock. In the case of a psychological reaction to an injury, the athlete should be instructed to lie down and avoid viewing the injury. The patient should be handled with patience and gentleness but also with firmness. Spectators should be kept away from the injured athlete. Reassurance is of vital concern to the injured individual. The person should be given immediate comfort through the loosening of clothing. Nothing should be given by mouth until a physician has determined that no surgical procedures are indicated.

THE SECONDARY SURVEY

After the primary survey has determined that no life-threatening injuries or illnesses exist, and the patient appears to be in stable condition, the athletic trainer should conduct an on-the-field secondary survey to assess the existing injury more precisely.[22]

Recognizing Vital Signs

The ability to recognize physiological signs of injury is essential to the proper handling of potentially critical injuries. When evaluating the seriously ill or injured patient, the athletic trainer or physician must be aware of nine response areas: level of consciousness, pulse, respiration, blood pressure, temperature, skin color, pupils, movement, and abnormal nerve response. The three primary vital signs are pulse, respiration, and blood pressure.[22]

> **Vital signs to observe:**
> - Level of consciousness
> - Pulse
> - Respiration
> - Blood pressure
> - Temperature
> - Skin color
> - Pupils
> - Movement
> - Abnormal nerve response

Level of Consciousness When recognizing vital signs, the examiner must always note the patient's level of consciousness. Normally, the individual is alert, is aware of the environment, and responds quickly to vocal stimulation. Head injury, heatstroke, and diabetic coma can alter the patient's level of conscious awareness.

The level of consciousness can be assessed by using several different scales: the AVPU scale, the ACDU scale, and the Glasgow Coma Scale. (See Chapter 27 for a discussion of the Glasgow Coma Scale.) The AVPU scale is widely used by EMTs for assessing the neurological status of trauma patients as originally taught in Advanced Trauma Life Support (ATLS). Both the AVPU and the ACDU scales are simpler to use than the Glasgow Coma Scale.

The AVPU scale is as follows:

- *A* for *alert* signifies that the patient is alert; awake; responsive to voice; and oriented to person, time, and place.

- *V* for *verbal* signifies that the patient responds to voice but is not fully oriented to person, time, or place.
- *P* for *pain* signifies that the patient does not respond to voice but does respond to a painful stimulus, such as a squeeze of the hand.
- *U* for *unresponsive* signifies that the patient does not respond to a painful stimulus.

The ACDU scale is as follows:

- Alert
- Confused
- Drowsy
- Unresponsive

Pulse The pulse is the direct extension of the functioning heart. In emergency situations, the pulse is usually determined at the carotid artery in the neck or the radial artery in the wrist (Figure 12–20). A normal pulse rate per minute for adults ranges between 60 and 100 beats, and in children, between 80 and 100 beats; however, well-conditioned athletes usually have slower pulses than the typical population.

> **Respiratory patterns:**
> - Apnea—temporary cessation of breathing
> - Tachypnea—rapid breathing
> - Bradypnea—slow breathing
> - Dyspnea—difficult breathing
> - Hyperventilation—labored breathing
> - Obstructed—blocked airway caused by either partial or complete obstruction

An alteration of a pulse from normal may indicate the presence of a pathological condition. For example, a rapid but weak pulse could mean shock, bleeding, diabetic coma, or heat exhaustion. A rapid and strong pulse may mean heatstroke or severe fright; a strong but slow pulse could indicate a skull fracture or stroke; and no pulse means cardiac arrest or death.[29]

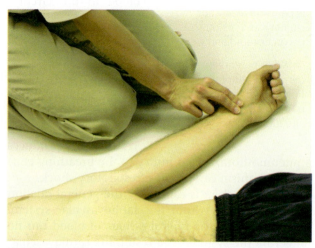

FIGURE 12–20 Pulse rate taken at the radial artery.

Respiration The normal breathing rate per minute is approximately 12 to 20 breaths in adults and 15 to 30 breaths in children. Breathing rate may be normal but breath may be shallow (indicating shock), labored, or noisy. Frothy blood being coughed up indicates a chest injury, such as a fractured rib, that has affected a lung. The athletic trainer should look, listen, and feel: look to ascertain whether the chest is rising or falling; listen for air passing into and out of the mouth, nose, or both; and feel where the chest is moving. If the victim is prone, look for the back to rise and fall with respiration.

Blood Pressure Blood pressure, as measured by the sphygmomanometer, indicates the amount of pressure exerted against the arterial walls. It is indicated at two pressure levels: systolic and diastolic. **Systolic blood pressure** occurs when the left ventricle contracts, thereby pumping blood, and **diastolic blood pressure** is the residual pressure present in the arteries when the heart is between beats. The resting blood pressure for 15 to 20-year-old males should be less than 120 **mm Hg** (systolic) and less than 80 mm Hg (diastolic). The normal blood pressure for females is usually 8 to 10 mm Hg lower than in males for both systolic and diastolic pressures. Between the ages of 15 and 20, a systolic pressure of greater than 120 mm Hg and a diastolic pressure of greater than 80 mm Hg may be excessive. Table 12–2 provides recommendations for blood pressure. A lowered blood pressure (hypotension) could indicate hemorrhage, shock, heart attack, or internal organ injury.[60]

> **systolic blood pressure** The pressure caused by the heart pumping.
> **diastolic blood pressure** The residual pressure when the heart is between beats.
> **mm Hg** Millimeters of mercury.

Blood pressure is measured by applying the cuff circumferentially around the upper arm just proximal to the elbow (Figure 12–21). For individuals who have large or muscular upper arms, an extra-large sleeve should be used to get an accurate reading. The stethoscope should be placed on the anterior surface at the crease of the elbow joint directly over the brachial artery. The cuff should be inflated to 200 mm Hg, which occludes blood flow in the brachial artery distal to the cuff in the cubital fossa. The sounds, heard through the stethoscope are referred to as Korotkoff sounds. The cuff should be slowly deflated with the stethoscope in place; the first beating sound is recorded as systolic pressure. The cuff continues to be deflated until the beating sound disappears; diastolic pressure is then recorded.

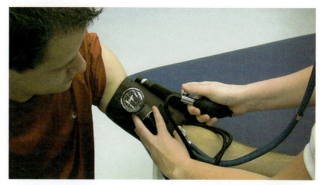

FIGURE 12–21 Blood pressure is measured using a sphygmomanometer and a stethoscope.

> Korotkoff sounds identify systolic and diastolic blood pressures

Temperature Body temperature is maintained by water evaporation and heat radiation. It is normally 98.2°F (36.8°C) to 98.6°F (37°C). Temperature is measured with a thermometer, which is placed under the tongue, in the armpit, against the tympanic membrane in the ear, or, in case of unconsciousness, in the rectum. Core temperature is most accurately measured in the rectum (see Focus Box 6–5: "Measuring rectal temperature"). The technique using tympanic membrane temperature measurement in the ear (Figure 12–22) is easily done and is becoming a more accurate indication of core temperature. However, it is difficult to achieve the same temperature in consecutive trials due to difficulty replicating the depth and angle of insertion. A digital oral

> To convert Fahrenheit to centigrade (Celsius):
> $°C = (°F − 32) ÷ 1.8$.
> To convert centigrade to Fahrenheit: $°F = (1.8 × °C) + 32$.

TABLE 12–2	American Heart Association Recommended Blood Pressure Levels[34]		
Blood Pressure Category	**Systolic (mm Hg)**		**Diastolic (mm Hg)**
Normal	Less than 120	and	Less than 80
Prehypertension	120–139	or	80–89
High			
Stage 1	140–159	or	90–99
Stage 2	160 or higher	or	100 or higher

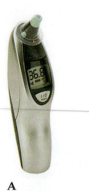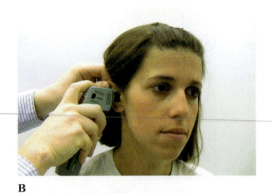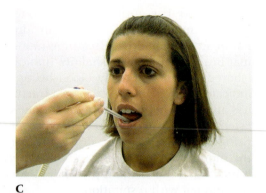

A   B   C

FIGURE 12–22   Measuring temperature. **(A)** Digital tympanic membrane thermometer. **(B)** Measuring tympanic membrane thermometer. **(C)** Digital oral thermometer temperature measurement.

thermometer can also provide a reasonably accurate temperature measure (Figure 12–22C). Changes in body temperature can be reflected in the skin. For example, hot, relatively dry skin might indicate disease, infection, or overexposure to environmental heat. Cool, clammy skin could reflect trauma, shock, or heat exhaustion; cool, dry skin is possibly the result of overexposure to cold.

A rise or fall of internal temperature may be caused by a variety of circumstances, such as the onset of a communicable disease, cold exposure, pain, fear, or nervousness. Characteristically, a lowered body temperature is accompanied by chills with chattering teeth, blue lips, goose bumps, and pale skin.

Skin Color For individuals who are lightly pigmented, the skin can be a good indicator of the state of health. Normal skin tone is pink. A flushed or red skin color may indicate heatstroke, sunburn, allergic reaction, high blood pressure, or elevated temperature. A pale, ashen, or white skin can mean insufficient circulation, shock, fright, hemorrhage, heat exhaustion, or insulin shock. Skin that is bluish in color (cyanotic), primarily in the lips and fingernails, usually means an airway obstruction or a respiratory insufficiency. A yellowish or jaundice color may indicate liver disease or dysfunction.

Assessing skin color in a dark-skinned individual is more difficult. These individuals normally have pink coloration of the nail beds and inside the lips, mouth, and tongue. When a dark-skinned person goes into shock, the skin around the mouth and nose will often have a grayish cast, and the tongue, the inside of the mouth, the lips, and the nail beds will have a bluish cast. Shock resulting from hemorrhage will cause the tongue and inside of the mouth to become a pale, grayish color instead of blue. Fever in these individuals can be noted by a red flush at the tips of the ears.[29]

Pupils The pupils of the eyes are extremely sensitive to situations affecting the nervous system.

Although most persons have pupils of regular outline and equal size, some individuals normally have pupils that are irregular and unequal. This disparity requires the athletic trainer to know which individuals deviate from the norm.

A constricted pupil may indicate the patient is using a central nervous system depressant drug. If one or both pupils are dilated, the patient may have sustained a head injury; may be experiencing shock,

> Some athletes normally have irregular and unequal pupils.

heatstroke, or hemorrhage; or may have ingested a stimulant drug (Figure 12–23). The pupils' response to light also should be noted. If one or both pupils fail to accommodate to light, there may be brain injury or alcohol or drug poisoning. When examining a patient's pupils, the examiner should note the presence of contact lenses. Pupil response is more critical than pupil size in an evaluation.

Movement The inability to move a body part can indicate a serious central nervous system injury that has involved the motor system. An inability to move one side of the body (hemiplegia) could be caused by a head injury or cerebrovascular accident (stroke). Bilateral tingling and numbness or sensory or motor deficits of the upper extremity may indicate a cervical spine injury. Weakness or inability to move the lower extremities could mean an injury below the neck, and pressure on the spinal cord could lead to limited use of the limbs.[23]

Abnormal Nerve Response The injured patient's pain or other reactions to adverse stimuli can provide valuable clues to the athletic trainer. Numbness or tingling in a limb with or without movement can indicate nerve or cold damage. Blocking of a main artery can produce severe pain, loss of sensation, or lack of a pulse in a limb. A complete lack of pain or of awareness of serious but obvious injury may be caused by shock, hysteria, drug usage, or a spinal

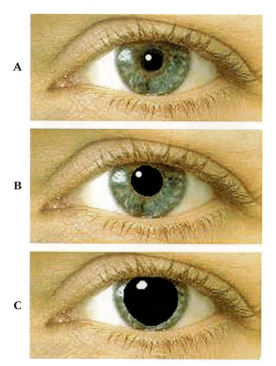

FIGURE 12–23 The pupils of the eyes are extremely sensitive to situations affecting the nervous system. (A) Constricted. (B) Normal. (C) Dilated.

cord injury. Generalized or localized pain in the injured region probably means there is no injury to the spinal cord.

Musculoskeletal Assessment

A logical process must be used to evaluate accurately the extent of a musculoskeletal injury.[52] The athletic trainer must be aware of the major signs that reveal the site, nature, and, above all, severity of the injury. Detection of these signs can be facilitated by understanding the mechanism or traumatic sequence and by methodically inspecting the injury.[13] Knowledge of the mechanism of an injury is extremely important in determining which area of the body is most affected. When the injury mechanism has been determined, the examiner proceeds to the next phase: physical inspection of the affected region. At this point, information is gathered by what is seen, heard, and felt.[34]

In an attempt to understand the mechanism of injury, a detailed *history* of the complaint must be taken. The patient is asked, if possible, about the events leading up to the injury and how it occurred and what he or she heard or felt when the injury took place.[6] Sounds occurring at the time of injury or during manual inspection yield pertinent information about the type and extent of pathology present. Such uncommon sounds as grating or harsh rubbing may indicate fracture. Such sounds as a snap, crack, or pop at the moment of injury

often indicate bone fracture or injury to ligaments or tendons. Joint sounds may be detected when either arthritis or internal derangement is present. Areas of the body that have abnormal amounts of fluid may produce crepitus when palpated or moved.

The athletic trainer should make a visual *observation* of the injured site, comparing it with the uninjured body part and looking for symmetry. The initial visual examination can disclose obvious deformity, swelling, and skin discoloration.

Finally, the region of the injury should be gently *palpated*. Feeling, or palpating, a part with trained fingers can, in conjunction with visual and audible signs, indicate the nature of the injury. Palpation is started away from the injury and gradually moved toward it. As the examiner gently feels the injury and surrounding structures with the fingertips, several factors can be revealed: the extent of point tenderness, the extent of irritation (whether it is confined to soft tissue alone or extends to the bony tissue), deformities that may not be detected by visual examination alone, and the presence of a pulse.[6]

Assessment Decisions After a quick on-site injury inspection and evaluation, the athletic trainer should make the following decisions:

1. The seriousness of the injury
2. The type of first aid and immobilization necessary
3. Whether the injury warrants immediate referral to a physician for further assessment
4. The manner of transportation from the injury site to the sidelines, athletic training room, or hospital

All information about the initial history, signs, and symptoms of the injury must be documented, if possible, so that they may be described in detail to the physician.

Immediate Treatment Musculoskeletal injuries are extremely common in sports. The athletic trainer must be prepared to provide appropriate first aid immediately to control hemorrhage and associated swelling. Every first-aid effort should be directed toward one primary goal—reducing the amount of swelling and inflammation resulting from the injury.[45] If swelling and inflammation can be controlled initially, the amount of time required for injury rehabilitation will be significantly reduced. Initial management of musculoskeletal injuries should

> **Decisions that can be made from the secondary survey:**
> - Seriousness of injury
> - Type of first aid required
> - Whether injury warrants physical referral
> - Type of transportation needed.

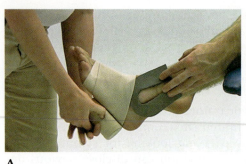 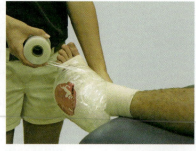 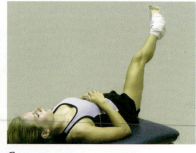

A B C

FIGURE 12–24   RICE technique. **(A)** A wet compression wrap should be applied over the horseshoe pad. **(B)** Ice bags should be secured in place by a dry compression wrap. **(C)** The leg should be elevated as much as possible during the initial treatment period.

include rest, ice, compression, and elevation (RICE) (see Figure 12–24).

Rest (Restricted Activity)   Rest after any type of injury is an extremely important component of any treatment program. Once a body part is injured, it immediately begins the healing process.[45] If the injured part is not rested and is subjected to external stresses and strains, the healing process never takes place. Consequently, the injured part does not heal, and the time required for rehabilitation is greatly increased. The number of days necessary for resting varies with the severity of the injury. Parts of the body that have experienced minor injury should rest for approximately 72 hours before a rehabilitation program is begun.

Ice (Cold Application)   The initial treatment of acute injuries should use cold.[36] Therefore, ice is used for most conditions involving strains, sprains, and contusions. Cold is most commonly used immediately after injury to decrease pain and promote local superficial constriction of the vessels (vasoconstriction), thus controlling hemorrhage and edema.[36] Cold applied to an acute injury will lower metabolism and tissue demands for oxygen and will reduce hypoxia.[45] This benefit extends to uninjured tissue, preventing injury-related tissue death from spreading to adjacent normal cellular structures. Cold is also used in chronic inflammatory conditions, such as bursitis, tenosynovitis, and tendonitis, conditions in which heat may cause additional pain and swelling. Cold is also used to reduce the muscle guarding that accompanies pain. Its pain-reducing (analgesic) effect is probably one of its greatest benefits. One explanation of the analgesic effect is that cold slows the speed of nerve transmission, so the pain sensation

> Rest, ice, compression, and elevation (RICE) are essential in the emergency care of musculoskeletal injuries.

is reduced. It is also possible that cold bombards pain receptors with so many cold impulses that pain impulses are lost. With ice treatments, the athlete usually reports an uncomfortable sensation of cold, followed by burning, then an aching sensation, and finally complete numbness.

Because the subcutaneous (under the skin) fat slowly conducts the cold temperature, applications of cold for short periods of time will be ineffective in cooling deeper tissues. For this reason, longer treatments of at least 20 minutes are recommended. However, prolonged application of cold can cause tissue damage.[45]

Cold treatments seem to be more effective in reaching deep tissues than most forms of heat are. Cold applied to the skin is capable of significantly lowering the temperature of tissues at a considerable depth. The temperature to which the deeper tissues can be lowered depends on the type of cold that is applied to the skin, the duration of its application, the thickness of the subcutaneous fat, and the region of the body to which it is applied.[37] Ice packs should be applied to the area for at least 72 hours after an acute injury. With many injuries, regular ice treatments may be continued for several weeks.

For best results, ice packs (crushed ice and towel) should be applied over a compression wrap. Frozen gel packs should not be used directly against the skin because they reach much lower temperatures than do ice packs. A good rule of thumb is to apply a cold pack to a recent injury for 30 to 60 minutes every 2 hours throughout the waking day. Depending on the severity and site of the injury, cold may be applied intermittently for one to 72 hours. For example, a mild strain will probably require 1 day of 20-minute periods of cold application, whereas a severe knee or ankle sprain might need 3 to 7 days of intermittent cold. If the severity of an injury is in doubt, the best approach is to extend the time that ice is applied.

Compression In most cases, immediate compression of an acute injury is considered to be at least as essential as cold and elevation and in some cases may be superior to them.[45] Placing external pressure on an injury assists in decreasing hemorrhage and hematoma formation by mechanically reducing the space available for swelling to accumulate. Fluid seepage into interstitial spaces is retarded by compression, and absorption is facilitated. However, applying compression to an anterior compartment syndrome in which swelling has significantly increased pressure in that area, or to certain injuries involving the head and neck, is contraindicated.

12–5 Clinical Application Exercise

A field hockey player trips over an opponent's stick, plantar flexing and inverting her ankle, and she falls to the turf with a grade 2 ankle sprain. She has immediate effusion and significant pain. On examination, there appears to be some laxity in the ankle joint. The athletic trainer transports the patient to the training room so that the ankle sprain can be managed properly.

? What specifically should the athletic trainer do to most effectively control the initial swelling associated with this injury?

Many types of compression are available. An elastic wrap that has been soaked in water and frozen in a freezer can provide both compression and cold when applied to a recent injury. Pads can be cut from felt or foam rubber to fit difficult-to-compress body areas. For example, a horseshoe-shaped pad placed bilaterally around the malleoli in combination with an elastic wrap and tape provides focal compression to reduce ankle edema.[45] Although cold is applied intermittently, compression should be maintained throughout the day and if possible throughout the night. Because of the pressure buildup in the tissues, the patient may find it painful to leave a compression wrap in place for a long time. However, it is essential to leave the wrap in place in spite of significant pain because compression is so important in the control of swelling. The compression wrap should be left in place for at least 72 hours after an acute injury. In many chronic overuse problems, such as tendinitis, tenosynovitis, and particularly bursitis, the compression wrap should be worn until almost all of the swelling is gone.

Elevation Along with cold and compression, elevation reduces internal bleeding. The injured part, particularly an extremity, should be elevated to eliminate the effects of gravity on blood pooling in the extremities.[45] Elevation assists the lymphatic system, which drains blood and other fluids from the injured area, returning them to the central

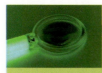

FOCUS 12–6 Focus on Treatment and Rehabilitation

Guidelines for proper splinting

- Put a dressing on any open wound before applying a splint.
- Splint the injury in the position in which it is found.
- Make sure the splint immobilizes the injury and doesn't permit movement.
- Immobilize the joints above and below the site of injury.
- Elevate the splinted extremity if possible.
- Apply a cold pack to the injury around the splint.
- Continuously check the color of the fingers and toes to make sure circulation is not impaired.

circulatory system. The greater the degree of elevation, the more effective the reduction in swelling. In an ankle sprain, for example, the leg should be placed so that the ankle is virtually straight up in the air. The injured part should be elevated as much as possible during the first 72 hours.

Emergency Splinting Any suspected fracture should be splinted before the patient is moved.[35] Transporting a person with a fracture without proper immobilization can

> A suspected fracture must be splinted before the patient is moved.

result in increased tissue damage, hemorrhage, and shock.[35] Conceivably, a mishandled fracture could cause death. Therefore, a thorough knowledge of splinting techniques is important. Applying splints should be a simple process using commercial emergency splints.[35,40] The athletic trainer usually does not have to improvise a splint because such devices are readily available in most sports settings. Whatever the type of splint used, the principles of good splinting remain the same. Two major concepts of splinting are to splint from one joint above the fracture to one joint below the fracture and to splint where the patient lies. If at all possible, do not move the patient until he or she has been splinted. *Focus Box 12–6:* "Guidelines for proper splinting" outlines the approach to be used.

Rapid form Vacuum Immobilizer The rapid form vacuum immobilizer is widely used by both EMTs and athletic trainers.[47] It consists of styrofoam chips contained inside an airtight cloth sleeve that is pliable. This splint can be molded to the shape of any joint or angulated fracture through the use of Velcro straps. A handheld pump sucks the air out of the sleeve, giving it a cardboardlike rigidity. This splint is most useful for injuries that are angulated and must be splinted in the position in which they are found (Figure 12–25A).

Air Splint An air splint is a clear plastic splint that is inflated with air around the affected part and can be used for extremity splinting, but its use requires some special training. This splint provides support and moderate pressure to the body part and affords a clear view of the site for X-ray examination. The inflatable splint should not be used if it will alter a fracture deformity (Figure 12–25B).

SAM® Splint A SAM® Splint is made with a thin sheet of soft, pliable aluminum covered by padding. The material can be cut with a pair of taping scissors. However, when shaped into structural curves, the SAM® Splint's aluminum core becomes rigid. The material is reusable and can be folded and unfolded repeatedly, allowing the same sheet of splint material to be reused as many times as desired (Figure 12–25C).

Half-Ring Splint For fractures of the femur, the half-ring traction splint offers the best support and immobilization but takes considerable practice to master. An open fracture must be carefully dressed to avoid additional contamination (Figure 12–25D).

Splinting of Lower-Limb Fractures Fractures of the ankle or leg require immobilization of the foot and knee. Any fracture involving the knee, thigh, or hip needs splinting of all the lower-limb joints and one side of the trunk.

Splinting of Upper-Limb Fractures Fractures around the shoulder complex are immobilized by a sling and swathe bandage, with the upper limb securely bound to the body. Upper-arm and elbow fractures must be splinted, with immobilization effected in a straight-arm position to lessen bone override. Lower-arm and wrist fractures should be splinted in a position of elbow flexion and should be supported by a sling. Hand and finger dislocations and fractures can be buddy-taped or may be splinted with tongue depressors, roller gauze, or aluminum splints.[50]

Splinting of the Spine and Pelvis Injuries involving a possible spine or pelvic fracture are best splinted and the patient moved using a spine board. Recently, a full body mattress vacuum splint immobilizer has been developed for dealing with spinal injuries

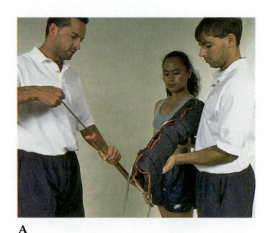

A

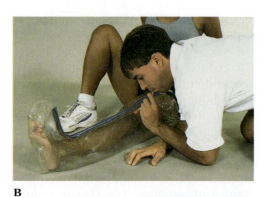

B

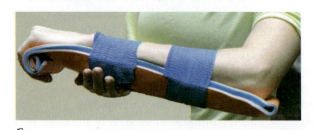

C

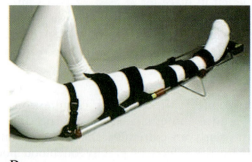

D

FIGURE 12–25 Examples of splints. **(A)** Rapid form vacuum immobilizer. **(B)** Air splint. **(C)** SAM® Splint (from SAM® Splint). **(D)** Half-ring splint (from Reel Research and Development).

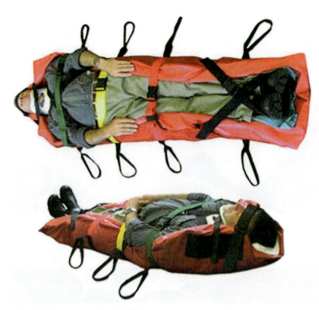

FIGURE 12–26   Full body mattress vacuum splint immobilizer. (From Neann, Victoria, Australia).

(Figure 12–26). The effectiveness of this piece of equipment as an immobilization device has yet to be determined.[47]

MOVING AND TRANSPORTING THE INJURED PATIENT

Moving, lifting, and transporting the injured patient must be executed with the use of techniques that will prevent further injury. Moving or transporting the patient improperly causes more additional injuries than does any other emergency procedure.[29,40] There is no excuse for poor handling of the injured patient. Planning should take into consideration all the possible transportation methods and the necessary equipment to execute them.[40] Capable and well-trained personnel, spine boards, stretchers, and a rescue vehicle may be needed to transport the injured patient. Special consideration must be given to extracting an injured swimmer from a pool.

> Great caution must be taken when transporting the injured athlete.

In 2001, an interassociation task force which included representatives from the NATA developed a consensus statement "Prehospital care of the spine injured athlete" http://www.nata.org/sites/default/files/PreHospitalCare4SpineInjuredAthlete.pdf).

In 2009, NATA developed a position statement "Acute management of the cervical spine injured athlete" (http://www.nata.org/sites/default/files/AcuteMgmtOfCervicalSpineInjuredAthlete.pdf). Links to both of these statements can be found at www.mhhe.com/prentice15e.

Placing the Patient on a Spine Board

In cases of suspected cervical spine injury, the athletic trainer should generally access the EMS and wait until the rescue squad arrives before attempting to move the patient. The only exception is if the patient is not breathing. Then the patient must be logrolled onto his or her back for CPR.

A suspected spinal injury requires extremely careful handling and is best left to properly trained paramedics or EMTs or to athletic trainers who are well trained and have access to the proper equipment for transport.[61] (See the inside back cover of this text for a list of emergency equipment that should be available on the sidelines.) If such personnel are not available, the patient should be moved under the express direction of a physician, and a spine board should be used (Figure 12–27). The most important principle in transporting an individual on a spine board is to maintain the head and neck in alignment with the long axis of the body.[5,18] In such cases, it is best to have one person whose sole responsibility is to ensure and maintain proper positioning of the head and neck until the head is secured to a spine board.[59]

Primary emergency care involves helping the patient maintain normal breathing, treating the patient for shock, and keeping the patient quiet and in the position found until medical assistance arrives. Ideally, transportation should not be attempted until a physician has examined the athlete and has given permission to move him or her. Neck stabilization must be maintained throughout transportation, first to the emergency vehicle, then to the hospital, and throughout the hospital procedure.[18]

These steps should be followed when moving a patient with a suspected neck injury:

1. The examiner should immediately maintain the position of the cervical spine[5] (Figure 12–27A).
2. The examiner must determine whether the patient is breathing and has a pulse.
   a. A spine board is retrieved for moving the patient.
   b. If the patient is lying prone, he or she must be logrolled onto his or her back for CPR or to be secured to the spine board.[43] If the patient is supine, the lift and slide technique is recommended over the logroll technique. A patient with a possible cervical fracture is transported face up. A patient with a suspected spinal fracture in the lower-trunk area may be transported face down.
3. If the patient is wearing a helmet with a face mask, the face mask should be removed to allow access to the airway prior to spine boarding. However if the patient is prone, he or she should be logrolled onto a spine board before removing the face mask.
   a. The spine board is placed close to the side of the patient (Figure 12–27B).

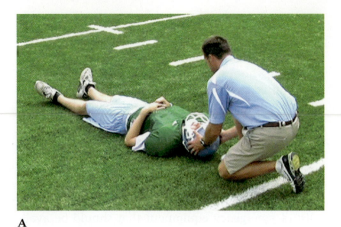

A

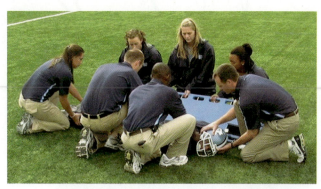

B

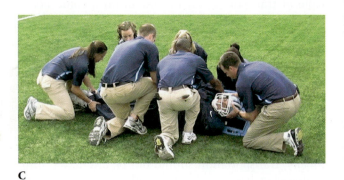

C

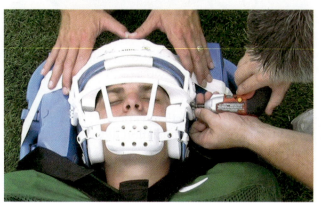

D

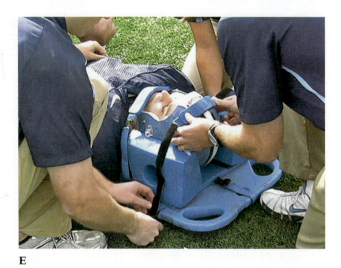

E

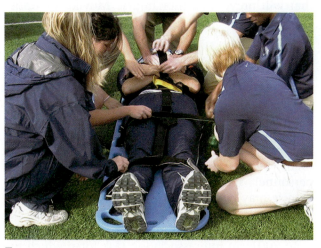

F

FIGURE 12–27 **(A)** When moving an unconscious athlete, first establish whether the athlete is breathing and has a pulse. An unconscious athlete must always be treated as having a serious neck injury. If the athlete is lying supine, the head and neck should be immediately stabilized. **(B)** If lying prone, the athlete must be turned over for CPR or be secured to a spine board for possible cervical fracture. One person (the "captain") should stabilize the athlete's neck and head. The spine board is placed as close to the athlete as possible. **(C)** Each assistant is responsible for one of the athlete's segments. When the athletic trainer gives the command "roll," the athlete is moved as a unit onto the spine board. **(D)** The face mask is cut away while the captain continues to stabilize the athlete's neck. **(E)** The head and neck are stabilized onto the spine board by means of a chin strap secured to metal loops. **(F)** The trunk and lower limbs are secured to the spine board by straps.

(continued)

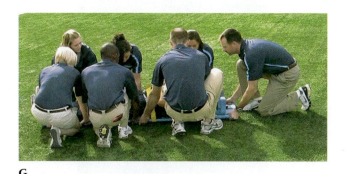

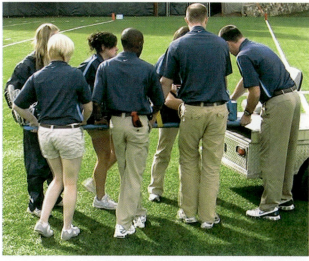

G

H

FIGURE 12–27 continued
(G) All carriers assume a position to stand. **(H)** Once the carriers are standing, the patient may be transported to a cart for removal from the field.

b. To roll the athlete over requires at least five persons, with the captain of the team protecting the patient's head and neck. The neck must be stabilized and must not be moved from its original position, no matter how distorted it appears.

c. All extremities are placed in an axial alignment.

d. Each assistant is responsible for one of the patient's body segments. One assistant is responsible for turning the trunk, another the hips, another the thighs, and the last the lower legs.

4. With the spine board close to the patient's side, the captain gives the command to logroll him or her onto the board as one unit (Figure 12–26C).

5. On the board, the patient's head and neck continue to be stabilized by the captain while the face mask is removed (Figure 12–26D).

6. Next, the head and neck are stabilized on the spine board by a chin strap, head strap, and side blocks (Figure 12–26E).[17]

7. Finally, the trunk and lower limbs are secured to the spine board by straps (Figure 12–27F).

8. The rescuers place themselves in a position to stand, and then, on the command of the person stabilizing the head, they collectively lift the patient on the spine board (Figure 12–27G).

9. The spine board can then be carried to a transport vehicle or cart for removal from the field (Figure 12–27H).

If the patient is supine, the lift and slide technique should be used to move the patient onto a spine board. Four or five persons are needed: a captain stationed at the patient's head and three or four assistants. One assistant is in charge of lifting the patient's trunk, one the hips, and one the legs. At the captain's lift command, the patient is lifted while the fourth assistant slides a spine board under the patient between the feet of the captain and the assistants (Figure 12–28A). One study has shown the lift and slide technique to be more effective in restricting motion in the head, reducing both lateral flexion and axial rotation, compared with the logroll technique.[18]

A scoop stretcher may also be used for transporting a patient with a potential injury to the spine, although it is not generally considered to be as safe as using a spine board (Figure 12–28B). A scoop stretcher has detachable hinges at each end and thus can be split into two halves (Figure 12–28C). Each half of the stretcher is placed on either side of the supine athlete. The athletic trainer can easily slide each half of the stretcher under the athlete until the hinges are locked together, in effect "scooping" the athlete onto the stretcher. The advantage in using a scoop stretcher is that it is not necessary to roll the injured athlete onto his or her side to get the stretcher underneath.

Ambulatory Aid

Ambulatory aid is support or assistance given to an injured patient who is able to walk (Figure 12–29). Before the patient is allowed to walk, he or she should be carefully scrutinized to make sure that the injuries are minor. Whenever serious injuries are suspected, walking should be prohibited. The patient should go from prone to supine or side lying to sitting and should sit for approximately 30 seconds before standing. Weight should be on the uninvolved extremity; the knee is bent;

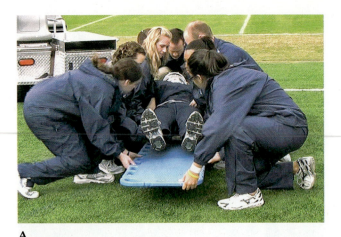

A

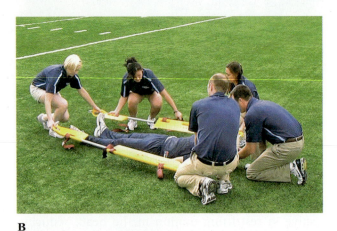

B

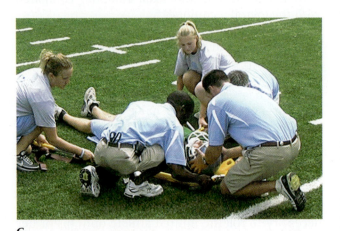

C

FIGURE 12–28　Alternative methods of placing the athlete on a spine board. **(A)** The lift and slide technique. **(B)** The scoop stretcher. **(C)** Latching the top of the scoop stretcher.

the athlete grasps the athletic trainer's hands and stands up. Two individuals who are approximately the same height should provide complete support on both sides of the patient. The patient's arms are draped over the assistants' shoulders, and their arms encircle his or her back.

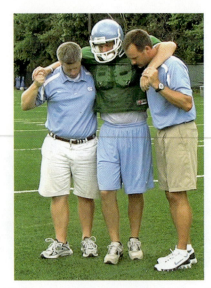

FIGURE 12–29　The ambulatory aid method of transporting a mildly injured athlete.

Manual Conveyance

Manual conveyance may be used to move a mildly injured individual a greater distance than the person could walk with ease (Figure 12–30). Any decision to carry the patient, such as a decision to use ambulatory aid, must be made only after a complete examination to determine the existence of potentially serious conditions. The most convenient carry is performed by two assistants.

Stretcher Carrying

Whenever a serious injury is suspected, the best and safest mode of transportation for a short

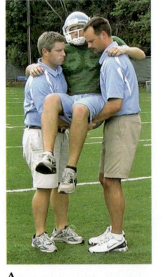

A

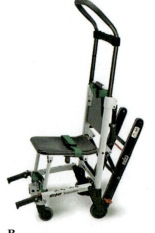

B

FIGURE 12–30　**(A)** Manual conveyance method for transporting a mildly injured athlete. **(B)** A stair chair can also be used if the athlete is too large for the athletic trainer to lift manually.

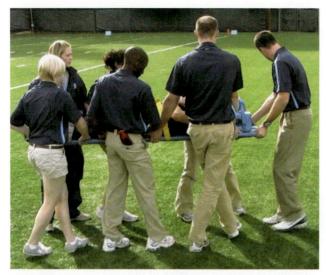

FIGURE 12–31 Whenever a serious injury is suspected, a stretcher is the safest method for transporting the patient. When loading the patient into a rescue vehicle, the head should go first.

distance is by stretcher. With each segment of the body supported, the patient is gently lifted and placed on the stretcher, which is carried adequately by a minimum of four assistants, two supporting each side (Figure 12–31). The stretcher carriers should face the direction of travel and carry the patient feet first. However, they should carry a patient head first if going uphill or upstairs, or when loading the stretcher into a rescue vehicle. Any person with an injury serious enough to require the use of a stretcher must be carefully examined before being moved.

A suspected fracture must be splinted properly before the patient is transported. Patients with shoulder injuries are more comfortably moved in a semisitting position, unless other injuries preclude such positioning. If injury to the upper extremity is such that flexion of the elbow is not possible, the individual should be transported on a stretcher with the limb properly splinted and carried at the side, with adequate padding placed between the arm and the body.

Pool Extraction

Removing an injured swimmer from a pool requires some special consideration on the part of the athletic trainer. Obviously, an athletic trainer who is providing coverage for athletes training or competing in a pool must be able to swim and should have water safety or lifeguard training. The athletic trainer should routinely have immediate access to both a rescue tube and an aquatic spine board in case an athlete sustains an injury while in the pool. A rescue tube should always be used to extract an injured swimmer from the pool.[3] The rescue tube

will not only serve as a flotation device but also can help prevent a swimmer who is distressed from grabbing the athletic trainer while in the water.

The following procedures are recommended for removing an injured swimmer from a pool:

1. When dealing with a swimmer who has sustained what appears to be a minor injury in the pool, if the swimmer is close to the edge of the pool, the athletic trainer can reach out to the swimmer with the rescue tube while standing on the pool deck and holding onto the shoulder strap with the other hand. The swimmer should grab the tube; then the athletic trainer can pull him or her to the edge of the pool (Figure 12–32A).[3]

2. If the swimmer is too far away from the pool deck, the athletic trainer should get into the water, approach the swimmer from the front, extend the rescue tube, have the swimmer grab the tube, and kick if possible, while the athletic trainer pulls the swimmer to the edge of the pool (Figure 12–32B).[3]

3. If a swimmer appears to be more severely injured, the athletic trainer should get into the water, approach the swimmer from behind, reach under the armpits, and grab the swimmer's shoulders while putting the rescue tube between the swimmer's back and the athletic trainer's chest. The athletic trainer should keep his or her head to either side to avoid being hit by the swimmer's head, should it fall backward. The athletic trainer should lean back, pulling the swimmer onto the rescue tube, which should support the swimmer, keeping the swimmer's mouth and face out of the water; the athletic trainer should pull the swimmer to the edge of the pool while attempting to keep him or her calm (Figure 12–33).[3]

4. Deciding to remove an injured swimmer from the water depends on several factors, including the swimmer's condition and size and the availability of help or how long until help arrives. For example, an injured swimmer requiring CPR should be removed immediately from the water; rescue

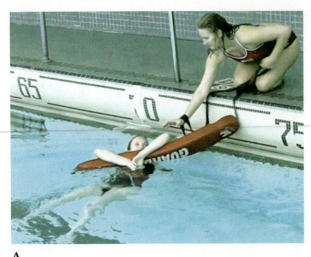
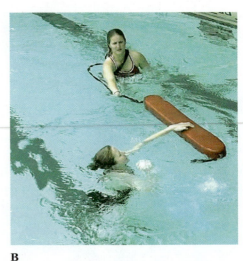

A

B

FIGURE 12–32   Techniques for pool rescue. **(A)** The swimmer is close to the edge of the pool. **(B)** The swimmer is in the middle of the pool, using a rescue tube.

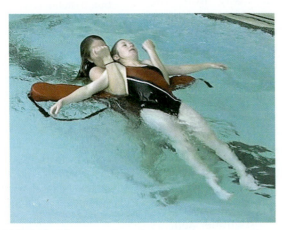

FIGURE 12–33   Technique for removing a severely injured swimmer from the water.

breathing should not be attempted in the water. A spine board should be used by two people to remove any swimmer from the water who is unable to get out on his or her own, even if a spinal injury is not suspected. The primary rescuer takes the injured swimmer to the side of the pool and turns him or her to face the pool deck. A second rescuer standing on the pool deck grabs the swimmer's opposite wrists and pulls the swimmer up, keeping the head above water and away from the edge of the pool (Figure 12–34A). The primary rescuer gets out of the water, grabs the spine board, then guides the spine board foot-end first down into the water between the swimmer and the edge of the pool (Figure 12–34B). The second rescuer then turns the swimmer so that his or her back rests against the spine board (Figure 12–34C). Each rescuer then grasps a wrist with one hand and the spine board with the other. The rescuers pull the spine board upward and backward, leveraging the board onto the pool deck (Figure 12–34D).[3]

5. A swimmer with a suspected head or cervical neck injury or a swimmer who is unconscious requires special precaution. A swimmer's cervical spine can be immobilized in the water by a single primary rescuer placing the victim's arms overhead and compressing them against the head. Squeezing the arms together stabilizes the spine and head. The swimmer may be held face up in the water in this position until help arrives (Figure 12–35A). While the primary rescuer continues stabilizing the head and neck, a second rescuer submerges the spine board, positioning it appropriately under the swimmer. The primary rescuer maintains stabilization of the neck. Rescue tubes may be used to help float the spine board. The second rescuer moves to the swimmer's head and assumes responsibility for stabilizing the swimmer's head. The primary rescuer then securely straps the chest, hips, thighs, and head to the spine board (Figure 12–35B&C). Both rescuers then remove the spine board from the pool, head first, by initially lifting the board onto the edge of the pool while still in the water. Then one rescuer gets on the pool deck while the other remains in the water to complete the pool extraction (Figure 12–35D).[3]

EMERGENCY EMOTIONAL CARE

Besides evaluating and responding to the emergency physical requirements of an injury, the athletic trainer must evaluate and respond

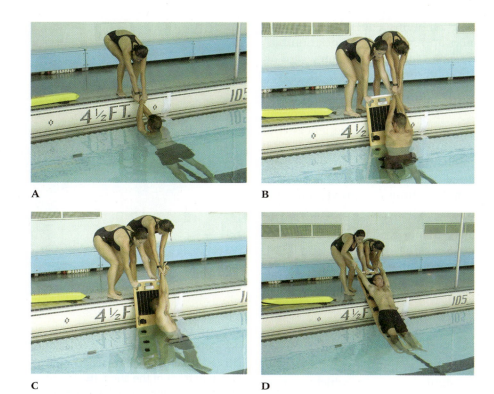

A

B

C

D

FIGURE 12–34 Technique for removing an athlete from the water who can't get out on his or her own.

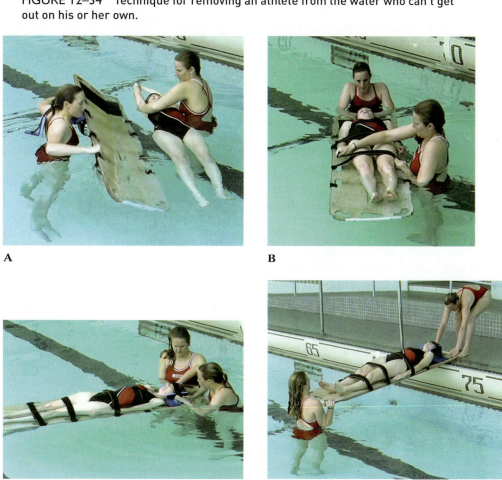

A

B

C

D

FIGURE 12–35 Technique for putting an athlete with a suspected spinal injury on a spine board and removing him or her from the pool.

appropriately to the emotions engendered by the situation. The American Psychiatric Association has set forth major principles for the emergency care of emotional reactions to trauma:

1. Accept everyone's right to personal feelings, because everyone comes from a unique background and has had unique emotional experiences. Do not tell the injured person how he or she should feel. Show empathy, not pity.
2. Accept the injured person's limitations as real.
3. Accept your own limitations as a provider of first aid.

In general, the athletic trainer dealing with an injured patient's emotions should be empathetic and calm and should make it obvious that the patient's feelings are understood and accepted (see Chapter 11).

PROPER FIT AND USE OF THE CRUTCH OR CANE

Weight bearing may be contraindicated for a patient with a lower-limb injury, in which case a crutch or cane should be used for ambulation. The athletic trainer must be responsible for properly fitting the crutch or cane to the injured patient and then for providing instruction in its use. If the crutch or cane is not properly fitted, the patient may experience discomfort in the axilla from excessive pressure as well as pain in the low back. Faulty mechanics in the use of the crutch or cane when ambulating and particularly when ascending or descending stairs can cause the patient to fall.

Fitting the Patient

The adjustable aluminum or wooden crutch is well suited to the patient. Before fitting, the athletic trainer should inspect the crutch tops and the bolts and wing nut to make sure they are neither worn nor defective. For a correct fit, the patient should wear low-heeled shoes and stand with good posture and the feet close together. The crutch length is determined first by placing the tip 6 inches (15 cm) from the outer margin of the shoe and 2 inches (5 cm) in front of the shoe. The underarm crutch brace is positioned 1 inch (2.5 cm) below the anterior fold of the axilla. Next, the hand brace is adjusted so that it is even with the patient's hand when the elbow is flexed at approximately a 30-degree angle (Figure 12–36).

Fitting a cane to the patient is relatively easy. Measurement is taken from the crease of the wrist to the floor while the patient is wearing street shoes. (Figure 12–37A). The patient holds the cane on the uninjured side and uses a 3-point gait to advance the cane 4 to 6 inches (10 to 15 cm) ahead of the uninjured foot while simultaneously bearing weight on the injured side on the cane (Figure 12–37B).

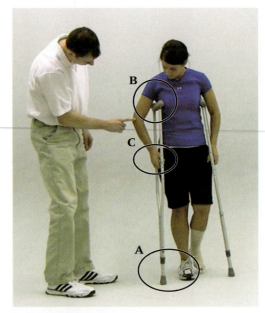

FIGURE 12–36   The crutch must be properly fitted to the patient. **(A)** The crutch tips are placed 6 inches (15 cm) from the outer margin of the shoe and 2 inches (5 cm) in front of the shoe. **(B)** The underarm crutch brace is positioned 1 inch (2.5 cm) below the anterior fold of the axilla. **(C)** The hand brace is placed even with the patient's hand, with the elbow flexed approximately 30 degrees.

Walking with the Crutch or Cane

Many elements of crutch walking correspond with normal walking. The technique commonly used is the tripod method. In this method, the patient swings through the crutches without making any surface contact with the injured limb or by partially bearing weight with the injured limb. The following sequence is performed:

> **Properly fitting a crutch or cane is essential to avoid placing abnormal stresses on the body.**

1. The patient stands on the uninjured leg with no weight or partial weight on the injured leg.
2. Placing the crutch tips 12 to 15 inches (30 to 37.5 cm) ahead of the feet, the patient leans forward, straightens the elbows, pulls the upper crosspiece firmly against the side of the

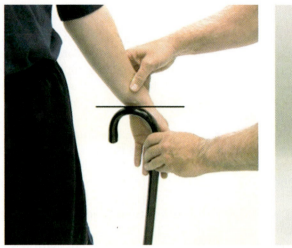
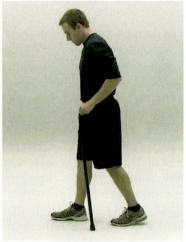

FIGURE 12–37   Using a cane. **(A)** Top of cane should be at the crease of the wrist.
(B) Patient should walk with cane on the uninjured side.

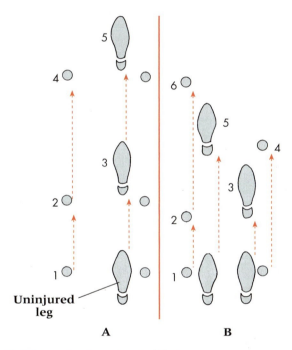

**Uninjured
leg**

FIGURE 12–38   Crutch gait. **(A)** Tripod method.
(B) Four-point gait.

chest, and swings or steps with the uninjured leg between the stationary crutches (Figure 12–38A). The patient should avoid placing the major support in the axilla.

3. After moving through, the patient recovers the crutches and again places the tips forward repeating the sequence. The crutches and the injured or non–weight-bearing leg always move together.

An alternative method is the four-point gait. In this method, the patient stands on both feet, moves one crutch forward, and steps forward with the opposite foot. The patient moves the crutch on the same side as the foot that moved forward, to just ahead of the foot, steps forward, using the opposite foot, followed by the crutch on the same side, and so on (Figure 12–38B).

The tripod gait that is used for crutch walking on a level surface is also used on stairs. In going up stairs, the uninjured support leg moves up one step while the body weight is supported by the hands on the crutches. The full weight of the body is transferred to the uninjured leg, and the crutch tips and injured leg are moved to that step. In going down stairs, the crutch tips and the injured leg move down one step, followed by the uninjured leg. If a handrail is available, the patient uses the tripod gait holding both crutches with the outside hand.

NOTE: The patient should exercise caution when ambulating on any wet surface.

Crutch walking will generally follow a progression from non–weight bearing (NWB) to touch-down weight bearing (TDWB), to partial weight bearing (PWB), to full weight bearing (FWB). The rate of progression will be dictated by the limitations of the injury as well as the capabilities of the patient.

When the injured patient needs to be partially weight bearing, a cane or a single crutch can be used to help with balance. In this case, the patient should hold the cane or crutch in the hand on the uninjured side and move the cane forward simultaneously with the uninjured leg. The patient should avoid leaning too heavily on the cane or crutch. If this is a problem, then the patient should use two crutches.

SUMMARY

- An emergency is defined as "an unforeseen combination of circumstances and the resulting state that calls for immediate action." The primary concern of emergency aid is to maintain cardiovascular function and, indirectly, central nervous system function. An emergency action plan should be activated whenever a patient is seriously injured.

- The athletic trainer must make a systematic assessment of the injured patient to determine appropriate emergency care. A primary survey assesses and deals with life-threatening situations. Once the patient is stabilized, the secondary survey makes a more detailed assessment of the injury.

- In adult CPR, the ratio of compression to breaths is 30 to 2, with 100 compressions per minute. An obstructed airway is relieved by using backblows, abdominal thrusts, the finger sweep of the throat, or all of these.

- Hemorrhage can occur externally and internally. External bleeding can be controlled by direct pressure, by applying pressure at pressure points, and by elevation. Internal hemorrhage can occur subcutaneously, intramuscularly, or within a body cavity.

- Shock can occur from a variety of situations. Shock can be hypovolemic, respiratory, neurogenic, psychogenic, cardiogenic, septic, anaphylactic, or metabolic. Symptoms include pale skin, dilated eyes, weak and rapid pulse, and rapid, shallow breathing. Management includes maintaining normal body temperature and slightly elevating the feet.

- Rest, ice, compression, and elevation (RICE) should be used for the immediate care of a musculoskeletal injury. Ice should be applied for at least 20 minutes every 1 to 1½ hours, and compression and elevation should be continuous for at least 72 hours after injury.

- Any suspected fracture should be splinted before the patient is moved. Commercial rapid form vacuum immobilizers and air splints are most often used as splints in an athletic training setting.

- Great care must be taken in moving the seriously injured patient. The unconscious patient must be handled as though he or she has a cervical fracture. Moving a patient with a suspected serious neck injury must be performed only by persons specifically trained to do so. A spine board should be used for transport to avoid any movement of the cervical region.

- Patients who are injured will respond emotionally to the situation. The athletic trainer must understand and fully accept their feelings.

- When removing an injured swimmer from a pool, the athletic trainer should make every effort to minimize movement of the head and cervical spine while placing the swimmer on a spine board in the water.

- The athletic trainer should be responsible for the proper fitting of and instruction in the use of crutches or a cane by a patient with an injury to the lower extremity.

WEB SITES

American Red Cross: www.redcross.org/en/aboutus
The American Red Cross offers many emergency services and training. This site describes those services, introduces the information provided in various training opportunities, and explains how to obtain that training.

American Heart Association: www.amhrt.org

Cervical Spine Stabilization: www.trauma.org/archive/spine/cspine-stab.html
This brief article describes the considerations with cervical spine stabilization.

First Aid with Parasol EMT: www.parasolemt.com.au
This site provides a comprehensive on-line first aid reference.

First Aid: www.mayohealth.org
This Web site on first-aid care is maintained by the Mayo Clinic.

National Safety Council: www.nsc.org
The National Safety Council is a membership organization with resources on safety, health, and environmental topics, training, products, publications, news, and more.

SOLUTIONS TO CLINICAL APPLICATION EXERCISES

12–1 Because of the mechanism of injury, the athletic trainer should suspect that the patient has a cervical neck injury, and the head should be stabilized throughout. Because the patient is prone and breathing, the trainer should do nothing until the patient regains consciousness. An on-field exam should determine the athlete's neurological status. Then the player should be carefully logrolled onto a spine board because CPR could be necessary at any time. The face mask should be removed in case CPR is required. The helmet and shoulder pads should be left in place. The patient should then be transported to an emergency facility. In this situation, the worst mistake the athletic trainer can make is not exercising enough caution.

12–2 If the equipment is available, the athletic trainer should administer supplemental oxygen, using a bag/valve mask and a pressurized oxygen cylinder to facilitate recovery.

12–3 The athletic trainer should encourage her to continue to cough to attempt to dislodge the gum. If she cannot breathe at all, the athletic trainer should perform a series of abdominal thrusts to help dislodge the gum, continuing the abdominal thrusts until the obstruction is ejected.

12–4 The patient may be going into hypovolemic shock secondary to hemorrhage and trauma, which can be a life-threatening situation. The athletic trainer should first direct someone to dial 911 to access the emergency medical system. Next, the athletic trainer must control the bleeding by using direct pressure, elevation, and pressure points. If bleeding is controlled and the rescue squad has not arrived, the forearm should be immobilized in a rapid form vacuum immobilizer. The patient should be supine, and his feet should be elevated in the shock position. His body temperature should be maintained.

12–5 The ankle should be wrapped with a wet elastic compression wrap. Ice should be applied to both sides of the joint over the compression wrap and secured. The ankle should be elevated so that the leg is above 45 degrees at a minimum. The compression wrap, ice, and elevation should be maintained

initially for at least 30 minutes, but not longer than an hour. The athletic trainer should also determine whether a fracture is suspected and make the appropriate referral.

12–6 A rapid form vacuum immobilizer will work well for this injury because of its ability to mold the splint to the joint without causing unnecessary movement. Therefore, the ankle can be immobilized in the current position before transporting the patient.

12–7 The athletic trainer should place the swimmer on a spine board and secure her before extracting her from the pool. Several people may be required to get the swimmer appropriately positioned on the spine board while still in the water. The swimmer should be given a brief neurological exam to determine the extent of the injury. The swimmer should then be transported to an emergency facility in a rescue vehicle.

12–8 The athletic trainer should instruct the patient in the tripod gait, in which the patient swings through the crutches without making any surface contact with the injured limb. The tripod gait is also used on stairs. In negotiating stairs, the rule of thumb is go up with the good leg first, followed by crutches, and to go down with the crutches first, followed by the good leg. If the stairs have a handrail, the patient can hold both crutches with his outside hand. Crutch walking will generally follow a progression: NWB to TDWB, to PWB, to FWB.

REVIEW QUESTIONS AND CLASS ACTIVITIES

1. What considerations are important in a well-planned system for handling emergency situations?
2. Discuss the rules for managing and moving an unconscious patient.
3. What are the life-threatening conditions that should be evaluated in the primary survey?
4. What are the ABCs of life support?
5. Identify the major steps in giving CPR and managing an obstructed airway. When might these procedures be used in a sports setting?
6. List the basic steps in assessing a musculoskeletal injury.
7. What techniques should be used to stop external hemorrhage?
8. Numerous types of shock can occur from a sports injury or illness; list them and their management.
9. What first-aid procedures are used to decrease hemorrhage, inflammation, muscle spasm, and pain from a musculoskeletal injury?
10. Describe the basic concepts of emergency splinting.
11. How should a patient with a suspected spinal injury be transported?
12. What techniques can be used to transport a patient with a suspected musculoskeletal injury?
13. Discuss the methods for extracting an injured swimmer from a pool.
14. Explain how to fit crutches properly.

REFERENCES

1. American Heart Association: 2010 American Heart Association guidelines for cardiopulmonary resuscitation and emergency cardiovascular care, *Circulation* 122:729–67, 2010.
2. American Red Cross: *CPR/AED for the professional rescuer participants manual*, Boston, 2006, American Red Cross.
3. American Red Cross: *Lifeguarding instructor's manual training*, San Bruno, CA, 2007, Staywell.
4. Andersen J, Courson R, Kleiner D: National Athletic Trainers' Association position statement: Emergency planning in athletics, *J Athl Train* 37(1):99, 2002.
5. Bailes, J: Management of cervical spine injuries in athletes, *J Athl Train* 42(1):126–34, 2007.
6. Baxter R: *Pocket guide to musculoskeletal assessment*, ed 4, St. Louis, 2003, WB Saunders.
7. Berry D, Miller M: Demonstrating external bleeding and shock, *Athletic Therapy Today* 11(4):22, 2006.
8. Berry, D, Seitz, R: Educating the educator: Teaching airway adjunct techniques in athletic training, *Athletic Training Education Journal*, 107–16, 2011.
9. Biddington C, Popovich M, Kupczyk N: Certified athletic trainers' management of emergencies, *J Sport Rehabil* 14(2):185, 2005.
10. Broglio S, Dillon M: Emergency management of head and cervical-spine injuries, *Athletic Therapy Today* 10(2):24, 2005.
11. Brukner P, Kahn K, Hunte G: Sporting emergencies. In Brukner P, editor: *Clinical sports medicine*, ed 2, Sydney, 2002, McGraw-Hill.
12. Cendoma M: Evaluating face mask removal techniques, *NATA News* 4:14, 2006.
13. Courson R, Clanton M, Patel H: Emergency assessment, *Athletic Therapy Today* 10(2):19, 2005.
14. Decoster L, Shirley C, Swartz E: Football face mask removal with a cordless screwdriver on helmets used for at least one season of play, *J Athl Train* 40(3):169, 2005.
15. Delano T, Petschauer M, Guskiewicz K, Prentice W: Removal of a men's lacrosse helmet is faster and produces less cervical movement compared with removal of the face mask, *J Athl Train* 41(S):S-57, 2006.
16. Delforge G: Sports injury assessment and problem identification. In Delforge G, editor: *Musculoskeletal trauma implications for sports injury management*, Champaign, IL, 2002, Human Kinetics.
17. Del Rossi G: Management of cervical-spine injuries, *Athletic Therapy Today* 7(2):46, 2002.
18. Del Rossi G, Horodyski M, Powers M: A comparison of spine-board transfer techniques and the effect of training on performance, *J Athl Train* 38(3):204–08, 2003.
19. Dezner J, Courson R, Roberts W: Inter-association as force recommendations on emergency preparedness and management of sudden cardiac arrest in high school and college athletic programs: a consensus statement, *Athl Train* 42(1):143, 2007.

20. Farrell RN: AEDs and cardiac resuscitation: Is prevention part of your plan? *Athletic Therapy Today* 6(3):46, 2001.

21. Flegel M: Primary survey and providing life support. In Flegel M, editor: *Sport first aid*, ed 4, Champaign, IL, 2008, Human Kinetics.

22. Flegel M: Secondary survey and first aid techniques. In Flegel M, editor: *Sport first aid*, ed 3, Champaign, IL, 2004, Human Kinetics.

23. Fincher AL: Managing medical emergencies, part 1, *Athletic Therapy Today* 6(3):44, 2001.

24. Gale S: The combined tool approach for face mask removal during on-field conditions, *J Athl Train*, 43(1):14-20, 2008.

25. Green BN: Important changes in the 2000 CPR guidelines, *J Sports Chiropractic and Rehabilitation* 15(2):80, 2001.

26. Herbert D: Emergency preparedness recommendations for high school and college athletic programs, *Exercise standards and malpractice reporter* 21(4):58, 2007.

27. Herbert D: Plan to save lives: Create and rehearse an emergency response plan, *ACSM's Health and Fitness Journal* 1(5):34, 1997.

28. Jenkins H, Valovich T, Arnold B: Removal tools are faster and produce less force and torque on the helmet than cutting tools during face mask retraction, *J Athl Train* 37(3):246, 2002.

29. Karren KJ, Hafen BQ: *First aid for colleges and universities*, Boston, 2011, Benjamin Cummings.

30. Kleiner DM: 10 questions about football helmet and face mask removal: A review of the recent literature, *Athletic Therapy Today* 6(3):29, 2001.

31. Kleiner D, Almquist J, Bailes J: *Prehospital care of the spine-injured athlete: A document from the Inter-Association Task Force for Appropriate Care of the Spine-Injured Athlete*, Dallas, 2001, National Athletic Trainers' Association.

32. Knox KE, Kleiner DM: The efficiency of tools used to retract a football helmet face mask, *J Athl Train* 32(3):211, 1997.

33. LaPrade RF, Schnetzler KA, Broxterman RJ: Cervical spine alignment in the immobilized ice hockey player: A computed tomographic analysis of the effects of helmet removal, *Am J Sports Med* 28(6):800, 2000.

34. Magee DL: *Orthopedic physical assessment*, Philadelphia, 2007, Elsevier Health Science.

35. Meredith RM, Butcher JD: Field splinting of suspected fractures: Preparation, assessment, and application. *Physician Sportsmed* 25(10):29, 1997.

36. Miller M, Berry D: *Emergency response management for athletic trainers*, Philadelphia, 2010, Lippincott, Williams & Wilkins.

37. National Athletic Trainers' Association: *Position stand: Helmet removal guidelines*, Dallas, 1998, National Athletic Trainers' Association.

38. National Collegiate Athletic Association: Guidelines for helmet fitting and removal. In Kiossner D, editor: *2011-2012 NCAA sports medicine handbook*, Indianapolis, National Collegiate Athletic Association.

39. National Federation of State High School Athletic Associations: Helmet removal guidelines. *Sports medicine handbook*, Indianapolis, 2011, National Federation of State High School Athletic Associations

40. National Safety Council: *Standard 2012. First aid and CPR and AED*, San Francisco, 2012, McGraw-Hill

41. Palumbo MA, Hulstyn MJ, Fadale PD: The effect of protective football equipment on alignment of the injured cervical spine: Radiographic analysis in a cadaveric model, *Am J Sports Med* 24(4):446, 1996.

42. Paluska, A: Laryngeal trauma in sport. *Current Sports Medicine Reports*, 7(1):16–21, 2008.

43. Petschauer M: Helmet fit and cervical spine motion in collegiate men's lacrosse athletes secured to a spine board, *Journal of Athletic Training*, 45(3): 215–21, 2010.

44. Potter B: Testing the emergency action plan in athletics, *Athletic Therapy Today* 14(6): 214, 2009.

45. Prentice WE: Considerations in designing a rehabilitation program., In Prentice WE, editor: *Rehabilitation techniques in sports medicine and athletic training*, St. louis, 2011, McGraw-Hill.

46. Ransone J, Dunn-Bennett LR: Assessment of first-aid knowledge and decision making of high school athletic coaches, *J Athl Train* 34(3): 267, 1999.

47. Ransone J, Kersey R, Walsh K: The efficacy of the rapid form cervical vacuum immobilizer in cervical spine immobilization of the equipped football player, *J Athl Train* 35(1):65, 2000.

48. Ray R, Luchies C, Frens M: Cervical spine motion in football players during 3 airway exposure techniques, *J Athl Train* 37(2):172, 2002.

49. Rothmier, J: The role of the automated external defibrillators in sports, *Sports Health: A Multidisciplinary Approach* 1(1):16, 2009.

50. Sailer SM, Lewis SB: Rehabilitation and splinting of common upper-extremity injuries in athletes, *Clin Sports Med* 14(2):411, 1995.

51. Schnirring L: AEDs gain foothold in sports medicine, *Physician Sportsmed* 29(4):11–19, 2001.

52. Starkey C, Ryan J: *Examination of orthopedic and athletic injuries*, Philadelphia, 2010, F.A. Davis.

53. Swartz, E: Cervical spine alignment during on-field management of potential catastrophic spine injuries, *Sports Health* 1(3):247–52, 2009.

54. Swartz, E: Emergency face mask removal effectiveness: A comparison of traditional and nontraditional football helmet face mask attachment systems. *J Athl Train*. 45(6): 560–69, 2010.

55. Swartz E, Armstrong C, Rankin J: A 3-dimensional analysis of face mask removal tools in inducing helmet movement, *J Athl Train* 37(2):178, 2002.

56. Swartz E, Boden B, Courson R, Decoster L, Horodysky M, et al: National Athletic Trainers' Association position statement: Acute management of the cervical spine-injured athlete, *J Athl Train* 44(3): 306–31, 2009.

57. Swartz E, Norkus S, Armstrong C: Face mask removal: Movement and time associated with cutting of the loop straps, *J Athl Train* 38(2):120, 2003.

58. Swartz E, Norkus S, Cappaert T: Football equipment design affects face mask removal efficiency, *AMJ Sports Med* 3(8):1210, 2005.

59. Swartz E, Nowak J, Shirley C: A comparison of head movement during back boarding by motorized spine-board and log-roll techniques, *J Athl Train* 40(3):162, 2005.

60. *Taber's cyclopedic medical dictionary*, Philadelphia, 2011, FA Davis.

61. Tator, C: Recognition and management of spinal cord injuries in sports and recreation, *Physical Medicine and Rehabilitation Clinics of North America*, 20(1):69–76, 2009.

62. Terry G, Kyle J, Ellis J: Sudden cardiac arrest in athletic medicine, *J Athl Train* 36(2):205, 2001.

63. Tierney R, Mattacola C, Sitler M: Head position and football equipment influence cervical spinal-cord space during immobilization, *J Athl Train* 37(2):185, 2002.

64. Toler, J: Comparison of 3 airway access techniques during suspected spine injury management in American football, *Clinical Journal of Sports Medicine* 20(2):92–97, 2010.

65. Walsh K: Thinking proactively: The emergency action plan, *Athletic Therapy Today* 6(5):57, 2001.

66. Waninger, K: Cervical spine injury management in the helmeted athlete, *Current Sports Medicine Reports* 10(1):45–49, 2011.

67. Waninger K, Rothman M, Foley J: Computed tomography is diagnostic in the cervical imaging of helmeted football players with shoulder pads, *J Athl Train* 39(3):2, 2004.

68. Waninger K; Management of the helmeted athlete with suspected cervical spine injury, *Am J Sports Med* 32(5):331, 2004.

ANNOTATED BIBLIOGRAPHY

American Red Cross: *CPR/AED For the Professional Rescuer Participants manual*, Boston, 2006, American Red Cross.

This text provides CPR information at the level that athletic trainers need to know to be a professional rescuer.

Karren KJ, Hafen BQ: *First aid for colleges and universities*, Boston, 2011, Benjamin Cummings.

A well-illustrated, simple approach to the treatment of emergency illness and injury.

Kleiner D, Almquist J, Bailes J: *Prehospital care of the spine-injured athlete: A document from the Inter-Association Task Force for Appropriate Care of the Spine-Injured Athlete*, Dallas, 2001, National Athletic Trainers' Association.

A well-referenced monograph that details consensus recommendations from NATA and a variety of other sports medicine organizations relative to the emergency care of an athlete with a suspected spinal injury from the time of injury until arrival at a medical care facility.

Leikin JB, Feldman BJ: *American Medical Association handbook of first aid and emergency care*, Philadelphia, 2004, Random House.

Covers urgent emergency situations as well as the common injuries and ailments that occur in every family, taking the reader step-by-step through basic first-aid techniques, the medical symptoms to recognize before an emergency occurs, and what to do when one does occur.

Magee DJ: *Orthopedic physical assessment*, Philadelphia, 2007, Elsevier Health Science.

An extremely well-illustrated book with excellent coverage. Its strength lies in its coverage of injuries commonly found during athletic training.

National Safety Council: *First aid CPR and AED*, San Francisco, 2012, McGraw-Hill

Well-written and extremely well-illustrated text that deals with first-aid and emergency procedures. Although most of the information is directed at the general population, the principles and techniques can certainly be applied to the injured athlete. An excellent resource for the athletic trainer.

Swartz E, Boden B, Courson R, Decoster C: National Athletic Trainers' Association position statement: Acute management of the cervical spine injured athlete, *J Athl Train* 44(3):306, 2009.

Provides athletic trainers, team physicians, emergency responders, and other health care professionals with recommendations on how to best manage a catastrophic cervical spine injury in the athlete.

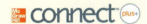

13

Off-the-Field Injury Evaluation

■ Objectives

When you finish this chapter you should be able to

- Discuss the athletic trainer's ability to make an accurate clinical diagnosis.
- Review the terminology used in injury evaluation.
- Apply the HOPS off-the-field evaluation scheme.
- Organize the process for documenting the findings of an off-the-field or progress evaluation.

- Recognize additional diagnostic techniques available to the athletic trainer through the team physician.
- Discuss how an ergonomic risk assessment can be performed to reduce workplace-related injuries.

■ Outline

■ Key Terms

biomechanics
pathomechanics
etiology
mechanism
pathology
symptom
sign
diagnosis

prognosis
sequela
syndrome
HOPS
active range of motion
passive range of motion
dermatome
myotomes

■ Connect Highlights connect plus+

Visit connect.mcgraw-hill.com for further exercises to apply your knowledge:

- Clinical application scenarios covering ability to make an accurate clinical diagnosis, HOPS off-the-field evaluation scheme, process for documenting findings, and using additional diagnostic techniques
- Click-and-drag questions covering ability to make an accurate clinical diagnosis, terminology and anatomy, HOPS off-the-field evaluation scheme, process for documentation findings, and using additional diagnostic techniques
- Multiple-choice questions covering terminology, HOPS, documentation, diagnostic techniques, and ergonomic risk assessment to reduce workplace-related injuries
- Selection questions covering terminology and anatomy
- Video identification of joint ranges of motion
- Picture identification of additional diagnostic techniques and terminology

Injury evaluation is an essential skill for the athletic trainer.[6] In athletic training, four distinct evaluations are routinely conducted: (1) The *preparticipation examination*, which was discussed in Chapter 2, is done prior to the start of preseason practice; (2) the initial *on-the-field injury assessment*, which was discussed in great detail in Chapter 12, is done immediately after acute injury to determine the immediate course of acute care, necessary first aid, and the approach to handling emergency situations; (3) a more detailed *off-the-field injury evaluation* is done in the athletic training clinic, a hospital or an outpatient clinic, an emergency room, or a physician's office after appropriate first aid has been rendered; and (4) a *progress evaluation* is done periodically throughout the rehabilitative process to determine the progress and effectiveness of a specific treatment regimen. This chapter concentrates on the off-the-field evaluation and the progress evaluation.

> Athletic trainers use their evaluation skills to make an accurate clinical diagnosis.

The setting in which the athletic trainer is employed determines the type of evaluation that is appropriate. An athletic trainer working in a hospital or an industrial setting is likely doing mostly off-the-field injury evaluations and progress evaluations. Athletic trainers who are employed in an athletic setting can expect to be arranging preparticipation exams, doing both on- and off-the-field evaluations, and writing progress evaluations throughout the course of rehabilitation.

CLINICAL EVALUATION AND DIAGNOSIS

Making a diagnosis is the use of scientific or clinical methods to establish the cause and nature of a patient's illness or injury and the subsequent functional impairment caused by the pathology. The diagnosis forms the basis for patient care.[39] Physicians are responsible for making a *medical* diagnosis, which is regarded as the ultimate determination of a patient's physical condition. Athletic trainers and other health care professionals use their evaluation and assessment skills to make a *clinical* diagnosis. The clinical diagnosis accurately identifies the pathology of injury, the limitations and the possible disabilities associated with a condition.[39] A certified athletic trainer has an academically based credential and in most states has some form of regulation that both recognizes the ability and empowers the athletic trainer to make an accurate clinical diagnosis. The term *diagnosis* is truly representative of what an athletic trainer actually does when evaluating an injury or illness.[39]

> Athletic trainers make a clinical diagnosis.

BASIC KNOWLEDGE REQUIREMENTS

The athletic trainer who is examining a patient with an injury must have a general knowledge of normal human anatomy and biomechanics and an understanding of the potential hazards inherent in a particular activity. Without this information, accurate assessment is impossible.

> To examine sports injuries, the athletic trainer must have a thorough knowledge of human anatomy and its function and of the hazards inherent in a particular activity.

Normal Human Anatomy

Surface Anatomy Understanding typical surface, or topographical, anatomy is essential when evaluating a possible injury.[28] Key surface landmarks provide the examiner with indications of the normal or injured anatomical structures lying underneath the skin.[13]

Body Planes and Anatomical Directions Associated with surface anatomy is the understanding of body planes and anatomical directions.[28] Body planes are used as points of reference from which positions of body parts are indicated. The three most commonly mentioned planes are the sagittal, transverse, and coronal (or frontal) planes (Figure 13–1). The sagittal plane runs vertically from front to back, or anterior/posterior, and divides the body into right and left sides. The transverse plane runs horizontally and divides the body into upper and lower parts. The coronal, or frontal, plane runs vertically from right to left and divides the body into front (anterior) and back (posterior). Anatomical directions refer to the position of one part in relation to another (Figure 13–2).

Abdominopelvic Quadrants and Regions The abdominopelvic *quadrants* are the four corresponding regions of the abdomen that are divided for evaluative and diagnostic purposes (Figure 13–3A). A second division system divides the abdominopelvic area into nine *regions* (Figure 13–3B). Clinicians use the quadrants and regions as reference points for locating underlying organs or abdominopelvic pain or abnormality (Figure 13–3C&D). The regions tend to be more specific relative to organ location, whereas the quadrants are simpler and generally more commonly used.

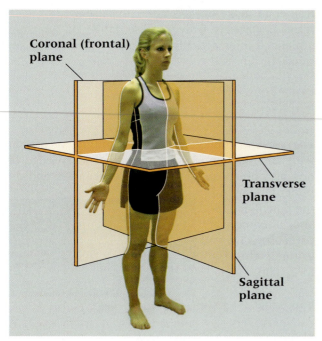

FIGURE 13–1 Knowledge of body planes helps provide points of reference.

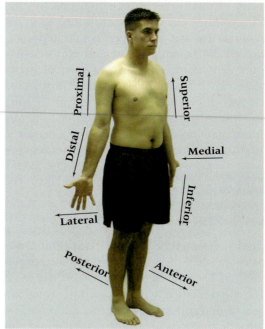

FIGURE 13–2 Anatomical directions refer to the position of one body part in relation to another.
anterior = in front of
posterior = in back of
superior = above
inferior = below
distal = farther away
proximal = closer to
medial = toward the middle
lateral = away from the middle

13–1 Clinical Application Exercise

A soccer player is taken down and lies on the field, holding her knee. The athletic trainer comes onto the field and quickly examines the knee. There does not appear to be any major instability, so the athlete is moved to the sideline, where the athletic trainer does a more careful evaluation. The athletic trainer is fairly certain that the soccer player has sustained a minor grade 1 medial collateral ligament (MCL) sprain and elects not to refer the patient to the physician. The next day the patient comes into the athletic training clinic with a very swollen knee. The athletic trainer now decides to refer the patient to the physician. On examination, the physician determines that the patient does have an MCL sprain but has also sustained a tear of the medial meniscus.

❓ How could the athletic trainer have handled this situation better?

Musculoskeletal System Anatomy Anyone examining the musculoskeletal system for injuries must have an in-depth knowledge of both structural and functional anatomy.[4] This knowledge encompasses the major joints and bony structures as well as skeletal musculature. A knowledge of neural anatomy is also of major importance, particularly that which is involved in movement control and sensation, along with the neural factors that influence superficial and deep pain.

Standard Musculoskeletal Terminology for Bodily Positions and Deviations When assessing the musculoskeletal system, the athletic trainer must use a standard terminology to convey precise information to other health care providers who may become professionally involved with the athlete. These terms are found in Table 13–1.

Biomechanics

The understanding of biomechanics is the foundation for the assessment of musculoskeletal injuries. **Biomechanics** is the application of mechanical forces, which may stem from within or outside the body, to living organisms. Of major concern is pathomechanics, which may precede an injury. **Pathomechanics** refers to mechanical forces that are applied to the body because of a structural body deviation, leading to faulty alignment. Pathomechanics often cause overuse syndromes.

biomechanics
Application of mechanical forces to living organisms.

pathomechanics
Mechanical forces that are applied to a living organism and adversely change the body's structure and function.

Understanding the Activity

Understanding the activity that the injured patient is involved in is critical if the athletic trainer is to be

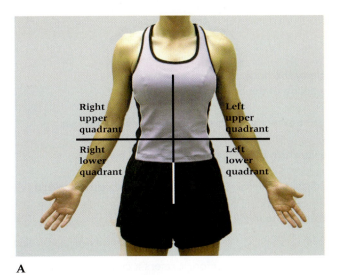

A

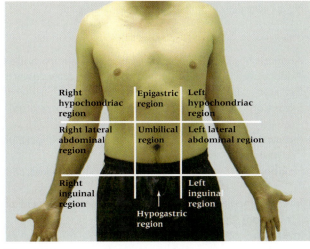

B

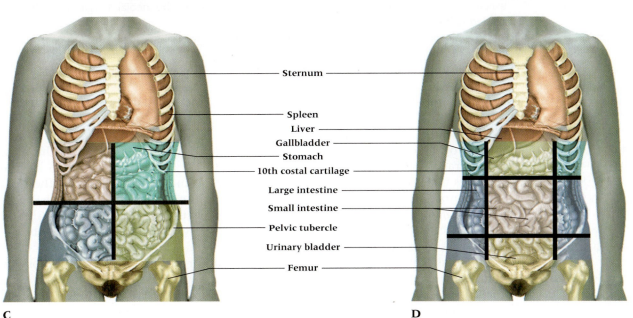

Sternum

Spleen
Liver
Gallbladder
Stomach
10th costal cartilage
Large intestine
Small intestine
Pelvic tubercle
Urinary bladder
Femur

C

D

FIGURE 13–3   Division of the abdomen into quadrants and regions. **(A&C)** Four quadrants. **(B&D)** Nine regions.

effective in determining the mechanism of injury, making an accurate clinical diagnosis, and designing a rehabilitation program that will address the functional aspects of returning to that activity. To fully understand injuries that occur in a particular activity, the athletic trainer must possess detailed knowledge and be able to apply the correct kinesiological and biomechanical principles that can correct faulty movement patterns. An athletic trainer overseeing a work hardening program must understand the ergonomics of a repetitive activity to correct the habits of a worker performing that job. An athletic trainer working with a ballet dancer needs to understand the physical demands of performing that artistic activity. The more the athletic trainer who evaluates a sports-related injury knows about how a sport is performed, the physical requirements of different positions within that sport, and

its potential for trauma, the better his or her injury assessment can be.[40]

Descriptive Assessment Terms

When evaluating injuries, examiners use certain terms to describe and characterize what is being learned about the condition. Student athletic trainers should become familiar with these terms.

Etiology refers to the cause of an injury or disease (for example, a patient rolls the foot inward when landing after jumping). In sports medicine, the term *mechanism of injury (MOI)* is often used interchangeably with *etiology*.

A **mechanism** is the mechanical description of the cause (for example, inversion and plantar flexion).

etiology
Cause of disease.

mechanism Mechanical description of the cause.

TABLE 13–1	Standard Orthopedic Definitions for Positions and Deviations
Term	**Definition**
Abduction	To draw away or deviate from the midline of the body.
Adduction	To deviate toward or draw toward the midline of the body.
Eversion	Turning outward.
Extension	To straighten; when the part distal to a joint extends, it straightens; joint angle decreases toward 0 degrees.
External (lateral) rotation	Rotary motion in the transverse plane away from the midline.
Flexion	To bend; when a joint is flexed, the part distal to the joint bends; joint angle increases toward 180 degrees.
Internal (medial) rotation	Rotary motion in the transverse plane toward the midline.
Inversion	Turning inward.
Pronation	Applied to the foot and assuming the foot is in a prone position, it refers a combination of eversion and abduction movements, resulting in a lowering of the medial margin of the foot; applied to the hand, the palm is turned downward.
Supination	To assume a supine position; applied to the foot, raising the medial margin of the foot; applied to the hand, turning the palm upward.
Valgus	Deviation of a part or portion of the extremity distal to a joint away from the midline of the body.
Varus	Deviation of a part or portion of an extremity distal to a joint toward the midline of the body.

pathology Structural and functional changes that result from injury.

symptom Change that indicates injury or disease.

sign Indicator of a disease.

diagnosis Name of a specific condition.

Pathology refers to the structural and functional changes that result from the injury process.

After developing an understanding of an injury's etiology, the athletic trainer ascertains symptoms and signs. **Symptom** refers to a *perceptible* change in a patient's body or its functions that indicates an injury or a disease. Symptoms are subjective; the patient describes them to the athletic trainer or physician. In comparison, a **sign** is objective, a definitive and obvious indicator of a specific condition. Signs are often determined when the patient is examined.

After it is inspected, an injury may be assigned a *grade*. Grade 1, 2, or 3 corresponds to an injury that is mild, moderate, or severe, respectively. Sometimes the term *degree* is used in place of *grade*, depending on the athletic trainer's preference.

Diagnosis denotes the name of a specific condition. To establish the diagnosis of a patient's injury or illness, the athletic trainer must study all aspects of the condition. A *differential diagnosis* is a systematic method of diagnosing a disorder that lacks unique symptoms or signs. The differential diagnosis is a list of possible injuries that cannot be ruled out until more information is obtained, typically through diagnostic tests. It involves a process of including, excluding,

and prioritizing possibilities by expecting the most serious injury first.[10] Prioritizing means to list the possible injuries from the most likely to the least likely. Applying the differential diagnosis technique, the athletic trainer first develops a list of possible injuries. By obtaining a history, observing, palpating, and conducting tests, the clinician can include or exclude some of the possible causes. Occasionally, the terms *working diagnosis* and *hypothesis* are also used to refer to the differential diagnosis. These terms also suggest a process for determining the most likely diagnosis for that condition. Once all the possible information has been gathered about the patient's condition, a **prognosis** is made. A prognosis is a prediction of the course of the condition. In other words, the patient is told what to expect as the injury heals. The amount of pain, swelling, or loss of function is discussed. *Prognosis* also refers to the projected outcome of an illness or injury and to the length of time predicted for complete recovery. For an athlete, prognosis translates into "the length of time before I can compete."

prognosis Predicted outcome of an injury.

Sequela refers to a condition following and resulting from a disease or an injury. Sequela is an additional condition developed as a complication of an existing disease or injury. For example, pneumonia might result from a bout with the flu, or osteoarthritis might follow a severe joint sprain.

sequela Condition resulting from disease or injury.

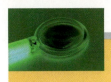

Off-the-field evaluation sequence

History

- Injuries to same body part
- Related injuries
- Present
- Mechanism of injury (MOI)
- Injury location
- Pain characteristics
- Joint responses
- Determining whether the injury is acute or chronic
- Past

Observation

- Demeanor
- Movement
- Posture
- Asymmetrics
- Deformity
- Swelling, redness, warmth

Palpation

- Bony palpation
- Soft-tissue palpation

Special Tests

Movement assessment
- Active range of motion
- Passive range of motion
- Resisted motions

Goniometric measurement of joint range

Testing accessory motions

Manual muscle testing

Testing joint stability
- Normal endpoints (end feels)
- Abnormal endpoints (endpoints)

Neurological examination
- Cerebral function
- Cerebellar function
- Cranial nerve function
- Sensory testing
- Reflex testing
- Determining projected/referred pain
- Motor testing

Postural examination

Anthropometric measurements

Volumetric measurements

Testing functional performance

---

syndrome Group of symptoms that indicate a condition or disease.

The term **syndrome** is refers to a group of symptoms and signs that, together, indicate a particular injury or disease.

The Off-the-Field Injury Evaluation Process

The on-the-field injury assessment discussed in detail in Chapter 12 is done on the field immediately after injury to rule out those injuries that may become life threatening, to assess musculoskeletal injuries, and to determine how the patient should be transported from the field. Once the patient has been transported from the site of initial injury, away from the excitement and confusion inherent in an athletic arena, a more detailed off-the-field injury evaluation is performed. This detailed evaluation may be performed on the sideline, in the athletic training clinic, in an emergency room, or in a sports medicine clinic. An injury may be evaluated immediately after the patient has been injured when it is still in an acute phase, or it may take place several hours or perhaps even days following traumatic injury.

The evaluation scheme is divided into four broad categories: history, observation, palpation, and a number of special tests that provide additional information about the extent of injuries. This evaluation scheme is sometimes referred to as the **HOPS** format. HOPS involves collecting information about an existing injury or illness and then making a decision about what the problem might be (see *Focus Box 13–1:* "Off-the-field evaluation sequence").

HOPS History, observation, palpation, and special tests.

The following discussion provides an overview of some of the steps and techniques that can be used in the evaluation process. (Chapters 18 through 27 provide specific injury assessment procedures.)

History

Obtaining as much information as possible about the history of the injury is perhaps the single most important aspect of the injury evaluation.[13] Understanding how the injury may have occurred (the mechanism of injury) and listening to the patient's complaints and answers to key questions can provide important clues to the exact nature of the injury. The athletic trainer

> Taking a detailed history from the athlete is perhaps the most critical aspect of the off-the-field evaluation.

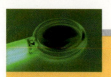

FOCUS 13-2 Focus on Clinical Evaluation and Diagnosis

History of musculoskeletal injuries

Information to obtain

- The mechanism of injury or trauma that caused the problem
- Chief complaints and present problems
- If pain is present, its location, character, duration, variation, aggravation, distribution or radiation, intensity, and course
- If the pain is increased or decreased by specific activities or stresses
- The existing environmental conditions when the injury occurred
- The type of equipment being worn at the time of the injury
- If the problem has occurred before and, if so, when and how it was treated and if the treatment was successful

becomes a detective in pursuit of as much accurate information as possible, which will lead to a determination of the true nature of the injury (see *Focus Box 13–2:* "History of musculoskeletal injuries"). From the history, the athletic trainer develops strategies for further examination and possible immediate and follow-up management.[4]

When obtaining a history, the athletic trainer should do the following:

- Be calm and reassuring.
- Ask open-ended questions that allow the patient to say anything that might be applicable rather than leading closed-end questions that require a yes or no response.
- Listen carefully to the patient's complaints.
- Maintain eye contact to try to see what the patient is feeling (remove sunglasses to get eye contact).
- Record exactly what the patient says without interpretation.
- Try to obtain the history as soon after injury as possible.[19]

Questions might be stated under specific headings in an attempt to get as complete a historical picture as possible. In many cases, a history becomes clear-cut because the mechanism, trauma, and pathology are obvious; in other situations, symptoms and signs may be obscured.

It is alright to observe the patient when taking a history but there should be no palpation while the patient is explaining what happened and what he or she is feeling.[11]

Present Injury If the patient is conscious and coherent, the athletic trainer should encourage him or her to describe the injury in detail.

Mechanism of Injury (MOI) If the athletic trainer did not see the injury happen, he or she should try to get the patient to describe in detail the mechanism of the injury by asking the following questions:

- What is the problem?
- How did it occur?
- When did it occur?
- Did you fall? How did you land?
- Which direction did your joint move?
- Did you hear or feel anything when it occurred?

If the patient is unable to describe accurately how the injury occurred, perhaps someone who observed the event can do so.

Injury Location The athletic trainer should ask the patient to locate the area of complaint by pointing to it with one finger only. If the patient can point to a specific pain site, the injury is probably localized. If the exact pain site cannot be indicated, the injury may be generalized.

Pain Characteristics The patient should describe as accurately as possible exactly what the pain feels like.

- What type of pain is it? Nerve pain is sharp, bright, or burning. Bone pain tends to be localized and piercing. Pain in the vascular system tends to be poorly localized, aching, and referred from another area. Muscle pain is often dull, aching, and referred to another area.[30]
- Where is the pain? Determining pain origin makes the evaluation of musculoskeletal injuries difficult. The deeper the injury site, the more difficult it is to match the pain with the site of trauma. This factor often causes treatment to be performed at the wrong site. Conversely, the closer the injury is to the body surface, the better the elicited pain corresponds with the site of pain stimulation.[3]
- Does the pain change at different times? Pain that subsides during activity usually indicates a chronic inflammation. Pain that increases in

a joint throughout the day indicates a progressive increase in edema. Does pain increase at night?

- Does the patient feel sensations other than pain? Pressure on nerve roots can produce pain or a sensation of "pins and needles" (paresthesia). What movement, if any, causes pain or other sensations?

Joint Responses

- If the injury is related to a joint, is there instability?
- Does the joint feel as though it will give way?
- Does the joint lock and unlock?

Positive responses may indicate that the joint has a loose body that is catching or that is inhibiting the normal muscular support in the area.

Determining Whether the Injury Is Acute or Chronic

The examiner should ask the patient how long he or she has had the symptoms and how often they appear.

History of Injury It is important to obtain information about the patient's previous or pre-existing injuries.[14] The athletic trainer who is working with a patient or group of patients on a daily basis often has the advantage of being familiar with their medical history. Nevertheless, an off-the-field injury evaluation requires asking.

- Has this ever happened before? If so, when?

Observation

The examiner gains knowledge and understanding of the patient's major complaint not only from a history but also through general observation, often done at the same time the history is taken. What is observed is commonly modified by the patient's complaints. The following are suggested as specific points to observe:

- Is there an obvious deformity?
- How does the patient move?
- Is there a limp?
- Are movements abnormally slow, jerky, and asynchronous?
- Is the patient unable to move a body part?
- Is the patient holding his or her body stiffly to protect against pain?
- Does the patient's facial expression indicate pain or lack of sleep?
- Are there any obvious body asymmetries?
- Does soft tissue appear swollen or wasted as a result of atrophy?
- Are there unnatural protrusions or lumps, such as occur with a dislocation or fracture?
- Is there a postural malalignment?

- Are there abnormal sounds, such as crepitus, when the athlete moves?
- Does a body area appear inflamed?
- Is there swelling, heat, or redness?

Palpation

Some examiners use palpation in the beginning of the examination procedure, whereas others use it only when they believe they have identified the specific injury site by other assessment means.[9,29] In some cases, palpation would be beneficial at both the beginning and the end of the examination. The two areas of palpation are bony and soft tissue. Like all examination procedures, palpation must be performed systematically.[32] The athletic trainer starts with very light pressure, followed by gradually deeper pressure, and usually begins away from the site of complaint and gradually moves toward it.

Bony Palpation Both the injured and noninjured sites should be palpated and compared. The sense of touch might reveal an abnormal gap at a joint, swelling on a bone, joints that are misaligned, or abnormal protuberances associated with a joint or a bone.

Soft-Tissue Palpation Through palpation, with the patient as relaxed as possible, the athletic trainer can assess normal soft-tissue relationships.[41] Tissue deviations, such as swelling, lumps, gaps, abnormal muscle tension, and temperature variations, can be detected. The palpation of soft tissue can detect where ligaments or tendons have torn. The athletic trainer can determine variations in the shape of structures, differences in tissue tightness and textures, and differentiation of tissue that is pliable and soft from tissue that is more resilient. Involuntary muscle twitching or tremors may also be felt. Excessive skin dryness and moisture can also be noted. The athletic trainer can become aware of abnormal skin sensations, such as diminished sensation (dysesthesia), numbness (anesthesia), or increased sensation (hyperesthesia). Like bony palpation, soft-tissue palpation must be performed on both sides of the body for comparison.[42]

Special Tests

Special tests have been designed for almost every body region to detect specific pathologies.[22] They are often used to substantiate what has been learned from the history, observation, and palpation portions of the evaluation process.[29] Special tests should be performed bilaterally beginning with the uninjured side to compare what is "normal" for that patient with what the injured side feels like. CAUTION: A joint should not be moved or stressed when a fracture is suspected.

Movement Assessment If a joint or soft-tissue lesion exists, the patient is likely to complain of pain on movement. Cyriax has developed a method for locating and identifying a lesion by applying tension selectively to each of the structures that might produce this pain.[9] Tissues are classified as contractile or inert. Contractile tissues include muscles and their tendons; inert tissues include bones, ligaments, joint capsules, fascia, bursae, nerve roots, and dura mater.

If a lesion is present in contractile tissue, pain will occur on active motion in one direction and on passive motion in the opposite direction. Thus, a muscle strain would cause pain on both active contraction and passive stretch. Contractile tissues are tested through the midrange by an isometric contraction against maximum resistance. The specific location of the lesion within the musculotendinous unit cannot be identified by the isometric contraction.[7]

A lesion of inert tissue elicits pain on active and passive movement in the same direction. For example, a sprain of a ligament results in pain whenever that ligament is stretched, through either active contraction or passive stretching. It is not possible to identify a specific lesion of inert tissue by looking at movement patterns alone; other special tests must be done to identify injured structures.[3]

Active Range of Motion Movement assessment should begin with **active range of motion**

> **Movement assessment:**
> - Active movement
> - Passive movement

> **Contractile tissue:**
> - Muscles and their tendons

> **Inert tissues:**
> - Bones
> - Ligaments
> - Joint capsules
> - Fascia
> - Nerves
> - Bursae
> - Nerve roots
> - Dura mater

(AROM). The athletic trainer should evaluate quality of movement, range of movement, motion in other planes, movement at varying speeds, and strength throughout the range but in particular at the endpoint. A complaint of pain on active motion will not distinguish contractile pain from inert pain, so the athletic trainer must proceed with an evaluation of both passive and resistive motion. A patient who seems to be pain free in each of these tests throughout a full range should be tested by applying passive pressure at the endpoint.

> **active range of motion (AROM)** Joint motion that occurs because of muscle contraction.

Passive Range of Motion When **passive range of motion (PROM)** is being assessed, the patient must relax completely and allow the athletic trainer to move the extremity to reduce the influence of the contractile elements. Particular attention should be directed toward the sensation of the patient at the end of the passive range. Cyriax has described *normal endpoints* and *abnormal endpoints*.[36] Normal endpoints have also been referred to as *end feels* and are what the examiner is looking for in passive range of motion testing.[23] Abnormal endpoints, sometimes referred to simply as *endpoints* are what the examiner feels during ligamentous stress tests.[9] The athletic trainer should categorize the "feel" of the endpoints as described in the following sections.[9]

> **passive range of motion (PROM)** Movement that is performed completely by the examiner.

Normal endpoints (end feels) Normal endpoints include the following:[25]

- Soft-tissue approximation—soft and spongy, a gradual, painless stop (e.g., knee flexion)
- Capsular feel—an abrupt, hard, firm endpoint with only a little give (e.g., endpoint of hip rotation)
- Bone to bone—a distinct and abrupt endpoint when two hard surfaces come in contact with one another (e.g., elbow in full extension)
- Muscular—a springy feel with some associated discomfort (e.g., end of shoulder abduction)

Abnormal endpoints (endpoints) Abnormal endpoints include the following:

- Empty feel—movement is definitely beyond the anatomical limit, and pain occurs before the end of the range (e.g., a complete ligament rupture)
- Spasm—involuntary muscle contraction that prevents motion because of pain; also called guarding (e.g., back spasms)
- Loose—occurs in extreme hypermobility (e.g., previously sprained ankle)
- Springy block—a rebound at the endpoint (e.g., meniscus tear)

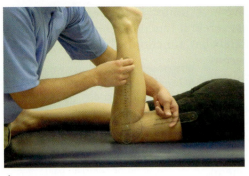 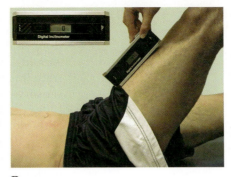 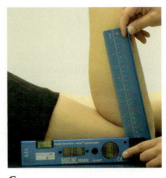

A   B   C

FIGURE 13–4   Measuring joint range of motion. **(A)** Goniometric measurement of knee joint flexion. **(B)** Inclinometer measurement of hip flexion. **(C)** Digital goniometer.

Throughout the passive range of movement, the athletic trainer is looking for limitation in movement and the presence of pain. A patient's report of pain before the end of the available range probably indicates acute inflammation, in which stretching and manipulation are both contraindicated as treatments. Pain occurring synchronous with the end of the range indicates that the condition is subacute and has progressed to some inert tissue fibrosis. If no pain occurs at the end of the range, the condition is chronic and contractures have replaced inflammation.[42]

Goniometric Measurement of Joint Range Goniometry, which measures joint range of motion, is an essential procedure during the early, intermediate, and late stages of injury. Full range of motion of an affected body part is a major criterion for a patient to return to activity. Active and passive joint range of motion can be measured using goniometry (Figure 13–4A).[34]

Although a number of different types of goniometers are on the market, the most commonly used are ones that measure 0 to 180 degrees in each direction. The arms of the instrument are usually 12 to 16 inches (30 to 40 cm) long, with one arm stationary and the other fully movable.[7,16]

When measuring joint range of motion, the goniometer should generally be placed along the lateral surface of the extremity being measured. The 0, or starting, position for any movement is identical to the standard anatomical position. The patient should move the joint either actively or passively through the available range to the endpoint. The stationary arm of the goniometer should be placed parallel with the longitudinal axis of the fixed reference part. The movable arm should be placed along the longitudinal axis of the movable segment. (NOTE: The axis of rotation will change throughout the range as movement occurs. Thus, the axis of rotation is located at the intersection of the stationary and movable arms.) A reading in degrees of motion should be taken and recorded as either active

or passive range of motion for that movement. Accuracy and consistency in goniometric measurement require practice and repetition. Digital inclinometers and goniometers are commonly used to provide a more accurate measure of joint range (Figures 13–4B and C).

The normal available range of motion for specific movements at individual joints is indicated in Table 13–2.

Digital Inclinometer The inclinometer is gradually replacing the goniometer as an instrument for measuring range of motion (Figure 13–4B). It measures the slope of elevation or the angle of movement relative to gravity. The inclinometer is placed on a body part and set to 0 degrees; it measures the total range of movement digitally. It provides accuracy, repeatability, and objective documentation of range of motion measurements. For this purpose, the digital inclinometer is considered to be a useful instrument because it is inexpensive and easy to use.

Manual Muscle Testing Manual muscle testing is an integral part of the physical examination process.[5,20] The ability of the injured patient to tolerate varying levels of resistance can indicate a great deal about the extent of the injury to the contractile units. For the patient, the limitation in muscular strength is generally caused by pain.[8] As pain diminishes and the healing process progresses, levels of muscular strength gradually return to normal. The development of isokinetic testing devices has enabled the athletic trainer to test levels of muscular strength objectively within the limitations of those devices.[21]

Manual muscle testing is usually performed with the patient positioned so that individual muscles or muscle groups can be isolated and tested through a full range of motion via the application of manual resistance. The ability of the patient to move through a full range of motion or to offer resistance to movement is subjectively graded by the athletic trainer according to various classification

TABLE 13–2 Range of Joint Motion

Joint	Action	Degrees of Motion
Shoulder	Flexion	180
	Extension	50
	Adduction	40
	Abduction	180
	Internal rotation	90
	External rotation	90
Elbow	Flexion	145
Forearm	Pronation	80
	Supination	85
Wrist	Flexion	80
	Extension	70
	Abduction	20
	Adduction	45
Hip	Flexion	125
	Extension	10
	Abduction	45
	Adduction	40
	Internal rotation	45
	External rotation	45
Knee	Flexion	140
Ankle	Plantar flexion	45
	Dorsiflexion	20
Foot	Inversion	40
	Eversion	20

systems and grading criteria. Table 13–3 indicates a commonly used grading system for manual muscle testing.

Neurological Examination The neurological examination usually follows manual muscle testing. Performing a detailed and accurate neurological exam is difficult for everyone, including physicians. The exam consists of six major areas: cerebral function, cranial nerve function, cerebellar function, sensory testing, reflex testing, projected or referred pain, and motor testing. In cases of musculoskeletal injury that

do not involve head injury, it is generally not necessary to assess cerebral function, cranial nerve function, and cerebellar function. The athletic trainer should concentrate instead on sensory testing, reflex testing, and motor testing to determine the involvement of the peripheral nervous system after injury.

> **Neurological examination:**
> - Cerebral function
> - Cranial nerve function
> - Cerebellar function
> - Sensory testing
> - Reflex testing
> - Projected or referred pain
> - Motor testing

Cerebral Function Tests for general cerebral function include questions that assess general affect, level of consciousness, intellectual performance, emotional status, thought content, sensory interpretation (visual, auditory, tactile), and language skills.

Cranial Nerve Function The function of the 12 cranial nerves can be quickly determined by assessing the quality of the following: sense of smell, eye tracking, imitation of facial expressions, biting down, balance, swallowing, tongue protrusion, and strength of shoulder shrugs. Table 13–4 lists the cranial nerves and their functions.

Cerebellar Function Because the cerebellum controls purposeful, coordinated movement, tests such as touching finger to nose, touching finger to finger of examiner, drawing alphabets in the air with the foot, and heel-toe walking will determine dysfunction.

> **13–4 Clinical Application Exercise**
>
> A baseball player complains of pain in his right shoulder. A manual muscle test for shoulder external rotation was a grade 3.
>
> **?** What does this evaluation indicate about the tissue? If the result of the manual muscle test was a grade 3, what is a possible conclusion for this evaluation?

TABLE 13–3 Manual Muscle Strength Grading

Grade	Percentage (%)	Qualitative Value	Muscle Strength
5	100	Normal	Complete range of motion (ROM) against gravity with full resistance
4	75	Good	Complete ROM against gravity with some resistance
3	50	Fair	Complete ROM against gravity with no resistance
2	25	Poor	Complete ROM with gravity omitted
1	10	Trace	Evidence of slight contractility with no joint motion
0	0	Zero	No evidence of muscle contractility

TABLE 13–4	Cranial Nerves and Their Functions
I. Olfactory	Smell
II. Optic	Vision
III. Oculomotor	Eye movement, opening of eyelid, constriction of pupil, focusing
IV. Trochlear	Inferior and lateral movement of eye
V. Trigeminal	Sensation to the face, mastication
VI. Abducens	Lateral movement of eye
VII. Facial	Motor nerve of facial expression; taste; control of tear, nasal, sublingual salivary, and submaxillary glands
VIII. Vestibulocochlear	Hearing and equilibrium
IX. Glossopharyngeal	Swallowing, salivation, gag reflex, sensation from tongue and ear
X. Vagus	Swallowing; speech; regulation of pulmonary, cardiovascular, and gastrointestinal functions
XI. Accessory	Swallowing, innervation of sternocleidomastoid muscle
XII. Hypoglossal	Tongue movement, speech, swallowing

Sensory Testing A major component of musculoskeletal assessment is determining the distribution of peripheral nerves and dermatomes (Figure 13–5). A **dermatome** is an area of skin that is innervated by the sensory fibers of a single spinal nerve or cranial nerve. The term *dermatome* is sometimes confused with **myotomes**, which are found in developing embryos. Segmental myotomes eventually develop into a muscle or a group of muscles that are innervated by motor fibers from a specific spinal nerve. Table 13–5 shows myotome patterns at muscle weakness that can occur with lesions to specific spinal nerve roots.

dermatome Area of skin innervated by a single nerve.

myotomes Muscle or groups of muscles innervated by a specific motor nerve.

Although peripheral nerve distribution varies with individuals, it is more predictable than dermatome distribution.[13] As the dermatome examination progresses, the examiner compares sensation from one side of the body to the other, using the following tests:

- Superficial sensation—touch dermatomes with cotton
- Superficial pain—touch dermatomes with a pin
- Deep pressure pain—squeeze a muscle (e.g., gastrocnemius)
- Sensitivity of temperature—touch dermatomes with ice cube
- Sensitivity of vibration—touch dermatomes with a tuning fork
- Position sense—move fingers or toes passively and ask athlete to indicate direction

Reflex Testing The term *reflex* refers to an involuntary response to a stimulus. In terms of the neurological examination, there are three types of reflexes: deep tendon (somatic) reflexes, superficial reflexes, and pathological reflexes.

A deep tendon reflex is caused by stimulation of the stretch reflex (see Chapter 4) and results in an involuntary contraction of a muscle when its tendon is stretched. Deep tendon reflexes can be elicited at the tendons of the biceps (C5), brachioradialis (C6), extensor digitorum (C6), triceps (C7), adductor (L2), patella (L4), Achilles (S1), and hamstring (S2). Table 13–6 shows a grading system for deep tendon reflexes.[19]

Superficial reflexes are elicited by stimulation of the skin at specific sites, which produces a reflex muscle contraction. Superficial reflexes include upper abdominal (T7, 8, 9), lower abdominal (T11, 12), cremasteric (T12, L1), plantar (S1, 2), and gluteal (L4, S3). An absence of a superficial reflex is indicative of some lesion in the spinal cord—specifically, the descending corticospinal tract in the spinal cord.

Most, but not all, pathological reflexes are also superficial reflexes. The presence of a pathological reflex indicates a lesion in the descending upper motor neuron, including the spinal cord; an absence indicates integrity. Babinski's sign, in which stroking of the lateral plantar surface produces extension and splaying of the toes, is an example of a pathological reflex.[19] Chaddock's, Oppenheim's, and Gordon's are additional reflexes that are alternatives for eliciting a Babinski's response. For

13–5 Clinical Application Exercise

A receiver in football has his feet taken out from under him by a tackler and lands flat on his low back with his legs above him. An on-the-field evaluation reveals unilateral decreased muscle strength, decreased sensation, and a decreased patellar tendon reflex in the right lower extremity.

? Based on the findings of the evaluation, how should the athletic trainer manage this injury?

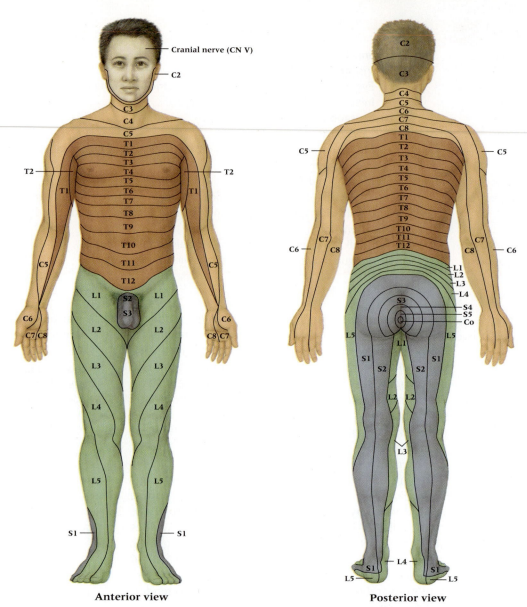

FIGURE 13–5 Dermatomes. Numbness, referred pain, and other nerve involvements often follow the segmental distribution of spinal nerves on the skin's surface.

TABLE 13–5	**Myotome Patterns of Weakness Resulting from Spinal Nerve Root Lesion**		
C1	None	L1	None
C2	Neck flexion	L2	Hip flexion
C3	Neck lateral flexion and extension	L3	Knee extension
C4	Shoulder shrug	L4	Ankle dorsiflexion
C5	Shoulder abduction	L5	Hallux extension
C6	Elbow flexion/wrist extension	S1	Plantar flexion/eversion/knee flexion/ hip extension
C7	Elbow extension/wrist flexion		
C8	Ulnar deviation/thumb extension	S2	Plantar flexion/knee flexion/hip extension
T1	None (finger abduction and adduction)	S3	None
		S4	Bladder, rectum

TABLE 13–6	Deep Tendon Reflex Grading		
	Grade	**Definition**	
Absence of a reflex	0	Areflexia	
Diminished reflex	1	Hyporeflexia	
Average reflex	2		
Exaggerated reflex	3	Hyperreflexia (increased but not pathological)	
Markedly hyperactive	4	Often associated with clonus, but clonus is not required for grade 4	

Chaddock's reflex, the lateral foot, from lateral malleolus to small toe, is stroked with a blunt instrument and there is extension of the great toe. For Oppenheim's reflex, the anterior tibia, from just below the patella to the foot, is firmly stroked with a knuckle and there is extension of the great toe. For Gordon's reflex, the calf muscles are squeezed and there is extension of the great toe or all of the toes.

In general, hyperactive reflexes, clonus (alternating contraction between antagonist muscle groups), Babinski's sign, and decreased superficial reflexes are all considered to be upper motor neuron signs and usually indicate a lesion somewhere in that tract as it courses through the brain, brain stem, and spinal cord.

Projected or Referred Pain As discussed in Chapter 10, a complaint of deep, burning pain, an ache that is diffused, or a painful area with no signs of disorder or malfunctioning is most likely referred pain.[7] Cyriax considers that the common sites for pain referral are, in order of importance, joint capsule, tendon, muscle, ligament, and bursa.[9] Pressures from the dura mater or nerve sheath can also produce referred pain or other sensory responses. Palpation of what is thought to be the area at fault often is misleading. Detecting the selective tension of the tissue at fault is one of the best means for gathering correct data. Some musculoskeletal pain is caused by myofascial trigger points, which are not related to deep, referred pain. Palpation is used to determine the presence or absence of tense tissue bands and tender trigger points.

Motor Testing The manual muscle tests discussed earlier in this chapter are used to test the function of the motor neurons in both the upper and lower extremities. Motor tests are done by evaluating strength in muscles that are innervated by a specific nerve root level to test neurological function of that nerve root.

Testing Joint Stability A number of specific tests for determining the integrity of the ligaments surrounding a particular joint are described in Chapters 18 through 25. Joint stability tests provide information about the grade of a sprain of a particular ligament and can determine the extent of the functional instability of the joint.

Testing Accessory Motions *Accessory motions* refers to the manner in which one articulating joint surface moves relative to another.[2] Normal accessory component motions must occur for full-range movement to take place. Accessory motions are limited by tightness of the joint capsule and/or ligaments that surround a joint. It is critical for the athletic trainer to closely evaluate the injured joint to determine whether motion is limited by tightness of the musculotendinous units or by limitation in accessory motion involving the joint capsule and ligaments. If accessory motion is limited by some restriction of the joint capsule or the ligaments, joint mobilization techniques should be incorporated into the treatment program.[24] Joint mobilization is discussed in detail in Chapter 16.

Testing Functional Performance Functional performance testing may be done as part of an initial evaluation to determine whether an injury is severe enough to keep the patient from activity. It may also be used to evaluate progress during a rehabilitation program. Decisions about when a patient is ready to return to full activity following injury should be based to a large extent on performance on functional tests.[22] Functional testing should proceed gradually from minimal stress to tests that mimic the actual stress that would normally come from full activity. The major concern is whether the patient has regained full strength, range of motion, speed, endurance, and neuromuscular control and is pain free.

> **Functional examination determines whether the athlete has full strength, joint stability, and coordination, and whether the part is pain free.**

Postural Examination As is discussed in Chapter 25, many cases of injuries can be attributed to body malalignments. Musculoskeletal assessment

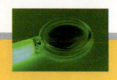

Constructing and using a volumetric tank

A volumetric tank (see Figure 13–6) is constructed of five 0.6-centimeter sheets of acrylic plastic molded together to form a container, which is mounted on a platform. The internal dimensions of the tank are length = 35.6 centimeters (14 in.), width = 17.8 centimeters (7 in.), and depth = 20.3 centimeters (8 in.). All the walls form right angles with each other as well as with the floor of the tank. The bottom of the tank has three adjustable leveling screws. Two of these screws are at one end of the tank base, and the third is centrally located on the opposite end. The end with one screw is classified as the front of the tank. A piece of acrylic plastic that measures 1.3 centimeters (0.5 in.) wide by 6 centimeters (2.4 in.) long is attached to the side of the tank, 4 centimeters (1.6 in.) from the back of the tank, to ensure consistent limb positioning in the tank.

A glass tube, 7.3 millimeters (0.29 in.) in diameter by 7.6 centimeters (3 in.) passes through the front of the tank. The tube extends 3.2 centimeters (1.25 in.) outside the front wall of the tank. The tube is 5.1 centimeters (2 in.) from the top of the front wall and is perpendicular to the wall of the tank. A 10.2-centimeter (4 in.) piece of rubber tubing is attached to the end of the glass tube. This tubing combination allows for displaced water to be collected. A centimeter ruler, a skin thermometer, and a 500- and 1,000-milliliter (19.7 in. and 39.4 in.) graduated cylinder is used for all measurements. A water collection container is used to catch the runoff when the tubing is unclamped.

Procedure for measuring water displacement

The volumetric tank is placed on the floor and leveled using the adjusting screws. The tank is then filled to the 17-centimeter (6.7 in.) mark on the ruler with 33.5°C (92.3°F) water. The subject places the limb against the back wall of the tank. The tank is then shaken gently to eliminate any air bubbles in the tank or on the surface of the limb. When the water is completely motionless, the tubing is unclamped and the runoff is collected in the container. Any water remaining in the tubing should be shaken out into the collection container. The amount of water collected in the runoff container is measured in the graduated cylinders and the measurements are noted.

---

might be one area of a postural examination. It is designed to test for malalignments and asymmetries by viewing the body compared with a grid or plumb line (see Figures 25–7 through 25–9).

Anthropometric Measurements Anthropometry is the science of measuring the human body. Anthropometric measurements include osteometry (measurement of the dimensions of the skeletal system), craniometry (measurement of the bones of the skull), skin-fold measurements to determine body composition (see Chapter 5), and height and weight measurements (see Chapter 2). Limb girth measurements taken during a rehabilitation program are also considered a type of anthropometric measurement. Anthropometric measurements are seldom used by athletic trainers in a sports medicine setting.

Volumetric Measurements Volumetric measurements can be taken to determine changes in limb volume caused by swelling, which can be attributed to hemorrhage, edema, or inflammation.[37] Limb volume may be measured in a volumetric tank that essentially measures the amount of water displaced by immersion of the limb in the tank (Figure 13–6). *Focus Box 13–3:* "Constructing and using a volumetric tank" describes the tank and the procedure for measuring limb volume.

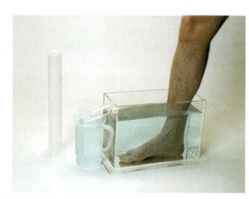

FIGURE 13–6 Tank for measuring limb volume.

PROGRESS EVALUATIONS

The athletic trainer who is overseeing a rehabilitation program must constantly monitor the progress of the patient toward full recovery throughout the rehabilitative process. In many instances, the athletic trainer will be able to treat the injured patient on a daily basis. This close supervision affords the athletic trainer the luxury of being able to continuously adjust or adapt the treatment program based on the progress made by the patient on a day-to-day basis.

The progress evaluation should be based on the athletic trainer's knowledge of exactly what is occurring in the healing process at any given time. The timelines of injury healing provide the framework that dictates the progress of the rehabilitation program. The athletic trainer must understand that the aggressive approach taken in rehabilitation does little to speed up the healing process. Progression will be limited by the constraints of that process.

Progress evaluations will be more limited in scope than the detailed off-the-field evaluation sequence described in this chapter. The off-the-field evaluation should be thorough and comprehensive. The athletic trainer should take time to systematically rule out information that is not pertinent to the present injury. Once the extraneous information has been eliminated, the subsequent progress evaluation can focus specifically on how the injury appears today compared with yesterday. Is the patient better or worse as a result of the treatment program rendered on the previous day?

To ensure that the progress evaluation will be complete, the athletic trainer still needs to go through certain aspects of history, observation, palpation, and special tests.

History

The athletic trainer should ask the patient the following questions:

- How is the pain today compared with yesterday?
- Are you able to move better and with less pain?
- Do you think that the treatment done yesterday helped or made you more sore?

Observation

The athletic trainer should make the following observations:

- Is the swelling today more or less than it was yesterday?
- Is the patient able to move better today?
- Is the patient still guarding and protecting the injury?
- How is the patient's affect? Is he or she upbeat and optimistic or depressed and negative?

Palpation

The athletic trainer should palpate the injured area to determine the following:

- Does the swelling have a different consistency today, and has the swelling pattern changed?
- Is the injured structure still as tender to the touch?
- Is there any deformity present today that was not obvious yesterday?

Special Tests

The athletic trainer should use special tests to make the following determinations:

- Does ligamentous stress testing cause as much pain? Has the athletic trainer's assessment of the grade of instability changed?
- How does a manual muscle test compare with yesterday?
- Has either active or passive range of motion changed?
- Does accessory movement appear to be limited?
- Can the athlete perform a specific functional test better today than yesterday?

DOCUMENTING INJURY EVALUATION INFORMATION

Complete and accurate documentation of findings from an evaluation is essential.[35] As stressed in Chapter 3, accurate documentation can be a strong ally, should the athletic trainer become involved in litigation. For the athletic trainer working in a clinical setting, clear, concise, accurate record keeping is necessary for third-party reimbursement. Although the process may seem at times cumbersome and time-consuming, the athletic trainer must develop proficiency not only in evaluation skills but also in generating an accurate report of the findings from that evaluation.

In documenting medical information, it is common practice for the clinician to use abbreviations for words that routinely appear in medical notes or evaluations.[18] Table 13–7 provides many terms and their corresponding abbreviations that an athletic trainer might use in documenting injury information during an evaluation.

SOAP NOTES

Documentation of acute injury can be effectively accomplished through a system designed to record subjective and objective findings and to document the immediate and future treatment plan for the patient.[27] The SOAP note format (subjective, objective, assessment, and plan) provides a standard

↑	increase		H/O	history of
↓	decrease		HA	headache
<	less than		HP	hot pack
>	greater than		HPI	history of present illness
Δ	change		ht	height; heart
c̄	with		HTN	hypertension
p̄	after		Hx	history
s̄ or w/o	without		IN	inversion
1°	primary		IPPA	inspection, percussion, palpation, and auscultation
2°	secondary		L	left
+tive	positive		LAT	lateral
A&O	alert & oriented		LBP	low back pain
abnor.	abnormal		LE	lower extremity
AC	acromioclavicular or acute		MAEEW	moves all extremities equally well
ADL	activities of daily living		MEDS	medications
ant.	anterior		mm	muscle; millimeter
ante	before		MMT	manual muscle testing
AOAP	as often as possible		MOD	moderate
AP	anterior-posterior; assessment and plans		N	normal, never, no, not
AROM	active range of motion		NC	neurological check; no complaints; not completed
ASAP	as soon as possible		NEG	negative
ASIS	anterior superior iliac spine		NKA	no known allergies
AT	athletic training		NP	no pain
B	bilateral		NPT	normal pressure and temperature
BID or bid	twice a day		NSA	no significant abnormality
C/O	complained of; complaints; under care of		NSAID	nonsteroidal antiinflammatory drug
CC	chief complaint; chronic complainer		NT	not tried
ck.	check		NWB	non–weight bearing
CP	cold pack; chronic pain		o	negative, without
CPR	cardiopulmonary resuscitation		O	objective finding
CWI	crutch walking instruction		OH	occupational history
D/C	discharge		ORIF	open reduction/internal fixation
DF	dorsiflexion		OT	occupational therapy
DOB	date of birth		P&A	percussion and auscultation
DTR	deep tendon reflex		p.o.	postoperatively
DVT	deep vein thrombosis		PA	posterior-anterior (X-ray); physician's assistant
Dx	diagnosis		PE	physical examination
E	edema		PF	plantar flexion
EENT	eyes, ears, nose, throat		PH	past history; poor health
ELOP	estimated length of program		PMH	past medical history
EMS	emergency medical services		PNF	proprioceptive neuromuscular facilitation
EMT	emergency medical technician		PNS	peripheral nervous system
EOA	examine, opinion, and advice		PPPBL	peripheral pulses palpable both legs
ES	electrical stimulation		PT	point tender
EV	eversion		PRE	progressive resistance exercise
exam.	examination		pre-op	preoperatively
FH	family history		prog.	prognosis
FROM	full range of movement		PROM	passive range of motion
FWB	full weight bearing		PT	physical therapy
Fx	fracture		Pt./pt.	patient
G1–4	grades 1 to 4		PWB	partial weight bearing
GA	general appearance		Px	physical exam; pneumothorax
H&P	history and physical		qd	once daily
			qid	four times a day

Continued

TABLE 13–7 continued

R	right	T	temperature
R/O	rule out	TENS	transcutaneous electrical nerve stimulation
rehab	rehabilitation	tid	three times a day
ROM	range of motion	TTWB	toe touch weight bearing
RROM	resistive range of motion	UE	upper extremity
RTP	return to play	UK	unknown
Rx	prescription, including therapy and treatment	US	ultrasound
S	subjective findings	WBAT	weight bearing as tolerated
SLR	straight leg raises	Whp	whirlpool
SOAP	subjective, objective, assessment, plan	WNL	within normal limits
stat	immediately	x	times
STG	short-term goals	y.o.	year old
Sx	signs; symptom	Y/O	years old

SOAP note format:

- Subjective
- Objective
- Assessment
- Plan

format for recording injury information obtained from on-site, sideline, or clinical evaluations. This method combines information provided by the patient and observations of the examiner.[26] Figure 13–7 presents a recommended injury report form that includes these components of documentation. This form also includes a provision to document findings arising from more definitive evaluation or from the examiner's subsequent evaluation.

S (Subjective) This component includes the subjective statements provided by the injured patient. History taking is designed to elicit the subjective impressions of the patient relative to time, mechanism, and site of injury. The type and course of the pain and the degree of disability experienced by the patient are also noteworthy.

O (Objective) Objective findings result from the athletic trainer's visual inspection, palpation, and assessment of active, passive, and resistive motion. Findings of special testing should also be noted here. Thus, the objective report would include assessment of posture, presence of deformity or swelling, and location of point tenderness. Also, limitations of active motion and pain arising or disappearing during passive and resistive motion should be noted. Finally, the results of special tests relative to joint stability or apprehension are also included.

A (Assessment) Assessment of the injury is the athletic trainer's professional judgment with regard to impression and nature of injury. Although the exact nature of the injury will not always be known initially, information pertaining to the suspected site and anatomical structures involved is appropriate. A judgment of severity may be included but is not essential at the time of acute injury evaluation.

P (Plan) The plan should include the first-aid treatment rendered to the patient and the athletic trainer's intentions relative to disposition. Disposition may include referral for more definitive evaluation or simply application of splint, wrap, or crutches and a request to report for reevaluation the next day. If the injury is chronic, the examiner's plan for treatment and therapeutic exercise would be appropriate. The treatment plan should establish specific short-term goals for the rehabilitation program and should provide criteria-based guidelines for accomplishing these goals (e.g., progress from touch-down gait on two crutches to weight bearing on one crutch). A specific long-term goal should also be clearly identified in the plan (e.g., normal gait without a limp).

Progress Notes

Progress notes should be routinely written after each progress evaluation done throughout the course of the rehabilitation program. Progress notes can follow the SOAP format, as indicated in the previous sections. They can

13–7 Clinical Application Exercise

A professional bull rider is thrown from the bull and, on landing, twists his knee. There is immediate swelling and pain. After evaluation, the athletic trainer is not sure what the injury is and sends the patient directly to the physician for a medical diagnosis. The physician decides that additional diagnostic tests are necessary to determine the exact pathology.

? What diagnostic tests is the physician likely to order to determine the exact nature and extent of the knee injury?

SUBJECTIVE: The patient is a _____-year-old athlete with the above diagnosis. The patient notes a _____ onset on _____. Past history for this condition is remarkable for _____ unremarkable. Diagnostic testing of _____ . Medications include _____. The patient's goals are to _____ . General medical history is remarkable for/unremarkable. The patient will follow with MD on _____.

OBJECTIVE: Measurable, Reproducible, Observable findings—Be Objective
OBSERVATION: Be descriptive
ROM: AROM/PROM—Measure with goniometer
STRENGTH: Strength to MMT—Use grading system 1 to 5
FLEXIBILITY: Try to document with goniometer if possible
PALPATION:
SENSATION:
SPECIAL TEST:
GAIT:
FUNCTIONAL TESTS:
TREATMENT:

ASSESSMENT: Your professional opinion of the patient's problem
The patient presents with the following problems (1) _____ , (2) _____ , (3) _____ , (4) _____ .

PLAN: Describe how you will manage the patient regarding frequency of treatment, what the treatment will include (i.e., modalities, therapeutic exercise, home program, and follow up with you).
Short-term goals include (1) _____ , (2) _____ , (3) _____ , (4) _____ .
Long-term goals include _____ .

Signature _____ ATC

FIGURE 13–7   SOAP note form.

be generated in the form of an expanded treatment note or done as a weekly summary. Information in the progress note should concentrate on the types of treatment received and the patient's response to that treatment, progress made toward the short-term goals established in the SOAP note, changes in the previous treatment plan and goals, and the course of treatment over the next several days.[1]

ADDITIONAL DIAGNOSTIC TESTS USED BY A PHYSICIAN

The physician, like the athletic trainer, often performs a detailed musculoskeletal examination on the injured patient. Often, the physician and the athletic trainer will discuss and compare their individual findings. Because the physician is charged with determining a medical diagnosis and deciding on a course of treatment, he or she may have to acquire and compare additional information. This information can come from imaging techniques, including plain film radiographs (X-rays), arthrography, arthroscopy, myelography, computed tomography, positron emission tomography, bone scanning, DEXA scans, magnetic resonance imaging, ultrasonography, and echocardiography.[33,41] Other tests include electrocardiography, electroencephalography, electromyography, nerve conduction velocity, synovial fluid analysis, blood testing, and urinalysis.[12,15,31]

Imaging Techniques

Plain Film Radiography (X-rays) An X-ray examination helps the physician identify fractures and dislocations or any bone abnormality that may be present. It may also be used to rule out serious disease, such as an infection or a neoplasm. A trained radiologist can detect some soft-tissue factors, such as joint swelling and ectopic bone development in ligaments and tendons (Figure 13–8A).[4]

Arthrography Arthrography is the visual study of a joint via X-ray after injection of an opaque dye, air, or a combination of air and opaque dye into the joint space. This procedure can show the disruption of soft tissue and loose bodies in the joint (Figure 13–8B).

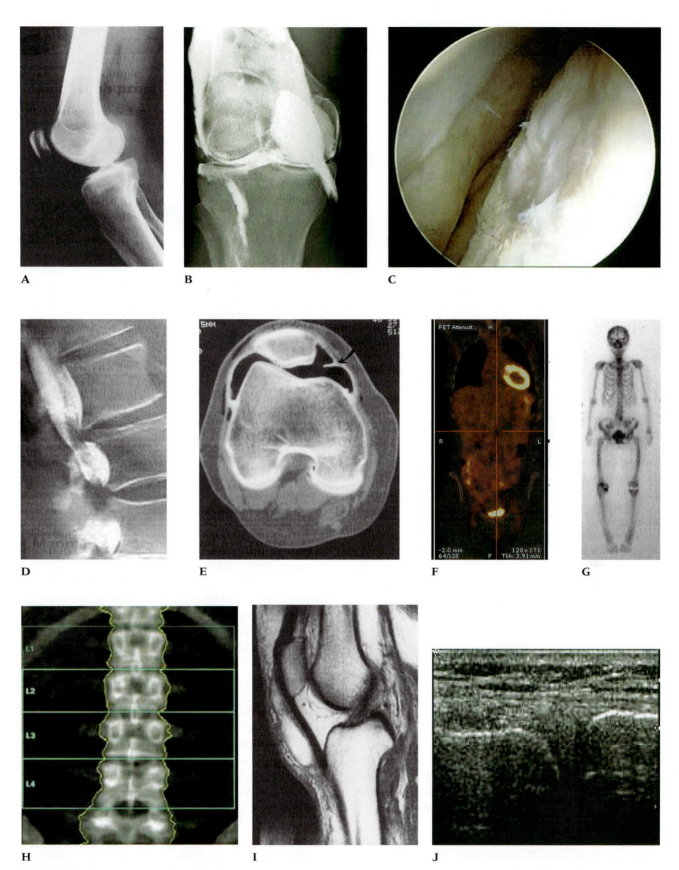

FIGURE 13–8 Imaging techniques (intended to provide examples of what these images look like, not intended to show specific pathologies). **(A)** X-ray of knee. **(B)** Arthrogram of knee. **(C)** Arthroscope of knee. **(D)** Myelogram of spine. **(E)** Computed tomography (CT) of knee **(F)** Positron emission tomography (PET) of thorax and abdomen. **(G)** Bone scan. **(H)** DEXA scan of spine. **(I)** MRI of knee. **(J)** Musculoskeletal ultrasound of knee.

(Continued)

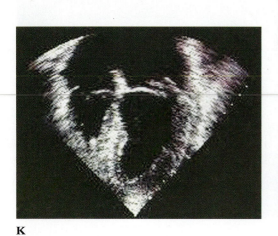

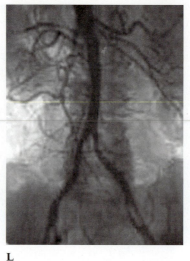

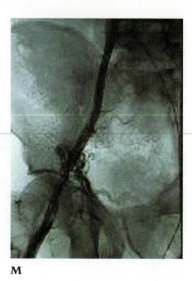

K   L   M

FIGURE 13–8   continued
(K) Echocardiogram of heart chambers. (L) Arteriogram of aorta. (M) Venogram of femoral vein.

Arthroscopy The fiber-optic arthroscope is widely used by orthopedists in surgery. It is considered more accurate than the arthrogram but is more invasive, requiring anesthesia and a small incision for the introduction of the arthroscope (endoscope) into the joint space. While the arthroscope is in the joint, the surgeon can perform surgical procedures, such as removing loose bodies and, in some cases, suturing torn tissues (Figure 13–8C).[33]

> Arthroscopy uses a fiber-optic arthroscope to view the inside of a joint.

Myelography During myelography, an opaque dye is introduced into the spinal canal (epidural space) through a lumbar puncture. While the patient is tilted, the dye is allowed to flow to different levels of the spinal cord. Using this contrast medium, physicians can detect conditions such as tumors, nerve root compression, and disk disease, as well as other diseases within the spinal cord (Figure 13–8D).

Computed Tomography Computed tomography (CT) penetrates the body with a thin, fan-shaped X-ray beam, producing a cross-sectional view of tissues. Unlike X-ray images, CT images allow the injured structure to be viewed from many angles. As the machine scans, a computer compares the many views; these electrical signals are then processed by a computer into a visual image (Figure 13–8E).

Positron Emission Tomography (PET) Positron emission tomography is a nuclear medicine imaging technique that uses an injection of a radioactive tracer chemical to produce a three-dimensional (3-D) image. A PET scan, unlike the other diagnostic imaging techniques that only confirm the presence of a mass, can help distinguish between living and dead tissue or between benign and malignant tissue. It can detect abnormal cellular activity in the very early stages, which is extremely valuable for oncology patients. A PET scan is often used in conjunction with an MRI and/or a CT to produce both anatomical and metabolic information (Figure 13–8F).

Bone Scan A bone scan involves the intravenous introduction of a radioactive tracer, such as technetium-99. By imaging the entire skeleton or part of a skeleton, bony lesions in which there is some inflammation, such as stress fractures, can be detected (Figure 13–8G).

DEXA Scan Dual-energy X-ray absorptiometry, or DEXA scanning, is currently the most widely used method to measure bone mineral density. For the test, a patient lies down on an examining table, and the scanner directs an X-ray toward the bone being examined. The greater the bone mineral density, the greater the signal picked up. DEXA scanning more precisely documents small changes in bone mass and is more flexible than a bone scan, because it can be used to examine both the spine and the extremities. DEXA scanning is less expensive, exposes the patient to less radiation, and is more sensitive and accurate at measuring subtle changes in bone density over time (Figure 13–8H).

Magnetic Resonance Imaging Magnetic resonance imaging (MRI) surrounds the body with powerful electromagnets, creating a field as much as 600,000 times as strong as that of the earth.[2] The magnetic current focuses on hydrogen atoms in water molecules and aligns them; when the current is shut off, the atoms continue to spin, emitting an energy that is detected by the computer. The hydrogen atoms in different tissues spin at different rates, thus producing different images. In many ways, MRI provides clearer images than does CT scanning. Despite the expense of MRI, it is currently physicians' test of choice for detecting soft-tissue lesions (Figure 13–8I).

MRI Arthrography MRI arthrography is an imaging study involving injection of a contrast agent into a joint prior to MRI to obtain more detail of the interior of the joint than standard MRI. The contrast agent is used to highlight certain areas of the body during imaging exams.

Ultrasonography Ultrasound imaging, also called *diagnostic ultrasound* or *sonography*, involves exposing part of the body to high-frequency sound waves to produce pictures of anatomical structures inside the body. Because ultrasound images are captured in real time, they can show the structure and movement of the body's musculoskeletal structures, internal organs, and blood flowing through blood vessels. Conventional ultrasound displays the images in thin, flat two-dimensional sections of the body. Advancements in ultrasound technology include 3-D ultrasound that formats the sound wave data into 3-D images.

Musculoskeletal Ultrasound Musculoskeletal ultrasound, or diagnostic ultrasound, is used for imaging and evaluating soft-tissue musculoskeletal disorders. It offers an excellent complementary imaging technique to traditional magnetic resonance imaging (MRI) or computed tomography (CT) studies. Imaging is accomplished by placing a transducer over the area to be visualized. Ultrasound is nonpainful and noninvasive, and it allows the patient to watch while his or her anatomical structures are being imaged on a video monitor. Compared with other cross-sectional modalities, diagnostic ultrasound is the most cost-effective imaging procedure available, other than plain X-ray (Figure 13–8J). Using a combination of physical and ultrasound data collected during the acute phase of sport-related muscle injury has been shown to be effective in helping to predict time until sport resumption.[17]

Doppler Ultrasonography This test uses ultrasound to examine the blood flow in the major arteries and veins in the arms and legs. It is done as an alternative to arteriography and venography and may help diagnose a blood clot, venous insufficiency, arterial occlusion (closing), or abnormalities in the blood flow caused by a narrowing of the vessels.

Echocardiography Echocardiography uses ultrasound to produce a graphic record of internal cardiac structures. An echocardiogram is most often used to visualize the cardiac valves and to determine the dimensions of the left atrium and both ventricles (Figure 13–8K).

Arteriogram Arteriography is a procedure in which a catheter is inserted into a specific blood vessel, contrast material is injected, and radiographs are taken, allowing the physician to see the vessel. An arteriogram can be used to examine almost any artery. In general, arteriograms give the best pictures of the body's blood vessels. Arteriograms are used to make specific diagnoses and to help determine the best treatment. Often, the treatment itself can be performed using the same type of catheters used in the arteriogram, instead of requiring a more extensive surgery in an additional procedure (e.g., angioplasty) (Figure 13–8L).

Venogram A venogram is a radiographic procedure used to image veins filled with a contrast medium. This imaging technique is most often used to detect thrombophlebitis. It provides a visual tracing of a venous pulse (Figure 13–8M).

Other Diagnostic Tests

Electrocardiography An electrocardiogram (ECG) records the electrical activity of the heart at various phases in the contraction cycle to determine whether impulse formation, conduction, and depolarization and repolarization of the atria and ventricles follows a normal pattern. It is of value in diagnosing causes of abnormal cardiac rhythm and myocardial damage. Figure 13–9 shows a visual representation of an ECG for a normal heart.

Electroencephalography The electroencephalogram (EEG) records electrical potentials produced in the brain on an instrument called an electroencephalograph. It is used to detect changes or abnormalities in brain wave patterns.

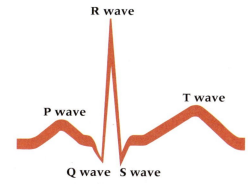

FIGURE 13–9 Electrocardiogram (ECG) tracing. This wave shows a graphic representation of the electrical activity in the heart at different points in the contraction cycle. P = atrial contraction, QRS = ventrical depolarization, T = ventrical repolarization.

Electromyography Electromyography (EMG) involves the graphic recording of a muscle contraction and the amount of electrical activity generated in a muscle using either surface or needle electrodes. Motor unit potentials can be observed on an oscilloscope screen or from a graphic recording called an electromyogram. Various muscular conditions can be evaluated.

Nerve Conduction Velocity Determining the conduction velocity of a nerve may provide key information to the physician about a number of neuromuscular conditions. After a stimulus is applied to a peripheral nerve, the speed with which a muscle action occurs is measured. Delays in conduction might indicate nerve compression or other muscular or nerve disease.

Pulse Oximetry A pulse oximeter is a device used for assessing breathing by indirectly measuring the oxygen saturation of arterial blood. Oxygen is transported in the blood by red blood cells, which are composed of hemoglobin molecules. Oxygen saturation (SpO_2) measures the amount of oxygen the blood is transporting as a percentage of the maximum amount that it can carry.[38] The simple example of how SpO_2 is calculated would be to take a single hemoglobin molecule that can bind with a maximum of eight oxygen atoms. If only six oxygen atoms are bound to a hemoglobin molecule, the oxygen saturation would be 75 percent. This is assuming that the hemoglobin molecule is not dysfunctional and that something other than oxygen has not binded to the hemoglobin, thus altering oxygen-carrying capabilities. Functional oxygen saturation is actually the amount of oxygen the hemoglobin is carrying as a percentage of the maximum amount that particular specimen could carry. Typically, that is about 1.34 mL of oxygen per gram of hemoglobin. In a fit, healthy athlete, the oxygen saturation should be between 95 and 99 percent.[44]

A pulse oximeter works by placing the device directly over a spot where there is a strong pulse, such as the tip of a finger (Figure 13–10). It emits two beams of light of different wavelengths, one red and one infrared, that pass through the finger to a photodetector. The photodetector is sensitive to the light absorption characteristics of hemoglobin that produce slight changes in the color of arterial blood, caused by differences in the amount of oxygen that is being carried by the hemoglobin.[38] The oximeter then calculates the ratio of red-to-infrared light that has passed through the finger and mathematically converts that ration to an SpO_2 value. A R:IR ratio of 0.5 equates to approximately 100 percent SpO_2 and a ratio of 1.0, to approximately 82 percent SpO_2.[44]

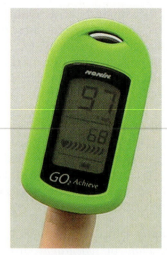

FIGURE 13–10   Pulse oximeter.

Pulse oximeters are commonly used in hospitals to monitor oxygen saturation and pulse rate in patients who have some type of respiratory difficulty (i.e. asthma, emphysema). In athletes, a pulse oximeter can help them be aware of their breathing rates and technique, which together can help maintain oxygen saturation levels above 95 percent during high-intensity training periods.[38]

Synovial Fluid Analysis The primary purpose of synovial fluid analysis is to detect the presence of an infection in the joint. The test also confirms the diagnosis of gout and differ-

> Analysis of synovial fluid and blood can be used to detect musculoskeletal infections.

entiates noninflammatory joint disease, such as degenerative arthritis, from inflammatory conditions, such as rheumatoid arthritis.[4]

Blood Testing The physician may decide to run a complete blood count (CBC) on a patient for many different reasons. The most common reasons are to screen for anemia (too few red cells) or infection (too many white cells).[43] Samples may be taken in a syringe from a vein in the arm or from a needle stick in the finger. A routine CBC addresses the following:

- The red blood cell count looks at the number of cells per unit volume to detect anemias, prolonged infections, iron deficiencies, internal bleeding, and certain types of cancers.
- Hemoglobin levels are closely associated with red blood cell count and tend to reflect overall blood volume.
- The hematocrit measures how much of the total blood volume is made up of red blood cells. A low hematocrit indicates certain types of anemias.

13-8 Clinical Application Exercise

An office worker who is participating in a corporate fitness program complains of feeling tired and run down. The athletic trainer suspects that she may be anemic and sends her to the physician for a blood test. After getting the results, the physician calls the athletic trainer and reports that her hematocrit was 36 percent and that her hemoglobin was 11 g/100 ml.

? Are these values normal? What should the athletic trainer conclude?

- The white blood cell count is used to determine the presence of bacteria. Differentiation of white cell types microscopically can identify specific types of infection.
- A deficiency in the platelet count can lead to dangerous internal bleeding.
- Blood testing can also measure levels of serum cholesterol. The recommended desirable range is <200 mg/dL.

Normal laboratory values for the CBC are summarized in Table 13–8. Normal laboratory values for blood electrolyte levels are summarized in Table 13–9.

Glucometer A glucometer is a small handheld device that is used to determine the approximate concentration of glucose in the blood (Figure 13–11). It is most commonly used by patients who have hypoglycemia or diabetes, to provide immediate feedback on levels of blood glucose. The skin must be pricked with a small lancet on the meter that draws a drop of blood, which is analyzed by the glucometer. In just a few seconds, the glucometer digitally displays the glucose level in mg/dl. A normal blood glucose level is less than 100 mg/dl when fasting and less than 140 mg/dl 2 hours after eating. Patients usually must repeat this test several times per day.

TABLE 13–9	Blood Electrolyte Levels (normal adult range)
Sodium	135–147 mEq/L
Potassium	3.5–5.2 mEq/L
Chloride	95–107 mEq/L
Calcium	8.8–10.3 mEq/dl
Phosphorus	2.5–4.5 mEq/dl
Carbon Dioxide (CO_2)	22–32 mEq/L
Bicarbonate	24–30 mEq/dl

Urinalysis Urinalysis is a common test that can yield a large quantity of information.[37] In most cases, a sample of urine in a small, dry container is all that is needed. If the urine will not be analyzed within 1 hour, the sample should be refrigerated. A routine urinalysis addresses the following:[43]

- Specific gravity indicates the ability of the kidney to concentrate and dilute fluids.
- The pH refers to how acid or alkaline the urine is. It may be acidic in cases of diabetes or dehydration. Alkaline urine is present in urinary tract infections and kidney disease. The presence of glucose may indicate diabetes.
- The presence of ketones, a by-product of fat metabolism, may also indicate diabetes.
- Hemoglobin may appear in urine after intense exercise or from kidney disease.
- The presence of protein indicates kidney disease.
- The presence of nitrate indicates infection.
- A small amount of urine is examined under a microscope to find red blood cells, white blood cells, and bacteria.
- If bacteria are present, a urine culture may be necessary to determine the specific bacteria causing an infection.
- Many additional tests may also be done on urine, including electrolytes, hormones, and drug levels.

TABLE 13–8	Normal Laboratory Values of a Complete Blood Count
Test	**Normal Values**
Red blood cell count	Males: 4.5–5.5 million/mm³
	Females: 4.0–4.9 million/mm³
White blood cell count	4,500–10,000/mm³
Platelet count	100,000–450,000/mm³
Hematocrit	Males: 41%–50%
	Females: 36%–44%
Hemoglobin	Males: 13.5–16.5 g/100 ml
	Females: 12–15 g/100 ml
Cholesterol	<200 mg/dl
HDL	30–70 mg/dl
LDL	65–180 mg/dl
Triglycerides	<160 mg/dl

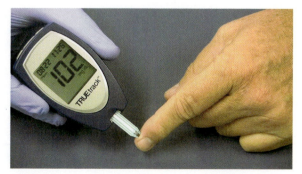

FIGURE 13–11 A glucometer is a device that measures blood glucose levels.

TABLE 13–10	Normal Laboratory Values of a Urinalysis
Test	**Normal Values**
Output	1,000–1,500 ml
Color	Yellow to amber and clear
Specific gravity	1.015–1.025
Osmolality	500–800 mosm/kg water
pH	4.6–4.8
Uric acid	250–750 mg/day
Urea	23–25 g/24 hr
Creatine	1–2 g/24 hr

Normal laboratory values for a standard urinalysis are listed in Table 13–10.

Urinalysis using dip-and-read test strips (such as Chemstrips) can provide fast, accurate results for a wide range of test parameters, such as specific gravity, leukocytes, nitrate, pH, protein, glucose, ketones, urobilinogen, bilirubin, and blood. Large test areas on each strip are impregnated with reagents that provide clear, easy-to-read color changes when dipped in urine. Color comparison charts are often located on the box.

Peak Flow Meter A peak flow meter is a small handheld device that quickly assesses a patient's peak expiratory flow rate or the ability to quickly expire or breathe air out of the lungs (Figure 13–12). These are most often used in patients who have some type of disease or condition that obstructs airflow through the bronchii. Asthma patients are typically evaluated using a peak flow meter. Peak expiratory flow is measured in l/min. There is a high degree of variability in peak flow measurement, thus readings should be taken using the same peak flow meter, by the same clinician.

ERGONOMIC RISK ASSESSMENT

In addition to performing injury evaluations, an athletic trainer working in a clinic, corporate, or industrial setting may be required to perform an *ergonomic risk assessment (ERA)*. An ergonomic risk assessment is the evaluation of factors within a job that increase the risk of someone suffering a workplace-related ergonomic injury and what aspects of, or movements within, that job should be focused on to reduce this risk. These factors include awkward postures, repetitive movements without variation, forceful movements, and vibration. The ERA aims at finding a solution through ergonomic control measures to make it safer for everyone performing that task. By combining information from the ERA with injury statistics, the physical demands of the job can be evaluated to prioritize ergonomic interventions.

Incorporating ergonomics into the introduction or design stage of a specific job task will prove a more efficient use of time and resources than dealing with the results of costly injuries and decreases in production at some point in the future. Likewise, when a process is being modified significantly, it is important to consider how the changes could impact the physical requirements to perform the work. Investigating complaints or concerns raised by the workers performing the work is a proactive step toward reducing the costly aspects of work-related injuries, lost time injuries, absenteeism, and workers compensation premiums. Workers who are tired or sore cannot produce at the same level of quality and productivity as healthy workers. Workers will know which jobs contain ergonomic risks. The discomfort or pain that workers experience is enough of an indicator that there is likely a better, safer, more efficient way of doing their work.

When an employee suffers a work-related injury, his or her body is reacting to an ergonomic stress. If the ergonomic risk is not identified and controlled, the possibility remains for another worker performing similar movements, or the same worker upon returning to an unmodified job, to develop a similar problem.

The first step in an ergonomic risk assessment is to identify the jobs most in need of attention. Prioritizing those jobs with the greatest potential for injury will assist in ensuring that the ergonomic interventions will have the greatest impact possible.

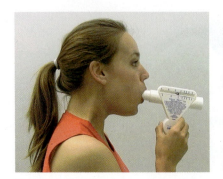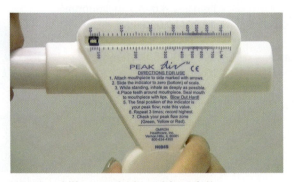

FIGURE 13–12　A peak flow meter assesses the ability to quickly and forcefully expire or breathe air out of the lungs.

Performing an ERA is an effective means of reducing the frequency and severity of workplace-related injuries. The workers need to be briefed on why the assessment is being completed and how they are involved in the solution process. This is done by reviewing injury statistics, worker concerns and complaints, and a physical demands analysis. An ergonomic risk assessment should include the following groups of employees:

- The *worker(s)* performing the job, so they understand what the ERA process is going to accomplish
- The worker's direct *supervisor*, who must understand why a job (or part of the job) needs to be modified and what the new expectations of work will be
- *Management*, so that they are aware of the costs associated with work-related musculoskeletal injuries and the benefits that the ERA can provide to the company
- Company support professionals, such as a nurse, an engineer, or safety personnel, because they will bring more resources to the group performing the ERA

Videotape can be an effective assessment tool; therefore, the athletic trainer should consider its use in the ERA. Videotape allows more people access to the assessment process than would be possible with everyone huddled around, watching the worker performing the job. Video can also be used for training purposes in addition to determining best work practices.

An ERA will result in a list of the ergonomic risk factors that exist in a specific job. The athletic trainer should identify risk factors to be controlled to minimize or eliminate the chance of a worker suffering from a workplace-related injury. These control measures should be decided in consultation with the workers affected, their supervisors, and management. The control measures can include making physical changes to the job (for example, providing a sit/stand option or tilting work surfaces) or making administrative changes (such as job rotation or a two-person lift policy). When either of these options is not reasonably practicable, personal protective equipment (such as antivibration gloves) may be beneficial. Proposed changes should also be subject to an ergonomic risk assessment to ensure that the original ergonomic risks are reduced and others are not being introduced.

SUMMARY

- Once the patient has been transported from the site of initial injury, a detailed off-the-field injury evaluation may be performed on the sideline, in the athletic training clinic, in an emergency room, or in a sports medicine clinic.
- Athletic trainers evaluate injuries and decide on a clinical diagnosis, whereas physicians are responsible for providing a medical diagnosis.
- To accurately evaluate an injury, the athletic trainer must possess a thorough background in human anatomy, including surface anatomy, body planes, and anatomical directions. The athletic trainer also needs an in-depth understanding of the musculoskeletal system, with special focus on adverse biomechanical forces, which become pathomechanical. After they are assessed, injuries must be described using appropriate terminology.

- The off-the-field evaluation scheme is divided into four broad categories: history, observation, palpation, and special tests that provide additional information about the extent of injuries.
- The progress evaluation focuses specifically on how the injury appears today compared with yesterday, and it is more limited in scope than the detailed off-the-field evaluation sequence.
- The SOAP note (subjective, objective, assessment, and plan) provides a standard format for documenting and recording injury information. Progress notes may also be recorded in the SOAP format.
- To make an accurate medical diagnosis, the physician may need to use a particular imaging technique or one of several additional tests.
- An ergonomic risk assessment can identify tasks performed in the workplace that can result in injury.

WEB SITES

SOLUTIONS TO CLINICAL APPLICATION EXERCISES

13–1 The athletic trainer must realize that the physician should have been consulted earlier in this case. Despite the fact that the athletic trainer correctly identified the MCL sprain, the meniscus tear was completely overlooked. Although the athletic trainer's actions were not inappropriate, it would have been better to refer the injured patient to the physician for medical diagnosis. In most cases, the athletic trainer's clinical diagnosis should reveal the same results as the physician's medical diagnosis.

13–2 The athletic trainer should first take a subjective history from the injured patient and follow that with an objective examination that includes observation, palpation, range of motion testing, manual muscle testing, a neurological examination, special tests, tests for joint stability, and a functional performance evaluation.

13–3 In this case, a ligamentous injury is more likely. A lesion of inert tissue will elicit pain on active and passive movement in the same direction. If a lesion is present in contractile tissue, pain will occur on active motion in one direction and on passive motion in the opposite direction. A sprain of a ligament will result in pain whenever that ligament is stretched either through active contraction or passive stretching.

13–4 A grade 3 manual muscle test suggests there is a gross lesion of contractile tissue in the shoulder, such as the rotator cuff. A weak and painful contraction indicates there may be a complete rupture of the tissue or a potential nervous system disorder.

13–5 Generally, injury to the spinal cord would result in bilateral symptoms. Unilateral changes are more indicative of peripheral nerve injury. However, any change in the neurological status of the athlete is cause for great concern. The athletic trainer should remove the patient from the playing field using a stretcher or, preferably, a spine board.

13–6 To ensure that the progress evaluation will be complete, the athletic trainer needs to go through history, observation, palpation, and special testing. The patient should be asked pertinent questions, such as "What types of exercises have you done for the past 3 months?" and "What type of pain, if any, are you still experiencing?" Observation of the symmetry to the other knee and palpation of the injured structures should be done. Range of motion, muscle strength, joint stability, and neuromuscular control should also be assessed.

13–7 Initially, it is likely that standard knee X-rays would be used to determine the presence of a fracture. An MRI is widely used by sports medicine physicians to determine injury to ligamentous, meniscal, and other soft tissues. On occasion, a diagnostic arthroscopy might be done to directly observe the injured structures.

13–8 Both the hematocrit and the hemoglobin levels are low and it is likely that the office worker does have anemia. However, depending on other signs and symptoms, the physician may need to order additional diagnostic tests to determine what may be causing this problem.

REVIEW QUESTIONS AND CLASS ACTIVITIES

1. Differentiate between a clinical diagnosis made by an athletic trainer and a medical diagnosis made by a physician.
2. What basic knowledge must the athletic trainer have before performing an injury assessment?
3. Explain the key terminology needed to communicate the results of an assessment.
4. Identify the various descriptive assessment terms.
5. How should an athletic trainer take a history? What questions should be asked?
6. Describe palpation and when and how it should be performed.
7. What can be ascertained from active, passive, and resisted isometric movement?
8. Explain how muscle testing, reflex testing, and sensory testing are performed.
9. What part do special tests play in injury assessment?
10. When should a functional evaluation be given?
11. What information should be included in a SOAP note?
12. What insights can a physician gain by having special laboratory tests performed? Describe each test in detail.
13. How can an ergonomic risk assessment be used to minimize the chances of workplace-related injuries?

REFERENCES

1. Arrigo C: Clinical documentation. In Konin J, editor: *Clinical athletic training*, Thorofare, NJ, 1997, Slack.
2. Barak T, Rosen E, Sofer R: Mobility: Passive orthopedic manual therapy. In Gould J, Davies G, editors: *Orthopedic and sports physical therapy*, St. Louis, 1997, Mosby.
3. Berry D, Miller M: Athletic and Orthopedic Injury Assessment: A Case Study Approach, 2010, Holcomb Hathaway Publishers.
4. Bickley L: *Bates' guide to physical examination and history taking*, Philadelphia, 2008, Lippincott, Williams and Wilkins.
5. Bohannon R: Manual muscle testing: does it meet the standards of an adequate screening test? *Clinical Rehabilitation* 19(6):662, 2005.
6. Booher J, Thibodeau G: *Athletic injury assessment*, San Francisco, 2001, McGraw-Hill.
7. Clarkson H, Gilewich G: *Musculoskeletal assessment: joint range of motion and manual muscle strength*, Philadelphia, 2000, Lippincott, Williams and Wilkins.
8. Cutter N, Kevorkian G: *Handbook of manual muscle testing*, New York, 1999, McGraw-Hill.
9. Cyriax J, Cyriax P: *Cyriax's illustrated manual of orthopaedic medicine*, London, 1996, Butterworth-Heinemann.
10. Delforge G: Sports injury assessment and problem identification. In Delforge G, editor: *Musculoskeletal trauma: implications for sports injury management*, Champaign, IL, 2002, Human Kinetics.
11. DeMont R: The place for palpation, *Athletic Therapy Today* 8(2):42, 2003.
12. Deyle G: Musculoskeletal imaging in physical therapist practice, *J Orthop Sports Phys Ther* 35(11):708, 2005.
13. Evans R: *Illustrated orthopedic physical assessment*, St. Louis, 2001, Mosby.
14. Gabbe B, Finch C, Bennell K: How valid is a self reported 12 month sports injury history? *British Journal of Sports Medicine* 37(6):545, 2003.
15. Garber, M: Diagnostic imaging and differential diagnosis in 2 case reports, *J Orthop Sports Phys Ther* 35(11):745, 2005.
16. Gottlieb J: *SOAP for orthopedics*, Philadelphia, 2005, Lippincott, Williams & Wilkins.
17. Guillodo Y: Value of sonography combined with clinical assessment to evaluate muscle injury severity in athletes, *J Athl Train*, 46(5):500–04, 2011.
18. Gylys B, Masters R: *Medical terminology simplified: A programmed learning approach by body systems*, ed 3, Philadelphia, 2009, F.A. Davis.
19. Hartley A: *Practical joint assessment*, St. Louis, 1995, Mosby.
20. Hilsop H, Montgomery J: *Daniels and Worthingham muscle testing*, San Diego, 2007, Elsevier Science.
21. Hoppenfeld S: *Physical examination of the spine and extremities*, New York, 1992, Appleton-Century-Crofts.
22. Hubbard T: How accurate is that clinical assessment test? *Athletic Therapy Today* 9(6):63, 2004.
23. Hurley W: Agreement of clinical judgments of end-feel between 2 sample populations, *J Sport Rehabil* 11(3):209, 2002.

24. Kaltenborn F, Evjenth O, Kaltenborn T: *Manual mobilization of the joints: the Kaltenborn method of joint examination and treatment: the extremities*, Minneapolis, 2002, Orthopedic Physical Therapy Products.

25. Kendall F, Kendall E: *Muscles testing and function*, Philadelphia, 2005, Lippincott, Williams and Wilkins.

26. Kettenbach G: *Writing SOAP notes with patient/client management formats*, Philadelphia, 2003, F.A. Davis.

27. Konin J: *Documentation for athletic training*, Thorofare, NJ, 2011, Slack.

28. Lumley J: *Surface anatomy—the anatomical basis of clinical evaluation*, Philadelphia, 2008, Churchill-Livingstone.

29. Mattacola CG: Introduction to clinical evaluation and testing, *Athletic Therapy Today* 8(2):24, 2003.

30. Magee DL: *Orthopedic physical assessment*, Philadelphia, 2007, Elsevier Health Sciences.

31. McKinnis L: *Fundamentals of musculoskeletal imaging*, Philadelphia, 2010, F.A. Davis.

32. McRae R: *Clinical orthopaedic examination*, Philadelphia, 2010, Elsevier Health Sciences.

33. Milbauer D: Principles of radiographic evaluation and imaging techniques. In Nicholas J, Hershman E, editors: *The lower extremity and spine in sports medicine*, St. Louis, 1995, Mosby.

34. Norkin C, White J: *Measurement of joint motion: A guide to goniometry*, Philadelphia, 2009, F.A. Davis.

35. Palmer ML, Epler MF, Adams M: *Fundamentals of musculoskeletal assessment techniques*, Philadelphia, 1998, Lippincott, Williams and Wilkins.

36. Petersen CM: Construct validity of Cyriax's selective tension examination: Association of end-feels with pain at the knee and shoulder, *J Orthop Sports Phys Ther* 30(9):512, 2002.

37. Peterson EJ, et al.: Reliability of water volumetry and the figure eight method on subjects with ankle joint swelling, *J Orthop Sports Phys Ther* 29(10):609, 1999.

38. Sinex J: Pulse oximetry: Principles and limitations, *The American Journal of Emergency Medicine*, 17(1):59–66, 1999.

39. Starkey C, Perriello V, Anderson S: Diagnosis appropriate? Physicians agree, *NATA News* 5:48, 2006.

40. Starkey C, Ryan J: *Evaluation of orthopedic and athletic injuries*, Philadelphia, 2009, F.A. Davis.

41. Suetens P: *Fundamentals of medical imaging*, Cambridge, 2009, Cambridge University Press.

42. Tixa S: *Atlas of palpatory anatomy of limbs and trunk*, Teteroboro, NJ, 2007, Icon Learning Systems.

43. Wurman R: *Medical access*, Los Angeles, 1985, Access Press.

44. Yamaya Y: Validity of pulse oximetry during maximal exercise in normoxia, hypoxia and hyperoxia, *Journal of Applied Physiology*, 92(1):162–68, 2002.

ANNOTATED BIBLIOGRAPHY

Booher JM, Thibodeau GA: *Athletic injury assessment*, ed 4, St. Louis, 2001, McGraw-Hill.

Addressed the practitioner in sports medicine or athletic training. It considers all aspects of musculoskeletal and internal sports injuries.

Cyriax J, Cyriax P: *Cyriax's Illustrated manual of orthopaedic medicine*, London, 1996, Butterworth-Heinemann.

A color-illustrated text designed for diagnosing and providing Cyriax management to musculoskeletal conditions.

Gross J, Fetto J, Rosen E: *Musculoskeletal examination*, Cambridge, MA, 2009, Blackwell.

An evaluation text is written primarily for physicians.

Hoppenfeld S: *Physical examination of the spine and extremities*, New York, 1992, Appleton-Lange.

Presents an easy-to-follow, methodical, and in-depth procedure for examining musculoskeletal conditions.

Konin J, Wiksten D, Isear J: *Special tests for orthopedic examination*, Stamford, CT, 2006, Thomson Learning.

A well-illustrated text that details examination techniques used in evaluating musculoskeletal injuries.

Magee DJ: *Orthopedic physical assessment*, Philadelphia, 2007, Elsevier Health Sciences.

An extremely well-illustrated book with excellent depth of coverage of injuries commonly found during athletic training.

Palmer ML, Epler MF, Adams M: *Fundamentals of musculoskeletal assessment techniques*, Philadelphia, 1998, Lippincott, Williams and Wilkins.

Contains contributions by many experts in the field of orthopedic examination. It covers each major joint in detail.

Starkey C, Ryan J: *Evaluation of orthopedic and athletic injuries*, Philadelphia, 2009, F.A. Davis.

A detailed, well-illustrated text addressing all aspects of injury assessment for the athletic trainer.

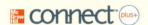

14

Infectious Diseases, Bloodborne Pathogens, and Universal Precautions

■ Objectives

When you finish this chapter you should be able to

- Discuss how infectious diseases are transmitted from person to person.
- Describe how the immune system neutralizes and eliminates an antigen that invades the body.
- Explain what bloodborne pathogens are and how they can infect patients and athletic trainers.
- Describe the transmission, symptoms, signs, and treatment of hepatitis B.
- Describe the transmission, symptoms, signs, and treatment of hepatitis C.

- Describe the transmission, symptoms, and signs of human immunodeficiency virus.
- Explain how human immunodeficiency virus is most often transmitted.
- List the pros and cons of athletes with hepatitis B virus, hepatitis C virus, or human immunodeficiency virus participating in sports.
- Evaluate universal precautions as mandated by the Occupational Safety and Health Administration and how they apply to the athletic trainer.

■ Outline

■ Key Terms

immune system   OSHA
retrovirus

■ Connect Highlights 🔲 connect™ (plus+)

Visit connect.mcgraw-hill.com for further exercises to apply your knowledge:

- Clinical application scenarios covering universal precautions and signs, symptoms, and transmission of disease
- Click-and-drag questions covering disease transmission, bloodborne pathogens, and disease identification
- Multiple choice questions covering signs, symptoms, and transmission of disease, immune system and transmission of infectious diseases

ike other health care providers, athletic trainers must be aware of and take universal precautions against the spread of infectious diseases and bloodborne pathogens.[4,29,40] It has always been important for the athletic trainer as a health care provider to be concerned with maintaining an environment in the athletic training room that is as clean and sterile as possible.[4] In our society, it has become critical for everyone to take measures to prevent the spread of infectious diseases.[13] Failure to do so may predispose any individual to life-threatening situations. The athletic trainer must take every precaution to minimize the potential for exposure to blood or other infectious materials. A link to the NATA official statement "Communicable and infectious diseases in secondary school sports" (http://www.nata.org/sites/default/files/Communicable InfectiousDiseasesSecondarySchoolSports.pdf) can be found at www.mhhe.com/prentice15e.

INFECTIOUS DISEASES

Infectious diseases are the invasion or infection of a *host* (person or animal) by microorganisms called *pathogens*.[13,17,27] A pathogen causes disease by either disrupting a vital body process or stimulating the immune system to mount a defensive reaction. An immune response against a pathogen, which can include a high fever, inflammation, and other damaging symptoms, can be more devastating than the direct damage caused by the pathogen itself. The most common pathogens are various bacteria, viruses, parasites, and fungi (Table 14–1).[22] A microorganism can live harmlessly in a host (such as an animal) without causing infection. Over time, these hosts gradually become resistant to the microorganisms. However, when a microorganism is somehow transmitted from that animal host to a human, it may cease being harmless and become a pathogen

TABLE 14–1	Common Infectious Diseases		
Viral infectious diseases			
AIDS	Hepatitis	Marburg haemor-	Viral
AIDS-related	A,B,C,D,E	rhagic fever	encephalitis
complex	Herpes simplex	Infectious	Viral
Chickenpox	Herpes zoster	mononucleosis	gastroenteritis
(varicella)	Human immuno-	Mumps	Viral meningitis
Common cold	deficiency disease	Poliomyelitis	Viral pneumonia
Cytomegalovirus	Human	Rabies	West Nile
infection	papillomavirus	Rubella	disease
Ebola	Influenza (flu)	SARS	Yellow fever
haemorrhagic	Type B	Smallpox	
fever	H1N1		
Hand, foot, and	Measles		
mouth disease			
Bacterial infectious diseases			
Anthrax	Lyme disease	Pneumococcal	Syphilis
Bacterial	MRSA	pneumonia	Tetanus
meningitis	(methacillin-	Rocky Mountain	Tuberculosis
Cat scratch	resistant staphy-	spotted fever	Typhoid fever
disease	lococcus aureus) infection	(RMSF)	Typhus
Cholera	Pertussis	Salmonellosis	Urinary tract
Diphtheria	(whooping	Scarlet fever	infections
Gonorrhea	cough)	Shigellosis	
Impetigo			
Parasitic infectious diseases			
Giardiasis	Pinworm infection	Trichinosis	
Malaria	Scabies	Tropical parasite	
Pediculosis	Toxoplasmosis	diseases	
Fungal infectious diseases			
Candidiasis	Histoplasmosis	Tinea pedis	

in the new host. Infectious disease requires an *agent* and a *mode of transmission*, as is the case when a mosquito is carrying malaria and injects that microorganism into the human. This microorganism becomes a pathogen and the person is now infected.[40]

An infectious disease is termed *contagious* if it is transmitted from one person to another. Transmission can be either direct or indirect. There are three types of direct transmission: contact between body surfaces (touching, sexual intercourse), droplet spread (inhalation of contaminated air droplets from someone who sneezes in close proximity), and fecal-oral spread (feces on the host's hands are brought into contact with the new host's mouth).[31]

Transmission does not have to occur through direct human contact. Indirect transmission from an infected person to an uninfected person occurs when infectious agents travel by means of inanimate objects, such as water, food, towels, clothing, and eating utensils. Infectious agents can also be indirectly transmitted through *vectors*, which are living things, such as insects, birds, or animals, that carry diseases from human to human. Airborne transmission of infected particles that have been suspended in an air source for an extended time can occur by sharing air with infected people who were in the same room earlier (such as passengers on an airplane).[40]

Pathogens can enter the body through the skin, respiratory system, digestive system, or reproductive system. Whether the pathogen will actually infect the new host is determined by factors such as acquired immunity, overall health, and health-related behavior.

When a pathogen infects a new host, a sequence of five stages predictably occurs. The *incubation* stage lasts from the time a pathogen enters the body until it multiplies to the point where signs and symptoms of a disease begin to appear. This stage can last from a few hours to many months, depending on the concentration of organisms, the virulence of the organisms, the level of the immune response in the host, and the presence of additional health problems. During this stage, a host may be infected but is not infectious. In the *prodromal* stage, a variety of signs and symptoms (watery eyes, runny nose, slight fever, malaise) may briefly develop. During this stage, the pathogenic agent continues to multiply and the host is capable of transferring pathogens to a new host. The person should be isolated to prevent transmission to others. In the *acute* stage, the disease reaches its greatest development, and the likelihood of transmitting the disease to others is highest. The body is resisting further damage from the pathogen. In the *decline* stage, the first signs of recovery appear, signaling that the infection is ending. However, patients can experience a relapse if they overextend themselves. The *recovery* stage is characterized by apparent recovery from the invading pathogen. However, because overall health has been compromised, the patient is susceptible to other pathogens. Following the recovery stage, subsequent exposure to that pathogen may not result in infection, because the body has built up immunity. It must be stressed that immunity is not necessarily permanent.[39]

The Immune System

The **immune system** consists of two lines of defense against invading pathogens: mechanical defenses and the cellular system defenses. *Mechanical defenses* separate the internal body from the external environment and include the skin, mucous membranes that line the respiratory and gastrointestinal tracts, nasal hairs, and cilia lining the airway that filter incoming air. When mechanical defenses are disrupted, the *cellular system* takes over, eliminating microorganisms, foreign proteins, and abnormal cells, collectively referred to as *antigens* (Figure 14–1). The immune system consists of two groups of cells, T cells and B cells, both of which are found within the bloodstream, the lymphatic tissues, and the intersititial fluid. An immune response requires that these components of the cellular system defend the body against specific antigens. The presence of an antigen triggers leukocytes and macrophages to locate and destroy the invading antigen. Macrophages activate T cells to assist in the immune response. Once T cells are activated, they then activate both killer T cells, which assist the macrophages in destroying the antigen, and B cells, which are transformed into specialized cells (plasma cells) capable of producing *antibodies*. Antibodies neutralize antigens by lysis and phagocytosis, by neutralizing toxins produced by bacteria, and by preventing the antigen from adhering to host cells. Simultaneously, memory T cells are being formed that record information about the invading antigen and the appropriate immune system response that successfully repressed the infection. Suppressor T cells allow the production of antibodies to be reduced when the immune system has neutralized the antigen.[31]

Immunity When the immune system successfully eliminates the effects of an invading antigen, it is

> **immune system**
> The body's defense system against invading microorganisms

Stages of pathogen infection:
- Incubation stage
- Prodromal stage
- Acute stage
- Decline stage
- Recovery stage

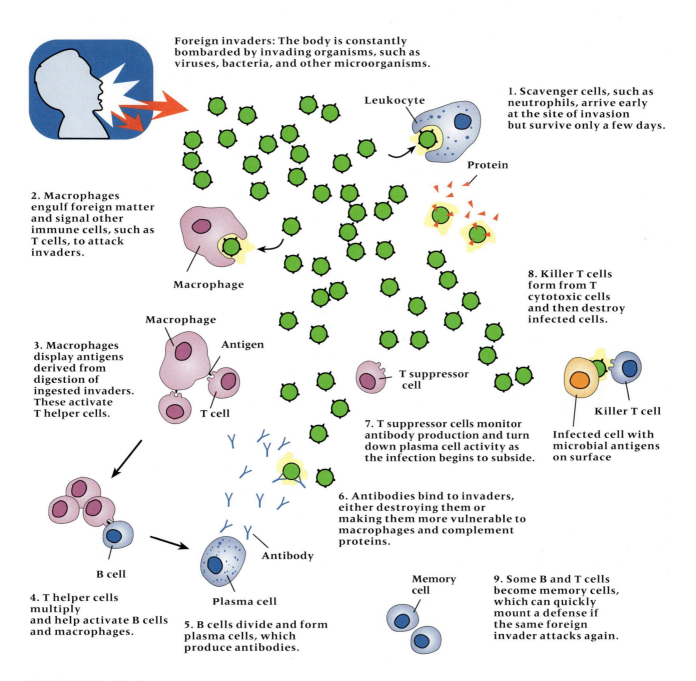

Foreign invaders: The body is constantly bombarded by invading organisms, such as viruses, bacteria, and other microorganisms.

Leukocyte

1. Scavenger cells, such as neutrophils, arrive early at the site of invasion but survive only a few days.

Protein

2. Macrophages engulf foreign matter and signal other immune cells, such as T cells, to attack invaders.

Macrophage

8. Killer T cells form from T cytotoxic cells and then destroy infected cells.

Macrophage

Antigen

3. Macrophages display antigens derived from digestion of ingested invaders. These activate T helper cells.

T cell

T suppressor cell

Killer T cell

Infected cell with microbial antigens on surface

7. T suppressor cells monitor antibody production and turn down plasma cell activity as the infection begins to subside.

Antibody

6. Antibodies bind to invaders, either destroying them or making them more vulnerable to macrophages and complement proteins.

B cell

Plasma cell

4. T helper cells multiply and help activate B cells and macrophages.

5. B cells divide and form plasma cells, which produce antibodies.

Memory cell

9. Some B and T cells become memory cells, which can quickly mount a defense if the same foreign invader attacks again.

FIGURE 14–1   The immune system response.

primed to respond quickly and effectively, should the same antigens appear again. Thus, the body has developed natural *acquired immunity*. Acquired immunity can also be developed either artificially, when the body is exposed to weakened pathogens through vaccination or immunization, or passively, when antibodies are injected to provide immediate protection until the body can develop natural immunity. Collectively, these forms of immunity can provide important protection against infectious disease.[11]

Immunizations Vaccinations against several potentially serious infectious conditions are available and should be given to everyone.[37] These include the following: diphtheria, pertussis (whooping cough), hepatitis B, haemophilus influenza type B, tetanus, rubella (German measles), measles (red measles), polio, mumps, and chickenpox. This immunization process has markedly reduced the incidence of several childhood communicable diseases and minimized the infection rate of hepatitis B, influenza, and tetanus.

Immunization has virtually eradicated many infectious diseases worldwide. Epidemiology is a tool used to study infectious disease in a population. For infectious diseases, it helps to determine whether a disease outbreak is *sporadic* (occasional occurrence),

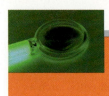

FOCUS 14–1 Focus on Injury/Illness Prevention and Wellness Protection

Suggestions for preventing the spread of infectious diseases

- Wash your hands frequently, especially after going to the bathroom.
- Keep immunizations up to date.
- Prepare/handle food carefully.
- Use antibiotics only for infections caused by bacteria.
- Be careful around all wild animals and unfamiliar domestic animals.
- Avoid insect bites.
- Protect yourself by using safer sex practices.
- Do not inject illegal drugs.
- Stay alert to disease threats when you travel or visit underdeveloped countries.
- Develop healthy habits, such as eating well, getting enough sleep, exercising, and avoiding tobacco and illegal substance use.

endemic (regular cases often occurring in a region), *epidemic* (an unusually high number of cases in a region), or *pandemic* (a global epidemic).

Preventing Spread of Infectious Diseases

The athletic trainer, like other health care professionals, must be diligent in efforts to minimize the chances of transmitting infectious diseases.[24,26]

> Handwashing is the single most important practice for preventing the spread of infectious diseases.

Without question, the most effective practice to accomplish this is for the athletic trainer to wash his or her hands frequently when treating patients, particularly after caring for a sick person, after using the bathroom, and after blowing the nose and/or using hands to cover sneezing or coughing. The athletic trainer should review medical histories of the patients being treated or cared for to make sure that all potential immunizations are up to date. The athletic trainer should also make sure that patients who are sick understand that taking antibiotics is not useful in treating infections caused by viruses and that antibiotics should be taken exactly as prescribed. Taking them unnecessarily will reduce their ability to combat subsequent bacterial infections. All patients should be routinely encouraged to develop healthy lifestyle

habits, such as eating well, getting enough sleep, exercising, and avoiding tobacco and substance abuse (see *Focus Box 14–1*: "Suggestions for preventing the spread of infectious diseases").

BLOODBORNE PATHOGENS

Despite the media attention given to bloodborne pathogens in recent years, many athletic trainers have only a moderate understanding of the magnitude of the problem (Figure 14–2).[20] Bloodborne pathogens are viruses transmitted through contact with blood or other body fluids. A virus is a submicroscopic parasitic organism that is dependent on the nutrients within cells.

> **Modes of transmission:**
> - Human blood
> - Semen
> - Vaginal secretions
> - Cerebrospinal fluid
> - Synovial fluid

A virus consists of a strand of either deoxyribonucleic acid (DNA) or ribonucleic acid (RNA). A virus contains one or the other, but not both. A virus consists of a shell of proteins surrounding genetic material. It is a parasite that depends on a host cell for metabolic and reproductive requirements. In general, viruses make their cell hosts ill by redirecting cellular activity to create more viruses (Figure 14–3).

Bloodborne pathogens are pathogenic microorganisms that can cause disease and are present in human blood and other body fluids, including semen, vaginal secretions, cerebrospinal fluid, synovial fluid, and any other fluid contaminated with blood

> **Bloodborne pathogens:**
> - Hepatitis B virus (HBV)
> - Hepatitis C virus (HCV)
> - Human immunodeficiency virus (HIV)

(Table 14–2). The three most significant bloodborne pathogens are the hepatitis B virus (HBV), the hepatitis C virus (HCV), and the human immunodeficiency virus (HIV).[1] Although HIV has been widely addressed in the media, HBV and HCV have

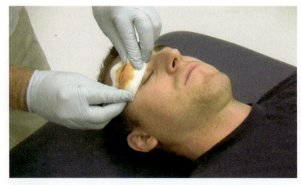

FIGURE 14–2 The athletic trainer must take precautions to prevent exposure to and transmission of bloodborne pathogens.

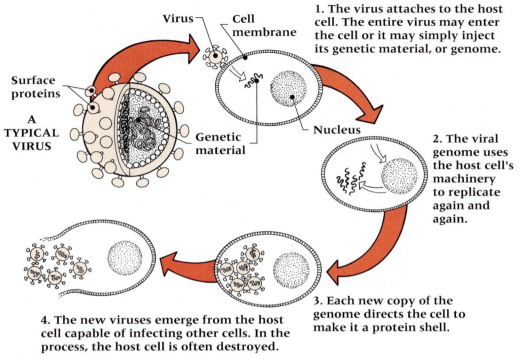

1. The virus attaches to the host cell. The entire virus may enter the cell or it may simply inject its genetic material, or genome.

2. The viral genome uses the host cell's machinery to replicate again and again.

3. Each new copy of the genome directs the cell to make it a protein shell.

4. The new viruses emerge from the host cell capable of infecting other cells. In the process, the host cell is often destroyed.

FIGURE 14–3   The reproducing virus.

TABLE 14–2	Body Fluids
Universal precautions should be practiced in any environment where individuals are exposed to bodily fluids, such as	Body fluids that do not require such precautions include
• Blood	• Feces
• Semen	• Nasal secretions
• Vaginal secretions	• Urine
• Synovial fluid	• Vomitus
• Amniotic fluid	• Perspiration
• Cerebrospinal fluid	• Sputum
• Pleural fluid	• Saliva
• Peritoneal fluid	
• Pericardial fluid	

a higher possibility for spread than does HIV, and thus athletic trainers should be more concerned about contracting HBV and HCV.[2,19,29] The hepatitis B virus is stronger and more durable than HIV and can be spread more easily via sharp objects, open wounds, and body fluids.[14]

Hepatitis B Virus

The hepatitis B virus attacks the liver, resulting in lifelong infection, cirrhosis (scarring) of the liver, liver cancer, liver failure, and death. Hepatitis B is not spread through food or water or by casual contact. HBV is spread when blood from an infected person enters the body of a person who is not infected. For example, HBV is spread through having unprotected sex (no condom) with an infected person, by sharing needles when "shooting" drugs, or in health care providers through needlesticks or sharps exposures on the job. Health care personnel who have received the hepatitis B vaccine and developed immunity to the virus are at virtually no risk of infection. An estimated 350 to 400 million people worldwide have chronic HBV infection (compared, with 40 million living with HIV). In the United States, it is estimated that 1.4 million have chronic hepatitis B and about 5,000 die per year of sickness caused by HBV.[5] An estimated 8,700 health care workers contract HBV each year, and as many as 200 of these cases end in death.[5]

Symptoms and Signs The symptoms and signs in a person infected with HBV include flulike symptoms, such as fatigue, weakness, and nausea; abdominal pain; headache; fever; dark urine; and possibly jaundice (yellowing of the skin or eyes). It is possible that an individual infected with HBV will exhibit no signs or symptoms, and the virus may go undetected. In these individuals, the HBV antigen will always be present. Thus, the disease may be unknowingly transmitted to others through exposure to blood or other body fluids or through intimate contact. Cases of chronic active hepatitis may occur because of a problem with the immune system that prevents the complete destruction of virus-infected liver cells.

An infected person's blood may test positive for the HBV antigen within 2 to 6 weeks after the symptoms develop. Approximately 85 percent of those infected recover within 6 to 8 weeks.

Prevention Good personal hygiene and avoiding high-risk activities are the best ways to avoid HBV.[32] Hepatitis B virus can survive for at least 1 week in dried blood or on contaminated surfaces and may be transmitted through contact with these surfaces. Caution must be taken to avoid contact with any blood or other fluid that potentially contains a bloodborne pathogen.[36] Several vaccines have been developed for preventing HBV. However vaccination does not help individuals already infected by HBV.

Management Vaccination against HBV must be made available by employers at no cost to any individual who may be exposed to blood or other body fluids and thus may be at risk of contracting HBV.[37] **All athletic trainers and any individual working in an allied health care profession should receive immunization**. The vaccine is given in three doses over a 6-month period. Approximately 87 percent of those receiving the vaccine are immune after the second dose, and 96 percent develop immunity after the third dose. Postexposure vaccination is available when individuals have come in direct contact with the body fluids of an infected person.[6]

Hepatitis C Virus

Originally referred to as non-A, non-B hepatitis, hepatitis C is both an acute and a chronic form of liver disease caused by the hepatitis C virus (HCV). HCV is the most common chronic bloodborne infection in the United States. At least 85 percent of those infected acutely with HCV become chronically infected, and 67 percent develop chronic liver disease. It is the leading indication for liver transplant. Three percent of those with chronic liver disease die from cirrhosis or liver cancer. It is estimated that 170 million people worldwide and 4.5 million Americans have been infected with HCV, of whom 2.7 million are chronically infected.[10]

Symptoms and Signs Eighty percent of those infected with HCV have no signs or symptoms. Those who are symptomatic may be jaundiced and/or have mild abdominal pain, particularly in the upper right quadrant, loss of appetite, nausea, fatigue, muscle or joint pain, and/or dark urine.

Prevention HCV is not spread by sneezing, hugging, coughing, food or water, eating utensils or drinking glasses, or casual contact. It is rarely spread through sexual contact. It is spread by contact with the blood of an infected person.[36] It is most commonly transmitted by sharing needles or syringes. However, it can also be transmitted by sharing personal care items that might have blood on them (razors, toothbrushes). Consider the risks of getting a tattoo or body piercing. Athletic trainers should always follow routine barrier precautions and safely handle needles and other sharp objects.

Management Unlike for HBV, presently there is no vaccine for preventing HCV transmission. Several blood tests can be done to determine whether a person has been infected with HCV. A physician may order just one or a combination of these tests. It is possible to find HCV within 1 to 2 weeks after being infected with the virus. A single positive test indicates infection with HCV. However, a single negative test does not prove that a person is not infected. When hepatitis C is suspected, even though an initial test is negative, the test should be repeated.[10]

HCV-positive persons should be evaluated by their doctor for liver disease. Interferon and ribavirin are two drugs used in combination that appear to be the most effective for the treatment of persons with chronic hepatitis C. Drinking alcohol can make liver disease worse.

Human Immunodeficiency Virus

Human immunodeficiency virus is a **retrovirus** that combines with a host cell. A number of cells in the immune system may be infected, such as T cells, B cells, and macrophages, which decreases their effectiveness in preventing disease. As of 2010, an estimated 34 million people worldwide were living with HIV/AIDS. Worldwide, approximately 11 of every 1,000 adults ages 15 to 49 are infected with HIV. An estimated 2.7 million new HIV infections occurred worldwide during 2010. That is about 7,500 infections each day. In 2010 alone, HIV/AIDS-associated illnesses caused approximately 1.9 million deaths worldwide.[41]

> **retrovirus** A virus that enters a host cell and changes its RNA to a proviral DNA replica.

Symptoms and Signs As is the case with HBV, HIV is transmitted by exposure to infected blood or other body fluids and by intimate sexual contact.[42] Symptoms of HIV include fatigue, weight loss, muscle or joint pain, painful or swollen glands, night sweats, and fever. Antibodies to HIV can be detected in a blood test within 1 year after exposure. As with HBV, people with HIV may be unaware that they have contracted the virus and may go for 8 to 10 years before developing any signs or symptoms. Unfortunately, most individuals who test positive for HIV will ultimately develop acquired immunodeficiency syndrome (AIDS). Table 14–3 summarizes information on HBV, HCV, and HIV.

Acquired Immunodeficiency Syndrome A syndrome is a collection of signs and symptoms that are recognized as the effects of an infection. An individual with AIDS has no protection against even the simplest infections and thus is extremely vulnerable to developing a variety of illnesses, opportunistic infections, and cancers (such as Kaposi's sarcoma and non-Hodgkin's lymphoma) that cannot be stopped.[25,34]

According to the Centers for Disease Control and Prevention (CDC), it is estimated that, as of 2011, 1.2 million U.S. residents are living with HIV infection and that approximately 50,000 new HIV infections occur each year. An estimated 1,108,611 people in the United States were living with AIDS, and since 1981 an estimated 594,500 people with AIDS in the United States have died.[8]

A positive HIV test cannot predict when the individual will show the symptoms of AIDS.[34] About 50 percent of people develop AIDS within 10 years of becoming HIV infected. Those individuals who develop AIDS generally die within 2 years after the symptoms appear.

Management Unlike HBV, there is no vaccine for HIV. Even though some drug therapy may extend their lives, there is currently no available treatment to cure patients with AIDS. Much research is being done to find a preventive vaccine and an effective treatment. Presently, the most effective treatment seems to be a therapy consisting of a combination of three drugs. One drug blocks the action of an enzyme that the virus needs to make some of the components for new virus cells. A second drug blocks the copying of viral genes that can enter the host cell's nucleus (a process called reverse transcription) and thus disables the synthesis of new viruses. A third drug helps protect the T cells and thus slows the progression of HIV.[31]

TABLE 14–3	Transmission of Hepatitis B and C Viruses and Human Immunodeficiency Virus		
Disease	**Symptoms and Signs**	**Mode of Transmission**	**Infectious Materials**
Hepatitis B virus	Flulike symptoms, jaundice	Direct and indirect contact	Blood, saliva, semen, feces, food, water, other products
Hepatitis C virus	Jaundice, upper right quadrant pain, loss of appetite, nausea, fatigue, dark urine	Direct and indirect contact with blood	Blood
Human immuno-deficiency virus/ acquired immuno-deficiency syndrome	Fever, night sweats, weight loss, diarrhea, severe fatigue, swollen lymph nodes, lesions	Direct and indirect contact	Blood, semen, vaginal fluid

Although new treatments have extended the healthy life span of many people with AIDS, HIV prevalence has continued to increase. As the number of AIDS cases declines because of these new treatments, the number of people with HIV will increase, which means there will be a greater need for both prevention and treatment services.

Prevention It is essential to understand that the greatest risk of contracting HIV is through intimate sexual contact with an infected partner.[31] Practicing safe sex is of major importance. Anyone engaging in sexual activities must choose nonpromiscuous sex partners and use condoms for vaginal or anal intercourse. Latex condoms provide a barrier against both HBV and HIV. Male condoms should have reservoir tips to reduce the chance of ejaculate being released from the sides of the condom. Condoms that are prelubricated are less likely to tear. Water-based, greaseless spermicides or lubricants should be avoided.[31] If the condom tears, a vaginal spermicide should be used immediately. The condom should carefully be removed and discarded.[31] Additional ways to reduce the risk of HIV infection can be found in *Focus Box 14–2*: "HIV risk reduction."

> **Human immunodeficiency virus is most often transmitted through intimate sexual contact.**

> **The use of latex condoms can reduce the chances of contracting HIV.**

Additional Hepatitis Viruses

Three additional viruses—hepatitis A, D, and E—exist, which, while related, are not generally considered to be bloodborne pathogens.

Hepatitis A Virus Hepatitis A (HAV) is a virus that causes inflammation of the liver but does not lead to chronic disease of the liver. HAV is transmitted by the fecal or oral routes, through close personal contact, or through ingestion of contaminated food or water. For example, it may be transmitted by an infected food preparer who doesn't wash his or her hands after going to the bathroom. In food, HAV is most commonly transmitted in milk, shellfish, salad, and sliced meat. HAV may show no outward symptoms or signs, but adults may have dark urine, light stools, fatigue, fever, and jaundice. HAV persists acutely for up to 21 days, but the effects last considerably longer. Death is rare with HAV infection.[5]

Hepatitis D Virus Hepatitis D (HDV), like HAV, causes inflammation of the liver and those infected are prone to developing hepatitis and cirrhosis. HDV may be transmitted by sexual activity, injected drugs,

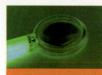

or needlesticks in health care workers. It is most likely to infect those individuals who are already infected with HBV. Symptoms are more severe than with HBV and there is at least a 2 percent mortality rate.[13]

Hepatitis E Virus Like HAV and HDV, hepatitis E (HEV) causes inflammation of the liver. It is transmitted through the fecal and oral routes.[11] Hepatitis E is a waterborne disease, and contaminated water and food supplies have been implicated in major outbreaks in foreign countries with poor sanitation standards. Person-to-person transmission is uncommon. There is no evidence for sexual transmission or for transmission by transfusion. HEV is a self-limiting viral infection followed by recovery, with mortality rates between 0.5 percent and 4.0 percent.[13]

Bloodborne Pathogens in Athletics

In general, the chances of transmitting HIV among athletes is low.[2,12,15,24,28] There is minimal risk of on-field transmission of HIV from one player to another in sports.[9] One study involving professional football estimated that the risk of transmission from player to player is less than 1 per 1 million games.[28] At this time there have been no validated reports of HIV transmission in sports.[29]

Some sports may have a higher risk of transmission because of close contact and the possibility of passing blood on to another person.[2] Sports such as the martial arts, wrestling, and boxing have more theoretical potential for transmission (see *Focus Box 14–3*: "Risk categories for HIV transmission in sports").[24]

Policy Regulation Athletes participating in organized sports are subject to procedures and policies

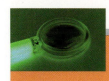

FOCUS 14-3 Focus on Immediate and Emergency Care

Risk categories for HIV transmission in sports

Although the risk of HIV transmission in athletics is minimal, the following classifications of sports indicate risks relative to one another:

- Highest risk: boxing, martial arts, wrestling, rugby
- Moderate risk: basketball, field hockey, football, ice hockey, judo, soccer, team handball
- Lowest risk: archery, badminton, baseball, bowling, canoeing/kayaking, cycling, diving, equestrianism, fencing, figure skating, gymnastics, modern pentathlon, racquetball, rhythmic gymnastics, roller skating, rowing, shooting, softball, speed skating, skiing, swimming, synchronized swimming, table tennis, volleyball, water polo, weight lifting, yachting

about the transmission of bloodborne pathogens.[35] The National Athletic Trainers' Association, U.S. Olympic Committee, National Collegiate Athletic Association, National Federation of State High School Athletic Associations, National Basketball Association, National Hockey League, National Football League, and Major League Baseball all have established policies to help prevent the transmission of bloodborne pathogens.[4,29] These organizations have also initiated programs to help educate athletes under their control. The Centers for Disease Control and Prevention is another useful resource for the athletic trainer seeking information and guidelines for medical assistance on disease control, epidemic prevention, and notification.

All institutions should take responsibility for educating their student-athletes about how bloodborne pathogens are transmitted.[35] In the case of a secondary-school athlete, efforts should also be made to educate the parents.[2,4] Professional, collegiate, and secondary-school athletes should be made aware that the greatest risk of contracting HBV or HIV is through their off-the-field activities, which may include unsafe sexual practices and

14–3 Clinical Application Exercise

A wrestler comes into the athletic training clinic very concerned that his wrestling partner got a bloody nose and that he came in contact with a few drops of that athlete's blood.

? What should the athletic trainer tell the athlete about the transmission of HIV from this type of contact?

sharing of needles, particularly in the use of steroids.[23] Athletes, perhaps more than other individuals in the population, think that they are immune and that infection will always happen to someone else. The athletic trainer should also assume the responsibility of educating and informing athletic training students about exposure control policies.

Each institution should implement policies and procedures concerning bloodborne pathogens.[16] A recent survey of NCAA institutions found that a large number of athletic trainers and other health care providers at many colleges and universities demonstrated significant deficits in following the universal guidelines mandated by OSHA. Universal precautions in a sports medicine or other health care setting protect both the athlete and the health care provider.[33]

Human Immunodeficiency Virus and Athletic Participation There is no definitive answer to whether asymptomatic HIV carriers should participate in sports.[21] Body fluid contact should be avoided, and the participant should avoid engaging in exhaustive exercise that may lead to an increased susceptibility to infection.[21]

The Americans with Disabilities Act of 1991 says that athletes infected with HIV cannot be discriminated against and may be excluded from participation only on a medically sound basis.[21] Exclusion must be based on objective medical evidence and must take into consideration the extent of risk of infection to others, the potential harm to the athlete, and what means can be taken to reduce this risk.[20]

14–4 Clinical Application Exercise

A female patient has had unprotected sex with a male she has dated only once previously. She knows that she should be tested for HIV but is so worried and embarrassed that she has avoided going to a medical facility to have a test. Finally, she goes to the athletic trainer and confides her concerns.

? What should the athletic trainer tell her about being tested for HIV?

Testing for Human Immunodeficiency Virus Testing for HIV should not be used as a screening tool to determine if an athlete can participate in sports.[21] Mandatory testing for HIV may not be allowed because of legal reasons related to the Americans with Disabilities Act and the Health Insurance Portability and Accountability Act (HIPAA).[18] In terms of importance, mandatory testing should be secondary to education to prevent the transmission of HIV.[36] Neither the NCAA nor the Centers for Disease Control and Prevention recommends mandatory HIV testing for athletes.[8,18]

Individuals who engage in high-risk activities should be encouraged to seek voluntary anonymous testing for HIV.[31] A blood test analyzes serum using an enzyme-linked immunosorbent assay (ELISA) or an enzyme immunoassay (EIA). These tests detect antibodies to HIV proteins. Positive EIA or ELISA tests should be repeated to rule out false-positive results. A second positive test requires the Western blot examination, which is a more sensitive test.[6] Detectable antibodies may appear from 3 months to 1 year after exposure. Testing, therefore, should occur at 6 weeks, 3 months, and 1 year.[6]

Home testing kits are also available in which an individual can collect a sample for testing in the privacy of his or her home and then send it to a laboratory for analysis. There are more than a dozen different HIV home test kits being advertised on the market today. Only the Home Access test system is FDA approved and legally marketed in the United States. This approved system uses a simple finger prick process for home blood collection, which results in dried blood spots on special paper. The dried blood spots are mailed to a laboratory with a confidential and anonymous personal identification number (PIN). The sample is then analyzed by trained clinicians in a certified medical laboratory using the same procedures that are used for samples taken in a doctor's office. The purchaser obtains results by calling a toll-free telephone number and using the PIN; posttest counseling is provided by telephone when results are obtained.[18]

> For additional information on HIV and AIDS care, contact the CDC National AIDS Hotline: 1 (800) 342-2437.

Many states have enacted laws that protect the confidentiality of the HIV-infected person. The athletic trainer should be familiar with state law and make every effort to guard the confidentiality and anonymity of HIV testing for athletes.

UNIVERSAL PRECAUTIONS IN AN ATHLETIC ENVIRONMENT

In 1991, the Occupational Safety and Health Administration **(OSHA)** established standards for an employer to follow that govern occupational exposure to bloodborne pathogens.[33]

> **OSHA** Occupational Safety and Health Administration.

The guidelines instituted by OSHA were developed to protect the health care provider and the patient against bloodborne pathogens.[30] OSHA has mandated that training programs for dealing with bloodborne pathogens be repeated each year to provide the most current information. It is essential that every program develop and carry out a bloodborne pathogen exposure control plan.[33] NATA has established specific guidelines for athletic trainers.[29] This plan should include counseling, education, volunteer testing, and the management of body fluids.[29]

> Throughout the remainder of this text, whenever there is a discussion of an injury or a technique of care that requires universal precautions, the biohazard icon will appear in the margin.

Universal precautions should be practiced by anyone coming into contact with blood or other body fluids (see Table 14–3).[3,30,38] Following are considerations specifically in the sports arena.

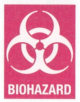

Preparing the Athlete

Before an athlete participates in practice or competition, all open skin wounds and lesions must be covered with a dressing that is fixed in place and does not allow for transmission to or from another athlete.[40] An occlusive dressing lessens the chances of cross-contamination. One example is the hydrocolloid dressing, which is considered a superior barrier. This type of dressing also reduces the chances that the wound will reopen because it keeps the wound moist and pliable.[24]

When Bleeding Occurs

As mandated by the NCAA and the USOC, open wounds and other skin lesions considered a risk for disease transmission should be given aggressive treatment. Athletes with active bleeding must be removed from participation as soon as possible and can return only when it is deemed safe by the medical staff.[18] Uniforms containing blood must be evaluated for infectivity. A uniform that is saturated with blood must be removed and changed before the athlete can return to competition. All personnel managing potential infective wound exposure must follow universal precautions.[18,36]

> A hospital-based sports medicine program must initiate and carry out a bloodborne pathogen exposure control plan.
>
> **?** What are the universal precautions, as proposed by OSHA, that must be followed?
>
> 14–5 Clinical Application Exercise

Personal Precautions

The health care personnel working directly with body fluids on the field or in the athletic training clinic must make use of the appropriate protective equipment in all situations in which there is

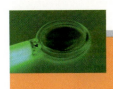

FOCUS 14-4 Focus on Immediate and Emergency Care

Glove use and removal

1. Avoid touching personal items when wearing contaminated gloves.
2. Remove the first glove and turn it inside out.
3. Place the first glove in the second gloved hand and then turn the second glove inside out so as to contain the first glove.
4. Remove the second glove, making sure not to touch soiled surfaces with the ungloved hand.
5. Discard gloves that have been used, discolored, torn, or punctured.
6. Wash hands immediately after glove removal.

potential contact with bloodborne pathogens. Protective equipment includes disposable nonlatex gloves, nonabsorbent gowns or aprons, masks and shields, eye protection, and disposable mouthpieces for resuscitation devices.[3] Equipment for dealing with bloodborne pathogens should be included in sideline emergency kits.[26] Disposable nonlatex gloves must be used when handling any potentially infectious material. Double gloving is suggested when there is heavy bleeding or sharp instruments are used. Gloves should always be removed carefully after use.

> **Nonlatex gloves should be worn whenever the athletic trainer handles blood or body fluids.**

In cases of emergency, heavy toweling may be used until gloves can be obtained[2] (see *Focus Box 14–4*: "Glove use and removal") (Figure 14–4).

Hand Washing Hands and all skin surfaces that come in contact with blood or other body fluids should be washed immediately with soap and water or other antigermicidal agents. Hands should also be washed between each patient treatment. If there is a possibility of body fluids becoming splashed, spurted, or sprayed, the mouth, nose, and eyes should be protected. Aprons or nonabsorbent gowns should be worn to avoid clothing contamination.

> **Hands should be washed frequently to minimize the spread of diseases.**

First-aid kits must contain protection for hands, face, eyes, and resuscitation mouthpieces. Kits should also contain towelettes for cleaning skin surfaces.[3]

Latex Sensitivity and Using Nonlatex Gloves It is recommended that athletic trainers use nonlatex, vinyl, or nitrile rubber gloves.[7] A number of manufacturers produce nonlatex gloves. Latex, a sap from the rubber tree, is composed of compounds that may cause an allergic reaction that can range from contact dermatitis to a systemic reaction. Recognizing the signs and symptoms of these reactions may help prevent a more severe reaction from occurring. Some individuals are more at risk of latex allergies due to repetitive exposure to latex through their career paths, multiple surgeries, other allergies, or respiratory conditions. Management of an acute reaction involves removing the irritant, cleansing the affected area, monitoring vital signs for changes, and seeking additional medical assistance as warranted.[7]

> **14–6 Clinical Application Exercise**
>
> During a basketball game, one of the players sustains a nosebleed. Blood is visible on the court and on the player's jersey and skin.
>
> **?** What actions need to take place before the game can resume?

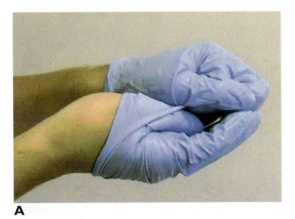
A

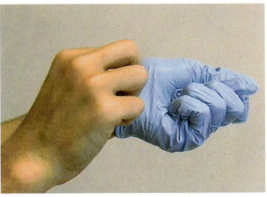
B

FIGURE 14–4 Technique for removing nonlatex gloves. **(A)** Grasp one gloved hand with the opposite hand and peel that glove off. **(B)** Ball up the removed glove and hold it in the opposite gloved hand then peel of the second glove trapping the first glove inside.

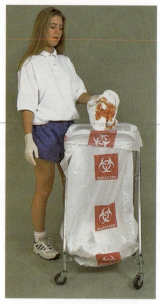

FIGURE 14–5   Soiled linens should be placed in a leakproof bag marked as a biohazard.

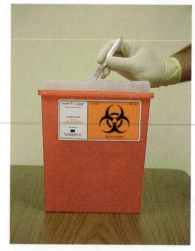

FIGURE 14–6   Sharps should be disposed of in a red or orange puncture-resistant plastic container marked as a biohazard.

Availability of Supplies and Equipment

In keeping with universal precautions, the sports program must have available chlorine bleach, antiseptics, proper receptacles for soiled equipment and uniforms, wound care bandages, and a designated container for disposal of sharp objects, such as needles, syringes, and scalpels.[18]

> Universal precautions minimize the risk of exposure and transmission.

Biohazard warning labels should be affixed to containers for regulated wastes, refrigerators containing blood, and other containers used to store or ship potentially infectious materials (Figure 14–5). The labels are fluorescent orange or red. Red bags or containers should be used for the disposal of potentially infected materials. If you're not sure whether a substance qualifies as biohazardous waste, the best practice is to use a biohazard bag to dispose of it.

Disinfectants   All contaminated surfaces, such as treatment tables, taping tables, work areas, and

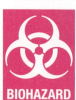

floors, should be cleaned immediately with a solution consisting of 1 part bleach to 10 parts water (1:10) or with a disinfectant approved by the Environmental Protection Agency.[36] Disinfectants should inactivate the HIV virus.

Contaminated Laundry   Towels and other linens that have been contaminated should be bagged and separated from other laundry. Soiled linen should be transported in red or orange containers or bags that prevent soaking or leaking and are labeled with biohazard warning labels (see Figure 14–4). Contaminated laundry should be washed in hot water (71°C/159.8°F for 25 minutes) using a detergent that deactivates the virus.[36] Laundry done outside the institution should be sent to a facility that follows OSHA standards. Gloves must be worn during bagging and cleaning of contaminated laundry.

Sharps   *Sharps* refers to sharp objects used in athletic training, such as needles, razor blades, and scalpels. Extreme care should be taken when handling and disposing of sharps to minimize the risk of puncturing or cutting the skin. Athletic trainers rarely use needles, but it is not unusual for them to use scalpels or razor

> **Sharps:**
> • Scalpels
> • Razor blades
> • Needles

blades. Whenever needles are used, they should not be recapped, bent, or removed from a syringe. Sharps should be disposed of in a leakproof and puncture-resistant container.[36] The container should be red or orange and should be labeled as a biohazard (Figure 14–6). Scissors and tweezers are not as likely to cause injury as sharps are, but they should be sterilized with a disinfecting agent and stored in a clean place after use.

Protecting the Athletic Trainer

OSHA guidelines for bloodborne pathogens are intended to protect the coach, athletic trainer, and other employees.[33] Coaches do not usually come in contact with blood or other body fluids from an injured athlete, so their risk is considerably reduced. It is the responsibility of the secondary school, college, professional team, or clinic to ensure the safety of the athletic trainer as a health care provider by instituting and annually updating policies for education on the prevention of transmitting bloodborne pathogens through contact with athletes. The institution must provide the necessary supplies and equipment to carry out these recommendations.

The athletic trainer has the personal responsibility of adhering to these policies and guidelines and enforcing them in the athletic training clinic. Athletic trainers may further minimize the risk of exposure in the athletic training setting by not eating, drinking, applying cosmetics or lip balm, handling contact lenses, or touching the face before washing hands. Food products should never be placed in a refrigerator containing contaminated blood.[33]

Protecting the Athlete from Exposure

Several additional recommendations may further help protect the athlete. The USOC supports the required use of mouthpieces in high-risk sports. It is also recommended that all athletes shower immediately after practice or competition. Athletes who may be exposed to HIV, HBV, or HCV should also be evaluated for immunization against HBV.

Postexposure Procedures

After a report of an exposure incident, the athletic trainer should have a confidential medical evaluation that includes documentation of the exposure route, identification of the source individual, a blood test, counseling, and an evaluation of reported illness. Again, the laws that pertain to the reporting and confidentiality of test results notification vary from state to state.[33]

SUMMARY

- Bloodborne pathogens are microorganisms that can cause disease and are present in human blood and other body fluids, including semen, vaginal secretions, cerebrospinal fluid, synovial fluid, and any other fluid contaminated with blood. Hepatitis B virus, hepatitis C virus, and HIV are bloodborne pathogens.
- A virus is a submicroscopic parasitic organism that contains either DNA or RNA, but not both. It is dependent on the host cell to function and reproduce.
- A vaccine is available to prevent HBV. Currently, no effective vaccine exists for HCV or HIV.
- An individual infected with HIV may develop AIDS, which is fatal.
- The risks of contracting HBV, HCV, or HIV may be minimized by avoiding exposure to blood and other body fluids and by practicing safe sex.

- The risk of an athlete being exposed to bloodborne pathogens on the field is minimal. Off-the-field activities involving risky sexual behaviors pose the greatest threat for transmission.
- Various national medical and sports organizations have established policies and procedures for dealing with bloodborne pathogens in the athletic population.
- The Occupational Safety and Health Administration has established rules and regulations that protect the health care employee.
- Universal precautions must be taken to avoid bloodborne pathogen exposure. All sports programs must carry out a plan for counseling, education, volunteer testing, and the management of exposure.

WEB SITES

Centers for Disease Control and Prevention:
   www.cdc.gov
Department of Health and Human Services:
   http://www.hhs.gov/
HIV/AIDS Prevention: cdc.gov/hiv

Occupational Safety and Health Administration
   (OSHA): www.osha.gov
National Institutes of Health: www.nih.gov

SOLUTIONS TO CLINICAL APPLICATION EXERCISES

14–1 During competition or practice, the athlete should be most concerned about coming in contact with blood from another athlete. There should be little or no concern about exposure to sweat or saliva. The chances of contracting HIV during athletic participation are minimal. Certainly, the athlete is most likely to be exposed to HIV during unprotected intimate sexual contact.

14–2 The participant complained of flulike symptoms, such as headache, fever, fatigue, weakness, nausea, and some abdominal pain. A blood test revealed the presence of the HBV antigen.

14–3 The greatest risk of contracting HIV is through intimate sexual contact with an infected partner. The athletic trainer should explain to the athlete that there is little chance of HIV transmission among athletes. There is a theoretical potential risk of transmission among athletes in close contact who pass blood from one to the other.

14–4 The athletic trainer should inform her that it is best if she waits for 6 weeks before being tested. The athletic trainer should strongly encourage her to seek testing and should explain to her that if she is uncomfortable with being tested

in a medical care facility, there is a home test available that has been approved by the FDA and provides confidentiality. The athletic trainer should add that if the athlete were to test positive on the home test, it would become imperative that she seek additional testing at a medical care facility.

14–5 Universal precautions should be practiced by anyone coming in contact with blood or other body fluids. This plan must include counseling, education, volunteer testing, and management of body fluids.

14–6 To prevent possible transmission of bloodborne pathogens, several precautions need to be followed. The athlete must be removed from the game until active bleeding has ceased and he or she has been cleared by the medical staff. The jersey must be removed and changed if the uniform is saturated with blood. Any blood on the skin must be cleaned off before the athlete can return to play. In addition, the basketball court needs to be properly cleaned and disinfected. The solution used to clean the court should be 1 part bleach to 10 parts water or a solution approved by the Environmental Protection Agency. All contaminated products need to be properly disposed of according to OSHA standards.

REVIEW QUESTIONS AND CLASS ACTIVITIES

1. What can the athletic trainer do to prevent the spread of infectious disease?
2. How are infectious diseases transmitted from person to person?
3. How does the immune system respond to an infectious antigen?
4. Define and identify the bloodborne pathogens.
5. Describe HBV and HCV transmission, symptoms, signs, prevention, and treatment.
6. Explain the pros and cons of allowing an athlete who is an HBV carrier to participate.
7. Describe HIV transmission, symptoms, signs, prevention, and treatment.
8. How is HIV transmitted, and why is it eventually fatal at this time?
9. Should an athlete who tests positive for HBV or HIV be allowed to participate in sports? Why or why not?
10. How can an athlete reduce the risk of HIV infection?
11. Define OSHA universal precautions for preventing bloodborne pathogen exposure.
12. What precautions would you, as an athletic trainer, take when caring for a bleeding wound on the field?

REFERENCES

1. American Academy of Orthopedic Surgeons: *Bloodborne pathogens*, 2011, Jones and Bartlett.
2. American Academy of Pediatrics: Human immunodeficiency virus and other bloodborne viral pathogens in the athletic setting, *Pediatrics*, 104(6):1400–03, 2009.
3. American Red Cross: *First aid: Responding to emergency*, San Bruno, CA, 2007, Staywell.
4. Arnold BL: A review of selected bloodborne pathogen position statements and federal regulations, *J Athl Train* 30(2):171, 1995.
5. Barreto M: Infectious diseases epidemiology, *Journal of Epidemiology and Community Health* 60(3):192, 2006.
6. Beers M, Porter R, Jones T: *The Merck manual of diagnosis and therapy*, ed 19, Whitehouse Station, NJ 2011, Merck.
7. Binkley H, Schroyer T, Catalfano J: Latex allergies: A review of recognition, evaluation, management, prevention, education, and alternative product use, *J Athl Train* 38(2):133, 2003.
8. Centers for Disease Control: HIV in the United States, http://www.cdc.gov/hiv/resources/factsheets/PDF/us.pdf, 2011.
9. Deere R, Stopka C, Curran K, Bolger C: Universal precautions for bloodborne pathogens: A checklist for your program, *Strategies* 14(6):18, 2001.
10. Dolan M: *The hepatitis C handbook*, Berkeley, CA, 1999, North Atlantic Books.
11. Gleeson M, Nieman D, Pedersen B: Exercise, nutrition and immune function, *Journal of Sports Sciences* 22(1):115, 2004.
12. Gutierrez R: Bloodborne infections and the athlete, *Dis Mon* 56(7):436–42, 2010.
13. Hamann B: *Disease: Identification, prevention, and control*, New York, 2006, McGraw-Hill.
14. Harrington, D: Viral hepatitis and exercise, *Medicine & Science in Sports and Exercise*, 32(7):422–30, 2000.
15. Harris, M: Infectious disease in athletes, *Current Sports Medicine Reports*, 10(2):84–89, 2011.
16. Hosey, R: Training room management of medical conditions: Infectious diseases, *Clinics in Sports Medicine*, 24(3):477–506, 2005.
17. Jaworski C: Infectious disease, *Clinics in Sports Medicine*, 30(3):575–90, 2011.
18. Klossner D: *National Collegiate Athletic Association 2011–2012 NCAA sports medicine handbook*, Indianapolis, 2012, National Collegiate Athletic Association.
19. Kordi R: Risk of hepatitis B and C infections in Tehranian wrestlers, *J Athl Train*, 46(4):445–50, 2011.
20. Kordi R: Blood borne infections in sport: Risks of transmission, methods of prevention, and recommendations for hepatitis B vaccination, *Br J Sports Med* 38:678–84, 2004.
21. Kukka C: Bloodborne Infections: Should they be disclosed? Is differential treatment necessary? *The Journal of School Nursing* 20(6): 324–30, 2004.
22. Landry G, Bernhardt D: Common infectious diseases. In Landry G: *Essentials of primary care sports medicine*, Champaign, IL, 2003, Human Kinetics.
23. Landry G, Bernhardt D: Sexually transmitted diseases and blood-borne infections. In Landry G: *Essentials of primary care sports medicine*, Champaign, IL, 2003, Human Kinetics.
24. Luke A: Prevention of infectious disease in athletes, *Clinics in Sports Medicine* 26(3):321–44, 2007.
25. LaPeniere A, Kiimas N, Major P: Acquired immune deficiency syndrome. In American College of Sports Medicine: *ACSM's exercise management for persons with chronic disease and disabilities*, Champaign, Ill. 2002, Human Kinetics.
26. Maloney G: Infectious disease update 2006: How to protect yourself and your patients. *Journal of Emergency Medical Services* 31(5):120, 2006.
27. Minoee A: Sports: The infectious hazards. In Schlossberg D: *Infections of leisure*, Philadelphia, 2009, ASM Press.
28. Midgley, A: Infection and the elite athlete: A review, *Research in Sports Medicine: An International Journal* 11(4):235–60, 2003.

29. National Athletic Trainers' Association: Blood-borne pathogens guidelines for athletic trainers. *J Athl Train* 30(3):203, 1995.

30. National Safety Council: *Bloodborne airborne pathogens*, New York, 2008, McGraw-Hill.

31. Payne W, Hahn D: *Understanding your health*, San Francisco, 2010, McGraw-Hill.

32. Pirozzolo J: Blood-borne infections, *Clinics in Sports Medicine* 26(3):425–31, 2007.

33. Ross C: Understanding the OSHA bloodborne pathogens standard and its impact upon recreational sports, *NIRSA* 19(2):12, 1999.

34. Sankaran G: HIV infection: Risk, right to know, and requirement to divulge, *Athletic Therapy Today*, 1(3):49, 1996.

35. Sankaran G, editor: *HIV/AIDS in sport: Impact, issues and challenges*, Champaign, IL, 1999, Human Kinetics.

36. Schultz SJ: Preventing transmission of bloodborne pathogens. In Schultz SJ, editor: *Sports medicine handbook*, Indianapolis, Ind., 2005, National Federation of State High School Associations.

37. Strikas RA: Immunizations: Recommendations and resources for active patients, *Physician Sportsmed* 29(10):33, 2001.

38. Thygerson A: *First aid. CPR, and AED Advanced*, Boston, 2011, Jones and Bartlett.

39. Tuberville S: Infectious disease outbreaks in competitive sports: A review of the literature, *Am J Sports Med* 34(11):1860, 2006.

40. Walsh K, Raedeke S: Infection and disease transmission in the athletic training setting, *Athletic Therapy Today* 9(3):11, 2004.

41. World Health Organization: Progress report 2011: Global HIV/Aids response http://www.who.int/hiv/pub/progress_report2011/summary_en.pdf.

42. Zinder S: National Athletic Trainers' Association position statement: Skin diseases, *J Athl Train*, 45(4): 411–28, 2010.

ANNOTATED BIBLIOGRAPHY

Beers M, Porter R, Jones T: *The Merck manual of diagnosis and therapy*, ed 19, Whitehouse Station, NJ, 2011, John Wiley and Sons.

This excellent guide discusses diagnosis, symptoms, signs, and treatment of bloodborne pathogens.

Dolan M: *The hepatitis C handbook*, Berkeley, Calif, 1999. North Atlantic Books.

This definitive guide outlines the course of the disease and associated symptoms. It discusses available treatment and lifestyle changes and contains an extensive section on herbs, vitamins, and nutritional supplements.

Hamann B: Disease: *Identification, prevention, and control*, St. Louis, 2006, McGraw-Hill.

This text is designed for health educators and covers in detail both AIDS and hepatitis.

Klossner D editor: *National Collegiate Athletic Association 2011–2012 sports medicine handbook*, Indianapolis, Ind., 2011, National Collegiate Athletic Association.

This text offers a complete discussion of bloodborne pathogens and intercollegiate athletic policies and administration.

National Safety Council: *Bloodborne pathogens*, Boston, 2011, Jones and Bartlett.

This manual is dedicated to presenting OSHA regulations specific to bloodborne pathogens.

Neilson RP: *OSHA regulations and guidelines: A guide to health care providers*, Clifton Park, NY, 2000, Delmar Learning.

Presents OSHA standards, with special emphasis on bloodborne pathogens and incident and injury reporting.

Zeigler T: *Management of bloodborne infections in sport*, Champaign, Ill., 1997, Human Kinetics.

Perhaps the most comprehensive single text available on dealing with bloodborne pathogens in an athletic population, this text contains procedure and policy statements from several different sport and health organizations on managing bloodborne pathogens in the athletic environment.

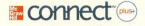

15

Using Therapeutic Modalities

■ Objectives

When you finish this chapter you should be able to

- Recognize the legal ramifications of treating a patient with therapeutic modalities.
- Explain how therapeutic modalities are classified according to the type of energy they produce.
- Describe the theoretical uses of the various types of modalities.
- Correctly demonstrate a variety of thermotherapy and cryotherapy techniques.

- Discuss the physiological basis and therapeutic uses of electrical stimulating currents.
- Examine the use of ultrasound in an athletic training setting.
- Describe how massage, traction, and intermittent compression can be used as therapeutic agents.

■ Outline

■ Key Terms

ischemia
conduction
convection
radiation
conversion

hunting response
cryokinetics
amperes
ohms
voltage

watts
frequency
tetany
attenuation
piezoelectric effect

effective radiating area
beam nonuniformity ratio (BNR)
coupling medium

effleurage
petrissage
friction
tapotement
vibration

■ Connect Highlights McGraw Hill connect™ plus+

Visit connect.mcgraw-hill.com for further exercises to apply your knowledge:

- Clinical application scenarios covering application of thermotherapy and cryotherapy techniques, use of ultrasound, use of electrical stimulating currents, and the use of massage, traction, and intermittent compression
- Click-and-drag questions covering thermotherapy and cryotherapy techniques, therapeutic modality nomenclature, and electrical stimulating currents
- Multiple-choice questions covering legal ramifications of the use of therapeutic modalities, theoretical use of modalities, and physiological uses of therapeutic modalities
- Picture identification of therapeutic modalities

Most athletic trainers routinely incorporate the use of therapeutic modalities into their rehabilitation programs.[9] When used appropriately, therapeutic modalities can be an effective adjunct to various techniques of therapeutic exercise. Rehabilitation protocols and progressions must be based primarily on the physiological responses of the tissues to injury and on an understanding of how various tissues heal. The decisions the athletic trainer makes on how and when therapeutic modalities may best be used should be based on his or her recognition of signs and symptoms as well as some awareness of the time frames associated with the various phases of the healing process. This chapter is an introduction to the therapeutic modalities that an athletic trainer may use: thermotherapy, cryotherapy, electrical stimulating currents, shortwave diathermy, low-level laser therapy, ultrasound, phonophoresis, traction, intermittent compression and massage.

LEGAL CONCERNS

Therapeutic modalities must be used with the greatest care possible; they should not be used indiscriminately. Specific laws governing the use of therapeutic modalities vary considerably from state to state. The athletic trainer must follow laws that specifically dictate how athletic trainers can use certain therapeutic modalities. An athletic trainer who uses any type of therapeutic modality must have a thorough understanding of the functions and the indications or contraindications for its use.[45]

> **The athletic trainer must carefully follow laws that prohibit him or her from the use of certain therapeutic modalities.**

The athletic trainer should avoid using a shotgun approach when deciding to incorporate therapeutic modalities into a treatment program. Selection of the appropriate modality should be based on an accurate clinical diagnosis of the injury and a decision about which modality can most effectively reach the desired target tissue to achieve specific results. The manufacturers of therapeutic modality equipment often provide recommended protocols for using their equipment in treating specific problems. The athletic trainer should certainly be familiar with these recommended treatment protocols. However, the athletic trainer does not necessarily have to follow the manufacturers' treatment protocols precisely. These are only recommendations. Decisions to alter recommended treatment protocols should be based on sound theory and previous experience. If used appropriately, modalities can be an integral part of a treatment and rehabilitation program.[45]

CLASSIFICATION OF THERAPEUTIC MODALITIES

There is considerable confusion among even the most experienced clinicians regarding the different forms of energy involved with the various therapeutic modalities. The forms of energy that are relevant to the use of therapeutic modalities are thermal conductive energy, electrical energy, electromagnetic energy, sound energy, and mechanical energy.[44]

Thermotherapy and cryotherapy techniques transfer thermal energy. The electrical stimulating currents and iontophoresis use electrical energy. Shortwave and microwave diathermy, infrared lamps, ultraviolet light therapy, and low-power lasers use electromagnetic energy. Ultrasound and extracorporal shockwave therapy use sound energy. Intermittent compression, traction, and massage use mechanical energy.

> **Classifications of modalities:**
> - Thermal conductive energy
> - Electrical energy
> - Electromagnetic energy
> - Sound energy
> - Mechanical Energy

When these different forms of energy come in contact with human biological tissue, they can be reflected, refracted, absorbed, or transmitted. In human tissue, the energy must be absorbed before any physiological effects can take place.[44]

Each of these therapeutic agents transfers energy in one form or another into or out of biologic tissues. Different forms of energy can produce similar effects in biologic tissues. For example, tissue heating is a common effect of several treatments that use different types of energy. Electrical currents that pass through tissues will generate heat as a result of the resistance of the tissue to the passage of electricity. Electromagnetic energy such as light waves will heat any tissues that absorb it. Ultrasound treatments will also warm tissues through which the sound waves travel. Although the electrical, electromagnetic, and sound energy treatments all heat tissues, the physical mechanism of action for each is different.[44]

The mechanism of action of each therapeutic modality depends on which form of energy is used during its application.

THERMAL CONDUCTIVE ENERGY MODALITIES

Thermotherapy

The application of heat to treat disease and injuries has been used for centuries. Athletic trainers working in all settings use thermotherapy.

Physiological Effects of Heat The body's response to heat depends on the type of heat energy applied, the intensity of the heat energy, the duration of application, and the unique tissue response to heat. For a physiological response to occur, heat must be absorbed into the tissue and spread to adjacent tissue. To effect a therapeutic change that results in normal function of the absorbing tissue, the correct amount of heat must be applied. With too little, no change occurs; with too much, the tissue may be damaged.

The desirable therapeutic effects of heat include increasing the extensibility of collagen tissues; decreasing joint stiffness; reducing pain; relieving muscle spasm; reducing inflammation, edema, and exudates in the postacute phase of healing; and increasing blood flow.[46]

Heat increases the extensibility of collagen tissue, thus permitting an increase in extensibility through stretching. Muscle fibrosis, the joint capsule, contractures and scar tissue can

> Heat has the capacity to increase the extensibility of collagen tissue.

all be effectively stretched after heating.[46] An increase in extensibility does not occur unless heat treatment is associated with stretching exercises.

Both heat and cold relieve pain via the gate control theory of pain modulation (see Chapter 10).[18] Muscle spasm caused by **ischemia** can be relieved by heat, which increases blood flow to the area of injury. Heat is also be-

ischemia Lack of blood supply to a body part.

lieved to assist the healing process by a number of mechanisms, such as raising temperature, increasing metabolism, reducing oxygen tension, lowering the pH level, increasing capillary permeability, and releasing histamine and bradykinin, which cause vasodilation. Histamine and bradykinin are released during acute and chronic inflammation.

Thermal energy is transmitted through conduction, convection, radiation, and conversion. **Conduction** occurs when heat is transferred from

conduction Heating through direct contact with a hot medium.

a warmer object to a cooler one. The ratio of this heat exchange depends on the temperature and the exposure time. Skin temperatures are influenced by the type of heat or cold medium, the conductivity of the tissue, the quantity of blood flow in the area, and the speed at which heat is being dissipated.[39] To avoid tissue damage, the temperature should never exceed 116.6°F (47°C). An exposure that includes close contact with a hot medium that has a temperature of 113°F (45°C) should not exceed 30 minutes. Examples of conductive therapeutic modalities are hydrocollator packs, paraffin baths, electric heating pads, ice packs, and cold packs.

Convection refers to the transference of heat through the movement of fluids or gases. Factors that influence convection heating are temperature, speed of movement, and the conductivity of the part.[46] The best example of modalities that use convection is hot and cold whirlpools. **Radiation** is the process whereby heat energy is transferred from one object through space to another object. Shortwave diathermy relies on the process of radiation for energy transfer. **Conversion** refers to the generation of heat from another energy form, such as sound, electricity, and chemical agents. The mechanical energy produced by high-frequency ultrasound sound waves changes to heat energy at tissue interfaces (ultrasound therapy).[46] The deep heat of shortwave diathermy can be produced by applying electrical currents of specific wavelengths to the skin. Chemical agents, such as liniments and balms, create a heating sensation through counterirritation of sensory nerve endings.[46]

convection Heating indirectly through medium, such as air or liquid.

radiation Transfer of heat through space from one object to another.

conversion Heating through other forms of energy.

Heat applied superficially to the skin directly increases the subcutaneous temperature and indirectly spreads to the deeper tissues. Muscle temperature increases through a reflexive effect on circulation and through conduction.[46] Comparatively, when heat is applied at the same temperature, moist heat causes a greater indirect increase in the deep-tissue temperature than does dry. Dry heat, in contrast to moist heat, can be tolerated at higher temperatures.

For the most part, moist heat aids the healing process in some local conditions by causing higher superficial tissue temperatures; however, joint and muscle circulation increase little in temperature. Superficial tissue is a poor thermal conductor, and temperature rises quickly on the skin surface as compared with the underlying tissues. The physiological responses to tissue heating are summarized in Table 15–1.

Hydrocollator Packs
Equipment Hydrocollator packs contain silicate gel in a cotton pad, which is

A construction worker has an elbow sprain that occurred 5 days ago. To this point he has been using cryotherapy treatment exclusively. His elbow is still tender with some minimal swelling. He says that he really hates the ice and wants to know if he can switch over to some form of heat, which he feels will be more comfortable.

? In the course of an injury rehabilitation program, when should the athletic trainer change from using cold to using heat?

TABLE 15–1	Physiological Responses to Thermotherapy
Variable	**Response to Therapy**
Muscle spasm	Decreases
Pain perception	Decreases
Blood flow	Increases
Metabolic rate	Increases
Collagen elasticity	Increases
Joint stiffness	Decreases
Capillary permeability	Increases
Edema	Increases

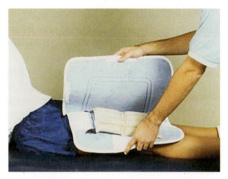

FIGURE 15–1 Protective layers of toweling or a commercially produced hydrocollator pack cover should be applied between the skin and a moist heat pack.

immersed in thermostatically controlled hot water at a temperature of 160°F (71.1°C) to 170°F (76.7°C). Each pad retains water and a constant heat level for 20 to 30 minutes. Multiple layers of toweling or a commercially produced hydrocollator pack cover should be used between the packs and the skin (Figure 15–1).

Indications The major value of the hydrocollator pack is that its use results in general relaxation and reduction of the pain-spasm-ischemia-hypoxia-pain cycle. There are limitations of the hydrocollator pack in that the deeper tissues, including the musculature, are usually not significantly heated because the heat transfer from the skin surface into deeper tissues is inhibited by the subcutaneous fat, which acts as a thermal insulator, and by the increased blood flow to the skin, which cools and carries away the heat externally applied.[40]

Application Remove the pack from water and allow it to drain for a few seconds. Cover the pack with six layers of dry toweling or commercial cover. Treat the area for 15 to 20 minutes. As the pack cools, remove layers of toweling to continue the heating.

Special Considerations The patient should not be lying on packs. Be sure the patient is comfortable at all times.

Whirlpool Baths

Equipment Whirlpool therapy is a combination of massage and water immersion. There are generally three types of whirlpools: the *extremity tank*, which is used for treating legs and arms; the *lowboy tank*, used for full-body immersion; and the *highboy tank*, which is designed for the hip or the leg.[6]

> The whirlpool bath combines heated water and massaging action.

The whirlpool is essentially a tank and a turbine motor, which regulates the movement of water and air. The amount of movement (agitation) is controlled by the amount of air that is emitted. The more air there is, the more water movement. The turbine motor can be moved up and down on a tubular column. It can also be rotated on the column and locked in place at a specific angle.

Indications The whirlpool provides both conduction and convection. Conduction is achieved by the skin's contact with the higher water temperature. As the water swirls around the skin surface, convection occurs (Figure 15–2).

This medium assists the body part by reducing swelling, muscle spasm, and pain. Because of the buoyancy of the water, active movement of the part is also assisted.

Application The water temperature should be set according to Table 15–2. As the volume of the body part submerged increases, the recommended water temperature should be decreased. A temperature that exceeds 104°F (40°C) should not be used for full body immersion. Some athletic trainers prefer to perform only cold-water treatments, whereas others

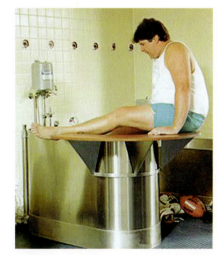

FIGURE 15–2 A whirlpool bath provides therapy through heat conduction and convection.

TABLE 15–2	Whirlpool Temperatures for Treatment of the Extremities
Descriptive Terms	**Temperature**
Very cold	>55°F (12.8°C)
Cold	55°F–65°F (12.8°C–18.3°C)
Cool	66°F–79°F (19°C–26°C)
Tepid	80°F–90°F (27°C–33.5°C)
Neutral	92°F–96°F (33.5°C–35.5°C)
Warm	96°F–98°F (35.5°C–36.5°C)
Hot	98°F–104°F (36.5°C–40°C)
Very hot	104°F–110°F (40°C–43°C)*

*Do not use water above 110°F.

prefer to increase the temperature according to the healing phase of an injury. Whirlpool use is contraindicated in acute injury because of the potential to increase swelling due to dependent positioning.[56] Chronic conditions normally require a higher water temperature.

Once the tank has been filled with water at the desired temperature, the patient is comfortably positioned so that the body part to be treated can be easily reached by the agitated water. In many cases, the water jet should not be placed directly on the body part but to the side of the tank. This placement is particularly relevant in the early stages of the acute injury.[56] In cases in which the stream is concentrated directly toward the injury site, the site should be at least 8 to 10 inches (20 to 25 cm) from the jet.

The duration of treatment is a major concern for the athletic trainer. The maximum length of treatment time for acute injuries should not exceed 20 minutes.

Special Considerations Caution should be taken anytime a patient is fully immersed in a whirlpool because of the possibility that the patient will experience lightheadedness.[40] Proper whirlpool maintenance is absolutely necessary to avoid infection—in particular, to prevent the spread of methicillin-resistant staphylococcus aureus (MRSA) (see Chapter 29). The whirlpool should be emptied and thoroughly disinfected after every patient. Both the inside and the outside of the tank as well as the turbine should be disinfected and dried.

Safety is of major importance in the use of the whirlpool. All electrical outlets should have a ground fault circuit interrupter. At no time should the patient turn the motor on or off. Ideally, the on/off switch should be a considerable distance from the machine.[40]

Paraffin Bath
Equipment Paraffin is a popular method for applying heat to the distal extremities. The commercial paraffin bath is a thermostatically controlled unit that maintains a temperature of 126°F to 130°F (52°C to 54°C). The paraffin mixture consists of a ratio of 25 kilograms of paraffin wax to 1 liter of mineral oil. Slats at the bottom of the container protect the patient from burns and collect the settling dirt. Also required for treatment are plastic bags, paper towels, and towels.

Indications The mineral oil acts to lower the melting point of the paraffin and thus the specific heat. Consequently, the ability to tolerate the heat from the paraffin is greater than it would be from water at the same temperature.

This therapy is especially effective in treating chronic injuries occurring to the more angular areas of the body, such as the hands, wrists, elbows, ankles, and feet.

> Paraffin bath therapy is particularly effective for injuries to the more angular body areas.

Application Therapy by means of the paraffin bath can be delivered in several ways. The body part can be dipped and wrapped in a plastic bag, or it can be dipped and reimmersed to form eight to ten layers. The paraffin can be painted on in several layers, or the body part can be soaked in the paraffin.

Before therapy, the body part to be treated is thoroughly cleaned and dried. Then the patient dips the affected part into the paraffin bath and quickly pulls it out, allowing the accumulated wax to dry and form a solid covering. The process of dipping and withdrawing is repeated 6 to 12 times until the wax coating is ¼ to ½ inch (0.6 to 1.25 cm) thick.

If the dip and wrap technique is used, the accumulated wax is allowed to solidify on the last withdrawal; then the wax is completely wrapped in a plastic material, which in turn is wrapped with a towel. The packed body part is placed in a position of rest for approximately 30 minutes or until heat is no longer generated. The covering is then removed and the paraffin is scraped back into the container.

If the soak technique is selected, the patient is instructed to soak the wax-coated part in the hot wax container for 20 to 30 minutes without moving it, after which the part is removed from the container and the paraffin on it is allowed to solidify. The part can be packed in towels following the soak, or the paraffin coating can be scraped back into the container immediately after it hardens. Once the paraffin has been removed from the part, an oily residue remains that provides an excellent surface for massage (Figure 15–3).

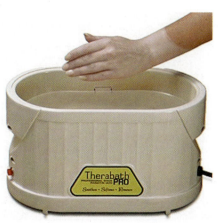

FIGURE 15–3   A paraffin bath is an excellent form of therapeutic heat for the distal extremities. After paraffin coating has been accomplished, the part is covered by a plastic material. When heat is no longer generated, the paraffin is scraped back into the container.

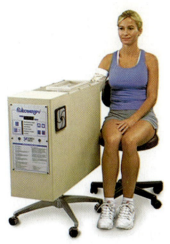

FIGURE 15–4   Fluidotherapy units contain fine cellulose particles in which warm air is circulated. (Courtesy Chattanooga Medical)

Special Considerations Avoid paraffin bath therapy on body areas that have open wounds or a decrease in normal circulation.

It is essential that the patient clean the body part thoroughly before therapy to avoid contaminating the mixture. In most cases, if this rule is closely adhered to, the mixture will only have to be replaced approximately every 6 months.[46]

Fluidotherapy Fluidotherapy creates a therapeutic environment with dry heat and forced convection through a suspended airstream.

Equipment Fluidotherapy units come in a variety of sizes, ranging from ones that treat distal extremities to ones that treat large body areas. The unit contains fine cellulose particles in which warm air is circulated. As the air is circulated, the cellulose particles become suspended, giving them properties that are similar to liquid.[42] Fluidotherapy allows the patient to tolerate much greater temperatures than would be possible using water or paraffin heat (Figure 15–4).

Indications Fluidotherapy is effective in decreasing pain, increasing joint range of motion, decreasing muscle guarding, and decreasing swelling.

Application Treatment temperature usually ranges from 100°F to 113°F (37.8°C to 45°C). Particle agitation should be controlled for comfort. Exercise can be performed while the patient is in the cabinet. The athlete should be positioned for comfort. Treatment duration is 15 to 20 minutes.

Cryotherapy

The application of cold for the first aid of trauma to the musculoskeletal system is a widely used practice in sports medicine. When applied intermittently after injury, along with compression, elevation, and rest, it reduces many of the adverse conditions related to the inflammatory or reactive phase of an acute injury.[28,34,38] Depending on the severity of the injury, rest, ice, compression, and elevation (RICE) may be used from the first day to as long as 2 weeks after injury.[34]

Physiological Effects of Cold In cryotherapy, the most common method for cold transfer to tissue is through conduction. The extent to which tissue is cooled depends on the cold medium that is being applied, the length of cold exposure, and the conductivity of the area being cooled.[39] In most cases, the longer the cold exposure, the deeper the cooling. At a temperature of 38.3°F (3.5°C), muscle temperatures can be reduced as deep as 1½ inches (4 cm). Cooling is dependent on the type of tissue. For example, tissue with a high water content, such as muscle, is an excellent cold conductor, whereas fat is a poor conductor. Because of fat's low cold conductivity, it acts as the body's insulator.[56] Tissue that has previously been cooled takes longer to return to a normal temperature than does tissue that has been heated.

When cold is applied to skin for 20 minutes or less at a temperature of 50°F (10°C) or less, vasoconstriction of the arterioles and venules in the area occurs. This vasoconstriction is caused in part by the reflex action of the smooth muscles.[46]

It has been hypothesized that when local temperature is lowered considerably for a period of about 30 minutes, intermittent periods of vasodilation occur, lasting 4 to 6 minutes. This phenomenon has come to be known as the **hunting response** and is said to be necessary to prevent local tissue

| **hunting response** |
| Causes a slight temperature increase during cooling. |

injury caused by cold. The hunting response has been accepted for a number of years as fact; in reality, however, it actually refers to measured temperature changes rather than circulatory changes. Some clinicians have taken the liberty of inferring that temperature changes produce circulatory changes, and this is simply not what the hunting response is. The hunting response is more likely a measurement artifact than an actual change in blood flow in response to cold.

Trauma is a result of compromised circulation, which decreases the amount of oxygen being delivered to the cells in the area of injury. The immediate use of ice after injury decreases the extent of ischemic injury to those cells on the periphery of the primary injury by slowing their metabolic rate.[38] This slowdown results in less damage to the tissues and thus decreases rehabilitation time.[34]

Because cold lowers the metabolic rate and produces vasoconstriction, swelling will be reduced in an acute inflammatory response. Cold does not reduce swelling that is already present.[38]

Cooling tissues can directly decrease muscle guarding by slowing metabolism in the area, thus decreasing the waste products that may have accumulated—waste products that act as muscle irritants and cause spasm.

Because the local application of cold can decrease acute muscle guarding, the muscle becomes more amenable to stretch. A gentle stretch of a muscle after an acute injury may be indicated; however, the stretching of long-standing contractures is contraindicated. The use of either cold or heat does not appear to help increase muscle length when used in combination with proprioceptive neuromuscular facilitation (PNF) stretching.[46] Cold tends to cause collagen stiffness.[46]

Cold decreases free nerve ending excitability as well as the excitability of peripheral nerves.[7] Analgesia is caused by raising the nerve's threshold.[46]

The extent of cooling depends on the thickness of the subcutaneous fat layer.

Nerve fiber response to cold depends mainly on the presence of myelination and the diameter of the fiber.[40] For example, most sensitive to cold are gamma efferent myelinated fibers to the muscle spindles.[46] The next most sensitive to cold are alpha motor nerves. The least sensitive to cold are the unmyelinated pain fibers and sympathetic nerves. During the application of cold, the patient experiences a progression of sensations from *cold*, to *burning*, to *aching*, and finally to *numbness* (CBAN). Table 15–3 indicates the usual outward sequential response to cold application.

Cold, in general, is more penetrating than heat. Once a muscle has been cooled through the

TABLE 15–3	Skin Response to Cold	
Stage	**Response**	**Estimated Time after Initiation**
1	Cold sensation	0 to 3 minutes
2	Mild burning, aching	2 to 7 minutes
3	Relative cutaneous numbness	5 to 12 minutes

TABLE 15–4	Physiological Variables of Cryotherapy
Variable	**Response to Therapy**
Muscle guarding	Decreases
Pain perception	Decreases
Blood flow	Decreases up to 10 minutes
Metabolic rate	Decreases
Collagen elasticity	Decreases
Joint stiffness	Increases
Capillary permeability	Increases
Edema	Controversial

subcutaneous fat layer, cold's effects last longer than heat effects do because fat acts as an insulator against rewarming.[46] The major problem is to penetrate the fat layer initially, so that muscle cooling occurs. In individuals with less than ½ inch (1.25 cm) of subcutaneous fat, significant muscle cooling can occur after 10 minutes of cold application. In persons with more than ⅘ inch (2 cm) of subcutaneous fat, muscle temperatures barely drop after 10 minutes (Table 15–4).[40]

Another unique quality of cooling is its ability to decrease muscle fatigue and increase and maintain muscular contraction. This ability is attributed to the decrease of the local metabolic rate and the tissue temperature.[46] Although adverse reactions to therapeutic cold application are uncommon, they do happen and are described in *Focus Box 15–1*: "Adverse reactions to cold."

The two most common means of delivering cold as therapy to the body are ice or cold packs and immersion in cool or cold water. The most effective type of pack contains wet ice rather than ice in a plastic container or in a commercial chemical pack (e.g., Cryogen).[46] Wet ice is a more effective coolant because of the extent of internal energy needed to melt the ice.[46] It has also been shown that ice that undergoes a phase change (i.e., ice melting to water) is more effective at lowering skin and intramuscular temperatures.[38]

Ice Massage

Equipment Water is frozen in a foam or waxed-paper cup, which forms a cylinder of ice. The foam

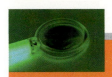

FOCUS 15–1 Focus on Injury/Illness Prevention and Wellness Protection

Adverse reactions to cold

- Cooling for an hour at 30.2°F to 15.8°F (−1°C to −9°C) produces redness and edema that lasts for 20 hours after exposure. Frostbite has been known to occur in subfreezing temperatures of 26.6° to 24.8°F (−3° to −4°C).[34]
- Immersion at 41°F (5°C) increases limb fluid volume by 15 percent due to placing the limb in the dependent position.
- Exposure for 90 minutes at 57.2°F to 60.8°F (14°C to 16°C) can delay resolution of swelling up to 1 week.[34]
- Some individuals are allergic to cold and react with hives and joint pain and swelling.[46]
- Icing through a towel or an elastic bandage limits the reduction in temperature, which could influence the effectiveness of the treatment.[57]

- Raynaud's phenomenon is a condition that causes vasospasm of digital arteries lasting for minutes to hours, which could lead to tissue death. The early signs of Raynaud's phenomenon are attacks of intermittent skin blanching or cyanosis of the fingers or toes, skin pallor followed by redness, and finally a return to normal color. Pain is uncommon, but numbness, tingling, or burning may occur during and shortly after an attack.
- Although it is relatively uncommon, the application of ice can cause nerve palsy. Nerve palsy occurs when cold is applied to a part that has motor nerves close to the skin surface, such as the peroneal nerve at the fibular head. Usually, the condition resolves spontaneously with no significant problem. As a general rule, ice should not be applied longer than 20 to 30 minutes at any one time.

---

is removed approximately an inch (2.5 cm) from the top of the cup. The remaining foam provides a handle for the athletic trainer to grasp while massaging. Another method is to fill a cup with water and insert a tongue depressor to act as a handle when the water is frozen. A towel should be present to absorb the water that is collected.

> **Cold therapy can begin immediately following injury.**

Indications Ice massage is commonly used over tendons, the belly of a muscle, bursae, or myofascial trigger points.

Application Ice massage is a cryotherapeutic method that is performed on a small body area. It can be applied by the athletic trainer and the patient. Grasping the ice cylinder, the athletic trainer rubs the ice over the patient's skin in overlapping circles in a 4- to 6-inch (10 to 15 cm) area for 5 to 10 minutes. The patient should experience the sensations of cold, burning, aching, and numbness. When analgesia has been reached, the patient can engage in stretching or exercise (Figure 15–5).

Special Considerations In a patient with normal circulation, tissue damage seldom occurs from cold application. The temperature of the tissue seldom goes below 59°F (15°C). However, when applying ice massage superficially, if an individual is going to have an adverse reaction to the cold, it tends to happen fairly early in the treatment.[34] The comfort of the patient must be considered at all times.

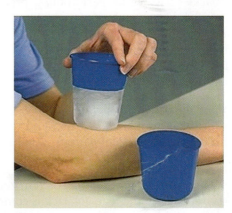

FIGURE 15–5 Ice massage can lead to analgesia, which can be followed by gentle muscle stretching.

Cold- or Ice-Water Immersion
Equipment Depending on the body part to be immersed, a variety of containers or basins can be used. In some cases, a small whirlpool can be used. Water and crushed ice are mixed together to reach a temperature of 50°F to 60°F (10°C to 15°C). Towels must be available for drying.

Indications Where circumferential cooling of a body part is desired, cold- or ice-water immersion is preferred.

Application The patient immerses the body part in the water and proceeds through the four stages of cold response. This process may take 10 to 15 minutes. When the pain cycle has been interrupted, the

---

A dancer has Achilles tendinitis.

? What different methods of cryotherapy can be used to control pain and inflammation for this condition? Describe the benefits of each application.

part is removed from the water, and normal movement patterns are conducted. When pain returns, the part is re-immersed. This procedure may be repeated three times. Cool water immersion used in combination with electrical stimulation has been shown to minimize edema formation.[8]

Special Considerations Because cold makes collagen tissue stiffer, caution should be taken in allowing the patient to return to activity immediately after receiving cold treatment. Overcooling can lead to frostbite. Any allergic response to cold should also be noted.

Ice Packs (Bags)

Equipment There are a number of types of ice packs. Wet ice packs provide the best cooling properties. Flaked or crushed ice can be encased in a wet towel and placed on the body part to be treated. An ice pack can be made by placing crushed or chipped ice in a self-sealing plastic bag. The packs easily fit the contour of the body part.

Indications The patient experiences cold, burning aching and finally numbness (CBAN) and then proceeds with normal movement patterns (Figure 15–6).

Application Two types of chemical cold packs are available. One is a gel pack that may be refrozen after use and is hypoallergenic. The gel pack is commonly used in many athletic training settings. The other type is a liquid bag within a bag of crystals. When the inner bag is ruptured, the chemicals mix, causing an endothermic reaction. If allowed contact with the skin, these chemicals can cause a chemical burn and a liability problem.[34] Plastic flexiwrap or an elastic wrap should be used to hold the pack firmly in place.

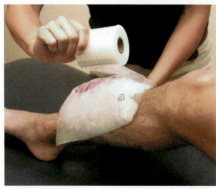

FIGURE 15–6 Ice packs are another way to apply cryotherapy. Use flexiwrap to hold the ice pack in place.

Special Considerations Excessive cold exposure must be avoided. With chemical gel packs, it is recommended that a single layer of toweling be used. Crushed or flaked ice packs may be applied directly to the skin. With any indication of allergy to cold or of abnormal pain, the treatment should be discontinued.

Vapocoolant Sprays

Equipment The most popular vapocoolant is fluori-methane, a nonflammable, nontoxic substance. Under pressure in a bottle, it gives off a fine spray when it is inverted and an emitter is pressed.

Indications The major value of a vapocoolant spray is its ability to reduce muscle guarding and increase range of motion. It is also a major treatment for myofascial pain and trigger points.[42]

> **Fluori-methane spray is used in the spray and stretch technique.**

Application When vapocoolant spray is used to increase the patient's range of motion in an area in which there is no trigger point, the following procedure is performed:

1. Hold the vapocoolant at a 30-degree angle, 12 to 18 inches (30 to 47 cm) from the skin.
2. Spray the entire length of the muscle from its proximal attachment to its distal attachment.
3. Cover the skin at a rate of approximately 4 inches (10 cm) per second; apply the spray two or three times as a gradual stretch is applied.

When dealing with a trigger point, the procedure is first to determine its presence, then to alleviate it. One method by which the athletic trainer can determine an active trigger point is to reproduce the injured patient's major pain complaint by pressing firmly on the site for 5 to 10 seconds. Another assessment technique is to elicit a jump response by placing the patient's muscle under moderate tension, applying firm pressure, and briskly pulling a finger across the tight band of muscle. This procedure causes the tight band of muscle to contract and the patient to wince.[46]

The spray and stretch method for treating trigger points and myofascial pain (Figure 15–7) using vapocoolant spray is performed as follows:[46]

1. Position the athlete in a relaxed but well-supported position. The muscle that contains the trigger point is stretched.
2. Alert the patient that the spray will feel cool.
3. Hold the fluori-methane bottle approximately 12 inches (30 cm) away from the skin to be sprayed.
4. Direct the spray at an acute angle in one direction toward the reference zone of pain.

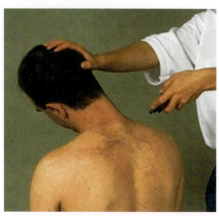

FIGURE 15–7 A vapocoolant spray, such as fluori-methane, can assist in reducing muscle spasm.

5. Direct the spray to the full length of the muscle, including the reference zone of pain.
6. Begin firm stretching that is within the patient's pain tolerance.
7. Continue spraying in parallel sweeps that are approximately ¼ inch (0.6 cm) apart at a speed of approximately 4 inches (10 cm) every second.
8. Cover the skin area one or two times.
9. Continue passive stretching while spraying. Do not force the stretch; allow time for the muscle to let go.
10. After the first session of spraying and stretching, warm the muscle with a hot pack or by vigorous massage.
11. If necessary, perform a second session after step 10.
12. When a stretch has been completed, have the patient actively but gently move the part in a full range of motion.
13. Do not overload a muscle with strenuous exercise immediately after a stretch.
14. After an initial spraying and stretching session, instruct the patient about stretch exercises that should be performed at home on a daily basis.

Cryokinetics

Indications **Cryokinetics** is a technique that combines cryotherapy, or the application of cold, with exercise.[34] The goal of cryo-

| cryokinetics Combines cryotherapy with exercise. |

kinetics is to numb the injured part to point of analgesia and then work toward achieving normal range of motion through progressive active exercise.

Equipment The technique uses ice immersion, cold packs, or ice massage.

Application The technique begins by numbing the body part. Patients report a feeling of numbness within 12 to 20 minutes. If numbness is not

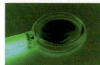

perceived within 20 minutes, the athletic trainer should proceed with exercise regardless. The numbness usually lasts for 3 to 5 minutes, at which point ice should be reapplied for an additional 3 to 5 minutes until numbness returns. This sequence should be repeated five times (see *Focus Box 15–2*: "Summary of cryokinetics"). Exercises are performed during the periods of numbness. The exercises selected should be pain free and progressive in intensity; the patient should concentrate on both flexibility and strength.[50]

Special Considerations Changes in the intensity of the activity should be limited by both the nature of the healing process and individual patient differences in perception of pain. However, progression always should be encouraged within the framework of those limiting factors; the ultimate goal is to return the athlete to full sport activities.[34]

ELECTRICAL ENERGY MODALITIES

Physical Properties of Electricity In general, electricity is a form of energy that displays magnetic, chemical, mechanical, and thermal effects on tissue.[21] It implies a flow of electrons between two points. Electrons are particles of matter that have a negative electrical charge and revolve around the core, or nucleus, of an atom.

An electrical current is a string of electrons that pass along a conductor, such as a nerve or wire. The volume or amount of the current is measured in **amperes** (A); 1 A equals the rate of flow of 1 coulomb (C) per second. A coulomb is a unit of electrical charge and is defined as the quantity of an electrical charge that can be transferred by 1 A in 1 second.

Resistance to the passing of an electrical current along a conductor is measured in **ohms** (Ω), and the force that moves the current along is called **voltage** (V). One volt is the amount of electrical force required to send a current of 1 A through a resistance of 1 Ω. In terms of electrotherapy, currents of 0 to 150 V are considered low-voltage currents, and currents above 150 V are considered high-voltage. The intensity of a current varies directly with the voltage and inversely with the resistance. Electrical power is measured in **watts** (amps × volts).[52]

An electrical current applied to nerve tissue at a sufficient intensity and duration to reach that tissue's excitability threshold will result in a membrane depolarization, or firing, of that nerve. There are three major types of nerve fibers: sensory, motor, and pain. As current intensity or duration is increased, the threshold for depolarization will be reached first for sensory fibers, then for motor fibers, and then for pain fibers. Thus, it is possible to produce different physiological responses by adjusting the treatment parameters.[25]

> **amperes** Measurement of volume or amount of electrical energy.
>
> **ohms** Measurement of resistance.
>
> **voltage** Force.
>
> **watts** Measurement of power.

Equipment Electrotherapeutic devices generate three types of current, which, when introduced into biological tissue, are capable of producing specific physiological changes.

> **Electrical currents include monophasic (DC), biphasic (AC), and pulsatile.**

These three types of current are monophasic (DC), biphasic (AC), and pulsatile.[25]

A great deal of confusion has developed about the terminology used to describe electrotherapeutic currents. All therapeutic electrical generators, regardless of whether they deliver biphasic, monophasic, or pulsatile currents through electrodes attached to the skin, are *transcutaneous electrical stimulators*. The majority of these generators are used to stimulate peripheral nerves and are correctly called *transcutaneous electrical nerve stimulators (TENS)* (Figure 15–8). Occasionally, the terms *neuromuscular electrical stimulator (NMES)* and *electrical muscle stimulator (EMS)* are used; however, these terms

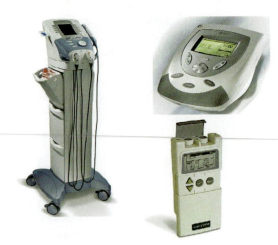

FIGURE 15–8 Many therapeutic electrical generators are transcutaneous electrical nerve stimulators (TENS). (Courtesy Chatanooga Medical)

are appropriate only when the electrical current is being used to stimulate muscle directly, as would be the case with denervated muscle in which peripheral nerves are not functioning. A type of transcutaneous electrical stimulator that uses current intensities too small to excite peripheral nerves has been called a *microcurrent electrical nerve stimulator (MENS)*, although this type is currently being referred to as a *low-intensity stimulator (LIS)*.[25]

Monophasic Current (DC) Monophasic current, also called direct current, flows in one direction only from the positive pole to the negative pole. DC may be used for pain modulation or muscle contraction or to produce ion movement. Specific physiological effects are determined by how the treatment parameters are set on the stimulating unit. Most electrical stimulators currently used in athletic training settings are monophasic units which deliver pulsed high-voltage currents.

Biphasic Current (AC) With biphasic current, also called alternating current, the direction of current flow reverses itself once during each cycle. Biphasic current may be used for pain modulation or muscle contraction.

Pulsatile Current Pulsatile currents usually contain three or more pulses grouped together. These groups of pulses are interrupted for short periods of time and repeat themselves at regular intervals. Pulsatile currents are used in interferential pre-modulated and so-called Russian currents.

Current parameters

Waveform A waveform is a graphic representation of the shape, direction, amplitude, and direction of a particular electrical current. Electrical stimulating units can take on various waveforms depending on the capability of the generator. Biphasic,

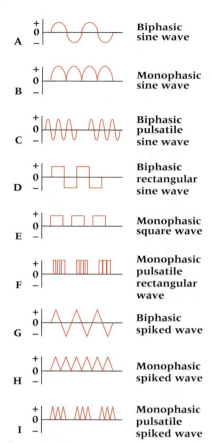

FIGURE 15–9 Waveforms of monophasic, biphasic, or pulsatile current may be either sine, rectangular, square, or spiked in shape.

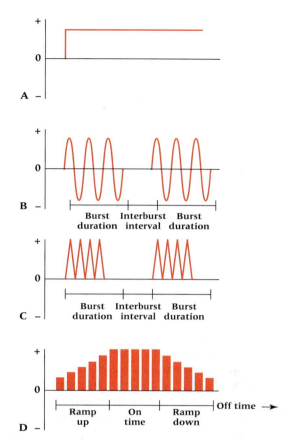

FIGURE 15–10 Current may be modulated using. **(A)** Continuous current. **(B)** Burst-modulated alternating current. **(C)** Burst-modulated pulsatile current. **(D)** Ramp-up and ramp-down modulation.

Current parameters:

- Waveform
- Modulation
- Intensity
- Duration
- Frequency
- Polarity
- Electrode setup

monophasic, and pulsatile units can produce currents with waveforms that are sine, rectangular, square, or spiked in shape (Figure 15–9).

Modulation Current modulation is the ability of the electrical stimulating unit to change the magnitude or duration of a waveform. Modulation may be continuous, bursts, or surging for biphasic, monophasic, and pulsatile currents (Figure 15–10).

Intensity Current intensity is the voltage output of the stimulating unit. Generators that produce voltage outputs of up to 150 V are low-voltage generators. Those that produce up to 500 V are high-voltage generators. Low-voltage generators are almost always monophasic; high-voltage generators may be either biphasic or monophasic. The majority of the electrical stimulators used in athletic training settings are high-voltage monophasic generators.

Duration *Duration* refers to the length of time that current is flowing. It is also referred to as pulse width or pulse duration. Duration is preset on most of the high-voltage monophasic stimulators.

Frequency **Frequency** refers to the number of waveforms being emitted by the electrical stimulating unit in 1 second. Frequency is identified in pulses per second (pps), cycles per second (cps), or hertz (Hz). Frequencies range from one pps to several thousand pps.

frequency Measured in pulses per second (pps), cycles per second (cps), and hertz (Hz).

Polarity Polarity is the direction of current flow toward either a positive or a negative pole.

Electrode setup In electrotherapy, electrode pads are affixed directly to the skin. Electrodes are of different sizes. Using a large *(dispersive)* electrode remote from the treatment area while placing a smaller *(active)* electrode as close as possible to the nerve or muscle motor point will give the greatest effect at the small electrode. The large electrode disperses the current over a large area; the small electrode concentrates the current in the area of the motor point. The physiological effects can occur anywhere between the two pads, but they usually occur at the active electrode because current density (the amount of current in a given area) is greater at this point.[20] Many newer electrical stimulating units have pads that are of equal size; thus, both electrodes are considered active electrodes.

Indications Monophasic, biphasic, and pulsatile currents may all be used to achieve a specific therapeutic effect.[25] Clinically, athletic trainers use electrical currents for several purposes: to produce the depolarization of sensory nerves to modulate pain, to produce a depolarization of motor nerve fibers to elicit a muscle contraction, to create an electrical field to the biological tissues to stimulate or alter the healing process at the cellular level, and to create an electrical field on the skin surface to transport ions beneficial to the healing process into deeper target tissues.[25]

Application

Pain Modulation Electrical stimulating currents can reduce pain associated with injury.[25] The neurophysiological mechanisms associated with pain modulation—including gate control, descending pathway pain control, and opiate pain control—were discussed in Chapter 10.

Gate control Electrical stimulation of sensory nerves will evoke the gate control mechanism and diminish awareness of painful stimuli. As long as the stimulation is causing the sensory nerves to fire, the gate to pain should be closed. If the stimulus stops, the gate is then open, and pain returns to perception. The following parameters can be used for gate control: Intensity should be adjusted to create a tingling sensation but should not cause a muscular contraction, and pulse duration and frequency should be set as high as possible so that a muscle contraction does not occur.[29]

Descending pathway pain control Intense electrical stimulation of the smaller pain fibers at trigger and acupuncture points for short time periods causes stimulation of descending neurons, which then affect the transmission of pain information by closing the gate at the spinal cord level. Current intensity should be very high, approaching a noxious level; pulse duration should be 10 microseconds (msec); frequency should be 80 pulses per second.[25]

Opiate pain control Electrical stimulation of sensory nerves stimulates the release of enkephalin from local sites throughout the central nervous system and the release of β-endorphins from the pituitary gland into the cerebrospinal fluid. Pain modulation is caused by applying an electrical current to areas close to the site of pain or to acupuncture or trigger points both local to and distant from the pain area. A point stimulator can be used, with current intensity set as high as tolerable; pulse duration should be set at the maximum possible on the machine; frequency should be set at 1 to 5 pps.[25]

Muscle Contraction The quality of a muscle contraction changes according to the changes in current parameters. As the frequency of stimulation increases, the muscle develops more tension because of progressive shortening of the muscle, until a tetanic contraction

| **tetany** Maximum muscle contraction. |

is achieved.[26] **Tetany** occurs for virtually all muscles

at approximately 50 pps. Increases in intensity spread the current over a larger area and increase the number of motor units

activated by the current. Increases in current duration also cause more motor units to be activated. A variety of therapeutic gains can be made by electrically stimulating a muscle contraction; these gains include muscle pumping contractions, muscle strengthening, retardation of atrophy, and muscle reeducation.

Muscle pumping This type of contraction is used to help stimulate circulation by pumping fluid and blood through the venous and lymphatic channels back to the heart. High-voltage monophasic current is recommended. Intensity should be increased to elicit a muscle contraction at a frequency of 20 to 40 pps, using a surged mode with on/off times set at 5 seconds each. The injured body part should be elevated, and active contraction should be encouraged. Treatment time is twenty to thirty minutes.[25]

Muscle strengthening Electrical stimulation can be used to facilitate strength gains. High-frequency biphasic current is recommended. Intensity should be increased at a frequency of 50 to 60 pps to elicit a tetanic muscle contraction using surging current set at 15 seconds on and 50 seconds off. Treatment should include 10 repetitions three times per week. For best results, the patient should combine this electrically induced tetanic contraction with maximal active contraction against some resistance.[25]

Retardation of atrophy Electrically induced muscle contraction can be used to minimize the atrophy and loss of muscle function that typically occurs with immobilization after injury. High-frequency biphasic current is recommended. Intensity should be increased to 30 to 60 pps to elicit a tetanic contraction using interrupted current mode. The athlete should incorporate voluntary isometric contraction. Treatment time should be 15 to 20 minutes.[25]

Muscle Reeducation Muscular inhibition after surgery or injury can be reduced by electrically stimulating a muscle. Intensity should be increased to a level necessary for a comfortable contraction at 30 to 50 pps using either interrupted or surged current. The athlete should watch and feel the contraction and attempt to initiate a voluntary contraction. Treatment time is 15 to 20 minutes; treatment is repeated several times daily.[25]

Iontophoresis

Iontophoresis is a therapeutic technique that involves the introduction of ions into the body tissues by means of a direct electrical current.[52]

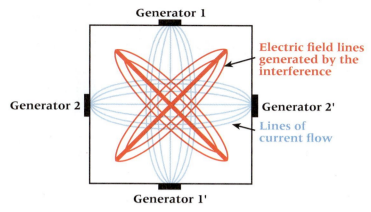

Generator 1

Generator 2

Electric field lines generated by the interference

Generator 2'

Lines of current flow

Generator 1'

FIGURE 15–11   Pattern created by interferential currents.

Equipment The iontophoresis generator must output continuous monophasic current to ensure the unidirectional migration of ions, which cannot be accomplished using a biphasic current. Current intensity ranges between 1 and 5 milliamps.

Indications Clinically, iontophoresis is used in the treatment of inflammatory musculoskeletal conditions; for analgesic effects, scar modification, and wound healing; and in treating edema, calcium deposits, and hyperhydrosis.[5]

Application A self-adhering, prepared electrode, either reusable or commercially produced, must be securely attached to the skin. There are three techniques of application: An active pad is applied over gauze that is saturated with a solution containing the ions (this pad is positioned as close as possible to the involved tissue); the active electrode is suspended in a container of the ion solution, and then the body part to be treated is immersed in the container; or a special active electrode with a reservoir into which a treatment ion can be injected and stored is positioned as close to the involved tissue as possible. In all cases, a large dispersive pad is applied to the patient. The manner in which ions move in solution forms the basis for iontophoresis. Positively charged ions are transported into the tissue from the positive pole, and negatively charged ions are transported under the negative pole. Treatment time varies from 10 to 20 minutes, depending on the intensity of the current or the current density at the active electrode, the duration of the current flow, and the concentration of ions in solution.[52] Dexamethasone and hydrocortisone are two of the most commonly used ions in iontophoresis.[5]

Special Considerations It is critical that the athletic trainer be knowledgeable in the selection of the most appropriate ions for treating specific conditions. Perhaps the single most common problem associated with iontophoresis is a chemical burn, which usually occurs as a result of the direct current itself, not because of the ion being used in treatment.

Interferential Currents

Equipment Interferential currents make use of two separate electrical generators that emit currents at two slightly different frequencies. Two pairs of electrodes are arranged in a square pattern such that the currents cross one another, creating an interference pattern at a central point of stimulation. The interference pattern creates a larger area of stimulation (Figure 15–11).[12]

Indications Interferential currents have been used for a variety of clinical conditions, including pain, joint pain with swelling, neuritis, retarded callus formation following fracture, and restricted mobility.

Application Positioning of the electrodes is critical to the success of the treatment. The athletic trainer must move the electrodes around until the patient indicates that the stimulation is centered over the area of pain. A frequency of stimulation should be selected with interferential currents that is similar to using other electrical stimulators: 20 to 25 pps for muscle contraction and 50 to 120 pps for pain management.

Special Considerations Although interferential currents are more complex from an engineering perspective than other electrical stimulating currents, the potential therapeutic effects are essentially the same.

Low-Intensity Stimulators

Equipment Low-intensity stimulators (LIS) were originally referred to as microcurrent electrical nerve stimulators, or MENS. Low-intensity stimulators deliver current to the patient at very low frequencies (1 pps) and at extremely low intensities (less than 1 milliamp) that are subsensory.

Indications This type of current is used to stimulate the healing process in both soft tissue and bone by altering the electrical activity to mimic a normal electrical field in normal individual cells. Specifically, it has been used to modulate pain and promote healing of wounds, nonunion fractures, and tendons and ligaments.

Application The electrical currents used by low-intensity stimulators are no different than those described previously. The athletic trainer need only turn the unit on and slightly increase the intensity. A large dispersive electrode keeps the current density low enough that threshold levels for depolarization of sensory nerves are not achieved.

Special Considerations The effectiveness of LIS therapy is currently based primarily on theory; there is little research information to support its use.[25]

ELECTROMAGNETIC ENERGY MODALITIES

Shortwave Diathermy

Physiological Effects of Diathermy Shortwave diathermy emits electromagnetic energy that is capable of producing temperature increases in the deeper tissues. Tissues with a higher water content (e.g., muscle) selectively absorb the heat delivered by shortwave diathermy.[48] The extent of muscle heating depends on the thickness of the subcutaneous fat layer.[48] Shortwave diathermy provides heat penetration similar to that of ultrasound. In contrast to shortwave diathermy, ultrasonic vibration is not absorbed by fat and is therefore not influenced by its thickness.[17]

Shortwave diathermy heats deeper tissues by introducing a high-frequency electrical current. Shortwave diathermy is in essence a radio transmitter; the Federal Communications Commission (FCC) has assigned a wavelength of 7.5 to 22 meters and a frequency of 13.56 or 27.12 megacycles per second for therapeutic purposes.[48]

Shortwave diathermy can be used in two ways: through a condenser that uses electrostatic field heating or through electromagnetic or induction field heating.[48] In electrostatic field heating, the patient is a part of the circuit. Heating is uneven because of different tissue resistance to energy flow, an application of Joule's law, which states that the greater the resistance, the more heat will develop. In electromagnetic field heating, the patient is not part of the circuit, but is heated by an electromagnetic field.[48]

Pulsed shortwave diathermy is a relatively new form of diathermy.[43] Pulsed diathermy is created by simply interrupting the output of continuous shortwave diathermy at consistent intervals.

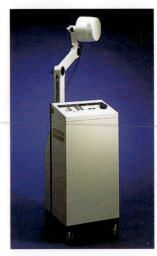

FIGURE 15–12 A shortwave diathermy unit: The Autotherm. (Courtesy Mettler Electronics)

Pulsing reduces the likelihood of any significant tissue temperature increase and reduces the patient's perception of heat. Generators that deliver pulsed shortwave diathermy typically use a drum type of electrode. Pulsed diathermy is claimed to have therapeutic value and to produce nonthermal effects with minimal thermal physiological effects, depending on the intensity of the application. When pulsed diathermy is used in intensities that create an increase in tissue temperature, its effects are no different from those of continuous shortwave diathermy.[40]

Shortwave Diathermy Treatments
Equipment In general, the shortwave diathermy unit consists of a power supply to a power amplifier and a frequency generator. It has an oscillator that produces high frequency (either 13.56 or 27.12 megacycles) and a power amplifier that converts biphasic current to monophasic current.[48] It also has a circuit that tunes in the patient automatically or manually as part of the circuitry (Figure 15–12).

The shortwave diathermy treatment applicators are either condensor or inductive types.[48] With the condensor, or field heating, the patient is a natural part of the circuit. The condensor applicator consists of electrodes formed by sheets of flexible or rigid metal covered by heavy insulation.

There are two types of inductive electrodes: the coil and the single drum unit. The inductive coil is a cable electrode that ranges from 6 to 16 feet (2 to 5 meters) long and is wound around the patient's injured part. Whereas the coil can heat generally, the single drum unit is designed to treat a more specific area.[30] Tissues with high water content, such as blood and muscle, are the most easily heated.

Indications Shortwave diathermy is used to treat bursitis, capsulitis, osteoarthritis, and muscle strains. The depth of the inductive technique can be as

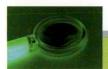
Precautions when using shortwave diathermy

- It is difficult to treat localized body areas.
- Dosage is subjective.
- Towels must be placed between the applicator and the skin. Towels absorb perspiration during treatment.
- When there is loss of sensation, shortwave diathermy should not be used.
- When metal objects, such as implants, pacemakers, jewelry, a metal table, intrauterine devices (IUDs), zippers on clothing, or glasses, are present, shortwave diathermy should not be administered.
- Avoid use when the patient is hemorrhaging, is pregnant, has open wounds, or wears contact lenses.

- Diathermy cables or coils must not touch one another or any metal.
- Avoid heating eyes, testicles, ovaries, bony prominences, and bone-growth areas.
- A deep, aching sensation during treatment may indicate overheating.
- In 2002, the FDA issued an advisory warning that shortwave diathermy in both heating and non heating modes can result in serious injury to an individual who has any type of implanted device or leads.

---

much as 2 inches (5 cm). The condensor technique penetrates from 1 to 2 inches (2.5 to 5 cm). Tissue temperature can reach 107°F (41.7°C).[48] Although shortwave diathermy has been used in connection with stretching, it is not clear whether using both diathermy and stretching increases flexibility more than stretching alone.[13,43]

Application If more superficial heating is desired, a condensor plate is used; when deeper therapy is desired, the induction coil should be used. A double-layered towel is placed between the applicator and the skin. When the patient is as comfortable as possible, he or she is tuned in with the oscillating circuit of the unit. In most cases, the treatment times range from 20 to 30 minutes (Table 15–5).[48] *Focus Box 15–3:* "Precautions when using shortwave diathermy" offers important information about this technique.

Special Considerations Shortwave diathermy and ultrasound are both considered to be deep-heating modalities. Shortwave diathermy has been shown to

be as effective as 1 Mhz ultrasound in increasing tissue temperature at a depth of $1^1/_8$ inches (3 cm). Although ultrasound is much more widely used than shortwave diathermy, shortwave diathermy would be the modality of choice in certain treatment situations. If the treatment area is large, diathermy is more effective than ultrasound in effectively heating it. If any condition exists in which pressure from an ultrasound transducer exacerbates pain, then shortwave diathermy is preferable. Unlike an ultrasound treatment, once a shortwave diathermy unit has been appropriately set up, it does not require constant monitoring by the athletic trainer.

Low-Level Laser Therapy

LASER is an acronym that stands for **l**ight **a**mplification by **s**timulated **e**mission of **r**adiation (Figure 15–13).[51]

Equipment Helium neon (HeNe, a gas) and gallium arsenide (GaAs, a semiconductor) lasers are two low-level lasers currently used in the United States and

---

TABLE 15–5	Sample Shortwave Diathermy Dosage	
Dosage	**Effect**	**Application**
Lowest dose (I)	Just below the point of any sensation of heat (acute inflammatory process)	20 to 30 minutes daily for 2 weeks
Low dose (II)	Mild heat sensation, barely felt (subacute, resolving inflammatory process)	20 to 30 minutes daily for 2 weeks
Medium dose (III)	Moderate but pleasant heat sensation (subacute, resolving inflammatory process)	20 to 30 minutes from 2 to 3 times weekly for 1 to 4 weeks
Heavy dose (IV)	Vigorous heating that causes a sensation that is well tolerated (chronic conditions): pain threshold should not be exceeded	20 to 30 minutes from 2 to 3 times weekly for 1 to 4 weeks

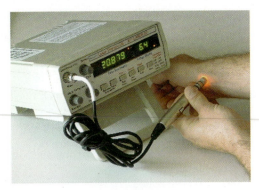

FIGURE 15–13 Low-level laser unit.

other countries for wound and soft-tissue healing and pain relief.[36] HeNe lasers deliver a characteristic red beam with a direct penetration of 0.07 to 0.5 inch (2 to 13 mm) and an indirect penetration of 0.4 to 0.6 inch (10 to 15 mm). GaAs lasers are invisible and have a direct penetration of 0.4 to 0.8 inch (1 to 2 cm) and an indirect penetration to 2 inches (5 cm).

Indications The proposed therapeutic applications of lasers in physical medicine include acceleration of collagen synthesis, decrease in microorganisms, increase in vascularization, and reduction of pain and inflammation.[51] Trigger or acupuncture points are also treated for painful conditions.

Application The technique of laser application ideally is done with gentle contact with the skin surface and should be perpendicular to the target surface.[31] Dosage appears to be the critical factor in eliciting the desired response, but exact dosimetry has not been determined. Dosage fluctuates by varying the pulse frequency and the treatment times. The laser is applied by developing an imaginary grid over the target area. The grid comprises 1 cm squares, and the laser is applied to each square for a predetermined time.

Special Considerations Although no deleterious effects have been reported, certain precautions and contraindications exist. Contraindications include lasing over cancerous tissue, directly into the eyes, and during the first trimester of pregnancy. Occasionally, pain may increase when laser treatments begin but does not indicate cessation of treatment. A low percentage of patients have experienced a syncope episode during laser treatment, but this is usually self-resolving.[27]

SOUND ENERGY MODALITIES

Therapeutic Ultrasound

Ultrasound is another widely used modality in athletic training. It is a valuable therapeutic tool in the rehabilitation of many different injuries because it stimulates the

> **Ultrasound can be applied either to the skin or through a water medium.**

repair of soft-tissue injuries and relieves pain.[14] Ultrasound is a deep-heating modality and is used primarily for elevating tissue temperatures. It is a form of acoustic rather than electromagnetic energy. Ultrasound is defined as inaudible, acoustic vibrations of high frequency that may produce either thermal or nonthermal physiological effects.[14] The use of ultrasound as a therapeutic agent may be extremely effective if the athletic trainer has an adequate understanding of its effects on biological tissues and of the physical mechanisms by which these effects are produced.[14]

The number of movements, or oscillations, in 1 second is referred to as the frequency of a sound wave and is known as a hertz (Hz) unit. More commonly, 1 Hz equals 1 cycle per second, 1 kHz equals 1,000 cycles per second, and 1 MHz equals 1 million cycles per second.[14] The human ear cannot detect sound greater than 20,000 Hz; therefore, inaudible sound is considered ultrasound. When sound scatters and absorbs as it penetrates tissue, its energy is decreased (**attenuation**). Absorption of sound increases with an increase in frequency.

> **attenuation** A decrease in intensity as sound enters deeper tissues.

Tissue penetration depends on impedance or acoustical properties of the media that are proportional to tissue density.[17] Sound reflection occurs when adjacent tissues have different impedance. The greater the impedance, the greater the reflection, and the more heat produced. The greatest heat is developed between bone and the adjacent soft-tissue interface.

Equipment The main piece of equipment for delivering therapeutic ultrasound is a high-frequency generator, which provides an electrical current through a coaxial cable to a transducer contained within an applicator. In the applicator or transducer are synthetic crystals, such as barium titanate or lead zirconate titanate, that possess the property of piezoelectricity. These crystals are in disks 0.07 to 0.1 inch (2 to 3 mm) thick and 0.4 to 1.2 inches (1 to 3 cm) in diameter.[14] The **piezoelectric effect** causes expansion and contraction of the crystals, which produce oscillation voltage at the same frequency as the sound wave.[14]

> **piezoelectric effect** Electrical current produced by applying pressure to certain synthetic crystals, such as quartz.

Frequency Therapeutic ultrasound has a frequency range between 0.75 and 3.0 MHz. The majority of ultrasound generators are set at a frequency between 1 and 3 MHz. A generator that can be set between 1 and 3 MHz affords the athletic trainer the greatest treatment flexibility. Ultrasound energy generated at 1 MHz is transmitted through the more superficial tissues and absorbed primarily in the deeper tissues at depths of 1.2 to 2 inches (3 to 5 cm).[11] A 1 MHz frequency is most useful in individuals with high percent body fat cutaneously and whenever the desired effects are in the deeper structures.[14,37] At 3 MHz the energy is absorbed in the more superficial tissues with a depth of penetration between 0.4 and 0.8 inch (1 and 2 cm).[15]

Ultrasound beam The portion of the surface of the ultrasound transducer that produces the sound wave is referred to as the **effective radiating area**. Energy is delivered to the tissues in a collimated cylindrical beam. The beam from ultrasound generated at 1 MHz is more divergent than at 3 MHz. Within this beam, the distribution of ultrasound energy is nonuniform. The amount of variability of intensity in the beam is indicated by the **beam nonuniformity ratio (BNR)**. The lower the BNR, the more uniform the energy output. Optimally, the BNR would be 1:1.

> **effective radiating area** The portion of the transducer that produces sound energy.
>
> **beam nonuniformity ratio (BNR)** The amount of variability in intensity of the ultrasound beam.

Intensity The intensity of the ultrasound beam is determined by the amount of energy delivered to the sound head (applicator). It is expressed in the number of watts per square centimeter (W/cm^2). As a therapeutic modality used in sports medicine, the intensity ranges from 0.1 to 3 W/cm^2.

Pulsed versus continuous ultrasound Virtually all therapeutic ultrasound generators can emit either continuous or pulsed ultrasound waves. If continuous ultrasound is used, the sound intensity remains constant throughout the treatment and the ultrasound energy is being produced 100 percent of the time. With pulsed ultrasound, the output is periodically interrupted and no ultrasound energy is produced during the off period. The percentage of time that ultrasound is being generated is referred to as the *duty cycle*. If the pulse duration is 1 millisecond and the total pulse period is 5 milliseconds, the duty cycle is 20 percent. Therefore, the total amount of energy being delivered to the tissues is only 20 percent of the energy that would be delivered if a continuous wave were being used.

> **Ultrasound can be continuous or pulsed.**

> **The duty cycle is the percentage of time that ultrasound is being generated.**

Continuous ultrasound is most commonly used to produce thermal effects. The use of pulsed ultrasound results in a reduced average heating of the tissues. Pulsed ultrasound or continuous ultrasound at a low intensity produces nonthermal or mechanical effects, which may be associated with soft-tissue healing.[49]

Indications

Thermal versus nonthermal effects Therapeutic ultrasound produces both *thermal* and *nonthermal effects.*[30] Traditionally, ultrasound has been used primarily to produce a tissue temperature increase. The clinical effects of using ultrasound to heat the tissues are similar to those of other forms of superficial heat, discussed in earlier sections. For the majority of these effects to occur, the tissue temperature must be raised to a level of 104°F to 113°F (40°C to 45°C) for a minimum of five minutes.[22] Temperatures below this range are ineffective, and temperatures above 113°F (45°C) may be damaging.[14] Ultrasound at 1 MHz with an intensity of 1 W/cm^2 can raise soft-tissue temperature by 0.2°C per minute; at 3 MHz, by as much as 0.6°C per minute.[14,22]

> **Ultrasound produces effects that are thermal or nonthermal.**

Whenever ultrasound is used to produce thermal changes, nonthermal changes also occur. However, if appropriate treatment parameters are selected, nonthermal effects can occur with minimal thermal effects.[60] The nonthermal effects of therapeutic ultrasound include *cavitation* and acoustic *microstreaming*. Cavitation is the formation of gas-filled bubbles that expand and compress because of ultrasonically induced pressure changes in tissue fluids.[30] Cavitation results in an increased flow in the fluid around these vibrating bubbles. Microstreaming is the unidirectional movement of fluids along the boundaries of cell membranes, resulting from the mechanical pressure wave in an ultrasonic field.[14] Microstreaming can alter cell membrane structure and function because of changes in cell membrane permeability to sodium and calcium ions important in the healing process. As long as the cell membrane is not damaged, microstreaming can be of therapeutic value in accelerating the healing process.[14] These nonthermal effects have been reported to alter membrane properties, alter cellular proliferation, and produce increases in proteins associated with inflammation and injury repair, implying that ultrasound can modify the inflammatory response.[30] The proposed *frequency resonance hypothesis* relates to the absorption of the mechanical energy of ultrasound by proteins and protein complexes, resulting in alterations to signaling mechanisms within the cell and disturbance of the cellular membrane and the molecular structures within the cell. This may help explain the mechanisms

> **Nonthermal effects include cavitation and microstreaming.**

responsible for changes in cell membrane permeability as well as an increase in protein production, which collectively may facilitate healing.

The nonthermal effects of therapeutic ultrasound in the treatment of injured tissues may be as important as the thermal effects and perhaps are even more important. The nonthermal effects—cavitation and microstreaming—can be maximized and the thermal effects minimized by using an intensity of 0.1 to 0.2 W/cm^2 with continuous ultrasound or 1.0 W/cm^2 at a duty cycle of 20 percent.

Acute conditions require frequent treatments over a short period of time, whereas chronic conditions require fewer treatments over a longer period of time.[13] Ultrasound treatments should begin as soon as possible after injury, ideally within hours but definitely within 48 hours, to maximize their effects on the healing process.[14] Acute conditions may be treated using low-intensity ultrasound once or twice daily for 6 to 8 days until acute symptoms, such as pain and swelling, subside. In chronic conditions, when acute symptoms have subsided, treatment may be done on alternating days for a total of 10 to 12 treatments.

Application There are a number of options for using ultrasound in sports medicine.

Direct skin application Because acoustic energy cannot travel through air and is reflected by the skin, there must be a **coupling medium** applied to the skin.[14] Coupling media include a variety of materials, such as mineral oil and water-soluble creams or gels.

> **coupling medium** Used to facilitate the transmission of ultrasound into the tissues.

The purpose of a coupling medium is to provide an airtight contact with the skin and a slick, low-friction surface. When a water-soluble material is used, the skin should first be washed and dried to prevent air bubbles from hampering the flow of acoustic energy into the skin (Figure 15–14). The use of topical analgesics as a coupling medium has also been recommended, although their effectiveness has not been clearly demonstrated.[42]

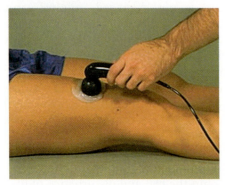

FIGURE 15–14 Ultrasound therapy, when applied directly to the skin, must be performed over a coupling medium because acoustic energy cannot travel through air.

Underwater application Underwater ultrasound is suggested for such irregular body parts as the wrist, hand, elbow, knee, ankle, and foot. The part is fully submerged in water; then the ultrasound head is submerged and positioned approximately 1 inch (2.5 cm) from the body part to be treated. The water medium provides an airtight coupling and allows sound waves to travel at a constant velocity. To ensure uninterrupted therapy, air bubbles that form on the skin must be continually wiped away. The sound head is moved slowly in a circular or longitudinal pattern.[14]

Underwater application should be done in a plastic or rubber (nonmetal), container to avoid reflection of energy off metal walls.

Gel pad technique If, for some reason, the treatment area cannot be immersed in water, a gel pad technique can be used. In this technique, a gel pad is applied to the treatment area, and the ultrasound energy is transmitted from the transducer to the treatment surface through this pad. Both sides of the pad should be coated with gel to ensure good contact.[4]

Moving the transducer Moving the transducer during treatment leads to a more even distribution of energy within the treatment area and can reduce the likelihood of developing hot spots. The transducer should be moved slowly at approximately 1½ inches (4 cm) per second. The transducer should be kept in maximum contact with the skin via some coupling agent throughout the treatment.

Movement of the transducer can be in a circular pattern or a stroking pattern. In the circular pattern, the transducer is applied in small, overlapping circles. In the stroking pattern, the transducer is moved back and forth, overlapping the preceding stroke by half. Both techniques are performed slowly and deliberately. The field covered should not exceed 3 to 4 inches (7.5 to 10 cm). The pattern is determined mainly by the skin area to be treated. For example, the circular pattern is best for highly localized areas, such as the shoulder, whereas the stroking pattern is best used in larger, more diffuse areas. When a highly irregular surface area is to be given therapy, the underwater method should be used.[14]

Dosage and treatment time Dosage of ultrasound varies according to the depth of the tissue treated and the state of injury, such as subacute or chronic.[14]

Basically, 0.1 to 0.3 W/cm² is regarded as low intensity, 0.4 to 1.5 W/cm² is medium intensity, and 1.5 to 3 W/cm² is high intensity. [22] The duration of treatment ranges from 5 to 10 minutes.

Special Considerations Although ultrasound is a relatively safe modality, certain precautions must be taken, and ultrasound should never be used in some situations. Great care must be taken when treating anesthetized areas because the sensation of pain is one of the best indicators of overdosage. Great precaution must be used in areas that have reduced circulation. In general, ultrasound must not be applied to highly fluid areas of the body, such as the eyes, ears, testes, brain, spinal cord, and heart. Reproductive organs and women who are pregnant must not receive ultrasound. Acute injuries should not be treated with thermal ultrasound, although nonthermal ultrasound is useful in managing acute injury. Epiphyseal areas in children should have only minimal ultrasound exposure. [14]

Ultrasound in combination with other modalities In an athletic training environment, it is not uncommon to combine modalities to accomplish a treatment goal. Ultrasound is frequently used with other modalities, including hot packs, cold packs, and electrical stimulating currents.

> Ultrasound is commonly used in conjunction with other modalities.

Hot packs and ultrasound are a useful combination because of the relaxing effects of hot packs in muscle spasm or muscle guarding. Hot packs produce more superficial heating, whereas ultrasound produces heating in the deeper tissues. The use of a hot pack and 1 MHz ultrasound treatments appears to have an additive effect on muscle temperature. [11]

Cold packs are frequently used before ultrasound application. However, if the treatment goal is an increase in deep-tissue temperature, the use of a cold pack before ultrasound interferes with heating and is not recommended. [14,16]

Ultrasound is often used with electrical stimulating currents and is thought to be particularly effective in treating trigger points and acupuncture points. Ultrasound increases the blood flow to the deep tissues, and the electrical currents produce a muscle contraction or modulate pain associated with an injury (Figure 15–15). [14]

15–4 Clinical Application Exercise

An athletic trainer is treating a woman who injured her back while picking up her 2-year-old. She has painful muscle spasms and guarding of the entire low back on both sides.

? How can the athletic trainer use ultrasound to treat this problem?

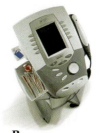
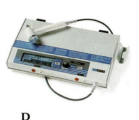

FIGURE 15–15 Combination ultrasound and electrical stimulator units. **(A)** Vectorgonic Combi. **(B)** Intellect Legend XT Combination System. **(C)** MedCon VC. **(D)** Theramini 3C.

Phonophoresis

Equipment Phonophoresis is a method of transporting medications through the skin using the mechanical vibrations produced by an ultrasound generator. [1]

Indications Phonophoresis is predominantly used to introduce hydrocortisone and an anesthetic into the tissues. Many clinicians prefer to use a 10 percent hydrocortisone ointment. [1] Sometimes lidocaine is added to the cortisone to provide a local anesthetic effect. This method has been proposed for treating painful trigger points, tendinitis, and bursitis. [14]

> Phonophoresis is a method of transporting molecules through the skin with ultrasound.

Application This medicine is massaged into the skin over an area of tendinitis, bursitis, or other chronic soft-tissue condition. A coupling gel is then spread over the medication, and the ultrasound is applied. Chempads are commercially produced pads that are impregnated with medication; they may be used instead of the traditional medicated ointment application. The effectiveness of phonophoresis as a treatment technique is questionable and needs further research. [1]

Special Considerations The techniques of phonophoresis and iontophoresis are often confused, and occasionally the two terms are erroneously interchanged. Both techniques are used to deliver chemicals to various biological tissues. Phonophoresis involves the use of acoustic energy in the form of ultrasound to transport whole molecules across the skin into the tissues, whereas iontophoresis uses an electrical current to transport ions into the tissues. Some athletic trainers prefer phonophoresis to iontophoresis, indicating that it is less hazardous to the skin and that there is greater penetration.[14]

MECHANICAL ENERGY MODALITIES

Traction

Traction is a drawing tension applied to a body segment. It is most commonly used in the cervical and lumbar regions of the spine.[24]

Physiological Effects Traction is used to produce separation of the vertebral bodies and in so doing can effect stretching of the ligaments and joint capsules of the spine, stretching of spinal and paraspinal muscles, increased separation of the articular facet joints, relief in pressure on nerves and nerve roots, decrease in the central pressure of the intervertebral disks. (allowing for the movement of herniated disk material back into the center of the disk), increases of and changes in joint proprioception, and relief of the compressive effects of normal posture.[24]

> Traction is commonly used in the cervical and lumbar spine.

Indications Traction is most commonly used for the treatment of spinal nerve root impingement, which has many causes, including vertebral disk herniation or prolapse and spondylolisthesis (see Chapter 25). It may also be used to decrease muscle guarding, treat muscle strain or sprain of the spinal ligaments, and relax discomfort resulting from normal spinal compression.

Application Traction may be applied to the spine through the use of manual techniques or mechanical traction, including table traction units, wall-mounted traction units, and inverted traction techniques.

Manual traction Manual traction is infinitely more adaptable and offers greater flexibility than mechanical traction. Changes in force, direction, duration, and patient position can be made instantaneously as the athletic trainer senses relaxation or resistance (Figure 15–16).

Mechanical traction For mechanical lumbar traction, a split table with a movable section to eliminate friction must be used to allow for smooth, nonrestricted traction. A nonslip traction harness applied directly to the skin is needed to transfer the traction force comfortably to the patient and to stabilize the trunk while the lumbar spine is placed under traction (Figure 15–17). For cervical traction, the patient

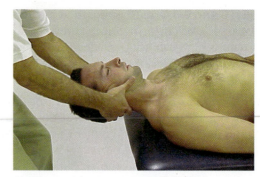

FIGURE 15–16   Manual cervical traction.

may be either in the supine or the sitting position. A nonslip cervical harness should be secured under the chin and back of the head.

Positional traction Positional traction is used on a trial-and-error basis to determine maximum position of comfort or to accomplish a specific treatment goal. For example, placing a patient with a lumbar disk problem in a back-lying position with the hips and knees flexed and supported at 90 degrees increases the opening of the foramen and takes pressure off the disk, thus minimizing pain and making the athlete more comfortable.[24]

Wall-mounted traction Cervical traction can be accomplished with a wall-mounted system. Plates, sand bags, or water bags can be used for weights. These units are relatively inexpensive and effective (Figure 15–18).

Inverted traction Specialized equipment or simply hanging upside down places the person in an inverted position. The spine is lengthened because of the stretch provided by the weight of the trunk (Figure 15–19).[10]

Special Considerations Good results have been achieved using both intermittent and sustained traction. In most cases of lumbar disk problems, sustained traction seems to be the treatment of choice.

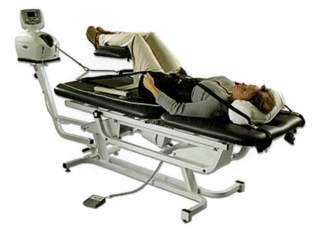

FIGURE 15–17   Lumbar traction using a split table and a traction machine.
(Courtesy Chattanooga Group)

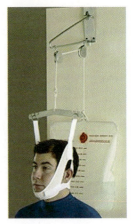

FIGURE 15–18   Cervical traction using a wall-mounted unit.

Intermittent traction is considered to be more comfortable.[24] Progressive traction increases the traction force gradually in a preselected number of steps, which allows the athlete to adapt slowly to the traction and helps him or her stay relaxed. Recommendations on length of treatment and on/off times vary depending on the specific problem to be treated. For the lumbar spine, a traction force equal to one-half the patient's body weight is a good guideline to use in selecting a force high enough to cause vertebral separation. Cervical traction forces can be adjusted from 20 to 50 pounds (9 to 23 kg), depending on patient comfort and response.

Intermittent Compression

Equipment Intermittent compression makes use of a nylon pneumatic inflatable sleeve applied around the injured extremity (Figure 15–20).[33] The sleeve can be inflated to a specific pressure that forces excessive fluid accumulated in the interstitial spaces into vascular and lymphatic channels, through which it is

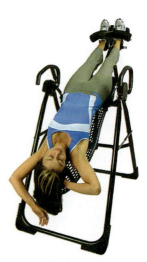

FIGURE 15–19   Inverted traction apparatus.
(Courtesy Teeter Hangups)

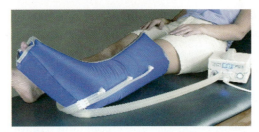

FIGURE 15–20   Intermittent compression devices are designed to reduce edema after injury.
(Courtesy Chattanooga Group)

removed from the area of injury. Compression facilitates the movement of lymphatic fluid, which helps eliminate the byproducts of the injury process.[35]

Indications Intermittent compression units are used for controlling or reducing swelling after one acute injury or for pitting edema, which tends to develop in the injured area several hours after injury.[23] The extremity should be elevated during treatment. It is also common to use electrical stimulating currents to produce muscle pumping, thus facilitating lymphatic flow.

Application Intermittent compression devices have three adjustable parameters: on/off time, inflation pressures, and treatment time. Recommended treatment protocols have been established through clinical trial and error, with little experimental data currently available to support any protocol.[51] On/off times are variable, including 1 minute on, 2 minutes off; 2 minutes on, 1 minute off; and 4 minutes on, 1 minute off. Again, these recommendations are not research based. Patient comfort should be the primary guide.

Recommended inflation pressures have been loosely correlated with blood pressures. The Jobst Institute recommends that pressure be set at 30 to 50 mm Hg for the upper extremity and at 30 to 60 mm Hg for the lower extremity. Because arterial capillary pressures are "approximately 30 mm Hg, any pressure that exceeds this level should encourage the absorption of edema and the flow of lymphatic fluid."[23] Clinical studies have demonstrated a significant reduction in limb volume after 30 minutes of compression.[2,23] Thus, a 30-minute treatment time seems to be efficient in reducing edema.

Special Considerations Some intermittent compression units have the capability of combining cold along with compression, which is more effective in reducing edema.[2,25] The *Cryo-Cuff* is a device that uses both cold and compression simultaneously (Figure 15–21A). The Cryo-Cuff is used both acutely following injury and postsurgically. It is made of a nylon sleeve that connects via a tube to a 1-gallon (3.8 L) cooler/jug. Cold water flows into the sleeve from the cooler. As the cooler is raised, the pressure in the cuff is increased. During the treatment, the water warms and can be rechilled by lowering the cooler to drain the cuff, mixing the warmer water with the colder water, and then again raising the jug to increase pressure in the cuff. The only drawback to this simple yet effective piece of equipment is that the water in the cuff must be continually rechilled. However, the Cryo-Cuff is portable, easy to use, and inexpensive. Other cold and compression units include the *Game Ready Accelerated Recovery System, VitalWrap,* and the *Polar Cub.*

15–6 Clinical Application Exercise

A patient who stepped off a curb comes to the hospital with a 2-day-old postacute ankle sprain. The initial injury was not managed appropriately; as a result, the patient has a considerable amount of swelling. He has little range of motion and is capable of only touch down weight bearing.

? The patient will have a difficult time regaining function until the swelling is reduced. What therapeutic modalities can reduce this postacute lymphedema?

The *Game Ready Accelerated Recovery System* consists of various soft wraps and a control unit designed to simultaneously deliver cold therapy and intermittent compression (Figure 15–21B). The wraps are made from flexible fabric designed to fit various body parts. The wraps fit snugly to apply consistent cooling and intermittent pressure to an injury. To operate the system, the control unit reservoir is filled with ice water, which is circulated through the wraps over the course of a standard treatment program, which can be customized for various time, temperature, and compression settings.

Massage

Massage is the systematic manipulation of the soft tissues of the body. The movements of gliding, compressing, stretching, percussing, and vibrating are regulated to produce specific responses in the patient.[19]

Indications Massage seems to be regaining popularity among athletic trainers as a treatment modality. Manipulation of soft tissue by massage is a useful adjunct to other modalities.[3] Massage causes mechanical, physiological, and psychological responses.[47]

Mechanical responses Mechanical responses to massage occur as a direct result of the graded pressures and movements of the hand on the body. Such actions encourage venous and lymphatic drainage and mildly stretch superficial and scar tissue.[61] Connective tissue can be stretched effectively by friction massage, which helps prevent rigidity in scar formation. When a patient is forced to remain inactive while an injury heals or when edema surrounds a joint, the stagnation of circulation may be prevented by using certain massage techniques.[20]

Physiological responses Massage can increase circulation and, as a result, increase metabolism to the musculature and aid in the removal of metabolites, such as lactic acid.[19] It also helps overcome venostasis and edema by increasing circulation at and around the

15–7 Clinical Application Exercise

A track and field athlete complains of pain in his left knee. The athletic trainer assesses the injury as patellar tendinitis.

? What type of massage may be indicated for this condition in the acute stage? What type of massage may be indicated for this condition after a few days?

Physiological responses to massage:

• Reflex effects
• Relaxation
• Stimulation
• Increased circulation

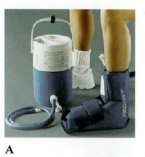
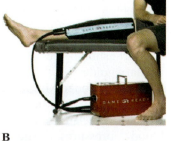
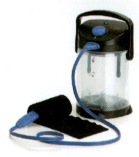
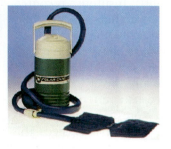

A   **B**

C   **D**

FIGURE 15–21 Portable compression and cold systems. **(A)** Cryo-Cuff. **(B)** Game Ready Accelerated Recovery System. **(C)** VitalWrap. **(D)** Polar Cub.

injury site, assisting in the normal venous blood return to the heart.[62]

The reflex effects of massage are processes that, in response to nerve impulses initiated through rubbing the body, are transmitted to one organ by afferent nerve fibers and then back to another organ by efferent fibers. Reflex responses elicit a variety of organ reactions, such as body relaxation, stimulation, and increased circulation.[47]

Relaxation can be induced by slow, superficial stroking of the skin. It is a type of massage that is beneficial for tense, anxious patients who may require gentle treatment.

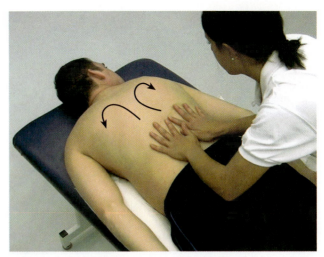

FIGURE 15–22   Effleurage: light stroking.

Stimulation is attained by quick, brisk action that causes a contraction of superficial tissue. The benefits derived by the patient are predominantly psychological. He or she feels invigorated after intense manipulation of the tissue.

Increased circulation is accomplished by mechanical and reflex stimuli. Together they cause the capillaries to dilate and be drained of fluid as a result of firm outside pressure, thus stimulating cell metabolism, eliminating toxins, and increasing lymphatic and venous circulation. In this way the healing process is aided.[62]

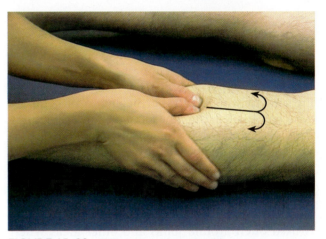

FIGURE 15–23   Effleurage: deep stroking.

Psychological responses The tactile system is one of the most sensitive systems in the human organism. From earliest infancy, humans respond psychologically to being touched. Because massage is the act of laying on of hands, it can be an important means for creating a bond of confidence between the athletic trainer and the patient.[47]

Application Massage strokes can be separated into five basic categories: effleurage, petrissage, friction, tapotement, and vibration.

Effleurage **Effleurage**, or stroking (Figure 15–22), is divided into light and deep methods. Light stroking is designed primarily to be sedative. It is also used in the early stages of injury treatment. Deep stroking is a therapeutic compression of soft tissue, which encourages venous and lymphatic drainage. A different application of effleurage may be used for a specific body part (Figure 15–23).

There are many variations in effleurage massage; some that are of particular value to sports injuries are pressure variations, the hand-over-hand

| **effleurage** Stroking. |

method, and the cross-body method.[19] Pressure variations range from very light to deep and vigorous stroking. Light stroking, as discussed previously, can induce relaxation or may be used when an area is especially sensitive to touch; on the other hand, deep massage is designed to bring about definite physiological responses. Light and deep effleurage can be used alternately when both features are desired. The hand-over-hand stroking method is of special benefit to those surface areas that are particularly unyielding. It is performed by an alternate stroke in which one hand strokes, followed immediately by the other hand, somewhat like shingles on a roof. The cross-body effleurage technique is an excellent massage for the low back region. The athletic trainer places a hand on each side of the patient's spine. Both hands first stroke simultaneously away from the spine; then both hands at the same time stroke toward the spine (Figure 15–24).

Petrissage Kneading, or **petrissage** (Figure 15–25), is a technique adaptable primarily to loose and heavy tissue areas, such as the trapezius, latissimus dorsi, and

| **petrissage** Kneading. |

15–8 Clinical Application Exercise

A javelin thrower has a muscle strain in his back. He comes into the sports medicine clinic on the sixth day after the initial injury, complaining of pain. He asks the athletic trainer whether anything can be done to help modulate his pain.

? What modalities can the athletic trainer use to modulate the pain?

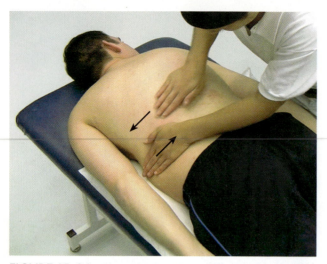

FIGURE 15–24   Cross-body effleurage.

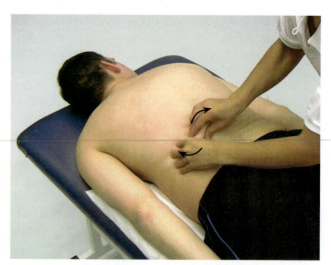

FIGURE 15–25   Petrissage (kneading).

triceps muscles. The procedure consists of picking up the muscle and skin tissue between the thumb and forefinger of each hand and rolling and twisting them in opposite directions. As one hand is rolling and twisting, the other begins to pick up the adjacent tissue. The kneading action wrings out the muscle, thus loosening adhesions and squeezing congestive materials into the general circulation. Picking up skin may cause an irritating pinch. Whenever possible, deep muscle tissue should be gathered and lifted.

Friction   The **friction** massage (Figure 15–26) is used often around joints and other areas where

| **friction** Heat-producing massage. |

tissue is thin and on tissues that are especially unyielding, such as scars, adhesions, muscle spasms, and fascia. The action is initiated by bracing with the heels of the hands, then either holding the thumbs steady and moving the fingers in a circular motion or holding the fingers steady

and moving the thumbs in a circular motion. Each method is adaptable to the type of area or articulation that is being massaged. The motion is started at a central point, and then a circular movement is initiated, with the hands moving in opposite directions away from the center point. The purpose is to stretch the underlying tissue, develop friction in the area, and increase circulation around the joint.[47]

Tapotement   The most popular methods of **tapotement**, or percussion,

are cupping, hacking, and pinching movements.

| **tapotement** Percussion. |

Cupping   The cupping action produces an invigorating and stimulating sensation. It is a series of percussion movements rapidly duplicated at a constant tempo. The hands are cupped to such an extent that the beat emits a dull and hollow sound, unlike the sound of the slap of the open hand. The hands move alternately, from the wrist, with the elbow flexed and the upper arm stabilized

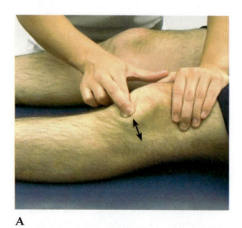

A

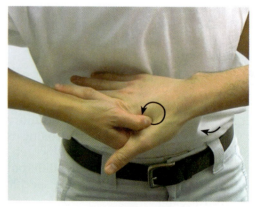

B

FIGURE 15–26   Friction massage. **(A)** Transverse friction technique–one finger crossed over another. **(B)** Circular friction technique using the thumb.

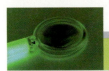
Guidelines for an effective massage

Besides knowing the different kinds of massage, the athletic trainer should understand how to give the most effective massage. The following rules should be used whenever possible:

1. Make the patient comfortable.
   a. Place the body in the proper position on the table.
   b. Place a pad under the areas of the body that are to be massaged.
   c. Keep the room at a constant 72°F (22.2°C) temperature.
   d. Respect the patient's privacy by draping him or her with a blanket or towel, exposing only the body parts to be massaged.

2. Develop a confident, gentle approach when massaging.
   a. Assume a position that is easy both on you and on the patient.
   b. Avoid using too harsh a stroke, or further injury may result.
3. To ensure proper lymphatic and venous drainage, stroke toward the heart whenever possible.
4. Know when not to use massage.
   a. Never give a massage if the patient may have a local or general infection. To do so may encourage the infection's spread or may aggravate the condition.
   b. Never apply massage directly over a recent injury; limit stroking to the periphery. Massaging over recent injuries may dislodge the clot organization and start bleeding.

(Figure 15–27A). The cupping action should be executed until the skin in the area develops a pinkish coloration.

Hacking Hacking can be used in conjunction with cupping to bring about a varied stimulation of the sensory nerves (Figure 15–27B). Hacking is similar to cupping except that the hands are rotated externally and the ulnar, or little finger, border of the hand is the striking surface. Only the heavy muscle areas should be treated in this manner.

Pinching Although pinching is not in the strictest sense percussive, it is categorized under tapotement because of the vigor with which it is applied. Alternating hands lift small amounts of tissue between the first finger and thumb in quick, gentle pinching movements (Figure 15–27C).

Vibration **Vibration** is rapid movement that produces a quivering or trembling effect. It is used in sports because of its ability to relax and soothe. Although

| **vibration** Rapid shaking. |

vibration can be done manually, the machine vibrator is usually the preferred modality.

Special Considerations Therapeutic massage performed by athletic trainers is usually confined to a specific area and is seldom given to the full body.[3] The time required for giving an adequate and complete body massage is excessive. It is not usually feasible to devote this much time to one patient; 5 minutes is usually all that is required for massaging a given area. *Focus Box 15–4*: "Guidelines for an effective massage" provides suggestions for giving an effective massage.

Massage lubricants To enable the hands to slide easily over the body, a friction-reducing medium must be used. Rubbing the dry body can cause gross skin irritation by tearing and pulling on the hair. Many media (e.g., fine powders, oil liniments, or almost any substance having a petroleum base) can be used as a lubricant.

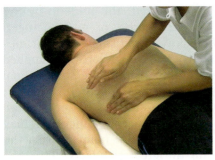
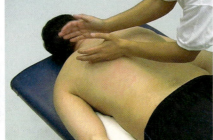
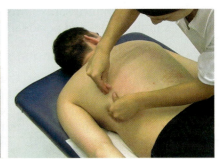

A   B   C

FIGURE 15–27 Tapotement. **(A)** Cupping. **(B)** Hacking. **(C)** Pinching.

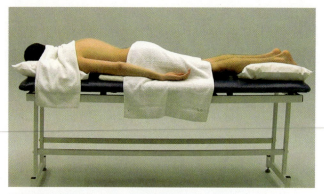

FIGURE 15–28 The patient should be placed in a position of comfort and appropriately draped with towels or sheets.

Positioning the patient It is important to position a patient properly for a massage. The injured body part must be easily accessible, the patient must be comfortable, and the part to be massaged must be relaxed (Figure 15–28).

Confidence Inexperienced hands can transmit a lack of confidence. Every effort should be made to think out the procedure to be used and to present a confident appearance to the patient.

Ensuring patient privacy and athletic trainer Integrity As is the case with a number of other therapeutic techniques, massage involves direct physical contact between the athletic trainer and the patient. It is critical that the athletic trainer be aware of and, if necessary, take the required precautions to ensure that this physical contact can in no way be construed or misinterpreted as being inappropriate. This is particularly important when dealing with a patient of the opposite sex or with patients who are under legal age. The athletic trainer should always make certain that only the body part or body region being treated is exposed and that the rest of the body is appropriately covered or draped. It is also advisable to perform the massage with another patient or athletic trainer physically present in the same room or to do the massage in plain view of others in the athletic training clinic. There is no good reason not to take these precautions, and failure to do so may create situations that unnecessarily threaten the athletic trainer's professional and personal integrity.

Deep Transverse Friction Massage

Indications The transverse, or Cyriax, method of deep friction massage is a specific technique for treating muscles, tendons, ligaments, and joint capsules. The major purpose of transverse massage is to move transversely across a ligament or tendon to mobilize

> Transverse massage is a method of deep transverse friction massage.

it as much as possible. This technique often precedes active exercise. Deep transverse friction massage restores mobility to a muscle in the same way that mobilization frees a joint.[19]

Application The position of the athletic trainer's hands is important in gaining maximum strength and control. Four positions are suggested: index finger crossed over middle finger, middle finger crossed over index finger, two fingers side by side, and opposed finger and thumb.

The massage must be directly over the site of lesion and pain. The fingers move with the skin and do not slide over it. Massage must be across the grain of the affected tissue. The thicker the structure, the more friction is given.[19] The technique is to sweep back and forth over the full width of the tissue.

Special Considerations Massage should not be given to acute injuries or over highly swollen tissues. A few minutes of this method will produce a numbness in the area, and exercise or mobilization can be instituted.

Acupressure Massage

Indications Acupressure is a type of massage based on the ancient Chinese art of acupuncture. Physiological explanations of the effectiveness of acupressure massage may likely be attributed to some interaction of the various mechanisms of pain modulation.

Application The athletic trainer uses acupuncture charts to select specific points that are described in the literature as having some relationship to the area of pain. The charts provide a general idea of where these points are located. Two techniques may be used to specifically locate acupressure points. Because it is known that electrical impedance is reduced at acupuncture points, an ohmmeter may be used to locate the points. Perhaps the easiest technique is for the athletic trainer simply to palpate the area until he or she feels either a small, fibrous nodule or a strip of tense muscle tissue that is tender to the touch.

Once the point is located, the athletic trainer begins massage with the index or middle finger, the thumb, or the elbow, using small, circular motions on the point. The amount of pressure applied to these acupressure points should be submaximal and determined by patient tolerance.

Effective treatment times range from one to five minutes at a single point per treatment. It may be necessary to massage several points during the treatment to obtain the greatest effects. If so, the athletic trainer should work distal points first and move proximally.

Special Considerations During the massage, the patient will report a dulling or numbing effect and will frequently indicate that the pain has diminished or subsided totally during the massage. The lingering effects of acupressure massage vary tremendously from patient to patient. The effects may last for only a few minutes in some but may persist in others for several hours.

MODALITIES NOT COMMONLY USED BY ATHLETIC TRAINERS

Several therapeutic modalities marketed as therapeutic devices are seldom used by athletic trainers. Magnet therapy has little evidence-based support in the professional literature, although a search of the Internet reveals significant anecdotal information about magnet use. Extracorporal shock wave therapy has been used for many years for a variety of purposes. This modality has been approved by the FDA, and there is considerable experimental evidence in the professional literature to support its use. Nevertheless, athletic trainers rarely use these modalities, and they are included here for informational purposes only.

Magnet Therapy

Magnet therapy has become popular among both competitive and recreational athletes. An increasing number of athletic trainers are using magnets as a treatment modality for a variety of musculoskeletal ailments. Although a wealth of anecdotal information on magnet therapy can be found in the popular literature, a careful review of the medical literature indicates few data-based research articles on the efficacy or potential therapeutic benefits of using magnets.

Magnet therapy is the application of a magnetic field to the human body. A magnet is a natural ferrous material with inseparable positively and negatively charged poles that characteristically attract particles of opposite charge and repel particles of similar charge. The strength of a magnetic field is measured in Gauss units. Most therapeutic magnets range between 300 and 1,000 Gauss. The explanations of the potential beneficial physiological effects of magnets include changes in polarity within a damaged cell, increased blood flow and thus increased oxygen saturation, increased muscle strength, increased hormone secretions, increased cell division rate, increased enzyme activity, increased lymphatic flow, and changes in blood pH. It has been shown that magnets do not appear to cause a local increase in tissue temperature.[54]

Although magnet therapy appears to be a relatively safe treatment modality, athletic trainers should use it with caution until some definitive basis for use has been determined scientifically.

Extracorporeal Shock Wave Therapy (ESWT)

Extracorporeal shock wave therapy (ESWT) is a pulsed, high-pressure, short-duration (<1 ms) acoustic sound wave that is produced by a generator and transmitted through a coupling medium over a large skin area to a specific target region with little attenuation.[53] This acoustic energy is concentrated in a focal area 0.08 to 0.3 inch (2 to 8 mm) in diameter. The treatment uses a sequence of 1,000 to 4,000 shock wave pulses at 1 to 4 pps. Focusing is checked every 200 to 400 shocks, and treatment lasts for 15 to 30 minutes. Shock wave therapy was first used for kidney stone fragmentation in the early 1980s.

Currently, because of its high cost, this modality is most likely to be found in a hospital, although there are a few athletic training facilities that have ESWT available. Imaging devices (e.g., ultrasound, X-ray) are sometimes used to target energy precisely but are not necessary in extremities.[55] Shock waves are applied to the point of maximal tenderness at the lowest energy setting. With direct patient feedback, the exact site of pain and pathology is identified. The intensity is slowly increased within the patient's level of tolerance. Anesthesia is sometimes used to minimize the pain associated with the treatment. However, anesthesia is not only unnecessary but also undesirable, because only the patient can verify that the correct site has been targeted. If the pain is not reproduced by the shock wave, the condition is unlikely to respond. Since the mid-1990s, ESWT has been approved for use in treating tennis elbow, plantar fasciitis, and nonunion fractures as well as for its analgesic effects. The mechanism of action is not well understood, but the healing that occurs with EWST has been attributed to enhanced metabolism, circulation, and revascularization.[59]

Because this is a relatively new modality, techniques for using ESWT have not yet been standardized. Precise dosages and optimal frequency of application have not been studied extensively. It has not been demonstrated whether shock waves should be directed to the target area by radiological or ultrasound imaging. Also, it is not yet clear whether local anesthetic injections should be used in the target area prior to treatment to reduce pain.[32]

RECORDING THERAPEUTIC MODALITY TREATMENTS

Athletic trainers who use a therapeutic modality in treatment need to record the procedure. The specifics of the modality treatment should be recorded on the original SOAP note, the progress note, and a therapeutic modalities treatment log like the one

Patient's Name _____

Diagnosis _____ Date of Injury _____

Athletic Trainer _____

Therapeutic Modality _____

Treatment Parameters

    Intensity/Output _____

    Frequency _____

    Duty Cycle _____

    Temperature _____

    Duration of Treatment _____

    Electrode Placement _____

Special Instructions:

Month/Year _____

Date Administered:

1234567891011121314151617181920212223242526272829303 1

FIGURE 15–29 Therapeutic modalities treatment log.

shown in Figure 15–29. Changes in the treatment parameters should be noted on the treatment log, so that anyone administering a treatment modality can consult the log to determine the appropriate parameters.

SAFETY IN USING THERAPEUTIC MODALITIES

When using any type of therapeutic modality, the athletic trainer must ensure that the equipment is used and maintained in an appropriate manner.[2,23] Manufacturers of therapeutic modality equipment usually provide written guidelines and recommendations for appropriate care and maintenance in the manuals that accompany new equipment. There is usually a regular maintenance schedule for each piece of equipment, designed to discover any defects or breakdowns that occur due to normal wear and tear. The athletic trainer should be familiar with and closely follow the manufacturer's recommendations for equipment maintenance. Failure to do so may make the athletic trainer legally negligent, should an incident occur that results in an unnecessary injury to a patient. The athletic trainer should arrange to have the maintenance done either by the manufacturer or by some other qualified agency. *Focus Box 15–5*: "Safe Use of Therapeutic Modalities" lists recommended safety practices for using and maintaining therapeutic equipment.

EVIDENCE-BASED DATA REGARDING THERAPEUTIC MODALITY USE

Despite the fact that therapeutic modalities are widely used by athletic trainers, as well as physical therapists, occupational therapists, and chiropractors, in general, their clinical effectiveness in treating a variety of conditions has yet to be established. For many years, health care professionals have tended to rely on information from therapeutic modality manufacturers, rather than on scientific evidence-based data generated by competent researchers from within the health care professions. A review of the relatively scarce evidence-based data in the scientific literature should lead the athletic trainer to seriously question how therapeutic modalities should be most appropriately incorporated into clinical treatment regimens. As health care professionals, athletic trainers have a responsibility to put the best available evidence to use when selecting clinical techniques for treating their patients.[29] Knowing that the evidence for the therapeutic effects of a particular modality is inadequate and applying it anyway presents a problematic level of accountability that the athletic trainer must consider.[29] Athletic trainers should work with equipment manufacturers to produce solid scientific data that determine the clinical efficacy of using a particular therapeutic modality as a treatment tool.

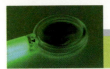

FOCUS 15–5 Focus on Treatment and Rehabilitation

Safe use of therapeutic modalities[25]

The following safety practices should be considered when using any type of electrical therapeutic modality:

- The entire electrical system of the building or athletic training room should be designed or evaluated by a qualified electrician. Problems with the electrical system may exist in older buildings or in rooms that have been modified to accommodate therapeutic devices (e.g., putting a whirlpool in a locker room where the concrete floor is always wet or damp).
- It should not be assumed that all three-pronged wall outlets are grounded. The ground must be checked.
- Ground fault interrupters (GFIs) should be used with all modalities that plug into a wall outlet. GFIs detect decreases in voltage output and can shut down electrical current automatically, should a problem occur.

- The athletic trainer should become very familiar with the equipment being used and with any potential or existing problems. Any defective equipment should be immediately removed from the clinic.
- The plug should not be jerked out of the wall by pulling on the cable.
- Extension cords or multiple adapters should never be used.
- Equipment should be calibrated yearly and should conform to *National Electrical Code* guidelines. If a clinic or an athletic training facility is not in compliance with this Code, then there is no legal protection in a lawsuit.
- Common sense should always be exercised when using electrotherapeutic devices. A situation that appears to be dangerous may, in fact, result in injury or death.

SUMMARY

- To avoid legal problems, athletic trainers must use therapeutic modalities with extreme care. Athletic trainers must be familiar with the laws of their state regarding therapeutic modality use. Before using any modality, the athletic trainer must have a thorough understanding of its function and when it should and should not be used.
- The forms of energy that are relevant to the use of therapeutic modalities are thermal conductive energy, electrical energy, electromagnetic energy, sound energy, and mechanical energy.
- Thermotherapy increases blood flow, increases collagen viscosity, decreases joint stiffness, and reduces pain and muscle spasm. When the body's temperature is raised, tissue metabolism is increased, vascular permeability is increased, and chemicals (such as histamine, bradykinin, and serotonin) are released.
- Heat energy is transmitted through conduction, convection, radiation, and conversion. Conduction occurs when heat is transferred from a warmer object to a cooler one. Convection heating occurs by means of fluid or gas movement. Radiation is heat energy that is transmitted through empty space. Conversion is heat that is generated when one type of energy is changed to another.
- Superficial therapeutic heat should not be applied when there is a loss of sensation, immediately after an acute injury, and when there is decreased arterial bleeding. Superficial therapeutic heat

should not be used over the eyes or genitals or over the abdomen of a pregnant woman. Types of superficial heat are moist heat packs, whirlpool baths, paraffin baths, and fluidotherapy.

- The use of cold for therapeutic purposes and as part of an emergency procedure is extremely popular in sports medicine. Cold penetrates more deeply than superficial heat. Therapy is usually performed when the tissue has reached a state of relative anesthesia. Cryotherapy decreases muscle spasm, pain perception, and blood flow. It increases the inelasticity of collagen fibers, joint stiffness, and capillary permeability. Common cryotherapy procedures and tools are ice massage, cold-water immersion, ice packs, vapocoolant sprays, and cryokinetics.
- The use of electrical stimulating currents is popular in sports medicine. Electrical stimulating units produce monophasic current (DC), biphasic current (AC), or pulsatile current. Both monophasic and biphasic current can be used for pain modulation and muscle contraction. Direct current can also be used for iontophoresis. The physiological effects of electrical current are determined by the treatment parameters and equipment selected. Current parameters include waveform, modulation, intensity, duration, frequency, polarity, and electrode setup. Interferential currents and low-intensity stimulators are two of the newest electrical stimulating currents available to the athletic trainer.

- Shortwave diathermy units produce heat through electromagnetic energy, whereas ultrasound produces heat through acoustic energy. The contraindications for the use of shortwave diathermy are the same as for superficial heating, with the additional restrictions of no implants, jewelry, or intrauterine devices.
- The low-level laser may be used to stimulate the healing process or to modulate pain.
- Ultrasound is a form of sound energy. It creates a mechanical vibration that is converted to heat energy within the body. Heating occurs in the denser tissues, such as bone and connective tissue. More heat is built up at tissue interfaces. Ultrasound has both thermal and nonthermal physiological effects. It can be combined with electrical stimulation or used to transport molecules through the skin with the method known as phonophoresis.
- Traction is used to produce separation of the vertebrae, most commonly for the treatment of spinal nerve root impingement and associated abnormalities. It is typically used in the cervical and lumbar spine and may involve either manual or mechanical traction.
- Intermittent compression devices are used to control swelling after acute injury and to reduce pitting edema.
- Massage is a useful modality for many sports-related injuries. Techniques include effleurage, petrissage, friction, tapotement, and vibration. Deep transverse massage is used on connective tissue.

WEB SITES

Cramer First Aider:
http://www.cramersportsmed.com/resources/first-aider

National Athletic Trainers' Association:
www.nata.org

SOLUTIONS TO CLINICAL APPLICATION EXERCISES

15–1 The decision is subjective to some extent. The athletic trainer must understand what is going on with the healing process. On the fifth day, the inflammatory process is ending and the fibroblastic stage is establishing itself. At this point it is still advisable to avoid any treatment that may increase swelling, which can interfere with healing. Heat would increase circulation, which might increase swelling. The athletic trainer would not likely exacerbate the injury by using heat, but it is recommended that cold be used during this time. A rule of thumb is that, when the tenderness is gone, it is safe to change to some form of heat.

15–2 Ice massage may be used for Achilles tendinitis and is beneficial, since this area of the body is small. Cold-water immersion is an alternative for cryotherapy. Ice-water immersion is indicated because the injury is in a distal area and the entire area can be iced easily. The athlete is also able to perform cryokinetics simultaneously with the cryotherapy. Another alternative for cryotherapy is the use of ice packs, which can be formed around the ankle.

15–3 At this point, some form of heat to increase blood and lymphatic flow to the injured area is warranted. Increased blood flow will help facilitate the process of healing, and an increased lymphatic flow will help remove the byproducts of the inflammatory process. Hot packs provide superficial heat and would not be effective in this case. Both diathermy and ultrasound would be recommended because they have a depth of penetration great enough to affect the injured area; ultrasound would be somewhat more effective. For best results, stretching and strengthening exercises should always be used along with modalities.

15–4 In this case, the best treatment is to not use ultrasound at all. A better decision would be to use either hydrocollator packs or diathermy, both of which are more useful in treating larger areas. If depth of penetration is a concern, then shortwave diathermy would be the treatment modality of choice.

15–5 The athletic trainer should try using manual lumbar traction techniques, which, if done properly, can be effective in isolating a specific ligament between two lumbar vertebrae. If the athletic trainer cannot manually generate enough traction force to stretch the ligament, a table traction unit or an inverted traction technique may prove to be more useful.

15–6 Proper initial management of the injury could have prevented a great deal of the swelling that has occurred. At this point, the athletic trainer should make use of ice to modulate pain; intermittent compression and electrical stimulating currents to induce a muscle pumping contraction (both of which can help the lymphatic system remove the swelling); and low-intensity ultrasound (>0.2 W/cm^2), which can help facilitate the healing process. In addition, the patient should continually wear a compressive elastic wrap. He must also progress to full weight bearing, concentrating on regaining a normal gait as soon as it can be tolerated.

15–7 Effleurage massage strokes are ideal during the initial stages of injury to help encourage venous and lymphatic drainage, especially if swelling is present. This method also is sedative for the athlete. Friction massage is beneficial for patellar tendinitis to increase circulation in the area and to develop friction.

15–8 The athletic trainer can use cryotherapy, heat, or electrical stimulating currents to help reduce pain. Electrical stimulating currents may be the most useful if the athletic trainer also wants to elicit a muscle contraction to help decrease muscle guarding. Massage also is useful for modulating pain and for relaxing muscles. Regardless of the modality chosen, the athlete should engage in some stretching and strengthening exercises after the treatment.

REVIEW QUESTIONS AND CLASS ACTIVITIES

1. Explain the legal factors that an athletic trainer should consider before using a therapeutic modality.
2. Give examples of modalities that heat through conduction, convection, radiation, and conversion.
3. What physiological changes occur when heat is applied to the body?
4. Discuss the physiological effects of using cryotherapy.
5. Demonstrate the proper technique for a variety of cryotherapeutic approaches.
6. Compare therapy delivered through heat to that delivered through cold. When would you use each?
7. What is a TENS unit?
8. Identify the potential treatment goals of an electrically stimulated muscle contraction.
9. What is shortwave diathermy used for?
10. Discuss how ultrasound can be used during a rehabilitation program.
11. Compare phonophoresis with iontophoresis.
12. List the mechanical effects of cervical and lumbar traction.
13. How is massage best used in a sports medicine setting?
14. Explain when and how intermittent compression can best be used as a treatment modality.

REFERENCES

1. Abrahams S: Phonophoresis of non-steroidal drugs: A review of the clinical evidence, *International Journal of Musculoskeletal Medicine* 30(1):37–41, 2008.
2. Angus J, Prentice W, Hooker D: A comparison of two external intermittent compression devices and their effect on post acute ankle edema, *J Athl Train* 29(2):178, 1994.
3. Archer PA: Three clinical sports massage approaches for treating injured athletes, *Athletic Therapy Today* 6(3):14, 2001.
4. Bishop S, Draper D, Knight K: Human tissue—temperature rise during ultrasound treatments with the Aquaflex gel pad, *J Athl Train* 39(2):126, 2004.
5. Brown C: Evidence-based guidelines for utilization of dexamethasone Iontophoresis, *Athletic Therapy and Training*, 16(4):33–36, 2011.
6. Burke D, Holt L, Rasmussen R: The effect of hot or cold water immersion and proprioceptive neuromuscular facilitation on hip joint range of motion, *J Athl Train* 36(1):16, 2001.
7. Costello J: Cryotherapy and joint position sense in healthy participants: A systematic review, *J Athl Train*, 45(3):306–16, 2010.
8. Dolan M, Mychaskiw A, Mendel F: Coolwater immersion and high-voltage electric stimulation curb edema formation in rats, *J Athl Train* 38(3):225–30, 2003.
9. Draper D: Are certified athletic trainers qualified to use therapeutic modalities? *J Athl Train* 37(1):11, 2002.
10. Draper D: Inversion table traction as a therapeutic modality, Part 1: Oh my aching back, *Athletic Therapy Today* 10(3):42, 2005.
11. Draper DO, Harris ST, Schulthies S, et al: Hot-pack and 1-MHz ultrasound treatments have an additive effect on muscle temperature, *J Athl Train* 33(1):21, 1998.
12. Draper D, Knight K: Interferential current therapy: Often used but misunderstood, *Athletic Therapy Today* 11(4):29, 2006.
13. Draper D, Miner L, Knight K: The carryover effects of diathermy and stretching in developing hamstring flexibility, *J Athl Train* 37(1):37, 2002.
14. Draper D, Prentice W: Therapeutic ultrasound. In Prentice W, editor: *Therapeutic modalities in rehabilitation*, ed 4, New York, 2011, McGraw-Hill.
15. Draper DO, Ricard M: Rate of temperature decay in human muscle following 3-Mhz ultrasound: the stretching window revealed, *J Athl Train* 30(4):304, 1995.
16. Draper D, Schulthies S, Sorvisto P: The effect of cooling the tissue prior to ultrasound treatment, *J Athl Train* 29(2):154, 1994.
17. Draper D, Sunderland S: Examination of the law of Grotthus Draper: Does ultrasound penetrate subcutaneous fat? *J Athl Train* 28(3):246, 1993.
18. French D: The effects of contrast bathing and compression therapy on muscular performance, *Med Sci Sport Exer* 40(7):1297–06, 2008.
19. Fritz S: *Mosby's fundamentals of therapeutic massage*, St. Louis, 2008, Elsevier Health Sciences.
20. Gazzillo LM: Therapeutic massage techniques for three common injuries, *Athletic Therapy Today* 6(3):5, 2001.
21. Holcomb W: A practical guide to electrical therapy, *J Sport Rehabil* 6(3):272, 1997.
22. Holcomb W, Joyce C: A comparison of temperature increases produced by 2 commonly used ultrasound units, *J Athl Train* 38(1):24, 2003.
23. Hooker D: Intermittent compression devices. In Prentice W, editor: *Therapeutic Modalities in Rehabilitation*, ed 4, New York, 2011, McGraw-Hill.
24. Hooker D: Traction as a specialized modality. In Prentice W, editor: *Therapeutic Modalities in Rehabilitation*, ed 4, New York, 2011, McGraw-Hill.
25. Hooker D, Prentice, W: Basic principles of electricity and electrical stimulating currents. In Prentice W, editor: *Therapeutic Modalities in Rehabilitation*, ed 4, New York, 2011, McGraw-Hill.
26. Hopkins J, Ingersoll C, Edwards J: Cryotherapy and transcutaneous electric neuromuscular stimulation decrease arthrogenic muscle inhibition of the vastus medialis after knee joint effusion, *J Athl Train* 37(1):25, 2002.
27. Hopkins J, McLoda T, Seegmiller J: Low-level laser therapy facilitates superficial wound healing in humans: A tripleblind, sham-controlled study, *J Athl Train* 39(3):223, 2004.
28. Hubbard T, Aronson S, Denegar C: Does cryotherapy hasten return to participation? A systematic review, *J Athl Train* 39(1):88, 2004.
29. Ingersoll C: It's time for evidence, *J Athl Train* 41(1):7, 2006.
30. Johns L: Nonthermal effects of therapeutic ultrasound, *J Athl Train* 37(3):293, 299, 2002.
31. Johnson DS: Low-level laser therapy in the treatment of carpal tunnel syndrome, *Athletic Therapy Today* 8(2):30, 2003.
32. Kaltenborn J: The efficacy of extracorporeal shock-wave treatment: A new perspective, *Athletic Therapy Today* 10(6):50, 2005.
33. Khanna A: Intermittent pneumatic compression in fracture and soft-tissue injuries healing, *British Medical Bulletin*, 88(1):147–56, 2008.
34. Knight K: Cryotherapy in sports injury management, Champaign, Ill.,1995, Human Kinetics.
35. McBrier, N: Low level laser therapy for stimulating muscle regeneration following injury, *Athletic Therapy Today* 14(3):104, 2009.
36. McLeod I: Low-level laser therapy in athletic training, *Athletic Therapy Today* 9(5):17, 2005.
37. Merrick M: Does 1-MHz ultrasound really work? *Athletic Therapy Today* 6(6):48, 2001.
38. Merrick M: Secondary injury after musculoskeletal trauma: A review and update, *J Athl Train* 37(2):209, 2002.
39. Merrick M, Jutte L, Smith M: Cold modalities with different thermodynamic properties produce different surface and intramuscular temperatures, *J Athl Train* 38(1):28, 2003.
40. Michlovitz SL, editor: *Modalities for therapeutic intervention* Philadelphia, 2012, FA Davis.
41. Myrer JW, Measom G, Durrant E, et al: Cold- and hot-pack contrast therapy: Subcutaneous and intramuscular temperature change, *J Athl Train* 32(3):238, 1997.
42. Myrer J, Measom G, Fellingham G: Intramuscular temperature rises with topical analgesics used as coupling agents during therapeutic ultrasound, *J Athl Train* 36(1):20, 2001.
43. Peres S, Draper D, Knight K: Pulsed shortwave diathermy and long-duration stretching increase dorsiflexion range of motion more than identical stretching without diathermy, *J Athl Train* 37(1):43, 2002.
44. Prentice W: The basic science of therapeutic modalities, In Prentice W, editor: *Therapeutic modalities in rehabilitation*, ed 4, New York, 2011, McGraw-Hill.
45. Prentice W: Preface. In Prentice W, editor: *Therapeutic modalities in rehabilitation*, ed 4, New York, 2011, McGraw-Hill.
46. Prentice W: Thermotherapy and cryotherapy. In Prentice W, editor: *Therapeutic modalities in sports medicine and athletic training*, ed 5, St. Louis, 2003, McGraw-Hill.

47. Prentice W: Therapeutic massage. In Prentice W, editor: *Therapeutic modalities in rehabilitation*, ed 4, New York, 2011, McGraw-Hill.

48. Prentice W, Draper, D: Shortwave and microwave diathermy. In Prentice W, editor: *Therapeutic modalities in rehabilitation*, ed 4, New York, 2011, McGraw-Hill.

49. Rubley, M: Thermal ultrasound: It's more than power and time, *Athletic Therapy Today* 14(1):62, 2009.

50. Rubley M, Denegar C, Buckley W: Cryotherapy, sensation, and isometric-force variability, *J Athl Train* 38(2):113, 2003.

51. Saliba E, Saliba S: Low-power laser. In Prentice W, editor: *Therapeutic modalities in rehabilitation*, ed 4, New York, 2011, McGraw-Hill.

52. Snyder-Mackler L, Robinson A: *Clinical electrophysiology: Electrotherapy and electrophysiology*, Baltimore, 2007, Lippincott, Williams and Wilkins.

53. Stemmans C: Low-energy extracorporeal shock-wave therapy, *Athletic Therapy Today* 8(2):44, 2003.

54. Sweeney K, Merrick M, Ingersoll C: Therapeutic magnets do not affect tissue temperature, *J Athl Train* 36(1):27, 2001.

55. Thigpen C: Extracorporal shockwave therapy. In Prentice W, editor: *Therapeutic modalities in rehabilitation*, ed 4, New York, 2011, McGraw-Hill.

56. Tomchuk D: The magnitude of tissue cooling during cryotherapy with varied types of compression, I 45(3):230–37, 2010.

57. Tsang K, Buxton B, Gulon W, et al: The effects of cryotherapy applied through various barriers, *J Sport Rehabil* 6(4):343, 1997.

58. Tsang K, Hertel J, Denegar C: Volume decreases after elevation and intermittent compression are negated by gravity-dependent positioning, *J Athl Train* 38(4):320, 2003.

59. Wang CJ, Chen HS: Shock wave therapy for patients with lateral epicondylitis of the elbow: A one- to two-year follow-up study, *Am J Sports Med* 30(3):422, 2002.

60. Watson T: Ultrasound in contemporary physiotherapy practice, *Ultrasonics*, 48(4):321–29, 2008.

61. Whitehill W: Massage and skin conditions: Indications and contraindications, *Athletic Therapy Today* 7(3):24, 2002.

62. Zainuddin Z, Newton M, Sacco P: Effects of massage on delayed-onset muscle soreness, swelling, and recovery of muscle function, *J Athl Train* 40(3):174, 2005.

ANNOTATED BIBLIOGRAPHY

Cameron M: *Physical agents in rehabilitation: From research to practice*, Philadelphia, 2008, WB Saunders.

A guide for the physical therapist using therapeutic modalities.

Denegar C: *Therapeutic modalities for athletic injuries*, Champaign, IL, 2009, Human Kinetics.

Focuses on the neurophysiological mechanisms of pain control as mediated by a variety of therapeutic modalities.

Knight KL: *Cryotherapy in sports injury management*, Champaign, IL, 1995, Human Kinetics.

Excellent coverage, both theoretical and practical, of one of the most widely used therapeutic approaches in sports medicine and athletic training—cryotherapy; clearly written and easily applied.

Knight KL, Draper DO: *Therapeutic modalities: The art and science*, 2008, Philadelphia, PA: Lippincott Williams & Wilkins.

Addresses all facets of therapeutic modality use.

Michlovitz SL, editor: Modalities for therapeutic intervention. Philadelphia, 2011, F.A. Davis.

An excellent text about understanding the foundations and use of thermal agents in sports medicine and athletic training. Provides detailed discussions of inflammation, pain, superficial heat and cold, and the therapeutic use of ultrasound and shortwave diathermy.

Prentice W: *Therapeutic modalities in rehabilitation*, New York, 2011, McGraw-Hill.

A comprehensive guide to using therapeutic modalities in treating a variety of patient populations. Contains pertinent case studies and laboratory activities.

Prentice W, editor: *Therapeutic modalities for sports medicine and athletic training*, ed 5, St. Louis, 2010, McGraw-Hill.

A comprehensive guide to the use of therapeutic modalities in the sports medicine setting. Addresses all aspects of modality use, including massage, traction, and intermittent compression. An excellent blend of theory and practical application.

Starkey C: *Therapeutic modalities for athletic trainers*, Philadelphia, 2004, F.A. Davis.

Discusses many of the modalities used by athletic trainers in a clinical setting.

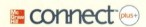

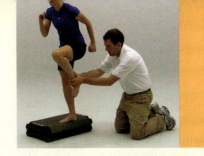

16

Using Therapeutic Exercise in Rehabilitation

■ Objectives

When you finish this chapter you should be able to

- Explain how the athletic trainer approaches rehabilitation.
- Contrast therapeutic exercise and conditioning exercise.
- Describe the consequences of sudden inactivity and injury immobilization.
- Recognize the primary components of a rehabilitation program.
- Discuss the concept of open versus closed kinetic chain exercises.
- Explain the importance of incorporating core stabilization training into a rehabilitation program.

- Evaluate the value of aquatic exercise in rehabilitation.
- Identify the techniques and principles of proprioceptive neuromuscular facilitation.
- Demonstrate the use of mobilization, traction, and Mulligan techniques for improving accessory joint motions.
- Discuss how muscle energy, myofascial release, strain/counterstrain, positional release, active release, and biofeedback techniques can be incorporated into a rehabilitation program.

■ Outline

■ Key Terms

proprioception   kinesthesia   buoyancy

■ Connect Highlights   McGrawHill connect plus+

Visit connect.mcgraw-hill.com for further exercises to apply your knowledge:

- Clinical application scenarios covering primary components of rehabilitation, core stabilization, aquatic exercises, and mobilization techniques
- Click-and-drag questions covering components of a rehabilitation program, rehabilitation exercises, and joint mobilization
- Multiple-choice questions covering core stabilization, aquatic rehabilitation, joint mobilization, traction, therapeutic exercises, conditioning, and consequences of inactivity

THE ATHLETIC TRAINER'S APPROACH TO REHABILITATION

The process of rehabilitation begins immediately after injury. Initial first-aid and management techniques can have a substantial impact on the course and ultimate outcome of the rehabilitative process. Thus, in addition to possessing a sound understanding of how injuries can be prevented, the athletic trainer must also be competent in providing correct and appropriate initial care when injury occurs. In a sports medicine setting, the athletic trainer generally assumes the primary responsibility for design, implementation, and supervision of the rehabilitation program for the injured patient.

> The athletic trainer is responsible for design, implementation, and supervision of the rehablitation program.

Designing programs for rehabilitation is relatively simple and involves several basic components: minimizing swelling, controlling pain, reestablishing neuromuscular control, establishing or enhancing core stability, restoring or increasing muscular strength and endurance, regaining or improving range of motion, regaining balance and postural control, and maintaining levels of cardiorespiratory endurance. Addressing each of these components is the easy part of supervising a rehabilitation program. The difficult part comes in knowing exactly when and how to change the rehabilitation protocols to most effectively accomplish both long- and short-term goals. Progression during the rehabilitation program should be based on specific criteria, and return to competition must be based on level of function and patient outcomes.

The approach to rehabilitation in an athletic environment is considerably different than in most other rehabilitation settings. The competitive nature of athletics necessitates an aggressive approach to rehabilitation. Because the competitive season in most sports is relatively short, the athletic patient does not have the luxury of simply sitting around and doing nothing until the injury heals. The goal is for the patient to return to activity as soon as safely possible. Thus, the athletic trainer who is supervising the rehabilitation program must perform a balancing act between not pushing the patient hard enough and being overly aggressive. In either case, a mistake in judgment on the part of the athletic trainer may hinder the patient's return to activity.

Decisions as to when and how to alter and progress a rehabilitation program should be based within the framework of the healing process. The athletic trainer must possess a sound understanding of both the sequence and the time frames for the various phases of healing and must realize that certain physiological events must occur during each of the phases.[62] Any actions taken during a rehabilitation program that interfere with this healing process will likely increase the length of time required for rehabilitation and slow the patient's return to full activity. The healing process must have an opportunity to accomplish what it is supposed to. At best, the athletic trainer can only try to create an environment that is conducive to the healing process. Little can be done to speed up the process physiologically, but many things can be done during rehabilitation to impede healing.[62]

Athletic trainers have many tools at their disposal that can facilitate the rehabilitative process. How the athletic trainer chooses to use those tools is often a matter of individual preference and experience. Additionally, each patient is different, and the responses to various treatment protocols vary. Thus, a cookbook approach to rehabilitation, with specific protocols that can be followed like a recipe, is impossible. In fact, the use of rehabilitation recipes is strongly discouraged. Instead, the athletic trainer must develop a broad theoretical knowledge base from which he or she can select and apply specific rehabilitation techniques to each athlete.

THERAPEUTIC EXERCISE VERSUS CONDITIONING EXERCISE

Exercise is an essential factor in fitness conditioning, injury prevention, and injury rehabilitation. To compete successfully at a high level, the athlete must be fit. An athlete who is not fit is more likely to sustain an injury. Improper conditioning is one of the major causes of sports injuries. It is essential that the athlete engage in training and conditioning exercises that minimize the possibility of injury while maximizing performance.

The basic principles of conditioning that were discussed in Chapter 4 also apply to therapeutic, rehabilitative, and reconditioning exercises for restoring normal body function following injury. The term *therapeutic exercise* is perhaps most widely used to indicate exercises that are used in a rehabilitation program.[46]

> Therapeutic exercises are concerned with restoring normal body function after injury.

SUDDEN PHYSICAL INACTIVITY AND INJURY IMMOBILIZATION

The human body is a dynamic, moving entity that requires physical activity to maintain proper physical function. When an injury occurs, two problems immediately arise that must be addressed. First is the generalized loss of physical fitness that occurs when activity is stopped, and second is the specific inactivity of the injured part, resulting from protective splinting of the soft tissue and, in some cases, immobilization by some external means.

Effects of General Inactivity

An individual who is highly conditioned will experience a rapid, generalized loss of fitness when exercise is suddenly stopped.[1] This sudden lack of activity causes a loss of muscle strength, endurance, and coordination. Whenever possible, the patient must continue to exercise the entire body without aggravating the injury.

> A sudden loss of physical activity leads to a generalized loss of physical fitness.

Effects of Immobilization

An injured body part that is immobilized for a period of time causes a number of disuse problems that adversely affect muscle, joints, ligaments and bones, and the cardiorespiratory system.

Muscle and Immobilization When a body part is immobilized for even as short a period as 24 hours, definite adverse muscular changes occur.

Atrophy and Fiber-Type Conversion Disuse of a body part quickly leads to a loss of muscle mass. The greatest atrophy occurs in the type I (slow-twitch) fibers. Over time, the slow-twitch fibers develop fast-twitch characteristics. Slow-twitch fibers also diminish in number without type II (fast-twitch) fibers lessening in number.[1] A muscle that is immobilized in a lengthened or neutral position tends to atrophy less. In contrast, immobilizing a muscle in a shortened position encourages atrophy and greater loss of contractile function.[1] Atrophy can also be prevented through isometric contraction and electrical stimulation of the muscles. As the unused muscle decreases in size because of atrophy, protein is also lost. When activity is resumed, normal protein synthesis is reestablished.

> Immobilization of a part causes atrophy of slow-twitch muscle fibers.

Decreased Neuromuscular Efficiency Immobilization causes motor nerves to become less efficient in recruiting and stimulating individual muscle fibers within a given motor unit.[4] Once immobilization ends, the original motor neuron discharge returns within about 1 week.

Joints and Immobilization The immobilization of joints causes a loss of normal compression, which in turn leads to a decrease in lubrication within the joint, causing degeneration. This degeneration occurs because the articular cartilage is deprived of its normal nutrition. The use of continuous passive motion, electrical muscle stimulation, or rehabilitative hinged braces (see Figure 7–30C) has in some cases retarded the loss of articular cartilage.[53]

> Joint immobilization decreases normal lubrication.

Ligament and Bone and Immobilization Both ligaments and bones adapt to normal stress by maintaining or increasing their strength. However, when stress is eliminated or decreased, ligament and bone become weaker.[58] Once immobilization has been removed, high-frequency, short-duration endurance exercise positively enhances the mechanical properties of ligaments. Endurance activities tend to increase both the production and the hypertrophy of the collagen fibers. Full remodeling of ligaments after immobilization may take 12 months or more.

Cardiorespiratory System and Immobilization Like other structures, the cardiorespiratory system is adversely affected by immobilization. The resting heart rate increases approximately one-half beat per minute each day of immobilization. The stroke volume, maximum oxygen uptake, and vital capacity decrease concurrently with the increase in heart rate.

MAJOR COMPONENTS OF A REHABILITATION PROGRAM

A well-designed rehabilitation program should routinely address several key components before an injured athlete can return to pre-injury competitive levels. Those components include minimizing swelling through appropriate first aid and management of initial injury, controlling pain, reestablishing neuromuscular control, establishing

> **Components of a rehabilitation program:**
> - Minimizing swelling
> - Controlling pain
> - Reestablishing neuromuscular control
> - Establishing or enhancing core stability
> - Regaining or improving range of motion
> - Restoring or increasing muscular strength and endurance
> - Regaining balance and postural control
> - Maintaining cardiorespiratory endurance
> - Incorporating functional progressions

or enhancing core stability, regaining or improving range of motion, restoring or increasing muscular strength and endurance, regaining balance and postural control, maintaining levels of cardiorespiratory endurance, and incorporating functional progressions.[58]

Minimizing Initial Swelling

The process of rehabilitation begins immediately after injury. The manner in which the injury is first managed unquestionably has a significant impact on the course of the rehabilitative process. The one problem all injuries, regardless of type, have in common is swelling. Swelling is caused by any number of factors, including bleeding, the production of synovial fluid, an accumulation of inflammatory byproducts, edema, or a combination of several factors. Once swelling has occurred, the healing process is significantly retarded. The injured area cannot return to normal until all the swelling is gone. Therefore, all first-aid management of these conditions should be directed toward controlling the swelling.[58] If the swelling can be controlled initially in the acute stage of injury, the time required for rehabilitation is likely to be significantly reduced. To control and significantly limit the amount of swelling, the RICE principle—rest, ice, compression, and elevation—should be applied (see Chapter 12).

Controlling Pain

When an injury occurs, the athletic trainer must realize that the patient will experience some degree of pain (see Chapter 10). The extent of the pain is determined by the severity of the injury, the patient's individual response to and perception of pain, and the circumstances under which the injury occurred. The athletic trainer can modulate acute pain by using the RICE technique immediately after injury.[61] A physician may also make use of various medications to help ease pain.

Persistent pain can make strengthening or flexibility exercises more difficult and thus interfere with the rehabilitation process. The athletic trainer should routinely address pain during each treatment session. Making use of appropriate manual therapy techniques and therapeutic modalities, including various techniques of cryotherapy, thermotherapy, and electrical stimulating currents, will help modulate pain throughout the rehabilitation process (see Chapter 15).[61,72]

Reestablishing Neuromuscular Control

After injury and subsequent rest and immobilization, the central nervous system "forgets" how to put together information coming from muscle and joint mechanoreceptors and from cutaneous, visual, and vestibular input.[26] *Neuromuscular control* is the mind's attempt to teach the body conscious control of a specific movement.[40] Successful repetition of a patterned movement makes its performance progressively less difficult and thus requires less concentration; eventually, the movement becomes automatic. Reestablishing neuromuscular control requires many repetitions of the same movement through a step-by-step progression from simple to more complex movements.[76] Strengthening exercises, particularly those that tend to be more functional, are essential for reestablishing neuromuscular control (Figure 16–1).[83]

Regaining neuromuscular control means regaining the ability to follow a previously established sensory pattern.[51] The central nervous system compares the intent and production of a specific movement with stored information, continually adjusting until any discrepancy in movement is corrected.[17] Four elements are critical for reestablishing neuromuscular control: (1) proprioceptive and kinesthesia, (2) dynamic stability, (3) preparatory and reactive muscle characteristics, and (4) conscious and unconscious functional motor patterns.[83]

Relearning normal functional movement and timing after injury to a joint may require several months. Addressing neuromuscular control is critical throughout the recovery process but may be most critical during the early stages of rehabilitation to avoid reinjury.[83]

Reestablishing proprioception and kinesthesia should also be of primary concern to the athletic trainer in all rehabilitation programs.[40] **Proprioception** is the ability to determine the position of a joint in space; **kinesthesia** is the ability to detect movement.[68] The ability to sense the position of a joint in space is mediated by mechanoreceptors found in both muscles and joints and by cutaneous, visual, and vestibular input. Neuromuscular control relies

proprioception The ability to determine the position of a joint in space.

kinesthesia The ability to detect movement.

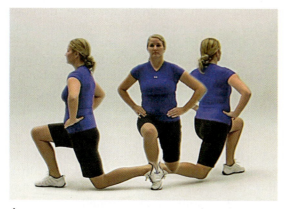 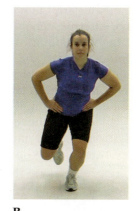

A

B

FIGURE 16–1 Reestablishing neuromuscular control involves performing multiple repetitions of the same functional strengthening movements. **(A)** Multiplanar lunges. **(B)** Single-leg squat.

Neuromuscular control produces coordinated movement.

on the central nervous system to interpret and integrate proprioceptive and kinesthetic information and then to control individual muscles and joints to produce coordinated movement.[68,73]

Joint Mechanoreceptors Joint mechanoreceptors are found in ligaments, capsules, menisci, labria, and skin:

- Ruffini's corpuscles in the joint capsules, ligaments, and skin are sensitive to touch, tension,

Joint mechanoreceptors include Ruffini's corpuscles, Pacinian corpuscles, Merkel's corpuscles, Meissner's corpuscles, and free nerve endings.

and possibly heat; these receptors are sensitive to changes in the position of the joint and to the rate and direction of movement of the joint. They are most active in the end ranges of motion.[61]

- Pacinian corpuscles in the skin respond to deep pressure.
- Merkel's corpuscles in the skin respond to deep pressure, but more slowly than Pacinian corpuscles.
- Meissner's corpuscles in the skin are activated by light touch.
- Free nerve endings are sensitive to extreme mechanical, thermal, or chemical energy. They respond to noxious stimuli—in other words, to impending or actual tissue damage (for example, sprains, cuts, and burns).

Before the 1970s, these receptors in the joint capsules and ligaments were thought to be primarily responsible for joint proprioception. Since then,

there has been considerable debate concerning the role of the joint mechanoreceptors in proprioception and whether joint mechanoreceptors and muscle mechanoreceptors do, in fact, interact with one another. At this point, it has become apparent that the joint mechanoreceptors are not solely responsible for determining joint position. The contemporary viewpoint is that, although joint and muscle mechanoreceptors work in a complementary manner, muscle mechanoreceptors play a more important role in signaling joint position.[76] Any single receptor working in isolation from the others is generally ineffective in signaling information about the movements of the body.[40]

Muscle Mechanoreceptors The function and role of muscle spindles and Golgi tendon organs were discussed in detail in Chapter 4. Muscle spindles, located in the muscle, are sensitive to changes in the length of that muscle,

Muscle mechanoreceptors include muscle spindles and Golgi tendon organs.

whereas Golgi tendon organs, found at the musculotendinous juncture, are sensitive to changes in muscle tension.[60]

Establishing or Enhancing Core Stability

A dynamic core stabilization training program should be an important component of all comprehensive strengthening and injury rehabilitation programs.[35] The *core* is defined as the lumbo-pelvic-hip complex. The core is where the center of gravity is located and where all movement begins. Twenty-nine muscles have their attachment to the lumbo-pelvic-hip complex. The key lumbar spine muscles are the transversospinalis group, erector spinae, quadratus lumborum, and latissimus dorsi.

The key abdominal muscles are the rectus abdominus, external oblique, internal oblique, and transverse abdominus. The key hip muscles are the gluteus maximus, gluteus medius, and psoas.[10]

A core stabilization program improves dynamic postural control, ensures appropriate muscular balance and joint movement around the lumbo-pelvic-hip complex, allows for the expression of dynamic functional strength, and improves neuromuscular efficiency throughout the body.[10] This permits optimal acceleration, deceleration, and dynamic stabilization of all of functioning interconnected segments of the entire body, referred to as the kinetic chain, during functional movements. It also provides proximal stability for efficient lower-extremity movements.[12]

> **Kinetic Chain** Series of functioning interconnected segments throughout the entire body.

Many individuals have developed the functional strength, power, neuromuscular control, and muscular endurance in specific muscles that enable them to perform functional activities. However, relatively few have developed the muscles required for stabilization of the spine (see Chapters 4 and 25). The body's stabilization system has to be functioning optimally to effectively use the strength, power, neuromuscular control, and muscular endurance that individuals have developed in their prime movers. If the extremity muscles are strong and the core is weak, then there will not be enough force created to produce efficient movements.[12] A weak core is a fundamental problem of inefficient movements that leads to injury.

A core stabilization training program is designed to help an individual gain strength, neuromuscular control, power, and muscle endurance in the lumbo-pelvic-hip complex.[35] This approach facilitates a balanced muscular functioning of the entire kinetic chain. Greater neuromuscular control and stabilization strength offer a more biomechanically efficient position for the entire kinetic chain, therefore allowing optimal neuromuscular efficiency throughout the kinetic chain.[77]

A comprehensive core stabilization training program should be systematic, progressive, and functional.[10] When designing a functional core stabilization training program, the athletic trainer should select the appropriate exercises to elicit a maximal training response. The exercises must be safe yet challenging, stress multiple planes, incorporate a variety of resistance equipment (physioball, medicine ball, bodyblade, weight vest, dumbbells, tubing, etc.), derive from fundamental movement skills, and be activity specific (Figure 16–2). The athletic trainer should follow a progressive functional continuum to allow optimal

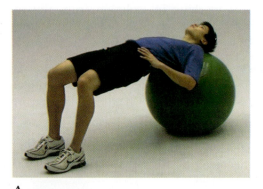

A

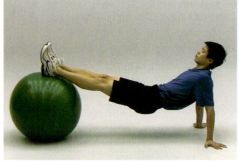

B

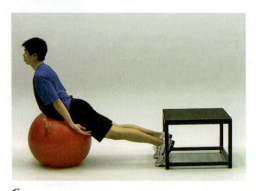

C

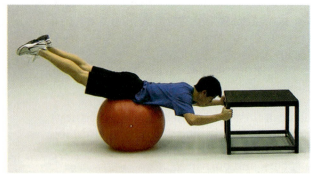

D

FIGURE 16–2 Core stabilization training exercises using a stability ball to increase strength and control in the lumbo-pelvic-hip complex.

adaptations. The patient starts with the exercises at the highest level at which he or she can maintain stability and optimal neuromuscular control. Patients then progress through the program as they achieve mastery of the exercises at each level.[10]

Regaining or Improving Range of Motion

Injury to a joint will always be associated with some loss of motion. That loss of movement may be attributed to contracture of connective tissue (i.e., ligaments, joint capsules), resistance to stretch of the musculotendinous unit (i.e., muscle, tendon, and fascia), or a combination of the two.

Physiological versus Accessory Movements Two types of movement govern range of motion about a joint. *Physiological movements* result from an active

Physiological movements:
• Flexion
• Extension
• Abduction
• Adduction
• Rotation

Accessory motions:
• Spin
• Roll
• Glide

muscle contraction that moves an extremity through flexion, extension, abduction, adduction, and rotation. *Accessory motions* refers to the manner in which one articulating joint surface moves relative to another; such motions are *spin, roll*, and *glide*.[31] Physiological movements are voluntary, and accessory movements normally accompany physiological movements. The two occur simultaneously. Normal accessory motions must occur for full-range physiological movements to take place. If any of the accessory component motions are restricted, normal physiological cardinal plane movements will not occur.[59]

Traditionally, rehabilitation programs tended to concentrate more on passive physiological move-

Restricted physiological movement requires stretching.

Restricted accessory motion requires joint mobilization.

ments and not pay much attention to accessory motions. It is critical for the athletic trainer to closely evaluate the injured joint to determine whether motion is limited because of physiological movement constraints involving musculotendinous units or because of limitation in accessory motion involving the joint capsule and ligaments. If physiological movement is restricted, the patient should engage in stretching activities designed to improve flexibility.[3] Stretching exercises should be used whenever there is musculotendinous resistance to stretch.[14]

If accessory motion is limited because of some restriction of the joint capsule or the ligaments, the athletic trainer should incorporate mobilization techniques into the treatment program. Mobilization techniques should be used whenever there are tight articular structures.[59]

Restoring or Increasing Muscular Strength and Endurance

Muscular strength is one of the most essential factors in restoring the function of a body part to pre-injury status. Isometric, progressive resistance, and isokinetic exercises can benefit rehabilitation. A major goal in performing strengthening exercises is for the patient to work through a full, pain-free range of motion.

Isometric Exercises Isometric exercises are commonly performed in the early phase of rehabilitation when a joint is immobilized for a period of time. They are useful when resistance training though a full range of motion may make the injury worse. Isometrics increase static strength and assist in decreasing the amount of atrophy. Isometrics can also lessen swelling by causing a muscle-pumping action to remove fluid and edema. Isometric exercise can be used to increase strength at whatever angle weakness exists.

Strength gains are limited primarily to the angle at which the joint is exercised. No functional force or eccentric work is developed. Other difficulties are motivation and measurement of the force that is being applied.

Progressive Resistance Exercises Progressive resistance exercises are the most commonly used strengthening technique in a reconditioning program. These exercises may be done using free weights, exercise machines, rubber tubing, or manual resistance (Figure 16–3).[75] Progressive resistance exercises use isotonic contractions, in which force is generated while the muscle is changing in length.

Concentric and Eccentric Muscle Contractions Isotonic contractions may be either concentric or eccentric. Traditionally, patients engaging in progressive resistance exercises have concentrated primarily on the concentric component, without paying much attention to the importance of the eccentric component. The use of eccentric contractions, particularly in the rehabilitation of various injuries related to sport, has received considerable emphasis in recent years.[57] Eccentric contractions are critical for deceleration of limb motion, especially during high-velocity dynamic activities. For example, a baseball pitcher relies on an eccentric contraction of the external rotators at the glenohumeral joint to decelerate the

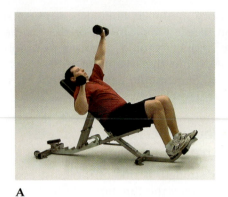

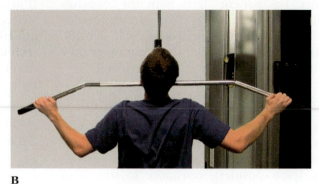

A B

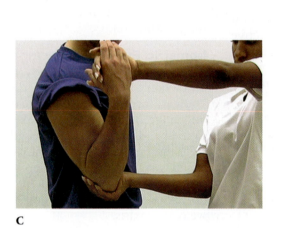

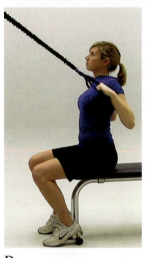

C D

FIGURE 16–3 Progressive resistance exercise techniques. **(A)** Free weights.
(B) Exercise machines. **(C)** Manual resistance. **(D)** Elastic bands or tubing.

humerus, which may be internally rotating at speeds as high as 8,000 degrees per second. Strength deficits or the inability of a muscle to tolerate these eccentric forces can predispose an athlete to injury. Eccentric contractions are used to facilitate concentric contractions in plyometric exercises and may be incorporated into functional proprioceptive neuromuscular facilitation strengthening exercises. Thus, the athletic trainer should include both eccentric and concentric strengthening exercises in a rehabilitation program.

Both concentric and eccentric contractions are possible with free weights, most isotonic exercise machines, and rubber tubing or an elastic band (Figure 16–3). A disadvantage of machines and free weights is that they do not allow exercises to be performed in diagonal or functional planes. It is also difficult to exercise at functional velocities without producing additional injuries. Conversely, resistance exercise using rubber tubing allows both concentric and eccentric resistance and is not encumbered by the design of an exercise machine. It offers a wide range of usefulness at an extremely low cost.

Isokinetic Exercises If isokinetic exercises are used in the rehabilitation process, they are most often

incorporated during the later phases.[54] Isokinetics uses a fixed speed with accommodating resistance to provide maximal resistance throughout the range of motion (Figure 16–4). Isokinetic devices are generally capable of calculating measures of torque, average power, and total work, and ratios of torque to body weight, each of which may be used diagnostically by the athletic trainer. Isokinetic measures are

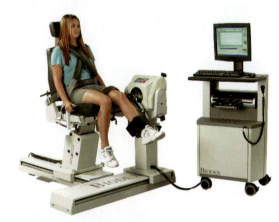

FIGURE 16–4 Isokinetics are primarily used as a diagnostic tool to determine levels of strength.

commonly used as a criterion for return of the athlete to functional activity after injury.

The speed of movement can be altered in isokinetic exercise. Gains in strength from training at slower speeds (60 to 120 degrees per second) are fairly specific to the angular velocity used in training. Isokinetic machines allow the athlete to exercise at speeds that are somewhat more functional. Training at faster speeds seems to produce more general improvement because increases in torque values can be seen at both fast and slow speeds. Isokinetic exercises performed at high speeds tend to decrease the joint's compressive forces. Fast exercises produce fewer negative effects on joints than do slow exercises. Short-arc submaximal isokinetic exercise spreads out synovial fluid, helping nourish the articular cartilage and preventing deterioration.[54] It also develops neuromuscular patterning for the functional speed and movements demanded by specific sports.

Testing Strength, Endurance, and Power Testing for improvement in muscular strength, endurance, or power can be accomplished through manual muscle tests, progressive resistance exercises, or isokinetic dynamometers. Isokinetic testing generally provides the most reliable objective measure of changes in strength.

Regaining Balance and Postural Control

Balance involves the complex integration of muscular forces, neurological sensory information received from the mechanoreceptors, and biomechanical information.[16] Achieving postural control involves positioning the body's center of gravity within the base of support. When the

> **Postural control involves the integration of muscular, neurological, and biomechanical information.**

center of gravity extends beyond the base of support, the limits of stability are exceeded, even though the base of support has not changed, and a corrective step or stumble is necessary to prevent a fall. Even when an individual appears to be motionless, the body is undergoing constant postural sway caused by reflexive muscle contractions, which correct and maintain dynamic equilibrium in an upright posture.[16] When balance is disrupted, the response to correct it is primarily reflexive and automatic.[3] The primary mechanisms for postural control occur in the joints of the lower extremity.[82]

The ability to balance and maintain postural control is essential to a patient who is acquiring or reacquiring complex motor skills.[16] Patients who show a decreased sense of balance or lack of postural control after injury may lack sufficient proprioceptive and kinesthetic information or muscular strength, either of which may limit the patient's ability to generate an effective correction response to disequilibrium.[3] A rehabilitation program must include functional exercises that incorporate balance and proprioceptive training to prepare the patient for return to activity. Failure to address balance problems may predispose the patient to reinjury (Figure 16–5).

Maintaining Cardiorespiratory Endurance

Although strength and flexibility are commonly regarded as essential components in any injury rehabilitation program, relatively little consideration is given to maintaining levels of cardiorespiratory endurance. An athlete spends a considerable amount of time preparing the cardiorespiratory system to be able to handle the increased demands made on it during a competitive season. When injury occurs and the athlete is forced to miss training time, levels of cardiorespiratory endurance may decrease

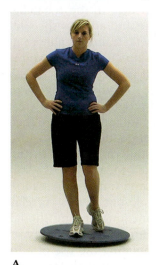
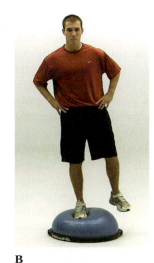
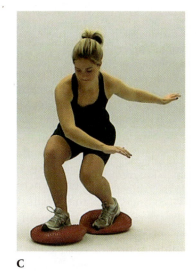

A   B   C

FIGURE 16–5 Balance training is essential in the rehabilitation program. Many balance training products are available. **(A)** BAPS Board. **(B)** Bosu Balance Trainer. **(C)** Dynadisc.

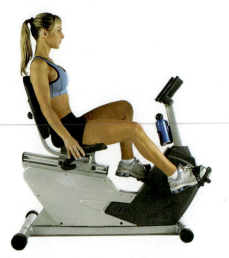

FIGURE 16–6 Stationary cycling provides a means of maintaining cardiorespiratory fitness during rehabilitation. (Courtesy LifeCore)

rapidly. Thus, the athletic trainer must design or substitute alternative activities that allow the individual to maintain existing levels of cardiorespiratory endurance during the rehabilitation period.

Depending on the nature of the injury, a number of possible activities are open to the athlete. For a lower-extremity injury, non–weight bearing activities should be incorporated. Pool activities provide an excellent means for injury rehabilitation. Cycling can also positively stress the cardiorespiratory system (Figure 16–6).

Incorporating Functional Progressions

The purpose of any rehabilitation program is to restore normal function after injury. Functional progressions involve a series of gradually progressive activities designed to prepare the individual for return to a specific sport.[17] Functional progressions should be incorporated into the treatment program as early as possible. Well-designed functional progressions will gradually assist the injured patient in achieving normal, pain-free range of motion, restoring adequate strength levels, and regaining neuromuscular control throughout the rehabilitation process.[59] Ultimately, the focus becomes a safe return to activity. Those skills necessary for successful participation in a given

activity are broken down into component parts, and the patient gradually reacquires those skills within the limitations of his or her progress.[17] The athletic trainer should transfer those skills observed in the performance of a specific activity into a progression of rehabilitative exercises.

Functional activities follow a consistent progression from simple to complex skills, slow to fast speeds, short to longer distances, or light to heavy activities.[81] The athletic trainer must monitor every new activity introduced to determine the athlete's ability to perform as well as his or her physical tolerance. If an activity does not produce additional pain or swelling, the level should be advanced; new activities should be introduced as quickly as possible. Thus, the injured patient would be gradually introduced to the stresses imposed by a particular demand until function is adequate for the patient to return to *sport-specific activity*.[17]

In the case of an athlete, the optimal functional progression program would be designed such that the athlete would have an opportunity to practice every possible skill that is required in a sport before he or she returns to competition. This program would minimize the normal anxiety and apprehension the athlete would experience on return to a competitive environment.[47] Supervised functional progression activities can be done during team practice sessions. This arrangement allows athletes to be around teammates and coaches, which should help them feel more accepted as team members.[47]

> Functional progressions incorporate sport-specific skills into the rehabilitation program.

Functional Testing Functional testing involves having the patient perform certain tasks appropriate to his or her stage in the rehabilitation process in order to isolate and address specific deficits.[63] As a result, the athletic trainer is able to determine the patient's current functional level and set functional goals. Functional testing can be used to determine risk of injury due to limb asymmetry, provide objective measure of progress during a treatment or rehabilitation program, and measure the ability of the individual to tolerate forces.[47]

Functional testing can provide the athletic trainer with objective data for review. Traditional rehabilitation programs and improvements in strength and range of motion do not always correlate with functional ability. Functional testing should have a better correlation with functional ability.

When contemplating the use of a functional test or battery of tests, the athletic trainer must evaluate the test(s) chosen. Validity and reliability must be considered. A test should measure what it intends to measure (validity) and should consistently provide similar results (reliability) regardless of the evaluator. Other factors must be considered before releasing a patient to full activity. These include a subjective evaluation of the injury, performance on functional tests, presence or absence of signs and symptoms, other recognized clinical tests (isokinetic testing, special tests, etc.), and the physician's approval. Functional testing should attempt to look at unilateral function and bilateral function in an attempt to determine whether the patient is compensating with the uninjured limb. Other considerations should include the stage of healing for the patient, appropriate rest time, and self-evaluation.[63]

Obviously, a patient who cannot complete the test(s) is not ready for a return to play. If the athletic trainer has normative values or has collected preinjury baseline values, comparison with postinjury testing values makes a return to activity decision easier. Usually, the athletic trainer has to make a subjective decision based on the test result. But if the normative data or preinjury data are available, the athletic trainer can make an objective decision. If a soccer player is able to complete a sprint test with a mean of 20 seconds but her preinjury time was 17 seconds, then she is only 85 percent functional. Without the preinjury data, the athletic trainer might be unable to determine the patient's functional level.[47]

For years, athletic trainers have used a variety of functional tests to assess a patient's progress, including sprinting tests, agility runs, figure eights, shuttle runs, carioca tests, side stepping, vertical jumps, hopping for time or distance, and balance tests. Functional testing should be an easy task for athletic trainers and should be equally simple for patients to understand. Cost efficiency, time demands, and space demands are important concepts when considering the tests to use.[17,47]

DEVELOPING A REHABILITATION PLAN

No rehabilitation program can be effective without a carefully designed plan. Athletic trainers overseeing a rehabilitation program must have a complete understanding of the injury, including knowledge of how the injury was sustained, the major anatomical structures affected, the grade of trauma, and the stage or phase of the injury's healing.

> **All exercise rehabilitation must be conducted as part of a carefully designed plan.**

Setting Long-term and Short-term Goals

Setting goals is the best way to achieve a successful rehabilitation outcome. The athletic trainer should work with patients to develop long-term and short-term measurable goals and insure that the goals agreed upon are realistic and attainable.[21] When beginning a rehabilitation program, the patient must have at least some idea of what he or she ultimately wants to accomplish at the end of the program. For an athlete, the long-term goal is almost always to return to practice and competition as soon as safely possible. For the office worker or the soccer mom who has been injured, the long-term goal may simply be to return to performing normal daily activities.

Short-term goals should be a means to help the patient achieve the long-term goal. For example, if a runner has sprained an ankle and the long-term goal for completing rehabilitation is to run a 5K road race, the early phases of rehabilitation should include two short-term goals: (1) walking once around a running track (400 yards) without a limp and then (2) jogging 1 mile in under 8 minutes without increased pain or swelling.

The short-term goals need to be linked to the problem that the patient is seeking help for, or the majority of patients will not stick with the program. When patients understand that their care has been customized for them and has been designed to restore the function that is important to them, two important things happen. First, they accept some ownership of the rehabilitation program because they were involved in the development of the plan. Patients are more likely to follow a procedure that they can see direct relevance in, and less likely to follow programs that they see as meaningless. Second, short-term goals provide the patient with a road map to follow. Because the goals are measurable, the patient is able to self-assess, and the plan provides the patient with a means of recognizing when he or she is on the expected path to full recovery.[21]

Generally, when designing an exercise program, it is better to have two or three simple exercises that are executed faithfully and correctly than to have an elaborate program that will not be done due to lack of time, understanding, or some other perceived barrier. Thus, another key element that goes hand-in-hand with the development of short-term goals is to keep the instruction simple.[47]

Exercise Phases

Rehabilitation progressions can be subdivided into three phases based primarily on the three stages of the healing process: phase 1, the acute inflammatory response phase; phase 2, the fibroblastic repair phase; and

> **Phases of rehabilitation:**
> - Preoperative phase
> - Phase 1—acute inflammatory response phase
> - Phase 2—fibroblastic repair phase
> - Phase 3—maturation-remodeling phase

phase 3, the maturation-remodeling phase (see Chapter 10). If surgery is necessary, a fourth phase, the preoperative phase, must also be considered. Depending on the type and extent of injury and the individual response to healing, phases will usually overlap. Each phase must include carefully considered goals and criteria for advancing from one phase to another.

Preoperative Exercise Phase The preoperative exercise phase applies only to those patients who sustain injuries that require surgery. If surgery can be postponed, exercise may be used as a means to improve its outcome. By allowing the initial inflammatory response phase to resolve and by maintaining or increasing muscle strength and flexibility, cardiorespiratory fitness, and neuromuscular control, the patient may be better prepared to continue the rehabilitation program after surgery.

> **Exercise performed during the preoperative phase can often assist recovery after surgery.**

Phase 1: Acute Inflammatory Response Phase Phase 1 begins immediately when injury occurs and may last as long as 4 days. This phase of the healing process is attempting to control and clean up the injured tissues, thus creating an environment that is conducive to the fibroblastic repair stage. The primary focus of rehabilitation during this phase is to control swelling and to modulate pain by using rest, ice, compression, and elevation (RICE) immediately after injury. Throughout this phase, ice, compression, and elevation should be used as much as possible.[58]

Rest of the injured part is critical during this phase. It is widely accepted that early mobility during rehabilitation is essential. However, if the athletic trainer becomes overly aggressive during the first 48 hours after injury and does not allow the injured part to rest during the inflammatory stage of healing, the inflammatory process never gets a chance to accomplish its purpose. Consequently, the length of time required for inflammation may be extended. Immobility during the first 2 days after injury is necessary to control inflammation.

Rest does not mean that the patient does nothing. The term *rest* applies only to the injured body part. During this period, the patient should work on cardiorespiratory endurance and should do strengthening and flexibility exercises for the parts of the body not affected by the injury. When immobilized, muscle tensing or isometrics may be used to maintain muscle strength.

By day 3 or 4, swelling begins to subside and eventually stops altogether. The injured area may feel warm to the touch, and some discoloration is usually apparent. The injury is still painful to the touch, and some pain is elicited when the injured part is moved. At this point, the patient may begin active mobility exercises, working through a pain-free range of motion. If the injury involves the lower extremity, the patient should be encouraged to bear progressively more weight.

A physician may choose to have the patient take nonsteroidal antiinflammatory drugs (NSAIDs) to help control swelling and inflammation. It is usually helpful to continue this medication throughout the rehabilitative process.

Phase 2: Fibroblastic Repair Phase Once the inflammatory response has subsided, the fibroblastic repair phase begins. During this stage of the healing process, fibroblastic cells are laying down a matrix of collagen fibers and forming scar tissue. This stage may begin as early as 4 days after the injury and may last for several weeks. At this point, swelling has stopped completely. The injury is still tender to the touch but is not as painful as during phase 1. Pain is also less with active and passive motion.[58]

As soon as inflammation is controlled, the athletic trainer should immediately begin to incorporate into the rehabilitation program activities that can help the patient maintain levels of cardiorespiratory endurance, restore full range of motion, restore or increase strength, and reestablish neuromuscular control.

Modalities in this phase, as in phase 1, should be used to control pain and swelling. Cryotherapy should be used during the early portion of this phase to reduce the likelihood of swelling. Electrical stimulating currents can help control pain and improve strength and range of motion.[61]

Phase 3: Maturation-Remodeling Phase The maturation-remodeling phase is the longest of the three phases and may last for several years, depending on the severity of the injury. The ultimate goal during this phase of the healing process is return to activity. The injury is no longer painful to the touch, although some progressively decreasing pain may still be felt on motion. The collagen fibers must be realigned according to tensile stresses and strains placed on them during functional sport-specific exercises.[48]

The focus during this phase should be on regaining activity-specific skills. Dynamic functional activities related to performance should be incorporated into the rehabilitation program. Functional training involves the repeated performance of a particular skill for the purpose of perfecting that skill. Strengthening exercises should progressively place stresses and strains on the injured structures that would normally be encountered during that activity. Plyometric strengthening exercises can be used to improve muscle power and explosiveness.[17] Functional testing should be done to determine specific skill weaknesses that need to be addressed before full return to activity.

At this point, some type of heating modality is beneficial to the healing process. The deep-heating modalities, ultrasound, or diathermy should be used to increase circulation to the deeper tissues. Massage and gentle mobilization may also be used to reduce spasm, increase circulation, and reduce pain. Increased blood flow delivers the essential nutrients to the injured area to promote healing, and increased lymphatic flow assists in the breakdown and removal of waste products.[61] As the maturation-remodeling phase begins, aggressive, active range of motion and strengthening exercises should be incorporated to facilitate tissue remodeling and realignment.

Engaging in exercise that is too intense or too prolonged can be detrimental to the progress of rehabilitation. Any increase in the amount of swelling, an increase in pain, a loss or plateau in strength, a loss or plateau in range of motion, an increase in the laxity of a healing ligament, or exacerbation of other clinical symptoms during or after a particular exercise or activity indicates that the load is too great for the level of tissue repair or remodeling.[17]

Adherence to a Rehabilitation Program

For a rehabilitation program to be successful, the injured patient must comply with and adhere to the plan of rehabilitation.[7,42] In the field of athletic injury, compliance is the biggest deterrent to successful rehabilitation.[24] The athletic trainer can take several steps to enhance adherence:

- The athletic trainer can provide the encouragement and positive reinforcement necessary for the patient to make a commitment. Patients who are committed to the rehabilitation program work harder and thus return to activity more quickly with better results than those who are not committed.[22,24,64]
- The athletic trainer can be creative in designing and varying the exercise routine to keep the patient interested and motivated.[41]
- Support from peers, family, and rehabilitation staff is important in influencing compliance. Those patients with support show a greater effort to fit the rehabilitation effort into their schedules.[20]
- The athletic trainer's attitude is another important consideration when dealing with injured patients. An athletic trainer who feels that a patient is not going to adhere to the treatment program is less likely to motivate the patient to comply with the program.[56]
- The patient is more likely to follow treatment plan instructions that are clearly explained verbally and then written down.[55]
- Encourage the coach to support the rehabilitation concept and to discipline the athlete if he or she does not participate in the rehabilitation process.
- Almost all rehabilitation should be pain free. Painful exercise not only is harmful but also reduces compliance, especially in the nonadherent patient. The athletic trainer should examine rehabilitation programs to determine the aspects that may be painful.[20]

Criteria for Full Return to Activity

All exercise rehabilitation plans must determine what is meant by complete recovery from an injury. Often, it means that the patient is fully reconditioned and has achieved full range of motion, strength, neuromuscular control, cardiovascular endurance, and activity-specific functional skills. Besides physical well-being, the patient must also have regained full confidence to return to his or her activity.

The decision to release a patient recovering from injury to a full return to activity is the final stage of the rehabilitation and recovery process. The decision should be carefully considered by each member of the sports medicine team involved in the rehabilitation process. The physician should be ultimately responsible for deciding that the patient is ready to return to practice or competition. The decision to return a patient to activity should address the following concerns:

- *Physiological healing constraints*—Has rehabilitation progressed to the later phases of the healing process?
- *Pain status*—Has pain disappeared, or is the patient able to function within his or her own levels of pain tolerance?

- *Swelling*—Is there still a chance that swelling will be exacerbated by a return to activity?
- *Range of motion*—Is the patient's range of motion adequate to allow him or her to perform both effectively and with minimized risk of reinjury?
- *Strength*—Is strength, endurance, or power great enough to protect the injured structure from reinjury?
- *Neuromuscular control/proprioception/kinesthesia*—Has the patient relearned how to use the injured body part?
- *Cardiorespiratory endurance*—Has the patient been able to maintain cardiorespiratory endurance at or near the level necessary for competition?
- *Sport-specific demands*—Are the demands of the activity or a specific position such that the patient will not be at risk of reinjury?
- *Functional testing*—Does the patient's performance on appropriate functional tests indicate that his or her extent of recovery is sufficient to allow successful performance?
- *Prophylactic strapping, bracing, padding*—Are any additional supports necessary for the injured patient to return to activity?
- *Responsibility of the patient*—Is the patient capable of listening to his or her body and recognizing a potential reinjury situation?
- *Predisposition to injury*—Is this patient prone to reinjury or to a new injury when he or she is not fully recovered?
- *Psychological factors*—Is the patient capable of returning to activity and competing at a high level without fear of reinjury?
- *Athlete education and preventive maintenance program*—Does the patient understand the importance of continuing to engage in conditioning exercises that can greatly reduce the chances of reinjury?

ADDITIONAL APPROACHES TO THERAPEUTIC EXERCISE IN REHABILITATION

Open versus Closed Kinetic Chain Exercises

The concept of the kinetic chain deals with the functional anatomical relationships that exist in the upper and lower extremities. In a weight-bearing position, the lower-extremity kinetic chain involves the transmission of forces among the foot, ankle, lower leg, knee, thigh, and hip. In the upper extremity, the hand as a weight-bearing surface transmits forces to the wrist, forearm, elbow, upper arm, and shoulder girdle.[57]

An open kinetic chain exists when the foot or hand is not in contact with the ground or some other surface.[27] In a closed kinetic chain, the foot or hand is weight bearing. Movements of the more proximal anatomical segments are affected by open and closed kinetic chain positions.[43] For example, the rotational components of the ankle, knee, and hip reverse direction when changing from an open to a closed kinetic chain activity.

> **An open kinetic chain occurs when the foot or hand is off the ground.**

> **A closed kinetic chain occurs when the foot or hand is on the ground.**

In a closed kinetic chain, the forces begin at the ground and work their way up through each joint. In a closed kinetic chain, forces must be absorbed by various tissues and anatomical structures rather than simply dissipating, as would occur in an open chain.[19]

The use of closed chain strengthening techniques has become the rehabilitation treatment of choice for many athletic trainers.[57] Because most activities involve some aspect of weight bearing with the foot in contact with the ground or with the hand in a weight-bearing position, closed kinetic chain strengthening activities are more functional than are open chain activities. Closed kinetic chain exercises are more sport- or activity-specific, involving exercise that more closely approximates the desired activity. Specificity of training must be emphasized to athletes for them to maximize carryover to functional activities on the playing field.[57] Therefore, the treatment program should incorporate rehabilitative exercises that emphasize strengthening the entire kinetic chain rather than an isolated body segment.[66]

Closed kinetic chain exercises use varying combinations of isometric, concentric, and eccentric contractions, which must occur simultaneously in different muscle groups within the chain. Isolation exercises typically make use of one type of muscular contraction to produce or control movement.[32] Consequently, there must be some neuromuscular adaptation to this type of strengthening exercise.

In the athletic training setting, several different closed kinetic chain exercises have gained popularity and have been incorporated into rehabilitation protocols.[29] Exercises commonly used for the lower extremity are minisquats, leg presses, forward and lateral step-ups, terminal knee extensions using tubing, and exercises that use equipment such as stair climbing or stepping machines, slide boards, and stationary bicycles.[57] Push-ups and weight-shifting exercises on a medicine ball are two of the more typically used upper-extremity exercises (Figure 16–7).[48,77]

Aquatic Exercise

Aquatic exercise is a popular rehabilitative tool. An athletic trainer who has access to a swimming pool is fortunate. Water submersion offers an excellent environment for

> Aquatic exercise provides an excellent means for rehabilitation.

beginning a program of exercise therapy, and it can complement all phases of rehabilitation.[28,72]

Because of **buoyancy** and water resistance, submersion in a pool presents a versatile exercise environment that can be varied easily according to individual needs.[2] With the proper technique, the patient can reduce muscle guarding; relax tense muscles; increase the range of joint motion; reestablish correct movement patterns; and, above all, increase strength, power, and muscular endurance.[28]

> **buoyancy** The tendency of a body to float or rise when placed in water.

Aquatic exercise uses the water's buoyancy and pressure; it can be described as assistive, supportive, and resistive.[74] As an assistive medium, the water's buoyancy can increase range of motion, strength, and control. The patient starts by placing the body part below the water level and allows the part to be carried passively upward, keeping within pain-free limits. As the patient gains strength, he or she

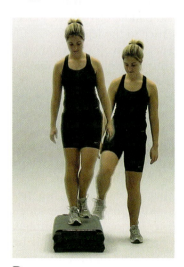

A

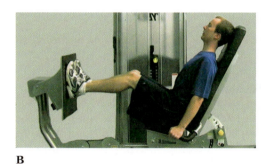

B

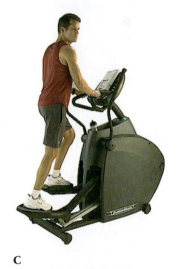

C

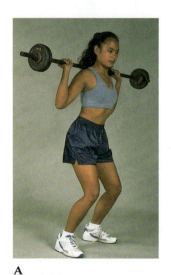

D

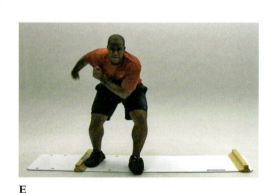

E

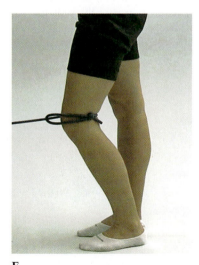

F

FIGURE 16–7 Closed kinetic chain exercises. **(A)** Minisquats. **(B)** Leg press. **(C)** Stepping machines. **(D)** Lateral step-ups. **(E)** Slide boards. **(F)** Terminal knee extensions using tubing.

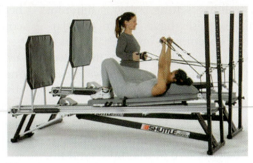

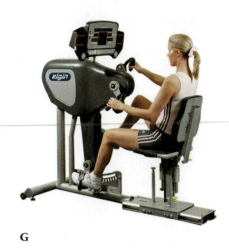

G

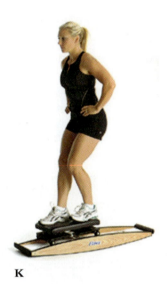

H

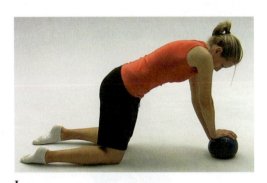

I

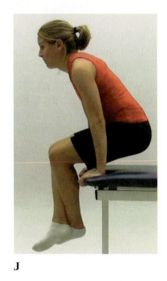

J

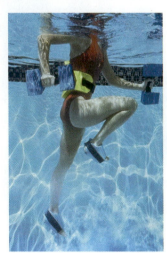

K

FIGURE 16–7   continued
(G) Stationary bicycling. (H) Shuttle 2000. (I) Weight shifting. (J) Seated push-ups. (K) Fitter.

actively engages in movement, again assisted by the buoyancy of the water. Progression of the movement can be initiated by increasing speed and by using the water above the body part as a resistive medium (Figure 16–8).[52]

A second use of water buoyancy is for support.[34] The limb normally will float just below the water's surface. In this position, the limb is parallel to the surface of the water. An increase in speed will make movement more difficult. Progression also can be accomplished if the part is less streamlined. In exercising the arm, for example, the athlete can increase the difficulty by moving across the water with the flat of the hand or by using a hand paddle or webbed glove. Flippers can increase resistance to the leg.

Resistance is the third use of water buoyancy.[34] The injured body part is moved downward against the upward thrust of the water. Maximum resistance is attained by keeping the limb at a right angle to the water's surface. Like the supportive technique, the resistive technique can be made progressively more difficult by the use of different devices. Extra resistance is added by pushing or dragging flotation devices down into the water.[5]

Besides engaging in specific exercises, the patient can practice sports skills, using the water's buoyancy and resistance to his or her advantage. For example, locomotor or throwing skills can be practiced to regain normal movement patterns.[49] The swimming pool can also be an excellent medium for retaining or restoring functional capacities as well as restoring cardiovascular endurance.

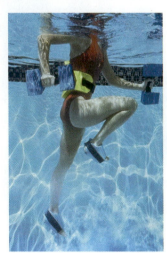

FIGURE 16–8   Using water's buoyancy and pressure for progressive exercise.

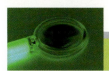
Suggested aquatic workouts

Swim workout*

Activity	Time
Warm-up (jog in place)	5 minutes
Scissors (abduction/adduction)	1 minute
Kicking (standing position with toes dorsiflexed—increase difficulty by plantar flexing toes)	1 minute
High knees	1 minute
Heels to butt	1 minute
Rest (passive)	45 seconds
Repeat sequence three times	
Running in place (sprinting)	10 times—30 seconds on, 15 seconds off
Active cool-down	3:30 minutes
	Total time: 30 minutes

Kick workout with a kickboard

Use flutter kick for this workout (prone to work hip flexors/knee extensors or supine to work hip extensors/knee flexors, using a kickboard).

Activity	Time
Warm-up	5 minutes
Prone	20 seconds hard, 10 seconds easy for 5 minutes
Rest (passive)	1 minute
Supine	20 seconds hard, 10 seconds easy for 5 minutes
Rest (passive)	1 minute
Sprint the middle 15 yards†	5 minutes
Active cool-down	5 minutes
	Total time: 27 minutes

*Increase difficulty by adding arm and leg buoys. Scissors and kicking should focus on both speed and a medium range of motion. Patient needs to be suspended in the water by a waist belt or tethered to the side of the pool. Patient should not worry about treading during the workout.

†Each lane is 25 yards. Have patient kick easy for the first 5 yards of the lap, kick hard for the middle 15 yards, and kick easy for the final 5 yards. Repeat for 5 minutes.

Wearing a flotation device around the waist, the patient can perform a variety of upper- and lower-limb movement patterns (Figure 16–9). Movements of straight-ahead running, backward running, side stepping, figure eights, and carioca can be performed by a patient bearing full weight while in 3 to 5 feet (0.9 to 1.5 m) of water.

Focus Box 16-1: "Suggested aquatic workouts" suggests aquatic workouts using a swim program and a kickboard program.

Proprioceptive Neuromuscular Facilitation Techniques

Proprioceptive neuromuscular facilitation (PNF) is an approach to therapeutic exercise that uses proprioceptive, cutaneous, and auditory input to produce functional improvement in motor output and can be a vital element in the rehabilitation process of many injuries.[37] These techniques have been

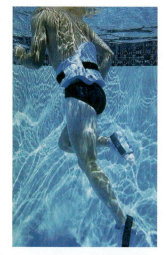

FIGURE 16–9 A wet vest can facilitate exercise programs in the water by making the patient more buoyant.

recommended and are widely used in sports medicine for increasing strength, flexibility, and coordination, as well as decreasing deficits in kinesthetic sense in response to demands placed on the neuromuscular system.[36,79] The principles and techniques of PNF are based primarily on the neurophysiological mechanisms involving the stretch reflex, which was discussed in detail in Chapter 4.[60] The PNF techniques are generally used in rehabilitation for facilitating strength and increasing range of motion. Flexibility is increased by the techniques of contract-relax, hold-relax, and slow-reversal-hold-relax. In contrast, strength can be facilitated by repeated contraction and the slow-reversal, rhythmic initiation, and rhythmic stabilization techniques.[60]

Strengthening Techniques To assist the patient in developing muscle strength, muscle endurance, and coordination, use the following techniques.[60]

> **PNF strengthening techniques:**
> - Rhythmic initiation
> - Repeated contraction
> - Slow reversal
> - Slow-reversal-hold
> - Rhythmic stabilization

Rhythmic Initiation Rhythmic initiation consists of a progressive series, first of passive movement, then of active assistive movement, followed by an active movement through an agonist pattern. This technique can be initiated within the first day following injury and is progressed over the next few days or weeks as the patient can tolerate. This approach helps patients with limited movement progressively regain strength through the range of motion.

Repeated Contraction Repeated contraction of a muscle or a muscle group is used for general weakness or weakness at one specific point. The patient moves isotonically against the maximum resistance of the athletic trainer until he or she experiences fatigue. At the time fatigue is felt, stretch is applied to the muscle at that point in the range to facilitate greater strength production. All resistance must be carefully accommodated to the strength of the patient. Because the patient is resisting as much as possible, this technique may be contraindicated for some injuries.

Slow Reversal The patient moves through a complete range of motion against maximum resistance. Resistance is applied to facilitate antagonist and agonist muscle groups and to ensure smooth and rhythmic movement. It is important that reversals of the movement pattern be instituted before the previous pattern has been fully completed. The major benefit of this PNF technique is that it promotes normal reciprocal coordination of agonist and antagonist muscles.

Slow-Reversal-Hold In this technique, the patient moves a body part isotonically, using agonist muscles, and immediately follows that movement with an isometric contraction. The patient is instructed to hold at the end of each isotonic movement. The primary purpose of this technique is to develop strength at a specific point in the range of motion.

> **PNF stretching techniques:**
> - Contract-relax
> - Hold-relax
> - Slow-reversal-hold-relax

Rhythmic Stabilization Rhythmic stabilization uses an isometric contraction of the agonists, followed by an isometric contraction of the antagonists. With repeated contraction of these muscles, strength is maximum at this point.

Stretching Techniques To produce muscle relaxation through an inhibitory response for increasing range of motion, the following PNF techniques may be used.

Contract-Relax The affected body part is passively moved until resistance is felt. The patient is then told to contract the antagonistic muscle isotonically. The athletic trainer resists the movement for 10 seconds or until the patient feels fatigued. The patient is instructed to relax for 10 seconds. The athletic trainer passively moves the limb to a new stretch position, and the exercise is repeated three times.

Hold-Relax The hold-relax technique is similar to contract-relax except that an isometric contraction is used. The patient moves the body part to the point of resistance and is told to hold that position. The athletic trainer isometrically resists the muscles for 10 seconds. The patient is then told to relax for 10 seconds, and the body part is moved to a new range, either actively by the patient or passively by the athletic trainer. This exercise is repeated three times.

Slow-Reversal-Hold-Relax The patient moves the body part to the point of resistance and is told to

> **16–7 Clinical Application Exercise**
>
> A patient was injured in karate and was immobilized in a cast for 6 weeks after a fracture of the olecranon process of the ulna. The cast was removed 3 weeks ago, and the patient has been working hard on stretching exercises to regain elbow extension. At this point, he is still lacking 16 degrees of extension and does not seem to be gaining any additional motion.
>
> **?** Because the stretching seems to be ineffective at this point, what can the athletic trainer do to help the patient regain range of motion?

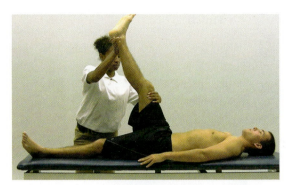

FIGURE 16–10 The slow-reversal-hold-relax stretching technique for the hamstring muscle.

hold that position. The athletic trainer isometrically resists the muscles for 10 seconds. The patient is then told to relax for 10 seconds, thus relaxing the antagonist while the agonist is contracted, moving the part to a new limited range (Figure 16–10).

Basic Principles of Using PNF Techniques These principles are the basis of PNF and must be used with any specific techniques. Application of the following principles may assist in promoting a desired response in the individual being treated.[37]

1. The patient must be taught, through brief, simple descriptions, the PNF patterns for sequential movements from starting position to terminal positions.
2. When learning the patterns, the patient should look at the moving limb for feedback on directional and positional control.
3. Verbal commands should be firm and simple—push, pull, or hold.
4. Manual contact with the hands can facilitate a movement response.
5. The athletic trainer must use correct body mechanics when providing resistance.
6. The amount of resistance given should facilitate a maximal response that allows smooth, coordinated motion.
7. Rotational movement is a critical component in all the PNF patterns.
8. The distal movements of the patterns should occur first and should be completed by no later than halfway through the pattern.
9. The stronger components are emphasized to facilitate the weaker components of a movement pattern.
10. Pressing the joint together causes increased stability, whereas traction pulls the joint apart and facilitates movement.
11. Giving a quick stretch causes a reflex contraction of that muscle.

PNF Patterns The PNF exercise patterns involve three component movements: flexion-extension, abduction-adduction, and internal-external rotation. Human movement is patterned and rarely involves straight motion because all muscles are spiral in nature and lie in diagonal directions.[37]

The PNF patterns involve distinct diagonal and rotational movements of upper extremity, lower extremity, upper trunk, lower trunk, and neck. The exercise pattern is initiated with the muscle groups in the lengthened or stretched position. The muscle group is then contracted, moving the body part through the range of motion to a shortened position.

The upper and lower extremities each have two separate patterns of diagonal movement for each part of the body, which are referred to as the diagonal 1 (D1) and diagonal 2 (D2) patterns. These two diagonal patterns are subdivided into D1 moving into flexion, D1 moving into extension, D2 moving into flexion, and D2 moving into extension. The patterns are named according to the movement occurring at either the shoulder or the hip.

Figures 16–11 and 16–12 are examples of PNF patterns that may be used for rehabilitating some sports injuries. PNF techniques for specific joints are discussed in Chapters 18 through 24.

Muscle Energy Techniques

Muscle energy techniques have been established to treat complex kinetic chain dysfunction.[18] *Muscle energy techniques (MET)* are manually applied stretching techniques that use principles of neurophysiology to relax overactive muscles and/or stretch chronically shortened muscles.[8] Muscle energy is a manual therapy technique that is a variation of the PNF contract-relax and hold-relax techniques. Like the PNF techniques, the muscle energy techniques are based on the same neurophysiological mechanisms involving the stretch reflex discussed in Chapter 4. Muscle energy techniques involve the voluntary contraction of a muscle in a specifically controlled direction at varied levels of intensity against a distinctly executed counterforce applied by the athletic trainer.[69] The patient provides the corrective *intrinsic* forces and controls the intensity of the muscular contractions, while the athletic trainer controls the precision and localization of the procedure. The amount of effort by the patient can vary from a minimal muscle twitch to a maximal muscle contraction.

Five components are needed to make muscle energy techniques effective:

1. Active muscle contraction by the patient
2. A muscle contraction oriented in a specific direction
3. Some control of contraction intensity by the patient

	Start	**Finish**	

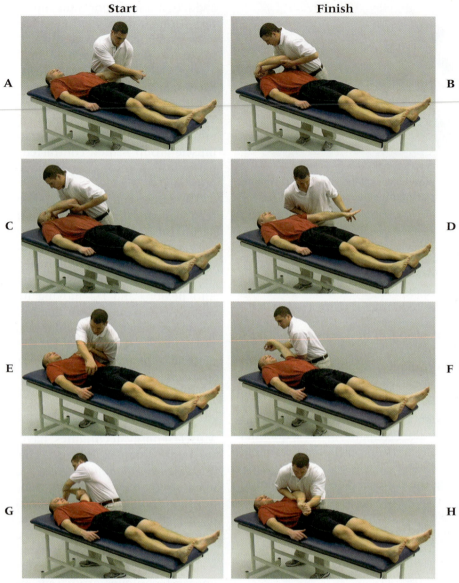

FIGURE 16–11   Upper-extremity PNF patterns. **(A&B)** D1 moving into flexion. **(C&D)** D1 moving into extension. **(E&F)** D2 moving into flexion. **(G&H)** D2 moving into extension.

4. Control of the joint position by the athletic trainer
5. Appropriate counterforce applied by the athletic trainer

The specific muscle energy technique begins by locating a point of resistance to stretch that is referred to as a *resistance barrier*. This is not necessarily a pathological barrier, but does represent the point in the range of motion at which movement will not occur without some degree of passive assistance.[23] Beginning at the resistance barrier, the patient is asked to contract the antagonist (muscle to be stretched) isometrically for 10 seconds. At this point, the patient is asked to relax completely and to inhale and exhale maximally. As the patient exhales, the athletic trainer moves the body part to the new resistance barrier. This process should be repeated three to five times or until there is no further gain in range of motion.[8]

Joint Mobilization and Traction

The techniques of joint mobilization are used to improve joint mobility and to decrease joint pain by restoring accessory movements to the joint, thus allowing for full, nonrestricted, pain-free range of motion.[59] Mobilization techniques may be used to attain a variety of treatment goals, such as the following: reducing pain; decreasing muscle guarding; stretching or lengthening tissue surrounding a joint, especially capsular and ligamentous tissue; either inhibiting or facilitating muscle tone or the stretch reflex; and proprioceptive effects that improve postural and kinesthetic awareness.

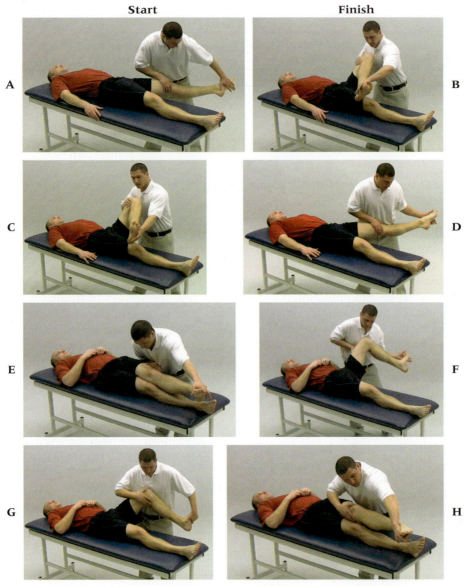

Start **Finish**

A

B

C

D

E

F

G

H

FIGURE 16–12 Lower-extremity PNF patterns. **(A&B)** D1 moving into flexion. **(C&D)** D1 moving into extension. **(E&F)** D2 moving into flexion. **(G&H)** D2 moving into extension.

Mobilization Techniques Mobilization techniques are used to increase the accessory motions about a joint.[59] Treatment techniques designed to improve accessory motion involve small-amplitude oscillating movements called *glides*, within a specific part of the range.[25,59] Mobilization should be done with both the patient and the athletic trainer in comfortable and relaxed positions. The athletic trainer should mobilize one joint at a time. The joint should be stabilized as near one articulating surface as possible; the other surface should be held with a firm, confident grasp.[59]

Maitland has categorized mobilization techniques into five grades as follows:[25]

> **Mobilization works to improve accessory motions.**

- Grade I—a small-amplitude glide at the beginning of the range of motion. It is used when pain and spasm limit movement early in the range of motion.
- Grade II—a large-amplitude glide within the midrange of movement. It is used when spasm limits movement sooner with a quick oscillation than with a slow one, or when slowly increasing pain restricts movement halfway into the range.
- Grade III—a large-amplitude glide up to the pathological limit in the range of motion. It is used when pain and resistance from spasm, inert tissue tension, or tissue compression limit movement near the end of the range.
- Grade IV—a small-amplitude glide at the end of the range of motion. It is used when resistance limits movement in the absence of pain and spasm.

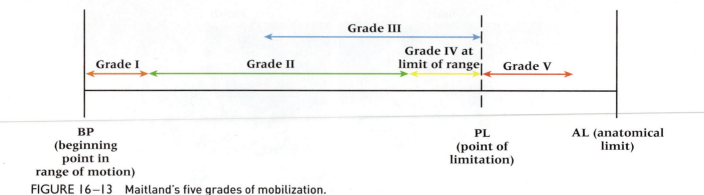

BP
(beginning
point in
range of motion)

PL
(point of
limitation)

AL (anatomical
limit)

FIGURE 16–13 Maitland's five grades of mobilization.

• Grade V—a small-amplitude, quick thrust delivered at the end of the range of motion, usually accompanied by a popping sound called a manipulation. It is used when minimal resistance limits the end of the range. Manipulation is most effectively accomplished by the velocity of the thrust rather than by the force of the thrust. Most authorities agree that manipulation should be used only by individuals trained specifically in these techniques because a great deal of skill and judgment is necessary for safe and effective treatment.

In Maitland's system, grades I and II are used primarily to treat pain, and grades III and IV are used to treat stiffness. It is necessary to treat pain first and stiffness second.[25] Figure 16–13 shows the various grades of oscillation that are used in a joint with some limitation of motion.

The shape of the articulating surfaces usually dictates the direction of the mobilization being performed.[59] Generally, one articulating surface may be considered to be concave and the other to be convex. When the concave surface is stationary and the convex surface is moving, the glide should be done in the opposite direction of the bone movement. If the convex surface is stationary and the concave surface is moving, the glide should be done in the same direction as the bone movement. If mobilization in the appropriate direction exacerbates complaints of pain or stiffness, the athletic trainer should apply the technique in the opposite direction until the patient can tolerate the application of the technique in the appropriate direction.

In many cases, traction can be combined with mobilization.[31] *Traction* is a technique in which one articulating segment is pulled to produce some separation of the two joint surfaces. Both mobilization and traction techniques use a translational movement of one joint surface relative to the other. This translation may be in one of two directions: either perpendicular or parallel to the *treatment plane*. The treatment plane falls perpendicular to, or at a right angle to, a line running from the axis of rotation

in the convex surface to the center of the concave articular surface (Figure 16–14). Mobilization techniques use glides that translate one articulating surface along a line parallel with the treatment plane. Traction techniques translate one of the articulating surfaces perpendicular to the treatment plane. Mobilization glides are done parallel to the treatment plane; traction is performed perpendicular to the treatment plane. Like mobilization techniques, traction may be used either to decrease pain or to reduce joint hypomobility.[31,38]

Figure 16–15 shows examples of joint mobilization techniques for some joints and body segments. Mobilizations for specific joints are discussed further in Chapters 18 through 24.

Mulligan Technique

The Mulligan technique combines passive accessory joint mobilization, applied by an athletic trainer, with active physiological movement by the patient for the purpose of correcting positional faults and returning the patient to normal

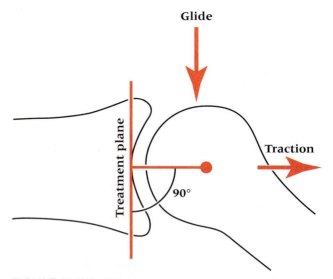

FIGURE 16–14 The treatment plane is perpendicular to a line drawn from the axis of rotation to the center of the articulating surface of the concave segment.

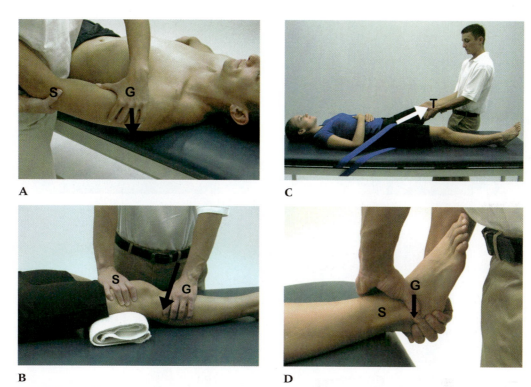

FIGURE 16–15 Joint mobilization and traction. **(A)** Posterior humeral glide (for increasing flexion and medial rotation). **(B)** Posterior tibial glide (for increasing flexion). **(C)** Inferior femoral traction (increases flexion and abduction). **(D)** Posterior talar glides (for increasing dorsiflexion). (S = stabilize, G = glide, T = traction)

pain-free function.[50] It is a noninvasive and comfortable intervention with applications for the spine and the extremities. Mulligan's concept uses what are referred to as either *mobilizations with movement (MWMs)* for treating the extremities or *sustained natural apophyseal glides (SNAGs)* for treating problems in the spine. Instead of the athletic trainer using oscillations or thrusting techniques, the patient moves in a specific direction as the athletic trainer guides the restricted body part. MWMs and SNAGs have the potential to quickly restore functional movements in joints, even after many years of restriction.[50]

Principles of Treatment The basic premise of the Mulligan technique for an athletic trainer choosing to make use of MWMs in the extremities or SNAGS in the spine is to never cause pain in the patient.[50] During assessment, the athletic trainer should look for specific signs, including a loss of joint movement, pain associated with movement, or pain associated with specific functional activities. A passive accessory joint mobilization is applied either parallel or perpendicular to the joint plane.[11] The athletic trainer must continuously monitor the patient's reaction to ensure that no pain is re-created during this mobilization. The athletic trainer experiments with various combinations of parallel or perpendicular glides until he or she discovers the appropriate treatment plane and grade of movement that

together significantly improve range of motion and/or significantly decrease or, better yet, eliminate altogether the original pain. Failure to improve range of motion or decrease pain indicates that the athletic trainer has not found the correct contact point, treatment plane, grade, or direction of mobilization. The patient then actively repeats the restricted and/or painful motion or activity while the athletic trainer continues to maintain the appropriate accessory glide. Further increases in range of motion or decreases in pain may be expected during a treatment session that typically involves three sets of 10 repetitions. Additional gains may be realized through the application of pain-free, passive overpressure at the end of available range.

An example of MWM might refer to a patient with restricted ankle dorsiflexion.[11] The patient stands on a treatment table with the athletic trainer manually stabilizing the foot (Figure 16–16). A nonelastic belt passes around both the distal leg of the patient and the waist of the athletic trainer, who applies a sustained anterior glide of the tibia by leaning backward away from the patient. The patient then performs a slow dorsiflexion movement until the first onset of pain or end of range. Once this end point is reached, the position is sustained for 10 seconds. The patient then relaxes and returns to the standing position, followed by release of the anteroposterior glide, followed by a 20 second rest period.

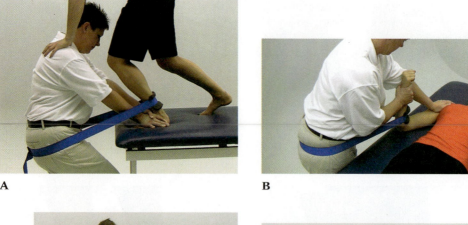

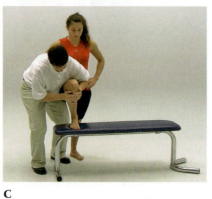

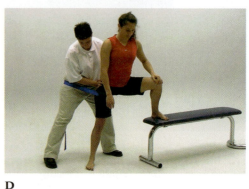

FIGURE 16–16   Mulligan technique. **(A)** Mobilization with manipulation (MWM) for restricted ankle dorsiflexion. **(B)** MWM for movement loss in the elbow. **(C)** MWM for restricted knee flexion. **(D)** MWM for restricted hip abduction.

Myofascial Release

Myofascial release refers to a group of techniques used to relieve soft tissue from the abnormal grip of tight fascia.[33] It is essentially a form of stretching that has been reported to have significant impact in treating a variety of conditions.[45] Some specialized training is necessary for the athletic trainer to understand specific techniques of myofascial release.[65] It is also essential to have an in-depth understanding of the fascial system.

Fascia is a type of connective tissue that surrounds muscles, tendons, nerves, bones, and organs. It is essentially continuous from head to toe and is interconnected in various sheaths or planes. Fascia is composed primarily of collagen along with some elastic fibers. During movement, the fascia must stretch and move freely. If there is damage to the fascia from injury, disease, or inflammation, it will affect not only local, adjacent structures but also areas far removed from the site of the injury. Thus, it may be necessary to release tightness in both the area of injury and distant areas. Tightness in these areas tends to soften and release in response to gentle pressure over a relatively long period of time.[44]

Myofascial release has also been referred to as *soft-tissue mobilization*, although technically all forms of massage involve the mobilization of soft tissue. Soft-tissue mobilization should not be confused with joint mobilization, although the two are closely related. Joint mobilization is used to restore normal joint arthrokinematics, and specific rules exist regarding direction of movement and joint position based on the shape of the articulating surfaces. Myofascial restrictions are considerably more unpredictable and may occur in many different planes and directions. Myofascial treatment is based on localizing the restriction and moving into the direction of the restriction, regardless of whether that follows the arthrokinematics of a nearby joint.[70] Thus, myofascial manipulation is considerably more subjective and relies heavily on the experience of the clinician.

Myofascial manipulation focuses on large treatment areas, whereas joint mobilization focuses on a specific joint. Releasing myofascial restrictions over a large treatment area can have a significant impact on joint mobility.[44] Once a myofascial restriction is located, the massage should be directly through the restriction. The progression of the technique is from superficial to deep. Once more superficial restrictions are released, the deep restrictions can be located and released without causing any damage to superficial tissues. Joint mobilization should follow myofascial release and will likely be more effective once soft-tissue restrictions are eliminated.

As the extensibility is improved in the myofascia, elongation and stretching of the musculotendinous unit should be incorporated.[45] In addition, strengthening exercises are recommended to enhance neuromuscular reeducation, which helps promote new, more efficient movement patterns.[70] As freedom of movement improves, postural reeducation may help to ensure the maintenance of the less restricted movement patterns.

Generally, acute cases tend to resolve in just a few treatments. The longer a condition has been present, the longer it will take to resolve. Occasionally, dramatic results occur immediately after treatment. It is usually recommended that treatment be done at least three times per week.

Graston Technique®

The Graston technique® is an instrument-assisted soft-tissue mobilization that enables clinicians to break down scar tissue and fascial restrictions as well as stretch connective tissue and muscle fibers (Figure 16–17).[15,30] The technique utilizes six handheld stainless steel instruments, shaped to fit the contour of the body, to scan an area and then to locate and treat the injured tissue that is causing pain and restricting motion.[30] A clinician normally palpates a painful area, looking for unusual nodules, restrictive barriers, or tissue tensions. The instruments help magnify existing restrictions, and the clinician can feel these through the instruments.[39] Then the clinician can use the instruments to supply precise pressure to break up scar tissue, which relieves the discomfort and helps restore normal function. The instruments, with a narrow surface area at their edge, have the ability to separate fibers.

A specially designed lubricant is applied to the skin prior to using an instrument, allowing the instrument to glide over the skin without causing irritation. Using a cross-friction massage in multiple directions, which involves using the instruments to stroke or rub against the grain of the scar tissue, the clinician creates small amounts of trauma to the affected area.[15] This temporarily causes inflammation, which increases the rate and amount of blood flow in and around the area. The theory is that this process helps initiate and promote the healing process of the affected soft tissues. It is common for the patient to experience some discomfort during the procedure and possibly some bruising. Ice application following the treatment may ease the discomfort. It is recommended that an exercise, stretching, and strengthening program be used in conjunction with the technique to help the injured tissues heal.[39]

Strain/Counterstrain

Strain/counterstrain is an approach to decreasing muscle tension and guarding that may be used to normalize muscle function. It is a passive technique that places the body in a position of greatest comfort, thereby relieving pain.[80]

In this technique, the athletic trainer locates "tender points" on the patient's body that correspond to areas of dysfunction in specific joints or muscles that are in need of treatment. These tender points are not located in or just beneath the skin, as

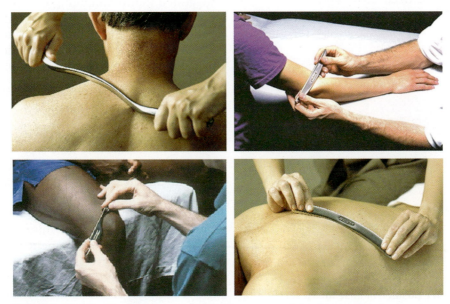

FIGURE 16–17   The Graston technique® uses a variety of curved instruments.

are many acupuncture points, but deeper in muscle, tendon, ligament, or fascia. They are characterized by tense, tender, edematous spots on the body; they are $^{3}/_{8}$ inch (1 cm) or less in diameter, with the most acute point $^{1}/_{10}$ of an inch (3 mm) in diameter, although they may be a few centimeters long within a muscle; there may be multiple points for one specific joint dysfunction; they may be arranged in a chain; and points are often found in a painless area opposite the site of pain and/or weakness.[80]

The athletic trainer monitors the tension and level of pain elicited by the tender point as he or she moves the patient into a position of ease or comfort. This is accomplished by markedly shortening the muscle.[71] When this position of ease is found, the tender point is no longer tense or tender. When this position is maintained for a minimum of 90 seconds, the tension in the tender point and in the corresponding joint or muscle is reduced or cleared. By slowly returning to a neutral position, the tender point and the corresponding joint or muscle remain pain free with normal tension. For example, with neck pain and/or tension headaches, the tender points may be found on either the front or back of the patient's neck and shoulders. The athletic trainer has the patient lie on his or her back and gently and slowly bends the patient's neck until that tender point is no longer tender. After the patient has held that position for 90 seconds, the athletic trainer gently and slowly returns the patient's neck to its resting position. Upon pressing that tender point again, the patient should notice a significant decrease in pain (Figure 16–18).[71]

The physiological rationale for the effectiveness of the strain/counterstrain technique can be explained by the stretch reflex. The stretch reflex was discussed in detail in Chapter 4. When a muscle is placed in a stretched position, impulses from the muscle spindles create a reflex contraction of the muscle in response to stretch. With strain/counterstrain, the joint or muscle is not placed in a position of stretch but rather a slack position. Thus, muscle spindle input is reduced and the muscle is relaxed, allowing for a decrease in tension and pain.[80]

Positional Release Therapy

Positional release therapy (PRT) is based on the strain/counterstrain technique. The primary difference between the two is the use of a facilitating force (compression) to enhance the effect of the positioning.[9]

Like strain/counterstrain, PRT is an osteopathic mobilization technique in which the body is brought into a position of greatest relaxation.[13] The athletic trainer finds the position of greatest comfort and muscle relaxation for a particular joint with the help of movement tests and diagnostic tender points. Once located, the tender point is maintained with the palpating finger at a subthreshold pressure.[67] The patient is then passively placed in a position that reduces the tension under the palpating finger and causes a subjective reduction in tenderness as reported by the patient. This specific position is adjusted throughout the 90-second treatment period. It has been suggested that maintaining contact with the tender point during the treatment period exerts a therapeutic effect.[9] This technique is one of the most effective and most gentle methods for the treatment of acute and chronic musculoskeletal dysfunction (Figure 16–19).[67]

Soft-Tissue Mobilization

Soft-tissue mobilization (active release technique, or ART®) is a relatively new type of manual therapy that has been developed to correct soft-tissue problems in muscle, tendon, and fascia caused by the formation of fibrotic adhesions as a result of acute injury, repetitive or overuse injuries, and constant pressure or tension injuries.[6] When a muscle, tendon, fascia, or ligament is torn (strained or sprained) or a nerve is damaged, the tissues heal with adhesions or scar tissue formation rather than the formation of brand new tissue. Scar tissue is weaker, less elastic, less pliable, and more pain

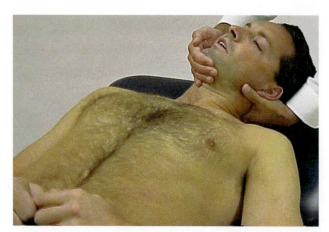

FIGURE 16–18 Strain/counterstrain technique. The body part is placed in a position of ease for 90 seconds and then slowly moved back to neutral position.

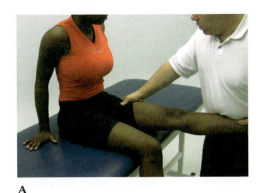
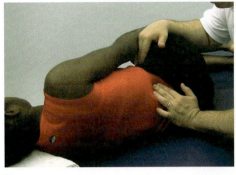

A **B**

FIGURE 16–19 Positional release therapy uses a position of comfort, with the finger or thumb exerting submaximal pressure on a tender point. **(A)** Quadriceps. **(B)** Quadratus lumborum.

sensitive than healthy tissue. These fibrotic adhesions disrupt the normal muscle function, which in turn affects the biomechanics of the joint complex and can lead to pain and dysfunction. Soft-tissue mobilization provides a way to diagnose and treat the underlying causes of cumulative trauma disorders that, left uncorrected, can lead to inflammation, adhesions/fibrosis, muscle imbalances that result in weak and tense tissues, decreased circulation, hypoxia, and symptoms of peripheral nerve entrapment, including numbness, tingling, burning, and aching.[6]

Soft-tissue mobilization is a deep-tissue technique used for breaking down scar tissue/adhesions and restoring function and movement. In soft-tissue mobilization, the athletic trainer should first locate through palpation those adhesions in the muscle, tendon, or fascia that are causing the problem. Once these are located, the athletic trainer traps the affected muscle by applying pressure or tension with the thumb or finger over these lesions in the direction of the fibers. Then the patient is asked to actively move the body part so that the musculature is elongated from a shortened position while the athletic trainer continues to apply tension to the lesion (Figure 16–20). This should be repeated three to five times per treatment session.

By breaking up the adhesions, the technique improves the patient's condition by softening and stretching the scar tissue, resulting in increased range of motion, increased strength, and improved circulation, which optimizes healing. Treatments tend to be uncomfortable during the movement phases as the scar tissue or adhesions tear apart. This is temporary and subsides almost immediately after the treatment. An important part of soft-tissue mobilization is for the patient to heed the athletic trainer's recommendations regarding activity modification, stretching, and exercise.

Biofeedback

In rehabilitation, athletic trainers use biofeedback to help a patient develop greater voluntary control for the purpose of enhancing either neuromuscular relaxation or muscle reeducation following injury.[78] A biofeedback unit is an electronic or electromechanical instrument that accurately measures, processes, and feeds back reinforcing information to the patient via auditory or visual signals (Figure 16–21). Perhaps the biggest advantage of biofeedback is that it provides the patient with immediate feedback on how effectively he or she is able to either contract or relax a muscle. Effective contraction or relaxation is immediately noted

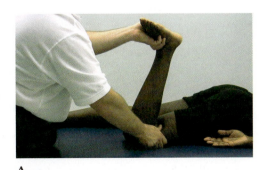
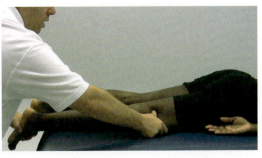

A **B**

FIGURE 16–20 Soft-tissue mobilization. **(A)** Starting position. **(B)** Muscle is elongated from a shortened position while static pressure is applied to the lesion.

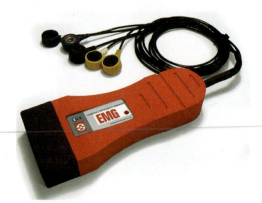

FIGURE 16–21 The biofeedback unit is connected via a series of electrodes to the skin over the contracting muscle and measures electrical activity in that muscle.

and rewarded so that eventually larger changes or improvements in these capabilities can be accomplished.[61]

Several types of biofeedback units are available for use in rehabilitation; EMG biofeedback is the most widely used in a clinical setting.[61] An EMG biofeedback unit measures the electrical activity produced by depolarization of a muscle fiber as an indicator of the quality of a muscle contraction. The EMG biofeedback unit detects small amounts of electrical energy generated during muscle contraction through active electrodes. The biofeedback unit processes and interprets this electrical activity and subsequently quantifies this information into either visual or auditory feedback that the patient can easily understand. Biofeedback information is displayed either visually using lights or meters or auditorily using tones, beeps, buzzes, or clicks.[78]

PURCHASING AND MAINTAINING THERAPEUTIC EXERCISE EQUIPMENT

The extent and variety of therapeutic exercise equipment available to use in injury rehabilitation can at times be overwhelming. Prices of rehabilitation equipment can range from $2 for a piece of resistance tubing to $4,000 for an electrical stimulating unit to $80,000 for certain computer-driven isokinetic or balance devices. It is certainly not necessary to purchase expensive exercise equipment to see good results. It is likely that an injured patient can achieve many of the same physiological benefits from using a $2 piece of surgical tubing as from exercising on an $80,000 isokinetic device. Many athletic trainers would argue that the most useful pieces of rehabilitation equipment available are the hands and the creativity of a well-trained and experienced clinician. Others maintain that the greater the extent and variety of rehabilitation equipment available, the more flexibility the athletic trainer has in devising rehabilitation programs.

For almost everyone, budgetary constraints, at least to some extent, will limit the pieces of rehabilitation equipment that can be purchased. Decisions to purchase pieces of rehabilitation equipment should be based on a realistic assessment of the usefulness and functionality of that piece of equipment, the extent to which it will be used, and its durability. Perhaps the most important question that should be asked when purchasing a new piece of equipment is whether this piece of equipment will help the patient reach the goals of the rehabilitation program.

Once rehabilitation equipment has been purchased, the athletic trainer should assume the responsibility of making sure that it is being used correctly and for the intended purpose as stated in the manufacturer's instructions for use. It is also essential that the athletic trainer apply the manufacturer's guidelines for the periodic inspection and maintenance of the equipment to ensure that it is operating safely.

SUMMARY

- When injuries occur, the athletic trainer usually assumes the primary responsibility for the design, implementation, and supervision of the rehabilitation program for the injured patient. Two major goals of rehabilitation are to prevent deconditioning and to restore the injured part to a preinjury state. Besides the physical aspect, the mental and emotional aspects of rehabilitation must always be considered.

- When an injured body part is immobilized for a period of time, a number of disuse problems adversely affect muscle, joints, ligaments, bones, cartilage, neuromuscular efficiency, and the cardiorespiratory system.

- Designing rehabilitation programs is relatively simple and involves several basic components: minimizing swelling, controlling pain, reestablishing neuromuscular control, establishing or enhancing core stability, regaining or improving range of motion, restoring or increasing muscular strength and endurance, regaining balance and postural control, maintaining cardiorespiratory endurance, and incorporating functional progressions. The long-term goal is to return the injured athlete to practice or competition as quickly and safely as possible.
- Rehabilitation programs can be subdivided into three phases, based primarily on the three stages of the healing process: phase 1, the acute inflammatory response phase; phase 2, the fibroblastic repair phase; and phase 3, the maturation-remodeling phase. If surgery is necessary, a fourth phase, the preoperative phase, must also be considered.
- The decision to release a patient recovering from injury to full activity is the final stage of the rehabilitation and recovery process. The decision should be carefully considered by each member of the sports medicine team involved in the rehabilitation process.
- An open kinetic chain exists when the foot or hand is not in contact with the ground or some other surface. In a closed kinetic chain, the foot or hand is weight bearing. The use of closed chain strengthening techniques is the rehabilitation treatment of choice for many athletic trainers. Closed kinetic chain strengthening activities are more functional than are open kinetic chain activities.
- Aquatic exercises can be an important rehabilitative tool for the athletic trainer, particularly with injuries involving the lower extremity. Aquatic exercises allow for resistance with motion without weight bearing.
- Proprioceptive neuromuscular facilitation is a manual therapy technique that can be used for strengthening muscle or increasing range of motion. The PNF movement patterns involve a sequential series of specific movements for the lower extremity, lower trunk, upper trunk, and upper extremity.
- Mobilization, traction, and Mulligan techniques are manual therapy techniques used to improve joint mobility or to decrease joint pain by restoring accessory movements to the injured joint, which allows full, pain-free range of motion.
- A variety of manual therapy techniques, including muscle energy, myofascial release, the Graston technique®, strain/counterstrain, positional release, soft-tissue mobilization, and biofeedback can be incorporated into a rehabilitation program.

WEB SITES

Archives of Physical Medicine and Rehabilitation: www.archives-pmr.org

Cramer First Aider: http://www.cramersportsmed.com/resources/first-aider

Journal of Sport Rehabilitation: http://journals.humankinetics.com/JSR

National Athletic Trainers' Association: www.nata.org
Accesses rehabilitation in the athletic training journals.

AOSSN Online Media Kit: www.sportsmed.org

The Physician and Sportsmedicine: www.physsportsmed.com
Search back issues and access the ones specifically geared toward weight training and rehabilitation.

SOLUTIONS TO CLINICAL APPLICATION EXERCISES

16–1 The components that should be addressed in any rehabilitation program are minimizing swelling, controlling pain, reestablishing neuromuscular control, establishing or enhancing core stability, regaining or improving range of motion, restoring or increasing muscular strength and endurance, regaining balance and postural control, maintaining cardiorespiratory endurance, and incorporating functional progressions. The approach to rehabilitation should be aggressive, and decisions as to when and how to alter and progress specific components within a rehabilitation program should be based on and are limited by the healing process.

16–2 After injury and subsequent rest and immobilization, it is not unusual for the patient to "forget" how to walk. The athletic trainer must help the patient relearn neuromuscular control, which means regaining the ability to follow some previously established motor and sensory pattern by regaining conscious control of a specific movement until that movement becomes automatic. Strengthening exercises, particularly those that tend to be more functional, such as closed kinetic chain exercises, are essential for reestablishing neuromuscular control. Addressing neuromuscular control is critical throughout the recovery process but may be most critical during the early stages of rehabilitation to avoid reinjury or overuse injuries to additional structures.

16–3 Anterior knee pain can result from many different causes. Strengthening the quadriceps can be helpful. If full-range-of-motion strengthening exercises increase pain, the patient should begin with positional isometric exercises done at different points in the range, progressing to full-range concentric and eccentric exercise as tolerated. Closed kinetic chain exercises, such as minisquats, stepping exercises, and leg presses, are excellent quadriceps-strengthening exercises and tend to be more functional than traditional open kinetic chain exercises.

16–4 The patient should have minimal signs of inflammation, such as pain and swelling. The appropriate healing time frame should also be reached before the patient progresses.

16–5 The athletic trainer can provide the encouragement and positive reinforcement necessary for the patient to make a commitment. Support from peers, coaches, and rehabilitation staff is important. The athletic trainer should clearly explain the instructions verbally to the athlete and then write them down. The rehabilitation program should fit into the patient's schedule. The athletic trainer must be creative in designing and varying the exercise routine. The rehabilitation program should be as pain free as possible. The coach needs to support the rehabilitation process.

16–6 Perhaps the best recommendation is to have the patient engage in an aquatic exercise program. In the water, the patient would not be weight bearing and could exercise the injured knee through a pain-free range of motion while working on maintaining levels of fitness by engaging in water-resisted conditioning exercises.

16–7 To achieve a full physiological range of motion, the joint must have normal accessory motions. Stretching techniques address motion restriction caused by tightness of the musculotendinous unit. The athletic trainer should incorporate joint mobilization techniques that address restriction of motion caused by some tightness of capsular and ligamentous structures that surround the affected joint.

16–8 To some extent, the answer depends on exactly what is causing her pain. In general, the athletic trainer may choose to use one of several or a combination of manual therapy techniques, including myofascial release, strain/counterstrain, positional release, and soft-tissue mobilization.

16–9 A biofeedback unit can help the patient relearn how to fire the quadriceps muscle. The biofeedback unit can provide both visual and auditory feedback to indicate the strength of a contraction as well as the timing of a contraction. Biofeedback can be used almost immediately following surgery.

REVIEW QUESTIONS AND CLASS ACTIVITIES

1. What occurs physiologically when an athlete is suddenly forced to stop physical activity?

2. Discuss the physiological effects of immobilization on muscles, ligaments, joints, bones, neuromuscular efficiency, and the cardiovascular system.

3. Discuss the similarities and differences between training and conditioning exercises and therapeutic exercise.

4. Why must an athlete condition the entire body while an injury heals?

5. Why is it important to modulate pain during a rehabilitation program?

6. Discuss the difference between proprioception and kinesthesia, and explain how they are related to neuromuscular control.

7. What is the significance of having the patient engage in core stabilization training during a rehabilitation program?

8. Critically compare the use of isometric, isotonic, and isokinetic exercises in rehabilitation.

9. How is range of motion restored after an injury?

10. How and when should functional progressions be incorporated into the rehabilitation program?

11. Describe how to determine whether a patient is ready to return to activity after injury.

12. What is the importance of developing a rehabilitation plan? Include the criteria for moving to various phases.

13. What are the important considerations during each of the three phases of rehabilitation?

14. Why are closed kinetic chain exercises more useful than open kinetic chain exercises in the rehabilitation of injuries?

15. How may aquatic exercise be incorporated into a rehabilitation program?

16. Proprioceptive neuromuscular facilitation includes stretching, strengthening, and movement-patterning techniques. How can these techniques apply to sports injuries?

17. How can a muscle energy technique be used to increase range of motion?

18. Explain why it is necessary to use stretching techniques to increase physiological movement and to use mobilization techniques to improve accessory motions.

19. How does a Mulligan technique help in treating pain and restricted motion?

20. How are the strain/counterstrain technique and positional release therapy related to one another?

REFERENCES

1. Anderson J: Effects of strength training on muscle fiber types and size; consequences for athletes training for high-intensity sport, *Scandinavian Journal of Medicine and Science in Sports* 20(Supplement):32–38, 2010.

2. Becker B: Aquatic Therapy: Scientific foundations and clinical rehabilitation applications, *Physical Medicine and Rehabilitation* 1(9):859–72, 2009.

3. Bernier MR: Perturbation and agility training in the rehabilitation of soccer athletes, *Athletic Therapy Today* 8(3):20, 2003.

4. Bialosky J: The mechanisms of manual therapy in the treatment of musculoskeletal pain, *Manual Therapy* 14(5):531–38, 2009.

5. Binkley H: Aquatic therapy in the treatment of upper extremity injuries, *Athletic Therapy Today* 7(1):49, 2002.

6. Blanchette M: Augmented soft tissue mobilization vs. natural history in the treatment of lateral epicondylitis, *Journal of manipulative and physiological therapeutics* 34(2):123–30, 2011.

7. Brewer B, Avondoglio J, Cornelius A: Construct validity and interrater agreement of the sport injury rehabilitation adherence scale, *J Sport Rehabil* 11(3):170, 2002.

8. Chaitlow L: *Muscle energy techniques*, Philadelphia, 2006, Churchill Livingstone.

9. Chaitlow L: *Positional release techniques*, Philadelphia, 2007, Elsevier Science.

10. Clark M: Core stabilization training in rehabilitation. In Prentice W, editor: *Rehabilitation techniques in sports medicine and athletic training*, St. Louis, 2010, McGraw-Hill.

11. Collins N, Teys P, Vicenzino B: The initial effects of a Mulligan's mobilization with movement technique on dorsiflexion and pain in subacute ankle sprains, *Manual Therapy* 2(May 9):77, 2004.

12. Colston M, Taylor T, Minnick A: Abdominal muscle training and core stabilization: The past, present, and future, *Athletic Therapy Today* 10(4):6, 2005.

13. D'Ambrogio K, Roth G: *Positional release therapy: Assessment and treatment of musculoskeletal dysfunction*, Philadelphia, 1997, Elsevier Science.

14. DeDeyne PG: Application of passive stretch and its implications for muscle fibers, *Phys Ther* 81:819, 2001.

15. DeLuccio J: Instrument assisted soft tissue mobilization utilizing Graston Technique: A physical therapist's perspective, *Orthopedic Physical Therapy Practice* 18(3):32–34, 2006.

16. DiStefano L: Evidence supporting balance training in healthy individuals: A systematic review, *Journal of Strength and Conditioning Research* 23(9):2718–31, 2009.

17. Ellenbecker T: *Effective functional progressions in sport rehabilitation*, Champaign, 2009, Human Kinetics.

18. Giammetto T, Giammetto S: *Integrative manual therapy: For biomechanics application of muscle energy and beyond technique*, vol. 3, Berkeley, CA, 2003, North Atlantic Books.

19. Glass R: The effects of open versus closed kinetic chain exercises on patients with

ACL deficient or reconstructed knees: A systematic review, *N Am J Sports Phys Ther.* 5(2):74–84, 2010.

20. Granquist M: Development of a measure of rehabilitation adherence for athletic training, *Journal of Sport Rehabilitation* 19: 249–67, 2010.

21. Halle J, Thomson B: Designing home exercise programs. In Hoogenboom B, Voight M, Prentice W, editors: *Musculoskeletal interventions techniques of therapeutic exercise,* New York, 2013, McGraw-Hill.

22. Hamson-Utley, J: Athletic trainers' and physical therapists' perceptions of the effectiveness of psychological skills within sport injury rehabilitation programs, *J Athl Train.* 43(3):258–64, 2008.

23. Harris AE, Worthy HA, Van Lunen BL, Vairo G: Immediate effects of static stretching and muscle energy technique on hamstring flexibility, *J Athl Train* 39 (2 Suppl):S-99, 2004.

24. Hedgepath E, Gieck J: Psychological considerations for rehabilitating the injured athlete. In Prentice W, editor: *Rehabilitation techniques in sports medicine and athletic training,* St. Louis, 2010, McGraw-Hill.

25. Hengeveld E: *Maitland's peripheral manipulation,* Waltham, MA, 2005, Butterworth-Heinemann.

26. Hertel J, Denegar C: A rehabilitation paradigm for restoring neuromuscular control following athletic injury, *Athletic Therapy Today* 3(5):12, 1998.

27. Hillman S: Principles and techniques of open kinetic chain rehabilitation, *J Sport Rehabil* 3(4):319, 1994.

28. Hoogenboom B, Lomax N: Aquatic therapy in rehabilitation. In Prentice W, editor: *Rehabilitation techniques in sports medicine and athletic training,* St. Louis, 2010, McGraw-Hill.

29. Hopkins JT, et al: An electromyographic comparison of 4 closed chain exercises, *J Athl Train* 34(4):353, 1999.

30. Hyde T: Graston technique: A soft tissue treatment for athletic injuries. *D.C. Tracts,* 15(3):2–4, 2003.

31. Kaltenborn F, Evjenth O, Kaltenborn B: *Manual mobilization of the joints: The Kaltenborn method of joint examination and treatment: The extremities,* vol. 1, and *The spine,* vol. 2, Minneapolis, 2003, Orthopedic Physical Therapy Products.

32. Karandikar N: Kinetic chains: A review of the concept and its clinical applications, *Physical Medicine and Rehabilitation,* 3(8):739–45, 2011.

33. Keirns M, editor: *Myofascial release in sports medicine,* Champaign, IL, 2000, Human Kinetics.

34. Kersey R, West S: Aquatic therapy, *Athletic Therapy Today* 10(5):48, 2005.

35. King M: Core stability: Creating a foundation for functional rehabilitation, *Athletic Therapy Today* 5(2):6, 2000.

36. Kitani I: The effectiveness of proprioceptive neuromuscular facilitation (PNF) exercises on shoulder joint position sense in baseball players, *J Athl Train* 39(2 Suppl):S-62, 2004.

37. Knott M, Voss EE: *Proprioceptive neuromuscular facilitation: Patterns and techniques,* ed 2, Philadelphia, 1985, Lippincott, Williams and Wilkins.

38. Konin J: Joint mobilization to decrease glenohumeral-joint impingement, *Athletic Therapy Today* 11(3):50, 2006.

39. Larkins P: Graston Technique, *Podiatry Management* 27(1):37–38, 2008.

40. Lephart S, Swanik C, Fu F: Reestablishing neuromuscular control. In Prentice W, editor: *Rehabilitation techniques in sports medicine and athletic training,* St. Louis, 2010, McGraw-Hill.

41. Levy A: Sport injury rehabilitation adherence: Perspectives of recreational athletes, *International Journal of Sport and Exercise Psychology* 7(2):212–29, 2011.

42. Levy A, Pullman R, Polman P: Mental toughness as a determinant of beliefs, pain, and adherence in sport injury rehabilitation, *J Sport Rehabil* 15(3):246, 2006.

43. Lim G: The effects of closed kinetic chain exercise and open kinetic chain exercise on knee position sense in normal adults, *Journal of International Academy of Physical Therapy Research* 1(2):126, 2010.

44. Manheim C: *Myofascial release manual,* Thorofare, NJ, 2008, Slack.

45. McClellan E, Padua D, Prentice W: Effects of myofascial release and static stretching on active range of motion and muscle activity, *J Athl Train* 39(2 Suppl):S-98, 2004.

46. McGee D: *Athletic and sport issues in musculoskeletal rehabilitation,* Philadelphia, 2010, Saunders.

47. McGee M: Functional progressions and functional testing in rehabilitation. In Prentice W, editor: *Rehabilitation techniques in sports medicine and athletic training,* St. Louis, 2010, McGraw-Hill.

48. McMullen J, Uhl TL: A kinetic chain approach for shoulder rehabilitation, *J Athl Train* 35(3):329, 2000.

49. Miller M, Berry D, Bullard S: Comparisons of land-based and aquatic-based plyometric programs during an 8-week training period, *J Sport Rehabil* 11(4):268, 2002.

50. Mulligan B: Manual therapy: NAGS, SNAGS, MWMS, etc., *Journal of Orthopedic and Sports Physical Therapy* 35(10)674–78, 2004.

51. Myers JB, et al: Proprioception and neuromuscular control of the shoulder after muscle fatigue, *J Athl Train* 34(4):362, 1999.

52. O'Neill DF: Return to function through aquatic therapy, *Athletic Therapy Today* 5(2): 14, 2000.

53. O'Sullivan, S: 2006. *Physical rehabilitation,* Philadelphia, F.A. Davis.

54. Perrin D: *Isokinetic exercise and assessment,* Champaign, IL, 1993, Human Kinetics.

55. Piccininni J, Drover J: Athlete-patient education in rehabilitation: developing a self-directed program, *Athletic Therapy Today* 4(6):51, 1999.

56. Pizzari T, Taylor N, McBurney H: Adherence to rehabilitation after anterior cruciate ligament reconstructive surgery: Implications for outcome, *J Sport Rehabil* 14(3): 201, 2005.

57. Prentice W: Closed kinetic chain exercise. In Prentice W, editor: *Rehabilitation techniques in sports medicine and athletic training,* St. Louis, 2010, McGraw-Hill.

58. Prentice W: The healing process and pathophysiology of musculoskeletal injury. In Prentice W, editor: *Rehabilitation techniques in sports medicine and athletic training,* St. Louis, 2010, McGraw-Hill.

59. Prentice W: Mobilization and traction techniques in rehabilitation. In Prentice W, editor: *Rehabilitation techniques in sports medicine and athletic training,* St. Louis, 2010, McGraw-Hill.

60. Prentice W: Proprioceptive neuromuscular facilitation techniques. In Prentice W, editor: *Rehabilitation techniques in sports medicine and athletic training,* St. Louis, 2010, McGraw-Hill.

61. Prentice W: *Therapeutic modalities in rehabilitation,* ed 4, New York, 2011, McGraw-Hill.

62. Prentice W: Understanding and managing the healing process through rehabilitation. In Prentice W, editor: *Rehabilitation techniques in sports medicine and athletic training,* St. Louis, 2010, McGraw-Hill.

63. Reiman M: 2009. *Functional testing in human performance,* Champaign, Human Kinetics.

64. Scherzer C, Brewer B, Cornelius A: Psychological skills and adherence to rehabilitation after reconstruction of the anterior cruciate ligament, *J Sport Rehabil* 10(3):165, 2001.

65. Sefton J: Myofascial release for athletic trainers, Part I, *Athletic Therapy Today* 9(1):40, 2004.

66. Smith D: Incorporating kinetic-chain integration, Part 2: Functional shoulder rehabilitation, *Athletic Therapy Today* 1(5):63, 2006.

67. Speicher T, Draper D: Top 10 positional release therapy techniques to break the chain of pain, Part 1, *Athletic Therapy Today* 1(5):60, 2006.

68. Stillman B: Making sense of proprioception: The meaning of proprioception, kinesthesia and related terms, *Physiotherapy* 88(11): 667–76, 2002.

69. Stone J: Muscle energy technique, *Athletic Therapy Today* 5(5):25, 2000.

70. Stone J: Myofascial release, *Athletic Therapy Today* 5(4):34, 2000.

71. Stone J: Strain-counterstrain, *Athletic Therapy Today* 5(6):30, 2000.

72. Swann E: Uses of manual-therapy techniques in pain management, *Athletic Therapy Today* 7(4):14, 2002.

73. Swanson K: Improving proprioception and neuromuscular control following shoulder injury, *Athletic Therapy Today* 3(5):30, 1998.

74. Thien-Brody L: *Aquatic exercise for rehabilitation and training,* Champaign, 2009, Human Kinetics.

75. Thomas M, Müller T, Busse M: Comparison of tension in thera-band and cando tubing, *J Orthop Sports Phys Ther* 32(11):576, 2002.

76. Tripp B: Integrating sensorimotor control into rehabilitation, *Athletic Therapy Today* 1(5):24, 2006.

77. Ubinger M, Prentice W, Guskiewicz K: Effect of closed kinetic chain training on neuromuscular control in the upper extremity, *J Sport Rehabil* 8(3):184, 1999.

78. Wasielewski N: Evaluation of electromyographic biofeedback for the quadriceps femoris: A systematic review, *J Athl Train* 46(5):543–54, 2011.

79. Westwater-Wood S: The use of proprioceptive neuromuscular facilitation in physiotherapy practice, *Physical Therapy Reviews* 15(1):23–28, 2010.

80. Wong C: Strain counterstrain: Current concepts and clinical evidence, *Manual Therapy* 17(1):2–8, 2012.

81. Yoke M: *Functional exercise progressions,* Monterey, CA, 2003, Healthy Learning.

82. Zech A: Balance training for neuromuscular control and performance enhancement: A systematic review, *J Athl Train* 45(4):392–403, 2010.

83. Zech A: Neuromuscular training for rehabilitation of sports injuries: A systematic review, *Medicine and Science in Sports and Exercise* 41(10):1831–41, 2009.

ANNOTATED BIBLIOGRAPHY

Brotzman S: *Clinical orthopedic rehabilitation*, Philadelphia, 2011, Elsevier Health Sciences.

Discusses the rehabilitation of injuries that occur in specific sports.

Chaitlow L: *Muscle energy techniques*, Philadelphia, 2006, Elsevier Health Sciences.

Discusses muscle energy techniques (manipulative treatments in which a patient engages a muscle against a counterforce) for osteopaths, chiropractors, athletic trainers, physical therapists, and massage therapists.

Chaitlow L: *Positional release techniques*, 2007, Churchill-Livingston.

Organizes the concept of strain/counterstrain and positional release into a systemic approach that is easy to use and document. Contains examples demonstrating each release position with an awareness of the clinician's body mechanics.

Edmond S: *Manipulation and mobilization: Extremity and spinal techniques*, New York, 2006, Mosby.

Provides the entry-level student and the practicing clinician with a comprehensive text on mobilization and manipulation techniques.

Ellenbecker T: *Effective functional progressions in sport rehabilitation*, Champaign, 2009, Human Kinetics.

Presents scientific principles and practical applications for using functional exercise to rehabilitate athletic injuries.

Kisner C, Colby A: *Therapeutic exercise: Foundations and techniques*, Philadelphia, 2007, F.A. Davis.

A clear, concise presentation of the field of therapeutic exercise well suited to sports medicine. Covers exercise for increasing range of motion and for treating soft tissue, bone, and postsurgical problems.

McGee D: *Athletic and sport issues in musculoskeletal rehabilitation*, Philadelphia, 2010, Saunders.

An extremely detailed, scientifically based, advanced text dealing with athletic injury rehabilitation.

Prentice W: *Mobilization and traction: Principles and techniques* (video, 33 minutes), St. Louis, 1993, Mosby/McGraw-Hill.

A thorough overview of mobilization and traction and includes detailed demonstrations of various techniques.

Prentice W: *Proprioceptive neuromuscular facilitation: Principles and techniques* (video, 26 minutes), St. Louis, 1993, Mosby/McGraw-Hill.

An introduction to PNF stretching and strengthening exercises, complete with a detailed, hands-on demonstration of specific techniques.

Prentice W: *Rehabilitation techniques in sports medicine and athletic training*, ed 4, St. Louis, 2010, McGraw-Hill.

A comprehensive text dealing with all aspects of rehabilitation used in a sports medicine setting.

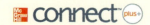

17

Pharmacology, Drugs, and Sports

■ Objectives

When you finish this chapter you should be able to

- Define the term *drug*.
- Identify the various methods by which drugs can be administered.
- Analyze pharmacokinetics relative to absorption, distribution, metabolism, and excretion.
- Explain the difference between administering and dispensing medications.
- Express legal concerns for administering medications to the athletic population.
- Apply the various protocols that the athletic trainer should follow for administering over-the-counter medications to patients.

- Categorize the various drugs that can be used to treat infection, reduce pain and inflammation, relax muscles, treat gastrointestinal disorders, treat symptoms of colds and congestion, and control bleeding.
- Recognize the problem of substance abuse in the athletic population.
- Describe the ergogenic aids used by athletes to improve performance.
- Discuss the abuse of alcohol, drugs, and tobacco by athletes.
- Evaluate drug-testing policies and procedures, and list the types of banned drugs.

■ Outline

■ Key Terms

pharmacology	drug vehicle	volume of	potency	half-life
drug	bioavailability	distribution	biotransformation	steady-state
pharmacokinetics		efficacy	metabolism	bioequivalent drugs

■ Connect Highlights connect plus+

Visit connect.mcgraw-hill.com for further exercises to apply your knowledge:

- Clinical application scenarios covering administering and dispensing medications, drug classifications and therapeutic uses, and the use of alcohol, drugs, and tobacco by athletes and banned substances for athletes
- Click-and-drag questions covering various methods by which drugs can be administered, regulating governing agencies for drugs, drug classifications and therapeutic uses, dispensing and application of medications, and banned drugs for athletes
- Multiple-choice questions covering various methods to administer/dispense drugs, legal concerns, drug classifications and therapeutic uses, substance abuse, ergogenic aids, and drug-testing policies and procedures
- Picture identification of various drug classifications and therapeutic uses

Pharmacology is the branch of science that studies the actions of drugs on biological systems, especially drugs that are used in medicine for diagnostic and therapeutic purposes.[30] Pharmaceutical care is the direct provision of medication-related care for the purpose of achieving definite outcomes that improve quality of life.[23] Medications of all types, both prescription and over-the-counter, are as commonly used by athletes as they are by others in the population.[1]

> **pharmacology** The study of drugs and their origin, nature, properties, and effects on living organisms.

Unfortunately, the abuse of various drugs and other substances for performance enhancement or for recreational mood alteration is also widespread among athletes. Thus, the athletic trainer must be knowledgeable about drug use and substance abuse within the population with which he or she works.[30]

WHAT IS A DRUG?

A **drug** is a chemical agent used in the prevention, treatment, or diagnosis of disease.[42] The use of substances for the express purpose of treating some infirmity or disease dates back to early history. The ancient Egyptians were highly skilled in making and using medications, treating a wide range of external and internal conditions.

> **drug** A chemical agent used in the prevention, treatment, or diagnosis of disease.

Many of our common drugs, such as aspirin and penicillin, are derived from natural sources. Historically, medications were composed of roots, herbs, leaves, or other natural materials that were identified as having, or were believed to have, medicinal properties. Today many medications that originally came from nature are produced synthetically.

PHARMACOKINETICS

Pharmacokinetics is the method by which drugs are absorbed, distributed, metabolized, and eliminated or excreted by the body. The term *pharmacodynamics* is often confused with *pharmacokinetics*. *Pharmacodynamics* refers to the actions or the effects of a drug on the body and will be discussed in more detail throughout this chapter.[9,42]

> **pharmacokinetics** The method by which drugs are absorbed, distributed, metabolized, and eliminated.

Administration of Drugs

To be effective therapeutically, a drug must first enter the system and then reach a receptor in a target tissue. The administration of medications can

> **Drugs can be administered internally or externally.**

be either internal or external and is based on the type of local or general response desired.

Internal Administration Drugs can be taken internally through inhalation, or they can be administered intradermally or subcutaneously, intramuscularly, intranasally, intraspinally, intravaginally, intravenously, orally, rectally, or sublingually and buccally.

Inhalation is a means of bringing medication or substances to the respiratory tract. This method is most often used in sports to relieve the athlete of the symptoms of respiratory illnesses, such as asthma. The vehicle for inhalation is normally water vapor, oxygen, or highly aromatic medications.

Intradermal (into the skin) or *subcutaneous* (under the cutaneous tissues) administration is usually accomplished through a hypodermic needle injection. Such introduction of medication is initiated when a rapid response is needed, but this method does not produce as rapid a response as intravenous injection offers.

Intramuscular injection means that the medication is given directly into the muscle tissue. The site for such an injection is usually the gluteal area or the deltoid muscle of the upper arm.

Intranasal application varies according to the condition that is to be treated. The introduction of a decongestant intranasal solution by using a dropper or an atomizer may relieve the discomfort of head colds and allergies.

Intraspinal injection may be indicated for any of the following purposes: introduction of drugs to combat specific organisms that have entered the spinal cord; injection of a substance, such as procaine, to anesthetize the lower limbs; or withdrawal of spinal fluid to be studied.

Intravaginal administration involves placement of a drug or drug-containing device inside the vagina. Drugs are readily absorbed through the vaginal mucosa.

Intravenous injection (into a vein) is given when an immediate reaction to the medication is desired. The drug enters the venous circulation and is spread rapidly throughout the body.

Oral administration of medicines is the most common method of all. Forms such as tablets, capsules, powders, and liquids are easily administered orally.

Rectal administration of drugs is limited. In the past, some medications have been introduced through the rectum to be absorbed by its mucous lining. Such methods have difficulties in regulating dosage.

Sublingual and *buccal* introductions of medicines usually consist of placing easily dissolved agents, such as troches (lozenges) or tablets, under the tongue. They dissolve slowly and are absorbed by the mucous lining.

TABLE 17–1   Drug Vehicles

Liquid preparations

Aqueous solution	Sterile water containing a drug substance.
Elixir	Alcohol, sugar, and flavoring with a drug dissolved in solution, designed for internal consumption.
Liniment	Alcohol or oil containing a dissolved drug, designed for external massage.
Spirit	A drug dissolved in water and alcohol or in alcohol alone.
Suspension	Undissolved powder in a fluid medium; must be mixed well by shaking before use.
Syrup	A mixture of sugar and water containing a drug.

Solid preparations

Ampule	A closed glass receptacle containing a drug.
Capsule	A gelatin receptacle containing a drug.
Ointment (emollient)	A semisolid preparation for external application of such consistency that it may be applied to the skin by inunction.
Paste	An inert powder combined with water.
Tablet	A solid pharmaceutical dosage compressed into a small oval, circle, square, or other form.
Plaster	A substance intended for external application, made of such materials and of such consistency as to adhere to the skin and thereby attach a dressing.
Powder	Finely ground drug plus vehicle or effervescent granules.
Suppository	A medicated gelatin molded into a cone for placement in a body orifice (e.g., the anal canal).

External Administration Medications administered externally include inunctions, ointments, pastes, plasters, transdermal patches, and solutions.

Inunctions are oily or medicated substances that are rubbed into the skin and result in a local or systemic reaction. Oil-based liniments and petroleum analgesic balms used as massage lubricants are examples of inunctions.

Ointments consisting of oil, petroleum jelly, or lanolin combined with drugs are applied for long-lasting topical medication.

Pastes are ointments with a nonfat base. They are spread on cloth and usually produce a cooling effect on the skin.

Plasters are thicker than ointments and are spread either on cloth or paper or directly on the skin. They usually contain an irritant, are applied as a counterirritant, and are used for relieving pain, increasing circulation, and decreasing inflammation.

Transdermal patches are patches resembling adhesive bandages that contain various types of slow-release medications that are absorbed gradually through the skin. Some patches may be left in place for only several hours, whereas others may be left on for several days.

Solutions can be administered externally and are extremely varied, consisting principally of bacteriostatics. Antiseptics, disinfectants, vasoconstrictors, and liquid rubefacients (alcohol, turpentine) are examples.

Drug Vehicles A **drug vehicle** is a therapeutically inactive substance that transports a drug. A drug is housed in a vehicle that may be either a solid or a liquid. Some of the more common drug vehicles are listed in Table 17–1.

> **drug vehicle** The substance in which a drug is transported.

Absorption of Drugs Once a drug is in the system, it must be dissolved before it can be absorbed. The rate and extent of absorption are determined by the chemical characteristics of the drug, the dosage form (e.g., tablet or solution), and the gastric-emptying time. Solutions in which the drug is already dissolved have the fastest absorption rate, and time-release medications have the slowest rate.[9]

Bioavailability Refers to how completely a particular drug is absorbed by the system and available to produce a response.[9] Bioavailability is most dependent on the characteristics of the drug and not on the dosage form, whereas absorption rate is largely determined by dosage form.

> **bioavailability** How completely a particular drug is absorbed by the system.

Distribution Once absorbed, the drug is transported through the blood to a specific target tissue. The drug will be distributed to other parts of the body

Chapter Seventeen ■ Pharmacology, Drugs, and Sports

as well. The **volume of distribution** is the volume plasma, or fluid, in which the drug is dissolved and indicates the extent of distribution of that drug. The **efficacy** of a drug is its capability of producing a specific therapeutic effect once it reaches a particular receptor site in a target tissue. **Potency** is the dose of the drug that is required to produce a desired therapeutic effect.[42]

volume of distribution
The volume of plasma in which a drug is dissolved.

efficacy A drug's capability of producing a specific therapeutic effect.

potency The dose of a drug required to produce a desired therapeutic effect.

Metabolism The **biotransformation** of drugs into water-soluble compounds that can be excreted is referred to as **metabolism**. Most of the metabolism takes place in the liver, with some occurring in the kidneys and blood. Metabolism of drugs in the liver transforms most active drugs into inactive compounds. Occasionally, when an active drug is metabolized, the metabolites (byproducts of this process) are toxic.[9]

biotransformation
Transforming a drug so that it can be metabolized.

metabolism Changing a drug into a water-soluble compound that can be excreted.

Excretion The excretion of a drug or its metabolites is controlled primarily by the kidneys. Drugs are filtered through the kidneys and are usually excreted in the urine, although some are reabsorbed. Some drugs are excreted in saliva, sweat, and feces.[9]

Drug Half-Life

The rate at which a drug disappears from the body—through metabolism, excretion, or a combination of the two—is called the drug's **half-life**. This rate is the amount of time required for the plasma drug level to be reduced by one-half. For most drugs, the half-life is measured in hours, but for some it is measured in minutes or days. Knowing the half-life of a drug is critical in determining how often and in what dosage a drug must be administered to achieve and maintain therapeutic levels of concentration. The dosage interval, or time between the administration of individual doses, may be equal to the half-life of that drug.[9]

half-life The rate at which a drug disappears from the body through metabolism, excretion, or both.

How often a drug will be administered is determined in part by the drug's **steady state**, which is reached when the amount that is taken is equal to the amount that is excreted. A steady state is usually reached after five half-lives of the drug have occurred.

steady state When the amount of the drug taken is equal to the amount that is excreted.

Drugs with long half-lives may take several days to weeks to reach a steady state.[9]

Effects of Physical Activity on Pharmacokinetics

In general, exercise decreases a drug's absorption after oral administration, whereas exercise increases absorption after intramuscular or subcutaneous administration because of an increased blood flow in the muscle.[9] Thus, exercise has an influence on the amount of a drug that reaches a receptor site, which significantly affects the pharmacodynamic activity of that drug.[9]

LEGAL CONCERNS IN ADMINISTERING VERSUS DISPENSING DRUGS

Administering a drug is defined as providing a single dose of medication for immediate use by the patient. Dispensing is providing the patient with a drug in a quantity sufficient for multiple doses.[24]

NOTE: The degree of variation between state laws and regulations is too vast to cover in this text. The athletic trainer should become familiar with the laws and regulations of the state in which he or she practices.

Dispensing Prescription Drugs

At no time can anyone other than a person licensed by law legally prescribe or dispense prescription drugs for a patient. An athletic trainer, unless specifically allowed by state licensure, is not permitted to dispense a prescription drug.[25] Failure to heed this fact can be a violation of federal laws and state statutes. Table 17–2 lists information about how medication dispensing is controlled. A violation of these laws could mean legal problems for the physician, athletic trainer, clinic, school, school district, or league.[24]

> At no time can anyone other than a person licensed by law legally prescribe or dispense prescription drugs for a patient.

A link to the NATA consensus statement "Managing prescription and nonprescription medication in the athletic training facility" (http://www.nata.org/sites/default/files/ManagingMedication.pdf) can be found at www.mhhe.com/prentice15e.

Administering Over-the-Counter Drugs

The situation is not as clear-cut for nonprescription drugs. Basically, the athletic trainer may be allowed to administer a single dose of a nonprescription medication. For example, most secondary schools do not allow the athletic trainer to administer nonprescription (over-the-counter [OTC])

TABLE 17–2 Agencies and Regulations That Govern the Provision of Pharmaceutical Care

Regulation	Enforced/Administered by	Purpose
Federal Food, Drug, and Cosmetic Act (FDCA) of 1938	Food and Drug Administration	Regulates the quality, strength, bioequivalence, and labeling of prescription and nonprescription drugs
Durham–Humphrey Amendment of 1951	Food and Drug Administration	Separates prescription from nonprescription drugs
Current Good Manufacturing Practice Regulations of 1962	Food and Drug Administration	Mandates standards for repackaging of medications
Federal Controlled Substances Act of 1970	Food and Drug Administration	Regulates controlled substances (drugs that have potential for abuse)
Poison Prevention Packaging Act (PPPA) of 1970	Food and Drug Administration	Regulates packaging of prescription and nonprescription drugs in child-resistant safety containers
Medical Device Act of 1976	Food and Drug Administration	Regulates classification and performance standards of medical devices
Federal Anti-Tampering Act of 1983	Food and Drug Administration	Mandates tamper-resistant packaging on all nonprescription drugs
Fair Packaging and Labeling Act	Food and Drug Administration	Mandates labeling of the contents of nonprescription drugs to assist consumers in identifying similar products
Prescription Drug Marketing Act of 1987	Food and Drug Administration	Mandates accountability of sample drugs from receiving through administering or dispensing
Anti–Drug Abuse Act of 1988	Drug Enforcement Authority	Regulates anabolic steroids as controlled substances
Omnibus Reconciliation Act of 1990 (OBRA '90)	Food and Drug Administration	Mandates drug review, patient medication records, and verbal patient education as part of dispensing of prescription medications
State pharmacy practice acts	Individual state boards of pharmacy	Regulates the provision of pharmaceutical care within each state; laws and regulations may vary considerably among states
State medical acts	Individual state boards of medicine	Regulates the practice within each state
Health Insurance Portability-Accountability Act of 1996 (HIPAA)	Department of Health and Human Services	Provides national standards to protect the privacy of personal health information
Anabolic Steroid Control Act of 2004	Drug Enforcement Administration	Added anabolic steroids and prohormones to the list of controlled substances regulated by the DEA.
Combat Methamphetamine Act 2005	Drug Enforcement Administration	Established retail sales and purchase transaction limits of pseudoephedrine products
Dietary Supplement & Nonprescription	Food and Drug Administration	Mandates reporting of serious adverse events for dietary supplements and Drug Consumer Protection Act 2006 nonprescription drugs
Affordable Care Act 2010	Department of Health and Human Services	Increases access to health coverage and introduce new protections for people with health insurance

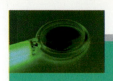

FOCUS 17–1 Focus on Organizational and Professional Health and Well-Being

General guidelines for administering medications

- Medications should be taken only as directed.
- Medications should not be used in combination before consulting a physician/pharmacist.
- Labels should not be removed from medication bottles or containers.
- Medications should not be used past the expiration date marked on the container.
- Oral medications should be taken with a full glass of water unless directed otherwise.
- Medications should be taken with food or on an empty stomach according to instructions.
- Specifically marked measuring spoons or caps should be used when measuring liquid medications.
- Containers should be childproof.
- Always consult individual states for rules and regulations governing the use of therapeutic medications.
- Check the banned substance status of all medications taken by athletes (according to the NCAA, IOC, and other governing bodies).

- Provide both verbal and written instructions for the use of medications.
- Make sure the patient reads the label information prior to taking a medication.
- Make sure the patient knows the dose schedule for the medications he or she is taking.
- Advise patients not to share medications with other people.
- Be aware of interactions between medications and exercise.
- NSAIDs are commonly used for their analgesic and antiinflammatory effects. Make sure patients understand the potential side effects and possible addiction to analgesics. They should be taken as prescribed.

From NATA Research and Education Foundation: *Guidelines for the use of therapeutic medications in sports*, Dallas, 2000, NATA.

---

drugs that the patient is to take internally, including aspirin and OTC cold remedies. Some secondary schools allow application of nonprescription wound medications under the category of first aid. On the other hand, some high-school athletic trainers in the United States are not allowed to apply even a wound medication in the name of first aid but can only clean the wound with soap and water. The patient must then be sent to the school nurse for medication. The dispensing of vitamins and even dextrose may be specifically disallowed by some school districts. At the college or professional level, minors are not usually involved, and the administration of nonprescription medications may be less restrictive. It is assumed that patients who are of legal age have the right to use whatever nonprescription drugs they choose. However, this right does not preclude the fact that the athletic trainer must be reasonable and prudent about the types of nonprescription drugs offered to the patient.[31]

A 2003 study indicated, that 9 years after a National Collegiate Athletic Association (NCAA) drug-distribution study of university athletic programs, many problem areas persisted, including unqualified personnel dispensing medications, inappropriately packaged and labeled medications, and a lack of record keeping.[25] In most athletic training clinics, athletic trainers (55.9 percent) and students (13.3 percent) still dispensed prescription drugs. In addition, in most athletic training clinics, athletic trainers (53.8 percent) administered any amount of

over-the-counter medication necessary, and many did not record the transaction (46.2 percent). In virtually every state, this practice is against the law. Athletic trainers should work in conjunction with members of the sports medicine team to review federal and state laws and revise institutional drug policies and procedures to comply with regulations to provide the best health care in a legal and safe manner.[25]

Generally, the administration of single doses of nonprescription medicines by a member of the athletic staff to any athlete depends on the philosophy of the school district and must be under the direction of the team physician.[43] In this area, as in all other areas of sports medicine and athletic training, the athletic trainer is obligated to act reasonably and prudently. See *Focus Box 17–1*: "General guidelines for administering medications."

Record Keeping

Those involved in any health care profession are acutely aware of the necessity of maintaining complete, up-to-date medical records, whether paper or electronic. The athletic training setting is no exception. The athletic trainer who administers medications must realize that maintaining accurate records of the types of medications administered is just as important as recording progress notes, treatments given, and rehabilitation plans.[37] The athletic trainer may be dealing with a number of different patients simultaneously while trying to get a team ready for practice or competition. Situations may become hectic, and stopping to record each time a medication is administered is difficult. Nevertheless, the athletic trainer should include the following information on the medication administration log:[24]

1. Name of the patient
2. Complaint or symptoms
3. Current medications
4. Any known drug allergies
5. Name of medication given
6. Lot number if available (identifies manufacturer, date, and place of production)
7. Expiration date
8. Quantity of medication given
9. Method of administration
10. Date and time of administration

Each athletic trainer should be aware of state regulations and laws that pertain to ordering, prescribing, distributing, storing, and dispensing or administering medications. Obtaining legal counsel, working with the state board of pharmacy or a student health clinic, working in cooperation with a physician, and establishing strict written policies are all actions that can minimize the chances of violating state laws that regulate the use of medications.[24,60]

Labeling Requirements OTC drugs are required to have directions for use and precautions that are adequate and readable. In 2011, the FDA finalized a regulation requiring OTC drugs to have clear and simple labeling. Standardized headings and subheadings make it easier for consumers to understand information about products, benefits, and risks, and how the drugs should be used most effectively.

The following "Drug Facts" must be included on the labels of prescription drugs:[51]

1. Name of the product
2. Active Ingredient(s)
3. Purpose
4. Use(s)
5. Warnings, such as contraindications to using the product and side effects that could occur
6. Directions for use including dosage and when, how, or how often to take
7. Other information
8. Inactive ingredients
9. Questions? (optional) followed by a telephone number

Additionally, the Food and Drug Administration Amendments Act of 2007 made it mandatory for human drug products to include a toll-free number for reporting adverse events. Nonprescription drugs may not be repackaged without meeting labeling criteria. All drugs dispensed from the athletic training room must be properly labeled. Legal violations may occur if a portion of a nonprescription drug is removed from an original, properly labeled package and dispensed to an athlete. This practice carries the same liability as does dispensing prescription drugs, because the athlete is not given the opportunity to review the label for name, contents, precautions, directions, and other information considered essential for the safe use of the product. Liability for any adverse patient outcome is therefore transferred to the dispenser of the improperly labeled OTC drug.[24]

An athletic trainer is covering a youth league soccer practice, and one of the soccer moms complains of a sore throat and stuffy head and asks the athletic trainer to give her some "drugs" to get rid of her problem.

? Is the athletic trainer legally allowed to give her any type of medication, and, if so, how should the athletic trainer give it to this individual?

17–1 Clinical Application Exercise

Safety in the Use of Pharmaceuticals

No drug can be considered completely safe and harmless. If a drug is potent enough to effect some physiological action, it is also strong enough, under some conditions, to be dangerous. All persons react individually to any drug.[27] A given amount of a specific medication may produce no adverse reaction in one person and a pronounced adverse response in another. Both the patient and the athletic trainer should be fully aware of any untoward effect a drug may have. It is essential that the patient be instructed clearly about when specifically to take medications, with meals or not, and what not to combine with the drug, such as other drugs or specific foods.[27] Some drugs can nullify the effect of another drug or can cause a serious antagonistic reaction. For example, calcium, which is found in a variety of foods and in some vitamins and medications, can nullify the effects of the antibiotic doxycycline.

Drug Responses Individuals react differently to the same medication, and different conditions may alter the effect of a drug on the athlete. Drugs themselves can be changed through age or improper preservation, as well as through the manner in which they are administered. Response variations also result from differences in each individual's size and age.

Alcohol should not be ingested with a wide variety of drugs, both prescription and nonprescription. Alcohol is a central nervous system depressant and can increase or decrease the effects of other drugs. Alcohol may intensify drowsiness if used in combination with

TABLE 17–3 General Body Responses Produced by Drugs

Addiction	Body response to certain types of drugs that produces both a physiological need and a psychological craving for the substance.
Antagonistic action	Result observed when medications, used together, have adverse effects or counteract one another.
Cumulative effect	Exaggerated drug effects, which occur when the body is unable to metabolize a drug as rapidly as it is administered; the accumulated, unmetabolized drug may cause unfavorable reactions.
Depressive action	Effect from drugs that slow down cell function.
Habituation	Individual's development of a psychological need for a specific medication.
Hypersensitivity	Allergic response to a specific drug; such allergies may be demonstrated by a mild skin irritation, itching, a rash, or a severe anaphylactic reaction, which could be fatal.
Idiosyncrasy	Unusual reaction to a drug; a distinctive response.
Irritation	Process, as well as effect, caused by substances that result in a cellular change; mild irritation may stimulate cell activity, whereas moderate or severe irritation by a drug may decrease cell activity.
Paradoxical reaction	A drug-induced effect that is the exact opposite of that which is therapeutically intended.
Potentiating agent	A pharmaceutical that increases the effect of another; for example, codeine is potentiated by aspirin, and therefore less of it is required to relieve pain.
Specific effect	Action usually produced by a drug in a select tissue or organ system.
Side effect	The result of a medication that is given for a particular condition but affects other body areas or has effects other than those sought.
Stimulation	Effect caused by drugs that speed up cell activity.
Synergistic effect	Result that occurs when drugs given together produce a greater reaction than when given alone.
Tolerance	Condition existing when a certain drug dosage is no longer able to give a therapeutic action and must therefore be increased.

another depressant. It is also important to realize that alcohol is used in many liquid preparations that are being used as medications. Warnings concerning the use of alcohol should be listed on the drug label.

Medications can affect certain physiological functions that are related to dehydration, such as sweating, urination, and the ability to control and regulate body temperature. Some medications cause fluid depletion that results in dehydration, which can increase the risk of heat illness. Other medications can make an individual more sensitive to sunlight, increasing the risk of sunburn or allergic reactions to sunlight. A fatty diet may decrease a drug's effectiveness by interfering with its absorption. Excessively acidic foods, such as fruits, carbonated drinks, and vegetable juice, may cause adverse drug reactions. Athletic trainers must thoroughly know the individuals with whom they work. The possibility of an adverse drug reaction is ever present and requires continual education and vigilance.

Table 17–3 is a list of general body responses sometimes produced by drugs and medications.

Buying Medications

One of the athletic trainer's best friends is the local pharmacist. The pharmacist can assist in the selection and purchase of nonprescription drugs, can save money by suggesting the lower-priced generic drugs, and can act as a general advisor on the effectiveness of drugs, the dose of a medicine, and even the dangers inherent in a specific drug.

All pharmaceuticals must be properly labeled, indicating clearly the content, the expiration date, and any dangers or contraindications for use. Pharmaceutical manufacturers place the expiration date on drugs, and athletic trainers should locate this date on the package. When storing medications;

1. Always keep both prescription and over-the-counter medications in a locked cabinet or secured place.
2. Keep them in the original container.
3. Store them away from heat, direct light, damp places, and extreme cold.
4. Keep over-the-counter medications in single-dose packs.[25]

Traveling with Medications

When traveling with a team or individually, the individual should be advised to do the following with regard to medications:

1. Medication should not be stored in a bag or luggage but carried by the athlete taking it.

2. A sufficient supply of medication should be packaged in case of emergency.
3. Make sure there is a source of medication while traveling.
4. Take copies of written prescriptions.
5. Keep medications in their original containers and in a secure place.
6. When traveling internationally, understand the restrictions of individual jurisdictions.

SELECTED THERAPEUTIC DRUGS

The use of medicines is widespread in the athletic population, as it is in society in general. Thousands of drugs, both prescription and nonprescription, are available for physicians and consumers to choose from, and new drugs are being constantly developed. Pharmaceutical laboratories develop compounds *in vitro* and then test, retest, and refine the drug *in vivo* before submitting it for Food and Drug Administration (FDA) approval.

> *In vitro* means in a laboratory; *in vivo* means in the body.

A number of texts and databases (e.g., *Physician's Desk Reference* and *Drug Facts and Comparisons*) are widely used as references for comparison of **bioequivalent drugs** (drugs that produce similar biological effects) relative to their appropriateness and effectiveness in treating a specific condition or illness.[38] Table 17–4 summarizes the classifications of drugs available.

> **bioequivalent drugs**
> Drugs that have similar biological effects.

The following sections discuss the most common pharmaceutical practices in athletic training to date and the specific drugs that are in use (Table 17–5). The discussions include both prescription and

TABLE 17–4	List of Drug Classifications and Definitions
Analgesics	Pain-relieving drugs.
Anesthetics	Agents that produce local or general numbness to touch, pain, or stimulation.
Antacids	Substances that neutralize acidity; commonly used in the digestive tract.
Anticoagulants	Agents that prevent the coagulation of blood.
Antibiotics	Drugs that kill bacteria or inhibit their growth.
Antidotes	Substances that prevent or counteract the action of a poison.
Antifungals	Drugs that kill fungi or inhibit their growth.
Antiinflammatories	Drugs that reduce and/or control inflammation.
Antipruritics	Agents that relieve itching.
Antipyretics	Drugs that reduce body temperature.
Antiseptics	Agents that kill bacteria or inhibit their growth and can be applied to living tissue.
Antispasmodics	Agents that relieve muscle spasm.
Antitussives	Agents that inhibit or prevent coughing.
Astringents	Agents that cause contraction or puckering action.
Bacteriostatics and fungistatics	Agents that retard or inhibit the growth of bacteria and fungi, respectively.
Carminatives	Agents that relieve flatulence (caused by gases) in the intestinal tract.
Cathartics	Agents used to evacuate substances from the bowels; active purgatives.
Caustics	Burning agents, capable of destroying living tissue.
Counterirritants	Agents applied locally to produce an inflammatory reaction for the relief of a deeper inflammation.
Depressants	Agents that diminish body functions or nerve activity.
Disinfectants	Agents that kill or inhibit the growth of microorganisms; should be applied only to nonliving materials.
Diuretics	Agents that increase the excretion of urine.
Emetics	Agents that cause vomiting.
Expectorants	Agents that suppress coughing.
Hemostatics	Substances that either slow down or stop bleeding.
Irritants	Agents that cause irritation.
Narcotics	Drugs that produce analgesic and hypnotic effects.
Sedatives	Agents that relieve anxiety.
Skeletal muscle relaxants	Drugs that depress neural activity within skeletal muscles.
Stimulants	Agents that excite the central nervous system.
Suppressants	Agents that reduce or control appetite.
Vasoconstrictors and vasodilators	Drugs that constrict and dilate blood vessels, respectively.

TABLE 17–5 Athletic Trainers' Guide to Frequently Used Medications

Generic Name	Trade Name	Primary Use of Drug/Precautions	Additional Considerations
Analgesics, antipyretics, and antiinflammatories (NSAIDs)			
Aspirin	Many trade names	Analgesic, antipyretic, antiinflammatory	Gastric irritation, nausea, tinnitus, prolonged bleeding if injured
Acetaminophen	Tylenol, others	Analgesic, antipyretic	Do not combine with alcohol. Hepatotoxicity with acute overdose; chronic daily dosing can result in liver damage
Flurbiprofen	Ansaid*	All are analgesic, antipyretic, antiinflammatory (NSAIDs).	Gastric irritation less common than with aspirin except for indomethacin. These medications should be used for reducing pain and inflammation; they should not be substituted for acetaminophen in cases of mild headache or low fever. Adequate hydration reduces the risk of adverse effects in the renal system
Ketoprofen	Orudis*		
Indomethacin	Indocin*	Notify doctor immediately for skin rash, itching, visual disturbances, weight gain, edema, black stools, dark urine, or persistent headache.	
Ibuprofen	Advil, Motrin		
Naproxen	Naprosyn,* Anaprox,* Aleve		
Diflunisal	Dolobid*		*NSAID hypersensitivity:* Because of cross-sensitivity. to aspirin and all other NSAIDs, do not give these agents to athletes in whom aspirin, iodides, or other NSAIDs have caused symptoms of asthma, rhinitis, rash, nasal polyps, bronchospasm, or other symptoms of allergic reactions.
Piroxicam	Feldene*	*Drug interactions:* salicylates, other NSAIDs, probenecid, cimetidine, diuretics, lithium, phenytoin, beta blockers, ACE inhibitors, anticoagulants, digoxin	
Tolmetin	Tolectin*		
Fenoprofen	Nalfon*		
Meclofenamate	Meclomen*		
Diclofenac	Voltaren,* Cataflam*		
Ketorolac	Toradol*		
Etodolac	Lodine*		
Mefenamic acid	Ponstel*		
Nabumetone	Relafen*		
Meloxicam	Mobic*		
Oxaprozin	Daypro*		
Sulindac	Clinoril*		
Celecoxib	Celebrex*		
Antifungal agents			
Ketoconazole	Nizoral*	Systemic (oral) antifungal	Should not be taken within 2 hours of antacids
		Drug has been associated with hepatic toxicity including fatalities.	May cause dizziness or drowsiness
		Notify doctor immediately for unusual fatigue, anorexia, nausea, jaundice, dark urine, pale stools, abdominal pain, fever, or diarrhea.	*Hypersensitivity:* Anaphylaxis has been reported.
Griseofulvin	Fulvicin P/G,* Gris-Peg*	Oral antifungal	Photosensitivity may occur: Patient should avoid prolonged exposure to sunlight or sunlamps.
		Notify doctor immediately for fever, sore throat, or skin rash.	
		Reduces the effectiveness of oral contraceptives	
Fluconazole	Diflucan*	Oral antifungal	
		Warnings: Hepatic injury, anaphylaxis, dermatological changes have been reported.	
		Notify doctor immediately for skin rash.	
		Drug interactions: cimetidine, rifampin, nonsedating antihistamines, phenytoin, theophylline, zidovudine	

Generic	Brand	Action / Uses / Drug interactions	Notes
Terbinafine	Lamisil*	Oral antifungal for treatment of toenails or fingernails, scalp, body, groin, or feet. Notify doctor immediately for skin rash, itching, aching joints, dark urine, difficulty swallowing, fever, chills, pale skin, pale stool, redness, blistering, peeling or loosening of skin, unusual tiredness, and yellowing of skin or eyes. Drug interactions: cimetidine, rifampin, caffeine	Weeks to months may be required to resolve infection. Alcohol consumption during treatment increases risk of liver toxicity.

Antibiotics

Generic	Brand	Action / Uses / Drug interactions	Notes
Penicillins	V-Cillin-K,* Pen Vee K,* Trimox	Drug interactions: beta blockers, erythromycin, tetracycline	If diarrhea occurs, do not give Imodium AD.
Cephalosporins	Keflex,* Ceftin*	Drug interactions: alcohol, probenecid	Patients allergic to penicillin may have cross-sensitivity to cephalosporins.
Macrolides	Ery-Tab,* Zithromax,* Biaxin*	Drug interactions: fluconazole, zidovudine, theophylline, nonsedating antihistamines, carbamazepine, ergot alkaloids, penicillins	
Fluoroquinolones	Cipro,* Noroxin,* Floxin,* Levaquin*	Notify doctor immediately for agitation, confusion, tremors, fever, and skin rash. Drug interactions: antacids, sucralfate, Pepto-Bismol, cimetidine, caffeine, probenecid, phenytoin, theophylline	Photosensitivity; avoid overexposure to sunlight or sunlamps. May cause dizziness. Rarely associated with pain, inflammation, or rupture of a tendon
Tetracyclines	Sumycin,* Vibramycin*	Drug interactions: antacids, anticoagulants, cimetidine, insulin, lithium, penicillins, sodium bicarbonate	Should not be taken with milk, antacids, or minerals because of reduced absorption. Photosensitivity may occur.

Drugs that affect the respiratory tract

Generic	Brand	Action / Uses / Drug interactions	Notes
Chlorpheniramine	Chlor-Trimeton	Antihistamine for allergies. Used primarily for treatment of allergic rhinitis; causes drowsiness and decreased coordination	
Cromolyn	Nasalcrom	Nasal allergy symptom controller; prevents and relieves nasal allergy symptoms such as Allergic rhinitis, seasonal allergies	
Oxymetazoline	Afrin, Dristan Long Lasting, Neosynephrine 12 Hour, Allerest	Adrenergic decongestant applied topically as spray or nose drops	Do not exceed recommended duration of treatment because of rebound congestion; may cause sneezing, dryness of nasal mucosa, and headache.
Pseudoephedrine	Sudafed, Oranyl, others	Adrenergic decongestant used orally	Produces stimulation of the central nervous system; topically applied decongestants work faster, but oral decongestants are preferred for long-term use. Federal and state laws require record keeping and accountability.
Diphenhydramine	Benadryl, Benylin cough syrup	Antihistamine used primarily for allergic reaction; also used for sleep	Produces drowsiness and dry mouth; found in over-the-counter sleeping medications

*Requires a prescription.

Continued

Generic Name	Trade Name	Primary Use of Drug/Precautions	Additional Considerations
Dextromethorphan	Robitussin DM, Benylin DMO, Sucrets lozenges	Nonnarcotic antitussive used for cough suppression	Very effective in cases of unproductive cough; rarely produces drowsiness and other side effects
		Drug interaction: newer antidepressants	
Cetirizine	Zyrtec	Antihistamine; effective for some allergic reactions	May cause some sedation but less than traditional antihistamines
Fexofenadine, loratidine	Allegra, Claritin	Antihistamines	Nonsedating
Benzonatate	Tessalon*	Peripherally acting antitussive that acts as an anesthetic	May cause dizziness; should not be chewed
Codeine	Robitussin AC*	Narcotic antitussive that depresses the central cough mechanism	Used in combination with expectorant; can produce sedation, dizziness, constipation, or nausea
Guaifenesin	Mucinex, Robitussin	Expectorant used for symptomatic relief of unproductive cough	Used for treating dry or sore throat; good hydration maximizes effects
Drugs that affect the gastrointestinal tract			
Sodium bicarbonate	Soda Mint	Antacid used for quick relief of upset stomach	Produces gas and belching; overuse may cause systemic alkalinity
Aluminum hydroxide	Amphogel, Dialume	Antacid used for upset stomach	May produce constipation
Calcium carbonate	Titralac, Mallamint, Tums	Antacid used for upset stomach and for calcium supplementation	May produce constipation and acid rebound; high acid neutralizing capacity
Magnesium hydroxide	Milk of Magnesia	Laxative used for constipation	May cause diarrhea
Cimetidine, nizatidine	Tagamet HB, Axid AR	Histamine-2 antagonists used for relief of upset stomach, heartburn, and acid indigestion Histamine-2 antagonists used for relief of upset stomach, heartburn, acid indigestion	Numerous drug interactions
Ranitidine Famotidine	Zantac 75 Pepcid AC		
Combination antacids	Alka-Seltzer, Digel, Gaviscon, Gelusil, Maalox, Mylanta, others	Combination drugs for controlling gastric upset	May produce either diarrhea or constipation
Promethazine	Phenergan*	Antiemetic used for preventing motion sickness, nausea, and vomiting	Produces sedation and drowsiness
Diphenoxylate HCL	Lomotil*	Narcotic antidiarrheals	Cause dry mouth, nausea, and drowsiness
Loperamide	Imodium AD	Nonnarcotic systemic antidiarrheal	Abdominal discomfort and drowsiness with large doses
Combination antidiarrheals	Donnagel, Kaopectate, Pepto-Bismol	Relief of diarrhea	Relatively safe with few side effects; effective for traveler's diarrhea
Proton pump inhibitor	Prilosec, Pepcid, Prevacid, others	Relief of heartburn; prevention of NSAID-induced ulcers	

*Requires a prescription.

nonprescription drugs, with emphases on what should most concern the athletic trainer and what the medications or materials are designed to accomplish.

Drugs to Combat Infection

Combating infection, especially skin infection, is of major importance in sports. Serious infection can cause countless hours of lost time and has even been the indirect cause of death.

> **Drugs used to combat infection include local antiseptics and disinfectants, antifungal agents, and antibiotics.**

Local Antiseptics and Disinfectants Antiseptics are substances that can be placed on living tissue for the express purpose of either killing bacteria or inhibiting their growth. Disinfectants are substances that combat microorganisms but should be applied only to nonliving objects. Types of antiseptics and disinfectants are germicides, which are designed to destroy bacteria; fungicides, which kill fungi; sporicides, which destroy spores; and sanitizers, which minimize contamination by microorganisms.

Many agents are used to combat infection. It is critical that agents have a broad spectrum of activity against infective organisms, including the human immunodeficiency virus (HIV).

Alcohol Alcohol is one of the most widely used skin disinfectants. Ethyl alcohol (70 percent by weight) and isopropyl alcohol (70 percent) are equally effective. They are inexpensive and nonirritating; they kill bacteria immediately, with the exception of spores. However, they have no long-lasting germicidal action. Besides being directly combined with other agents to form tinctures, alcohol acts independently on the skin as an antiseptic and astringent. In a 70 percent solution, alcohol can be used for disinfecting instruments. Because of alcohol's rapid rate of evaporation, it produces a mild anesthetic action. Combined with 20 percent benzoin, it is used as a topical skin dressing to provide a protective skin coating and astringent action.

> **Antiseptics and disinfectants include alcohol, phenol, halogens, and oxidizing agents.**

Phenol Phenol was one of the earliest antiseptics and disinfectants used by the medical profession. From its inception to the present, phenol has been used to control disease organisms, both as an antiseptic and as a disinfectant. It is available in liquids of varying concentrations and in emollients. Substances that are derived from phenol and that cause less irritation are now used more extensively. Some of these derivatives are resorcinol, thymol, and the common household disinfectant Lysol.

Halogens Halogens are chemical substances (chlorine, fluoride, and bromine) that are used for their antiseptic and disinfectant qualities. Iodophors, or halogenated compounds, a combination of iodine and a carrier, create a much less irritating preparation than tincture of iodine is. A popular iodophor is povidone-iodine complex (Betadine), which is an excellent germicide commonly used as a surgical scrub. Betadine as an antiseptic and germicide in athletic training has proved extremely effective on skin lesions, such as lacerations, abrasions, and floor burns.

Oxidizing Agents Oxidizing agents, as represented by hydrogen peroxide (3 percent), are commonly used in athletic training. Hydrogen peroxide is an antiseptic that, because of its oxidation, affects bacteria but readily decomposes in the presence of organic substances, such as blood and pus. For this reason, it has little effect as an antiseptic. Contact with organic material produces an effervescence, during which no great destruction of bacteria takes place. The chief value of hydrogen peroxide in the care of wounds is its ability to cleanse the infected cutaneous and mucous membranes. Application of hydrogen peroxide to wounds results in the formation of an active, effervescent gas that dislodges particles of wound material and debris and, by removing degenerated tissue, eliminates the wound as a likely environment for bacterial breeding. Hydrogen peroxide also possesses compounds that are widely used as antiseptics. Because it is nontoxic, hydrogen peroxide may be used for cleansing mucous membranes. A diluted solution (50 percent water and 50 percent hydrogen peroxide) can be used for treating inflammatory conditions of the mouth and throat.

Antifungal Agents Many medicinal agents on the market are designed to treat fungi, which are commonly found in and around athletic facilities. The three most common fungi are *Epidermophyton*, *Trichophyton*, and *Candida albicans*.

In recent years, antifungal agents such as terbinafine (Lamisil), ketoconazole (Nizoral), amphotericin B (Fungizone), and griseofulvin have been developed and used. Both ketoconazole and amphotericin B seem to be effective against deep-seated fungus infections, such as those caused by *Candida albicans*. Ketoconazole, fluconazole, and griseofulvin, all of which can be administered orally, produce an effective fungistatic action against the specific fungus species of *Microsporum*, *Trichophyton*, and *Epidermophyton*, all of which are associated with common athlete's foot. Given over a long period of time, griseofulvin becomes a functioning part of the cutaneous tissues, especially the skin, hair, and nails, producing a prolonged and continuous fungistatic action. Any patient taking an oral antifungal agent must be carefully monitored by a clinician. Terbinafine (Lamisil), miconazole (Micatin), clotrimazole (Lotrimin), and tolnaftate (Tinactin, which does not treat *Candida* infections) are topical medications for a superficial fungus infection caused by *Trichophyton* and other fungi.

WARNING: Ketoconazole has been associated with hepatoxicity, including some fatalities; use with caution in patients with impaired hepatic function, and perform periodic liver function tests. High doses of ketoconazole may depress adrenocortical function.

Antibiotics Antibiotics are bacteriostatic (inhibiting bacterial growth) or bacteriocidal (destroying bacteria). Their useful action is primarily a result of their interference with the necessary metabolic processes of pathogenic microorganisms. The physician can use antibiotics as either topical dressings or systemic medications. The indiscriminate use of antibiotics can produce extreme hypersensitivity or idiosyncrasies and can prevent the development of natural immunity to subsequent infections. The use of any antibiotic must be carefully controlled by the physician, who selects the drug on the basis of the suspected bacterial organism, most desirable type of administration, and the least amount of toxicity to the patient.

The antibiotics mentioned here are just a few of the many available. New types continue to be developed, mainly because, over a period of time, many microorganisms become resistant to a particular antibiotic, especially if it is indiscriminately used. Some of the more common antibiotics are penicillins and cephalosporins, bacitracin, tetracycline, erythromycin, and sulfonamides, and quinolones.[36]

> Antibiotics include penicillins and cephalosporins, bacitracin, tetracyclines, macrolides, sulfonamides, and quinolones.

Penicillins and Cephalosporins Penicillins and cephalosporins as prescription medications are probably the most important of the antibiotics; they are useful in a variety of skin and systemic infections. In general, penicillins and cephalosporins interfere with the metabolism of the bacteria.

Bacitracin Bacitracin has a broad spectrum of effectiveness as an antibacterial agent. Bacitracin plus polymixin (Polysporin) also has a broad spectrum of effectiveness as an antibacterial agent. Adding neomycin to the product (Neosporin) does not increase effectiveness, and some individuals are allergic to neomycin.

Tetracyclines Tetracyclines consist of a wide group of antibiotics that have a broad antibacterial spectrum. Their application, which is usually oral, modifies the infection rather than eradicating it completely. Tetracyclines cause sensitivity to sun exposure.

Macrolides Macrolides, such as erythromycin and azithromycin, are most often used for streptococcal infection and mycoplasma pneumoniae. Macrolides have the same general spectrum as penicillin and are a useful alternative in the penicillin-allergic patient.

Sulfonamides Sulfonamides are a group of synthetic antibiotics. In general, sulfonamides make pathogens vulnerable to phagocytes by inhibiting certain enzymatic actions. They are often used to treat urinary tract infections and skin infections.

Quinolones Quinolones have a broad spectrum of activity. Patients taking these antibiotics must be carefully monitored for adverse effects.

Drugs for Asthma

Asthma is a chronic inflammatory lung disorder characterized by obstruction of the airways as a result of complex inflammatory processes, smooth muscle spasm, and hyperresponsiveness to a variety of stimuli.[18] Asthma triggers include exercise, viral infection, animal exposure, dust mites, mold, air pollutants, weather, and NSAIDs as well as other drugs. The National Asthma Education and Prevention Program (NAEPP) has established international guidelines for the diagnosis and management of asthma.[32,33] The goals of asthma therapy are to prevent chronic and troublesome symptoms, maintain normal lung function and activity levels, prevent asthma exacerbations, provide optimal pharmacotherapy with minimal adverse effects, and meet athletes' expectation of and satisfaction with asthma care.[22]

Exercise-induced bronchospasm (EIB), also referred to as exercise-induced asthma (EIA), is a limiting and disruptive experience. Any asthma patient is subject to EIB. A bronchospastic event caused by loss of heat, water, or both from the lungs during exercise or exertion, EIB results from hyperventilation of air that is cooler and dryer than that in the respiratory tract.[56] EIB occurs during or minutes after physical activity, reaches its peak in 5 to 10 minutes after stopping the activity, and usually resolves in 20 to 30 minutes. In some asthma patients, exercise is the only precipitating factor.

17–2 Clinical Application Exercise

An aerobics instructor has a recurrent breathing problem, especially during high-intensity fitness training. Since the weather has gotten warmer, her symptoms have gotten worse.

? What should the athletic trainer expect is wrong with this patient and how should her condition be managed?

TABLE 17–6	Medications Recommended for the Management of Asthma	

Long-Term Control	Quick Relief
Inhaled corticosteroids (antiinflammatories)	Short-acting beta$_2$ agonists
Beclomethasone (Beclovent, Vanceril)	Albuterol (Proventil), Ventolin, Pro-Air
Budesonide (Pulmicort)	Pirbuterol (Maxair)
Fluticasone propionate (Flovent)	Levalbuterol (Xopenex)
Triamcinolone acetonide (Azmacort)	Metaproterenol (Alupent)
Mast cell stabilizers (antiinflammatories)	Terbutaline oral tablets only in the United States
Cromolyn nebulized solution	Anticholinergics
	Ipratropium bromide (Atrovent)
Long-acting beta$_2$ agonists (bronchodilators)	Oral Corticosteroids
Salmeterol (Serevent)	Methylprednisolone (Medrol)
Albuterol sustained release (VoSpire ER)	Prednisolone (various generics)
Formoterol (Foradil Aerolizer)	Prednisone (various generics)
Leukotriene modifiers	
Zafirlukast (Accolate)	
Zileuton (Zyflo).	
Montelukast (Singulair)	
Monoclonal antibody	
Omalizumab (Xolair)	
Combinations (antiinflammatory and bronchodilator)	
Fluticasone plus salmeterol (Advair)	
Budesonide plus formoterol (Symbicort)	
Mometasone plus formoterol (Dulera)	
Theophylline (bronchodilator)	

The individual who has asthma must be monitored carefully. The NAEPP recommends measurements of the following: asthma signs and symptoms, pulmonary function (peak flow or spirometry), quality of life/functional status, history of asthma exacerbations, patient satisfaction, and pharmacotherapy.[33] Table 17–6 identifies medications recommended in asthma management. A link to the NATA position statement "Management of asthma in athletes" (http://www.nata.org/sites/default/files/MgmtOfAsthmaInAthletes.pdf) can be found at www.mhhe.com/prentice15e.

Using an Inhaler The use of inhalers by individuals who have asthma and/or exercise-induced bronchospasm is common. Portable, handheld inhalers are convenient in that they deliver medicine directly to the lungs very rapidly. A variety of inhalers have been developed to relieve or control asthma symptoms. The two most common devices are *metered-dose inhalers (MDIs)* and *dry powder inhalers (DPIs)*. A metered-dose inhaler includes a pressurized canister with measured doses of medication inside.[57] The patient squeezes the top of the canister. The pressure within the canister converts the medication into a fine powder. To use an MDI, the individual places the mouthpiece of the inhaler between the teeth and closes the mouth around the mouthpiece. The person then breathes in slowly and presses down on the top of the inhaler. Using a metered-dose inhaler calls for coordinating two actions: squeezing the canister and inhaling the medication (Figure 17–1). Many individuals who use the metered-dose inhaler use it improperly; however, with careful and repeated instruction, more than 90 percent of people can use it correctly.[57] Metered-dose inhalers can use a spacer, which is a tube, 4 to 8 inches (10 to 20 cm) long, that attaches to the inhaler that allows time to inhale more slowly. The spacer acts as a holding chamber that keeps medication from escaping into the air.

Dry powder inhalers are not pressurized but rather release medication when the patient rapidly inhales. This type of inhaler requires the individual to place the lips on the mouthpiece and inhale more rapidly than with a traditional metered-dose inhaler. Generally, dry powder inhalers are easier to use than the conventional pressurized metered-dose inhalers because hand-lung coordination is not required. Spacers can't be used with dry powder inhalers.

People with asthma can rely too much on inhaled bronchodilators. Because these fast-acting medications can relieve symptoms quickly, there is a tendency, particularly among physically active individuals, to use them too often, leading to an overdose.[32] Signs of an overdose include irregular heartbeat, tremor, seizure, headache, nausea, and vomiting.

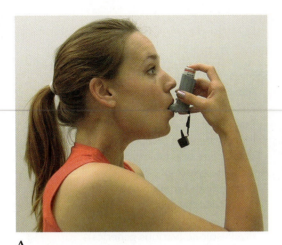
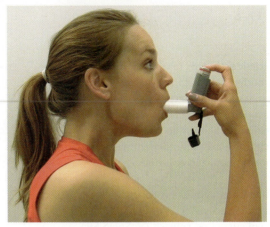

A   B

FIGURE 17–1 **(A)** Metered-dose inhalers are commonly used by patients who have asthma. **(B)** A spacer helps keep medication from dissipating into the air.

A device called a *nebulizer,* a compressor-driven pump that converts medication into a mist, is used by individuals who are not able to use an inhaler.

Using an inhaler is just one part of an asthma treatment plan. The treatment plan may also include checking lung function with a peak flow meter, eliminating asthma triggers, and exercising.

Drugs That Inhibit Pain and Inflammation

Pain Relievers Controlling pain can involve innumerable drugs and procedures, depending on the beliefs of the athletic trainer or physician. As discussed in Chapter 9, the reason pain is positively affected by certain methods is not clearly understood; however, some of the possible reasons are as follows:

> Drugs used to inhibit pain or inflammation include counterirritants and local anesthetics, narcotic analgesics, and nonnarcotic analgesics and antipyretics.

- The excitatory effect of an individual impulse is depressed.
- An individual impulse is inhibited.
- The perceived impulse is decreased.
- Anxiety created by pain or impending pain is decreased.

Counterirritants and Local Anesthetics Analgesics give relief by causing a systemic and topical analgesia. Many chemical reactions on the skin can inhibit pain sensations by rapid evaporation, which causes a cooling action, or by counterirritating the skin. Irritating and counterirritating substances act as rubefacients (skin reddeners) and skin stimulants, although their popularity has

> Counterirritants include spray coolants, alcohol, cold, menthol, and local anesthetics.

decreased in recent years. Their application causes local increase in blood circulation, redness, and rise in skin temperature. Frequently, mild pain can be reduced by a counterirritant, which produces a stimulus to the skin of such intensity that the athlete is no longer aware of the pain. Some examples of counterirritants are liniments, analgesic balms, heat, and cold.

Spray Coolants Spray coolants, because of their rapid evaporation, act as topical anesthetics to the skin. Several commercial coolants are presently on the market. Fluorimethane is one of the most commonly used spray coolants. Cooling results so quickly that superficial freezing takes place, inhibiting pain impulses for a short time. Athletic trainers disagree on the effectiveness of spray coolants. Some athletic trainers use them extensively for strains, sprains, and contusions. In most cases, spray coolants are useful only when other analgesics are not available.

Alcohol Alcohol evaporates rapidly when applied to the skin, causing a refreshingly cool effect that gives a temporary analgesia.

Menthol Menthol is an alcohol taken from mint oils and is principally used as a local analgesic, counterirritant, and antiseptic. Menthol is used most often with a petroleum base for treating cold symptoms and in analgesic balms.

Cold Cold applications immediately constrict blood vessels and numb sensory nerve endings. Applications of ice packs or submersion of a part in ice water may completely anesthetize an area. If extreme cold is used, caution must be taken that tissue damage does not result.

Local Anesthetics Local anesthetics are usually injected by a physician in and around injury sites for minor surgical procedures or to alleviate the pain of movement. Lidocaine hydrochloride is used extensively as a local anesthetic.

Narcotic Analgesics Most narcotics used in medicine are derived directly from opium or are synthetic opiates. They depress pain impulses and the respiratory center.

> **Narcotic analgesics include codine and morphine which are no longer recommended for treatment of pain.**

Codeine Codeine resembles morphine in its action but is less potent. Codeine is effective in combination with nonnarcotic analgesics. In small doses, it is a cough suppressant found in many cough medicines. Hydrocodone (Vicodin) is an example of this type of drug.

Morphine Morphine depresses pain sensations to a greater extent than most other drugs. It is also the most dangerous drug because of its ability to depress respiration and because of its habit-forming qualities. Morphine is never used before a diagnosis has been made by the physician or when the patient is unconscious, there is a head injury, or there is a decreased rate of breathing. It is never repeated within 2 hours.

Nonnarcotic Analgesics and Antipyretics Nonnarcotic analgesics are drugs designed to suppress all but the most severe pain, without the patient's losing consciousness. In most cases, these drugs also act as antipyretics, regulating the temperature-control centers.

> **Acetaminophen is a nonnarcotic analgesic.**

Acetaminophen Acetaminophen (Tylenol) is an effective analgesic and antipyretic but has no antiinflammatory activity. Because it does not irritate the gastrointestinal system, it is often a replacement for aspirin in noninflammatory conditions. Overingestion could lead to liver damage. Chronic daily dosages have resulted in liver damage in some patients. Heavy alcohol users may be at risk of liver damage when taking more than the recommended dose of acetaminophen. Many products used to treat cold and flu symptoms have a combination of ingredients, including acetaminophen. It is important to make sure that the total daily acetaminophen dose is not exceeded. The total daily dose has been lowered from 4 grams per day to 3 grams per day by some manufacturers of acetaminophen.

Drugs to Reduce Inflammation

Physicians have a wide choice of drugs at their disposal for the treatment of inflammation. A great variety of OTC drugs also claim to deal effectively with inflammation of the musculoskeletal system.

The problem of proper drug selection is tenuous, even for a physician, because new drugs are continually coming to the forefront. The situation is compounded by highly advertised OTC preparations. Any drug selection, especially drugs designed to treat the inflammatory process, must be effective and appropriate for the individual, and must not create any adverse reactions.[6] These points are addressed by the following discussions of the more generally accepted antiinflammatory drugs.

> **Antiinflammatories include acetylsalicylic acid (aspirin), NSAIDs, and corticosteroids**

Acetylsalicylic Acid (Aspirin) Aspirin is one of the most widely used analgesics, antiinflammatories, and antipyretics.[14] A number of medications that have salicylates reduce pain, fever, and inflammation. Aspirin has been associated with various adverse reactions that are primarily centered in the gastrointestinal region. Those reactions include difficulty in food digestion (dyspepsia), nausea, vomiting, and gastric bleeding.

Overingestion of aspirin can lead to serious side effects.[14] Adverse reactions to aspirin, especially in high doses, are ear ringing or buzzing (tinnitus) and dizziness. A major problem that can arise in individuals under 18 years of age is Reye's syndrome (fatty infiltration of the liver, kidneys, or heart). The administration of aspirin to a child during chickenpox or influenza can induce Reye's syndrome. Its etiology is unknown.

Severe allergic response resulting in an anaphylactic reaction can occur in individuals who have an intolerance to aspirin. Asthmatic patients may be at greater risk of allergic reactions to aspirin. Aspirin use should be avoided by athletes in contact sports because it prolongs blood-clotting time.

Nonsteroidal Antiinflammatory Drugs (NSAIDs)
Nonsteroidal antiinflammatory drugs (NSAIDs) have antiinflammatory, antipyretic, and analgesic properties.[13] They are strong inhibitors of prostaglandin synthesis and are effective for such chronic problems as rheumatoid arthritis and osteoarthritis. Nonsteroidal antiinflammatory drugs are used primarily for reducing the pain, stiffness, swelling, redness, and fever associated with localized inflammation.[13] Their antiinflammatory capabilities are thought to

be equal to those of aspirin; their advantages are fewer side effects and relatively longer duration of action.[62] NSAIDs are effective for patients who cannot tolerate aspirin because of the gastrointestinal distress associated with aspirin use. Even though NSAIDs have analgesic and antipyretic capabilities, they should not be used in place of aspirin or acetaminophen in cases of mild headache or increased body temperature. However, they can be used to relieve many other mild to moderately painful somatic conditions, such as menstrual cramps and soft-tissue injury. Table 17–7 lists the commonly used NSAIDs.[1]

The NSAIDs can produce adverse reactions and should be used cautiously.[28,53] Individuals who have the aspirin allergy triad of nasal polyps, associated bronchospasm or asthma, and history of anaphylaxis should not receive any NSAID. The NSAIDs can cause gastrointestinal tract reactions, headache, dizziness, depression, tinnitus, and a variety of other systemic reactions. Taking ibuprofen with heavy alcohol use may increase the risk of stomach bleeding.

WARNING: NSAIDs are associated with an increased risk of adverse cardiovascular events, including heart attack, stroke, and new onset or worsening of preexisting hypertension. Risk may be increased with duration of use or preexisting cardiovascular risk factors of disease. Carefully evaluate individual cardiovascular risk profiles prior to prescribing. Use caution with fluid retention, congestive heart failure, or hypertension. Concurrent administration of ibuprofen, and potentially other nonselective NSAIDs, may interfere with aspirin's cardioprotective effect. Use the lowest effective dose for the shortest duration of time, consistent with individual patient goals, to reduce risk of adverse cardiovascular events; alternate therapies should be considered for patients at high risk.

WARNING: NSAIDs may increase risk of gastrointestinal irritation, ulceration, bleeding, and perforation. These events may occur at anytime during therapy and without warning. Use caution with a history of gastrointestinal (GI) disease (bleeding or ulcers), concurrent therapy with

TABLE 17–7 Frequently Used NSAIDs

Generic Name	Drug/Trade Name	Dosage Range (mg) and Frequency	Maximum Daily Dose (mg)
Celecoxib	Celebrex	100–200 mg twice a day	200
Aspirin	Aspirin	325–650 mg every 4 hours	4,000
Diclofenac	Voltaren	50–75 mg twice a day	200
Diclofenac	Cataflam	50–75 mg twice a day	200
Diflunasil	Dolobid	500–1,000 mg followed by 250–500 mg 2 or 3 times a day	1,500
Fenoprofen	Nalfon	300–600 mg 3 or 4 times a day	3,200
Ibuprofen	Motrin	400–800 mg 3 or 4 times a day	3,200
Indomethacin	Indocin	5–150 mg a day in 3 or 4 divided doses	200
Ketoprofen	Orudis	75 mg 3 times a day or 50 mg 4 times a day	300
Mefenamic acid	Ponstel	500 mg followed by 250 mg every 6 hours	1,000
Naproxen	Naprosyn	250–500 mg twice a day	1,250
Naproxen	Anaprox	550 mg followed by 275 mg every 6 to 8 hours	1,375
Piroxicam	Feldene	20 mg a day	20
Sulindac	Clinoril	200 mg twice a day	400
Tolmetin	Tolectin	400 mg 3 or 4 times a day	1,800
Nabumatone	Relafen	1,000 mg once or twice a day	2,000
Flurbiprofen	Ansaid	50–100 mg 2 or 3 times a day	300
Keterolac	Toradol	10 mg every 4 to 6 hours for pain; *not to be used for more than 5 days*	40
Etudolac	Lodine	200–400 mg every 6 to 8 hours	1,200
Meloxicam	Mobic	7.5 mg once a day	15
Oxaprosin	Daypro	1,200 mg once a day	1,800

aspirin, use of anticoagulants and/or corticosteroids, smoking, and use of alcohol; use caution as well with the elderly and debilitated patients. Use the lowest effective dose for the shortest duration of time, consistent with individual patient goals, to reduce risk of GI adverse events; alternate therapies should be considered for patients at high risk.

Corticosteroids Corticosteroids, of which cortisone is the most common, are used primarily for chronic inflammation of musculoskeletal and joint regions. Cortisone is a synthetic glucocorticoid that is usually given orally or by injection. More caution is taken in the use of corticosteroids than was practiced in the past. Prolonged use of corticosteroids can produce the following serious complications:

- Fluid and electrolyte disturbances (e.g., water retention caused by excess sodium levels)
- Musculoskeletal and joint impairments (e.g., bone thinning and muscle and tendon weakness)
- Dermatological problems (e.g., delayed wound healing)
- Neurological impairments (e.g., vertigo, headache, convulsions)
- Endocrine dysfunctions (e.g., menstrual irregularities)
- Ophthalmic conditions (e.g., glaucoma)
- Metabolic impairments (e.g., negative nitrogen balance, muscle wasting)

Cortisone is primarily administered by injection. Other methods of administration are iontophoresis and phonophoresis (see Chapter 15). Studies have indicated that cortisone injected directly into tendons, ligaments, and joint spaces can lead to weakness and degeneration. Strenuous activity may predispose the treated part to rupturing. Tennis elbow and plantar fasciitis have benefited from corticosteroid treatment.

Drugs That Produce Skeletal Muscle Relaxation

Drugs that produce skeletal muscle relaxation include methocarbamol (Robaxin), cyclobenzaprine (Flexeril), and carisoprodol (Soma). There is growing speculation among physicians that because centrally acting muscle relaxants also act as sedatives or tranquilizers on the higher brain centers, these drugs are less specific to muscle relaxation than was once believed. Another major side effect is that they cause drowsiness.

Muscle spasm and guarding accompany many musculoskeletal injuries. Elimination of spasm and guarding should facilitate programs of rehabilitation. In many situations, centrally acting oral muscle relaxants are used to reduce spasm and guarding. However, to date the efficacy of using muscle relaxants has not been substantiated, and they do not appear to be superior to analgesics or sedatives in either acute or chronic conditions.

Drugs Used to Treat Gastrointestinal Disorders

Disorders of the gastrointestinal tract include upset stomach or formation of gas because of food incompatibilities and acute or chronic hyperacidity, which leads to inflammation of the mucous membrane of the intestinal tract. Poor eating habits may lead to digestive tract problems, such as diarrhea or constipation. Drugs that elicit responses within the gastrointestinal tract include antacids, antiemetics, carminatives, cathartics (laxatives), antidiarrheals, histamine-2 blockers, and proton pump inhibitors.

> Drugs used to treat gastrointestinal disorders include antacids, antiemetics, carminatives, cathartics (laxatives), antidiarrheals, histamine-2 blockers, and proton pump inhibitors.

Antacids The primary function of an antacid is to neutralize acidity in the upper gastrointestinal tract by raising the pH and inhibiting the activity of the digestive enzyme pepsin, thus reducing its action on the gastric mucosal nerve endings. Antacids are effective not only for the relief of acid indigestion and heartburn but also in the treatment of peptic ulcer. Antacids available on the market possess a wide range of acid-neutralizing capabilities and side effects.

One of the most commonly used antacid preparations is sodium bicarbonate, or baking soda. Other antacids include alkaline salts, which neutralize hyperacidity but are not easily absorbed in the blood. The ingestion of antacids containing magnesium tends to have a laxative effect. Those containing aluminum or calcium seem to cause constipation. Consequently, many antacid liquids and tablets are combinations of magnesium and either aluminum or calcium hydroxides. Overuse can cause electrolyte imbalance and other adverse effects.

Antiemetics Antiemetics are used to treat nausea and vomiting. Antiemetics act either locally or centrally. The locally acting drugs, such as most OTC medications (e.g., Pepto-Bismol), reportedly work by affecting the mucosal lining of the stomach. However, their effects of soothing an upset stomach may be more of a placebo effect. The centrally acting drugs affect the brain by making it less sensitive to irritating nerve impulses from the inner ear or stomach. A variety of prescription antiemetics can be used for controlling nausea and vomiting, including phenothiazines (Phenergan), antihistamines, anticholinergic drugs for preventing motion sickness, and sedative drugs. The primary side effect of these medications is drowsiness. Ondansetron (Zofran) is a very effective, nonsedating antiemetic that acts both centrally and peripherally by affecting select serotonin receptors. It is generally well tolerated with few side effects.

Carminatives Carminatives are drugs that give relief from flatulence (gas). Their action on the digestive canal is to inhibit gas formation and aid in its expulsion. Simethicone is the most commonly used carminative.

Cathartics (Laxatives) The use of laxatives in sports should always be under the direction of a physician. Constipation may be symptomatic of a serious disease condition. Indiscriminant use of laxatives may render an individual unable to have normal bowel movements. It may also lead to electrolyte imbalance. There is little need for healthy, active individuals to rely on artificial means for stool evacuation.

Antidiarrheals Diarrhea may result from many causes, but it is generally considered to be a symptom rather than a disease. It can occur as a result of emotional stress, allergies to food or drugs, adverse drug reactions, or many different types of intestinal problems. Diarrhea may be acute or chronic. Acute diarrhea, the most common, comes on suddenly and may be accompanied by nausea, vomiting, chills, and intense abdominal pain. It typically runs its course rapidly, and symptoms subside once the irritating agent is removed from the system. Chronic diarrhea, which may last for weeks, may result from more serious disease states.

Medications used for control of diarrhea are either locally acting or systemic. The locally acting medications most typically contain kaolin, which absorbs other chemicals, and pectin, which soothes irritated bowel. Some contain substances that add bulk to the stool. The systemic agents, which are generally antiperistaltic or antispasmodic medications, are considered to be much more effective in relieving symptoms of diarrhea, but most, except loperamide (Imodium AD), are prescription drugs. The systemic medications are either opiate derivatives or anticholinergic agents, both of which reduce peristalsis. Common side effects of the systemic antidiarrheals include drowsiness, nausea, dry mouth, and constipation. It is not advisable to treat antibiotic-induced diarrhea because diarrhea may be a protective symptom in antibiotic-induced pseudomembranous colitis.

Histamine-2 Blockers Histamine-2 blockers (H2 blockers) reduce stomach acid output by blocking the action of histamine on certain cells in the stomach. They are used to treat peptic and gastric ulcers and other gastrointestinal hypersecretory conditions. Cimetidine (Tagamet) and ranitidine (Zantac) are examples.

Proton Pump Inhibitors The mechanism of action of proton pump inhibitors (PPIs) is to suppress the gastric acid secretion by inhibition of the H+/K+-ATPase in the gastric parietal cell.

PPIs are used for treatment of erosive esophagitis, for maintaining symptom resolution and healing of erosive esophagitis, for treatment of symptomatic gastroesophageal reflux disease (GERD), as part of a multidrug regimen for *Helicobacter pylori* eradication in patients with duodenal ulcer disease, for prevention of gastric ulcers in patients at risk associated with continuous NSAID therapy, and for long-term treatment of pathological hypersecretory conditions. Omeprazole (Prilosec) is an over-the-counter example.

Drugs Used to Treat Colds and Allergies

Drugs on the market designed to affect colds and allergies are almost too numerous to count. In general, they fall into four categories, all of which deal with the symptoms of the condition and not

> **Drugs used to treat colds and allergies include nasal decongestants, antihistamines, cough suppressants, and sympathomimetics.**

the cause. Those categories are drugs that deal with nasal congestion, with histamine reactions, with cough, and with exercise-induced bronchospasm.

Nasal Decongestants Topical nasal decongestants that contain mild vasoconstricting agents, such as oxymetazoline (Afrin), xylometazoline (Otrivin), and phenylephrine (neosynephrine) are on the market. These agents are relatively safe. However, prolonged use can cause rebound congestion and dependency.

An effective oral decongestant is pseudoephedrine hydrochloride (Sudafed). Repeated dosing does not lead to rebound congestion. The Combat Methamphetamine Epidemic Act bans over-the-counter retail sales of cold medicines that contain the ingredient pseudoephedrine, which is commonly used to make methamphetamine in illegal "meth labs." The sale of cold medicine containing pseudoephedrine is limited to behind the counter. The amount of pseudoephedrine that an individual can purchase each month is limited, and individuals are required to present photo identification to purchase products containing pseudoephedrine. In addition, stores are required to keep personal information about purchasers for at least 2 years. This law became effective September 30, 2006.

In addition to these requirements, in order to comply with federal law, regulated sellers are mandated to complete a self-certification process that includes training their employees on the regulations and procedures. The final stage in the self-certification process is for regulated sellers to complete an online application on the Drug Enforcement Administration (DEA) Diversion Web site. Once this application is submitted, DEA sends a confirmation e-mail, which generates a self-certification certificate. Because the athletic training environment is not a "retail sales" operation, it is difficult to apply the federal law. Individuals must become familiar with individual state laws related to the provision of pseudoephedrine and develop procedures in compliance with state and federal regulations. Many states have enacted laws to limit the amount of pseudoephedrine that can be acquired, but the regulations vary from state to state.

Antihistamines Histamine is a protein substance contained in animal tissues that, when released into the general circulation, causes the reactions of an allergy. Histamine causes dilation of arteries and capillaries, skin flushing, and a rise in temperature. An antihistamine is a substance that opposes histamine action. Antihistamines offer little benefit in treating the common cold. They are beneficial in treating allergies, and antihistamines are often added to nasal decongestants. Examples are diphenhydramine hydrochloride (Benadryl), chlorpheniramine (Chlor-Trimeton), and loratidine (Claritin).

Antihistamines, as well as decongestants and diuretics, can decrease the peripheral mechanisms of sweating that impair the body's ability to dissipate heat and thus predispose the athlete to heat-related illness. The nonsedating antihistamines, such as loratidine (Claritin), may pose less risk of heat-related illnesses.

Cough Medicines Cough medicines either suppress the cough (antitussives) or increase the production of fluid in the respiratory system (expectorants). Antitussives are available in liquid, capsule, troche, and spray forms. Narcotic antitussives contain codeine (Robitussin AC); nonnarcotic antitussives contain diphenhydramine (Benylin cough syrup), dextromethorphan (Benylin DM, Sucrets), or benzonatate (Tessalon). The advantage of nonnarcotic antitussives is that they have few side effects and are not addictive. There is little evidence that expectorants (guaifenesin) are any more effective in the control of coughing than is simply drinking water.

Sympathomimetics Exercise-induced bronchospasm (EIB) is a spasm of smooth muscle in the bronchioles and shortness of breath. Drugs used to treat EIB are called sympathomimetics. An example is albuterol

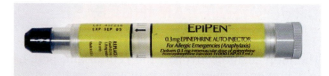

FIGURE 17–2 An EpiPen can be used to treat severe allergic reactions.

(Proventil, Ventolin). Bronchodilators generally reverse the symptoms. Sympathomimetics may cause heat-related problems if used in a hot environment.

Epinephrine In some states, the athletic trainer may receive instructions and certification for the administration of epinephrine via an injective device (EpiPen) to treat anaphylaxis resulting from insect stings. Once it is clear that an individual is having an anaphylactic reaction, the EpiPen can be used to safely and easily inject medication into the thigh (Figure 17–2).

Drugs Used to Control Bleeding

Various drugs and medicines, including vasoconstrictors, hemostatic agents, and anticoagulants, cause selective actions on the circulatory system.

> Drugs used to control bleeding include vasoconstrictors, hemostatic agents, and anticoagulants.

Vasoconstrictors Vasoconstrictors are most often administered externally to sites of profuse bleeding. The drug most commonly used for this purpose is epinephrine (adrenaline), which is applied directly to a hemorrhaging area. It acts immediately to constrict damaged blood vessels and is extremely valuable in cases of epistaxis (nosebleed) in which normal procedures are inadequate.

Hemostatic Agents Drugs that immediately inhibit bleeding are currently being investigated. There are products such as zeolite granules (QuikClot) and chitosan (HemCon) that can be used as specialized dressings to temporize hemorrhage outside of the operating room, such as in a rescue or battlefield situations. These may be used by a physician in an athletic setting.

Anticoagulants The most common anticoagulants used by physicians are heparin and coumarin derivatives. Heparin prolongs the clotting time of blood but will not dissolve a clot once it has developed. Heparin is used primarily to control extension of a thrombus (clot) that is already present. Warfarin (Coumadin) acts by suppressing the formation of prothrombin in the liver. Given orally, it is used to slow clotting time in certain vascular disorders.

DRUGS THAT CAN INCREASE THE RATE OF HEAT ILLNESS

Thermoregulation involves the central and peripheral nervous system and circulatory mechanisms.[7] Drugs that affect neurotransmitters in these systems could affect temperature regulation. Table 17–8 lists drugs that can predispose peoples to heat-related problems. Anticholinergics and antihistamines can decrease the peripheral mechanism of sweating and therefore eliminate the body's ability to lose heat from this mechanism. Sympathomimetic amines, including decongestants, are vasoconstrictors that can predispose an athlete to heat illness. Phenothiazines affect both hot and cold temperature regulation. Tricyclic antidepressants have been shown to affect hypothalamic heat control and to have anticholinergic activity. Diuretics can prevent volume expansion and limit cutaneous vasodilation.

Lithium carbonate can increase the risk of heatstroke by its effects on potassium levels. It is important that the athletic trainer recognize medications that can increase the risk of heat-related problems, especially when individuals are taking any of these medications and exercising in a warm climate.

PROTOCOLS FOR USING OVER-THE-COUNTER MEDICATIONS

There is a major difference between prescription and nonprescription drugs. Drugs that require a prescription may pose a greater risk to the patient and therefore require the clinical skills and judgment of individuals trained and licensed to prescribe drugs. In most cases, the athletic trainer will be concerned only with nonprescription medications.

Focus Box 17–2: "Protocols for the use of over-the-counter drugs for athletic trainers" presents guidelines for treating a number of minor illnesses or conditions seen frequently in the athletic population. The authors and publisher have exerted every effort to ensure that the drug selection and dosage set forth in this text are in accord with current recommendations and practice at the time of publication. However, in view of ongoing research, changes in government regulations, and the constant flow of information relating to drug therapy and drug reactions, the reader is urged to check the package insert for each drug for any change in indications and dosage and for added warnings and precautions. Reading the package insert is especially important when the recommended agent is a new or infrequently used drug.

SUBSTANCE ABUSE AMONG ATHLETES

Perhaps no other topic related to pharmacology has received more attention from the media during recent years than the use and abuse of drugs, especially by athletes. Much has been written regarding the use of performance-enhancing drugs among Olympic athletes and the widespread use of street drugs by collegiate and professional athletes. Clearly, substance abuse has no place in the athletic population.[44]

Although much of the information being disseminated to the public by the media may be based on hearsay and innuendo, the use and abuse of

---

TABLE 17–8	Drugs Reported to Predispose to Heat Illness

Sympathomimetics	Phenothiazines
Amphetamines	Prochlorperazine
Epinephrine	Chlorpromazine hydrochloride
Ephedrine	Promethazine hydrochloride
Cocaine	Butyrophenones
Norepinephrine	Haloperidol
Pseudoephedrine	Cyclic antidepressants
Anticholinergics	Amitriptyline hydrochloride
Atropine sulfate	Imipramine hydrochloride
Scopolamine HBr	Nortriptyline hydrochloride
Benztropine mesylate	Protriptyline hydrochloride
Belladonna and synthetic alkaloids	Monoamine oxidase inhibitors
Antihistamines	Phenelzine
Diuretics	Tranylcypromine sulfate
Furosemide	Alcohol
Hydrochlorothiazide	Lysergic acid diethylamide (LSD)
Bumetanide	Lithium

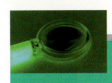

Protocols for the use of over-the-counter drugs for athletic trainers

The athletic trainer is often responsible for the initial screening of individuals who have various illnesses or injuries. Frequently, the athletic trainer must make decisions regarding the appropriate use of over-the-counter medications. Subjective findings, such as onset, duration, medication taken, and known allergies, must be included in the screening evaluation.

The following protocols should be viewed as guidelines. The protocols are aimed at clarifying the use of over-the-counter drugs in the treatment of common problems encountered by the athletic trainer while covering an event or traveling with a team. These guidelines do not cover every situation the athletic trainer encounters in assessing and managing the patient's physical problems. Therefore, physician consultation is recommended whenever there is uncertainty in making a decision regarding the appropriate care of the athlete.

Existing illness or injury	Appropriate Treatment Protocol
Temperature	
Greater than or equal to 102°F orally	Consult physician ASAP.
Less than 102°F but more than 99.5°F orally	Patient may be given acetaminophen. *See acetaminophen administration protocol.*
	Limit exercise of athlete. Do not allow participation in practice.
	If fever decreases to less than 99.5°F, the athlete may participate in practice.
	If patient is to be involved in an intercollegiate event, consult with a physician concerning participation.
Less than or equal to 99.5°F orally	Follow management guidelines for fever lower than 102°F, but allow patient to practice and/or compete.
Throat	
History	Advise saline gargles (½ tsp. salt in a glass of warm water).
Sore throat	Patient may also be given Cepastat®/Chloraseptic® throat lozenges.
No fever	Before administering, determine: Is the patient allergic to Cepastat®/
No chills	Chloraseptic® lozenges (which contain phenol)? If yes, do not administer.
Sore throat	Determine temperature. If fever, manage as outlined in temperature
Fever	protocol, and consult physician ASAP.
Sore throat and/or fever and/or swollen glands	Consult physician ASAP.
Nose	
Watery discharge	Patient may be given pseudoephedrine (Sudafed®) tablets. See *pseudoephedrine administration protocol.*
Nasal congestion	Patient may be given oxymetazoline HCl (Afrin®) nasal spray. See *oxymetazoline administration protocol.*
Chest	
Cough	You may administer Robitussin DM® (generic guaifenesin with dex-
Dry, hacking or clear, mucoid sputum	tromethorphan). Before administering, determine:
	Is the patient going to be involved in practice or a game within 4 hours of administration of medication?
	If yes, do not give Robitussin DM®.
	If indicated, you may administer one dose, 10 ml (2 tsp.). Inform the patient that drowsiness may occur. Repeat doses may be administered every 6 hours. Push fluids; encourage patient to drink as much as possible.
Green or rusty sputum	Consult physician ASAP.
Severe, persistent cough	Consult physician ASAP.
Ears	
Discomfort due to ears popping	Patient may be given pseudoephedrine (Sudafed®) tablets and/or oxymetazoline HCl (Afrin®) nasal spray. *See pseudoephedrine administration protocol and/or oxymetazoline protocol.*
Earache (external otitis)	Patient may be given acetaminophen. Consult physician ASAP. *See acetaminophen administration protocol.*
Recurrent earache	Consult physician ASAP.

Continued

Protocols for the use of over-the-counter drugs for athletic trainers—Cont'd

Prevention of Motion Sickness

Complaint: history of nausea, dizziness, and/or vomiting associated with travel

Patient may be given dimenhydrinate (Dramamine®) or diphenhydramine (Benadryl®). Before administering, determine:

Is the patient sensitive or allergic to Dramamine®, Benadryl®, or any other antihistamine? If yes, do not administer.

Has the patient taken any other antihistamines (e.g., Actifed®, Chlor-Trimeton®, various cold medications) or other medications that cause sedation within the last 6 hours? If yes, do not administer.

Does the patient have asthma, glaucoma, or enlargement of the prostate gland? If yes, do not administer.

Is the patient going to be involved in practice or game within 4 hours from administration of medication? If yes, do not administer.

Administer Dramamine® or Benadryl® dose based on body weight, 30 to 60 minutes before departure time: Under 125 lbs: one Dramamine® 50 mg tablet. Over 125 lbs: two Dramamine 50 mg tablets.

Benadryl® dose: Under 125 lbs: one 25 mg capsule. Over 125 lbs: two 25 mg capsules.

Inform the patient that drowsiness may occur for 4 to 6 hours after taking this medication. Avoid alcoholic beverages. Avoid driving for 6 hours after taking. If travelling time is extended, another dose may be administered 6 hours after the first dose.

Nausea, Vomiting

Prolonged and severe

Consult physician ASAP.

Nausea, Gastric Upset, Heartburn, Butterflies in the Stomach, Acid Indigestion

Associated with dietary indiscretion or tension

You may administer an antacid as a single dose, as defined by label of particular antacid (e.g. Riopan®, Gelusil®, Maalox®, Pepto-Bismol®, Titralac®), or a histamine (H2) antagonist (Pepcid AC®, Tagamet HB®, Axid A®, Zantac 75®). *See histamine-2 blocker protocol. Pepto-Bismol® warning: Contains salicylates. Do not give to children or teenagers who have or are recovering from chickenpox or flu because of the risk of Reye's syndrome. Do not use this product with aspirin.*

Associated with abdominal or chest pain

Consult physician ASAP.

Vomiting, nausea—no severe distress

Monitor symptoms. Patient may be given dimenhydrinate (Dramamine®) or diphenhydramine (Benadryl®) orally. Same as instructions and precautions for motion sickness.

Vomiting: projectile, coffee ground, febrile

Consult physician ASAP.

Diarrhea

Associated with abdominal pain or tenderness and/or dehydration, bloody stools, febrile, recurrent diarrhea

Consult physician ASAP.

Frequent, loose stools not associated with any of the above signs or symptoms

Encourage clear liquid diet. Encourage avoidance of dairy products and high-fat foods for 24 hours (BART diet—bananas, apples, rice, toast). If it persists, consult physician ASAP.

Patient may be given loperamide (Imodium AD®). Before administering, determine: How long has patient had diarrhea? If longer than 24 hours, see physician.

You may administer one dose (two caplets) of loperamide (Imodium AD®, 2 mg per caplet). One caplet may be administered after each loose stool not to exceed 8 mg (four caplets) per 24 hours. Inform the patient that dizziness or drowsiness may occur within 12 hours after taking this medication. Avoid alcoholic beverages. Use caution while driving or performing tasks requiring alertness.

Constipation

Prolonged or severe abdominal pain or tenderness, nausea or vomiting

Consult physician ASAP.

Continued

Protocols for the use of over-the-counter drugs for athletic trainers—Cont'd

Constipation—Continued

Discomfort associated with dietary change or decreased fluid intake

You may administer milk of magnesia, 30 ml as a single dose. Before administering, determine: Does the patient have chronic renal disease? If yes, do not administer.

Recommend increased fluid intake, increased intake of fruits, bulk vegetables, or cereals.

Headache

Pain associated with elevated BP, temperature elevation, blurred vision, nausea, vomiting, or history of migraine

Consult physician ASAP.

Pain across forehead (mild headache)

Patient may be given acetaminophen or NSAID. *See acetaminophen administration or* NSAID *administration protocol.*

Tension headache, occipital pain

Patient may be given acetaminophen. *See acetaminophen administration protocol.*

Pain in antrum or forehead associated with sinus or nasal congestion

Patient may be given pseudoephedrine (Sudafed®) tablets and acetaminophen. *See protocols for pseudoephedrine and acetaminophen administration.*

Musculoskeletal Injuries

Deformity

Consult physician ASAP.

Localized pain and tenderness, impaired range of motion

First aid to start as soon as possible:
Ice
Compression—Ace bandage
Elevation
Protection—crutches or sling and/or splint

Pain with swelling discoloration, no impaired movement or localized tenderness

If this injury interferes with the patient's normal activities, consult a physician within 24 hours.

Patient may be given acetaminophen or NSAID.
See acetaminophen administration or NSAID *administration protocol.*

Skin

Localized or generalized rash accompanied by elevated temperature, enlarged lymph nodes, sore throat, stiff neck, infected skin lesion, dyspnea, wheezing

Consult physician ASAP.

Mild, localized, nonvesicular skin eruptions accompanied by pruritis

Hydrocortisone 1.0% cream may be applied.
Before administering, determine:
Is the patient taking any medication? If yes, do not administer. Refer to physician.
Are eyes or any large area of the body involved? If yes, do not administer. Refer to physician.
Is there any evidence of lice infestation?
The cream may be repeated every 6 hours if needed.
Do not use more than three times daily.

Abrasions

Control bleeding. Clean with antibacterial soap and water. Apply appropriate dressing and antibiotic ointment. Monitor for signs of infection. Dressing may be changed 2 or 3 times a day if needed.

Localized erythema due to ultraviolet rays

Advise application of compresses soaked in a solution of cold water.

Jock itch or athlete's foot

Advise 10- to 15-minute application of compresses soaked in cool water to relieve intense itching.

Patient may be given terbinafine (Lamisil) or miconazole (Micatin®) cream topically. Before administering, determine:
Is the patient sensitive or allergic to miconazole or terbinafine? If yes, do not administer. Consult physician ASAP.
Is the patient receiving other types of treatment for rash in same area? If yes, do not administer. Consult physician ASAP.
Instruct patient to wash and dry area of rash, and then apply ¼- to ½-inch ribbon of cream. Give patient the cream on a clean gauze pad and rub gently on the infected area. Spread evenly and thinly over rash. The dose may be repeated in 8 to 12 hours (twice a day). Consult physician within 24 hours.

Continued

Protocols for the use of over-the-counter drugs for athletic trainers—Cont'd

Skin Wounds

Lacerations	Control bleeding. Cleanse area with antibacterial soap and water. Apply steristrips. Consult physician immediately if there is any question about the necessity for suturing.
Extensive lacerations or other severe skin wounds	Control bleeding. Protect area with dressing. Refer to physician immediately.

Wound Infection

Febrile, marked cellulitis, red streaks, tender or enlarged nodes	Consult physician ASAP.
Localized inflammation, afebrile, absence of nodes and streaks	Warm soaks to affected area. Consult physician ASAP.

Burns

First-degree erythema of skin, limited area	Apply cold compresses to affected area. Dressing is not necessary on first-degree burns. If less than 45 minutes have elapsed since burn injury, clean gently with soap and water. Patient may be given acetaminophen. *See acetaminophen administration protocol.*
First-degree with extensive involvement over body	Consult physician ASAP.
Second-degree erythema with blistering	Consult physician ASAP.
Third-degree pearly white appearance of affected area, no pain	Consult physician ASAP.

Allergies

Patient with known seasonal allergies who forgot to bring own medication	Patient may be given 10 mg tablet of loratidine (Claritin®). Before administering, determine:
	Is the patient sensitive to loratidine? If yes, do not administer. Consult physician ASAP.
	Does the patient have liver or kidney disease? If yes, do not administer. Consult physician ASAP.
	Has the patient taken any other antihistamines (e.g., Chlorpheniramine, Dramamine®, various cold medications) or other medications that cause drowsiness within the last 6 hours? If yes, do not administer. Consult physician ASAP.
	You may administer one dose of loratidine (10 mg) every 24 hours. Avoid alcoholic beverages. Contact physician if symptoms do not abate.

Contact Lens Care

Note: There are three types of contact lenses: hard, gas permeable, soft.

Solutions are labeled for use with a particular type of lens and should not be used for any other type of lens.

Do not use solutions preserved with thimersol or chlorhexidine because of possible allergy or irritation.

Lens needs rinsing/wetting before insertion	Hard lens: use all-purpose wetting/soaking solution (e.g., Wet-N-Soak®).
	Gas permeable lens: use all-purpose wetting/soaking solution (e.g., Wet-N-Soak®).
	Soft lens: use rinsing/soaking solution (e.g., Soft Mate ps®).
Lens needs soaking/storage	Hard lens: use all-purpose wetting/soaking solution (e.g., Wet-N-Soak®).
	Gas permeable lens: use all-purpose wetting/soaking solution (e.g., Wet-N-Soak®).
	Soft lens: use rinsing/soaking solution (e.g., Soft Mate ps®).
Lens needs cleaning	Hard lens: use cleaning solution (e.g., EasyClean®).
	Gas permeable lens: use cleaning solution (e.g., Easy Clean®).
	Soft lens: use cleaning solution (e.g., Lens Plus Daily Cleaner®).

Eye Care

Foreign body—minor: sand, eyelash, etc.	Use eye wash irrigation solution (Dacriose®).
Irritation—minor	Use artificial tears. Do not use with contact lens in eye.
Severe irritation, foreign body not easily removed, trauma	Consult physician ASAP.

Continued

Protocols for the use of over-the-counter drugs for athletic trainers—Cont'd

Red Eye

Only one eye affected	Consult physician ASAP.
Change in vision	Consult physician ASAP.
Pain in eye	Consult physician ASAP.
Sensitivity to light	Consult physician ASAP.
Thick discharge from eye, especially with lids sealed shut in morning	Consult physician ASAP.
Patient wears contacts	Consult physician ASAP.
Redness, tearing, both eyes itch	1. Apply cold compresses. 2. Instill one or two drops of antihistamine/decongestant eye drop (e.g., Vasocon-A®) into each eye four times a day. (Do not use one bottle for more than one patient.) 3. If condition does not improve or worsens, consult physician ASAP. 4. If condition has not improved in 24 hours or persists for more than 48 hours, consult physician ASAP.
Redness, tearing, both eyes itch in patient with known allergies who forgot to bring own medication	1. Apply cold compresses 2. Instill one or two drops of antihistamine/decongestant eye drop (e.g., Vasocon-A®) into each eye four times a day. (Do not use one bottle for more than one patient.) 3. *See also allergies treatment protocol.* 4. See No. 4 above.

Administration protocols for common over-the-counter drugs used in sports medicine Acetaminophen protocol (Tylenol®)

Before *administering*, determine:

Is the patient allergic to acetaminophen? If yes, do not give acetaminophen.

You may *administer* acetaminophen 325 mg, two tablets. Repeat doses may be *administered* every 4 hours if needed. If *dispensing* occurs, use labeled 2/pack only. Patient instructions must accompany *dispensing*. The maximum dose must not exceed 4 g (4,000 mg) in 24 hours.

Pseudoephedrine protocol (Sudafed®)

Before *administering*, determine:

Is the patient allergic or sensitive to pseudoephedrine? If yes, do not give pseudoephedrine.

Does the patient have high blood pressure, heart disease, diabetes, urinary retention, glaucoma, or thyroid disease? If yes, do not give pseudoephedrine.

Does the patient have problems with sweating? If yes, do not give pseudoephedrine.

Do not administer 4 hours before practice or game.

Do not administer if patient is involved in postseason play.

You may *administer* pseudoephedrine (Sudafed®) 30 mg, two tablets. Repeat doses may be *administered* every 6 hours up to four times a day. If *dispensing* occurs, use labeled 2/pack only. Patient instructions must accompany *dispensing*.

Oxymetazoline protocol (Afrin®)

Before *administering*, determine:

Is the patient allergic or sensitive to Afrin® or Otrivin®? If yes, do not administer.

Does the patient react unusually to nose sprays or drops? If yes, do not administer.

You may *administer* two or three sprays of oxymetazoline (Afrin®) 0.05% nasal spray into each nostril. Repeat doses may be administered every 12 hours. (The container can be marked with the patient's name and maintained by the athletic trainer for repeat administration or dispensed to the patient. Patient instructions must accompany *dispensing*.)

Do not use the same container for different patients.

Do not use for more than 3 days without MD supervision.

Use small package sizes to reduce risk of overuse/rebound congestion.

NSAID Protocol (ibuprofen: Advil®, naproxen sodium: Aleve®, ketoprofen: Orudis KT®)

Before *administering*, determine:

Is the patient allergic to aspirin, (e.g., asthma, swelling, shock, or hives associated with aspirin use)? If yes, do not give ibuprofen because, even though ibuprofen contains no aspirin or salicylates, cross-reactions may occur in patients allergic to aspirin.

Does the patient have renal disease or gastrointestinal ulcerations? If yes, do not administer ibuprofen.

You may *administer* ibuprofen 200 mg (Advil®), one or two tablets. Repeat doses may be *administered* every 6 hours if needed. Do not exceed six tablets in a 24-hour period without consulting an MD. Do not administer if patient is less than 12 years of age.

Continued

Protocols for the use of over-the-counter drugs for athletic trainers—Cont'd

or

You may *administer* naproxen sodium 220 mg (Aleve®), one tablet every 8 to 12 hours or two tablets to start followed by one tablet 12 hours later. Do not exceed three tablets in a 24-hour period without consulting a physician. Do not administer if patient is less than 12 years of age.

or

You may *administer* ketoprofen 12.5 mg (Orudis KT®, Actron®), one tablet or caplet every 4 to 6 hours if needed. If pain or fever persists after 1 hour, one more 12.5 mg tablet or caplet may be given. Do not exceed six tablets or caplets in a 24-hour period without consulting a physician. Do not administer if the patient is less than 16 years of age.

The patient should take the NSAID with a full glass of water and food if occasional and mild heartburn, upset stomach, or mild stomach pain occurs. Consult MD if these symptoms are more than mild or persist. Discontinue drug if patient experiences skin rash; itching; dark, tarry stools; visual disturbances; dark urine; or persistent headache. Instruct patient to avoid concurrent aspirin or alcoholic beverages.

Histamine-2 Blocker Protocol (ranitidine: Zantac 75®, nizatidine: Axid AR®, famotidine: Pepsid AC®, cimetidine: Tagamet-HB®)

Before *administering*, determine:

Is the patient less than 12 years of age? If yes, do not give histamine-2 blocker. Does the patient have difficulty swallowing or persistent abdominal pain? If yes, do not give histamine-2 blocker.

You may *administer* ranitidine (Zantac 75®), one 75 mg tablet with water up to two times a day. Do not administer more than two tablets in a 24-hour period.

or

You may *administer* nizatidine (Axid AR®), one 75 mg tablet with water up to two times a day. Do not administer more that two tablets in a 24-hour period.

or

You may *administer* famotidine (Pepcid AC®), one 10 mg tablet with water up to two times a day. Do not administer more than two tablets in a 24-hour period.

or

You may *administer* cimetidine (Tagamet-HB®), one 10 mg tablet with water up to two times a day. Do not administer more than two tablets in a 24-hour period. Do not administer cimetidine if the patient is taking phenytoin (Dilantin®) or theophyllin (Theodur®).

---

many different types of drugs can have a profound impact on athletic performance. To say that many experts in the field of sports medicine regard drug abuse among athletes with growing concern is a gross understatement. The athletic trainer must be knowledgeable about substance abuse in the athletic population and should be able to recognize signs that indicate when an individual is engaging in substance abuse[2] (see *Focus Box 17–3*: "Identifying the substance abuser").

Performance-Enhancing Substances (Ergogenic Aids)

Ergogenic aid is a term used to describe any method, legal or illegal, used to enhance athletic performance.[48] Athletic trainers should have a primary concern about the use of various pharmacological agents for enhancing performance. The NATA has prepared an official statement on this topic (*Focus Box 17–4*: "Steroids and performance-enhancing substances").

Stimulants People may ingest a stimulant to increase alertness, reduce fatigue, or increase competitiveness and even hostility. Some individuals respond to stimulants with a loss of judgment that may lead to personal injury or injury to others.

Two major categories of stimulants are psychomotor-stimulant drugs and adrenergic (sympathomimetic) drugs. Psychomotor stimulants are of two general types: amphetamines (e.g., methamphetamine) and nonamphetamines (e.g., methylphenidate and cocaine). The major actions of psychomotor stimulants result from the rapid turnover of catecholamines, which have a strong effect on the nervous and cardiovascular systems, metabolic rates, temperature, and smooth muscle.

Sympathomimetic drugs act directly on adrenergic receptors, or those that release catecholamines (i.e., epinephrine and norepinephrine) from nerve endings, and thus act indirectly on catecholamines. Ephedrine is an example of this type of drug and can, in high doses, cause mental stimulation and

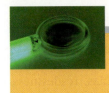

FOCUS 17–3 Focus on Clinical Evaluation and Diagnosis

Identifying the substance abuser

The following are signs of drug abuse:

- Sudden personality changes
- Severe mood swings
- Changing peer groups
- Decreased interest in extracurricular and leisure activities
- Worsening grades
- Disregard for household chores and curfews
- Feelings of depression most of the time
- Breakdown in personal hygiene habits
- Increased sleep and decreased eating
- Smell of alcohol or marijuana on clothes and skin
- Sudden weight loss
- Lying, cheating, stealing
- Arrests for drunk driving or for possessing illegal substances
- Truancies from school
- Frequent loss or change of jobs
- Defensiveness at the mention of drugs or alcohol
- Increased isolation (spends time in room)
- Deteriorating family relationship
- Drug paraphernalia (needles, empty bottles, etc.)
- Observations by others about negative behavior
- Signs of intoxication
- Missed appointments
- Falling asleep in class or at work
- Financial problems
- Missed assignments or deadlines
- Diminished productivity

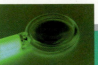

FOCUS 17–4 Focus on Organizational and Professional Health and Well-Being

NATA official statement on steroids and performance-enhancing substances

Members of the National Athletic Trainers' Association are on the front line in the battle against drug use and abuse in athletics. Athletic trainers know first hand the negative effects steroids and performance-enhancing drugs can have on healthy athletes. Certified athletic trainers (ATCs) are medical professionals who specialize in the prevention, assessment, treatment and rehabilitation of injuries and illnesses that occur to athletes and physically active people. Athletic trainers in the professional, college/university and high-school settings often are the first to identify athletes with potential drug abuse problems. ATCs are involved in research on the effects of steroids and performance-enhancing drugs. In addition, they provide drug education and are involved in the drug testing process.

The National Athletic Trainers' Association and its members are working to eliminate drug use and abuse from athletics and schools.

From Steroids and performance enhancing substances (2005), http://www.nata.org/sites/default/files/SteroidsPerformanceEnhancingSubstances.pdf.

increased blood flow. As a result, it may also cause elevated blood pressure and headache, increased and irregular heartbeat, anxiety, and tremors.

Amphetamines and cocaine are the psychomotor drugs most commonly used. Cocaine is discussed in the section on recreational drug abuse in this chapter. Sympathomimetic drugs present an extremely difficult problem in sports medicine because they are commonly found in cold remedies.[55] The U.S. Olympic Committee (USOC) has approved some substances to be used by asthmatics who develop exercise-induced bronchospasms. These substances are selective B_2 agonists, consisting of albuterol (Proventil), salmeterol (Serevent), and formoterol (Foradil). Before an athlete engages in Olympic

> **Common ergogenic aids include stimulants, beta blockers, narcotic analgesics, diuretics, anabolic steroids, human growth hormone, and blood doping.**

competition, his or her physician must notify the USOC Medical Subcommission in writing about the patient's use of these drugs.[59]

Amphetamines Amphetamines are synthetic alkaloids that are extremely powerful and dangerous drugs. They may be injected, inhaled, or taken as tablets. Amphetamines are among the most abused of those drugs used to enhance performance. In ordinary doses, amphetamines can produce euphoria, with an increased sense of well-being and heightened mental activity, until fatigue sets in (from lack of sleep), accompanied by nervousness, insomnia, and anorexia. In high doses, amphetamines reduce mental activity and impair the performance of complicated motor skills. The patient's behavior may become irrational. The chronic user may be "hung up"—that is, stuck in a repetitious behavioral sequence. This perseveration may last for hours and become increasingly more irrational. The long-term or even short-term use of amphetamines can lead to amphetamine psychosis, manifested by auditory and visual hallucinations and paranoid delusions. Physiologically, high doses of amphetamines can cause mydriasis (abnormal pupillary dilation), increased blood pressure, hyperreflexia (increased reflex action), and hyperthermia.

Many athletes believe that amphetamines improve performance by promoting quickness and endurance, delaying fatigue, and increasing confidence, thereby causing increased aggressiveness. Studies indicate that there is no improvement in performance, but there is an increased risk of injury, exhaustion, and circulatory collapse.[16]

Caffeine Caffeine is found in coffee, tea, cocoa, and cola and is readily absorbed into the body (Table 17–9).[5] Caffeine is a central nervous system stimulant and diuretic, and it stimulates gastric secretion. One cup of coffee can contain from 100 to 150 milligrams of caffeine. In moderation, caffeine causes stimulation of the cerebral cortex and medullar centers, resulting in wakefulness and mental alertness. In larger amounts and in individuals who ingest caffeine daily, it raises blood pressure, decreases and then increases the heart rate, and increases plasma levels of epinephrine, norepinephrine, and renin. It affects coordination, sleep, mood, behavior, and thinking processes.[5]

In terms of exercise and sports performance, caffeine is controversial. Like amphetamines, caffeine can affect some athletes by acting as an ergogenic aid during prolonged exercise. The USOC considers caffeine a stimulant if the concentration in the athlete's urine exceeds 12 micrograms per milliliter. Some adverse effects of caffeine ingestion are tremors, nervousness, headaches, diuresis, arrhythmias, restlessness, hyperactivity, irritability, dry mouth, tinnitus, ocular dyskinesia (involuntary eye movement), scotomata (blind spots), insomnia, and depression.[5] A habitual user of caffeine who suddenly stops may experience withdrawal, including headache, drowsiness, lethargy, rhinorrhea, irritability, nervousness, depression, and loss of interest in work. Caffeine also acts as a diuretic when hydration may be important.[5]

Narcotic Analgesic Drugs Narcotic analgesic drugs are derived directly from opium or are synthetic opiates. Morphine and codeine (methylmorphine) are examples of substances made from the alkaloid of opium. Narcotic analgesics are used for the management of moderate to severe pain. Users risk physical and psychological dependency as well as many other problems stemming from the use of narcotics. It is believed that slight to moderate pain can be controlled effectively by drugs other than narcotics.

Beta Blockers The *beta* in beta blockers refers to the type of sympathetic nerve ending receptor that is blocked.[40] Medically, beta blockers are used primarily for hypertension and heart disease. Beta blockers have been used in sports that require steadiness, such as marksmanship, sailing, archery, fencing, ski jumping, and luge.[40] Beta blockers are one class of adrenergic agents that inhibit the action of catecholamines released from sympathetic nerve endings. Beta blockers produce relaxation of blood vessels. This relaxation in turn slows heart rate and decreases the contractility of heart muscle, thus decreasing cardiac output.

Diuretics Diuretic drugs increase kidney excretion by decreasing the kidney's resorption of sodium. The excretion of potassium and bicarbonate may also be increased. Therapeutically, diuretics are used for a variety of cardiovascular and respiratory conditions (e.g., hypertension) in which the elimination of fluids from tissues is necessary. Sports participants have misused diuretics mainly in two ways: to reduce body weight quickly and to decrease a drug's concentration in the urine (increasing its excretion to avoid the detection of drug misuse). In both cases, there are ethical and health grounds for banning certain classes of diuretics from use during competition.

Anabolic Steroids Anabolic steroids are synthetically created chemical compounds whose structure closely resembles naturally occurring sex hormones—in particular, the male hormone testosterone.[19,20] Anabolic steroids have both androgenic

TABLE 17–9	Examples of Caffeine-Containing Products
Product	**Dose**
Coffee (1 cup)	100.0 mg
Diet Coke (12 oz)	45.6 mg
Diet Pepsi (12 oz)	36.0 mg
No-Doz (1)	100.0 mg
Anacin (1)	32.0 mg
Excedrin (1)	65.0 mg
Midol (1)	32.4 mg
Jolt (12 oz)	200.0 mg
Mountain Dew (12 oz)	54.0 mg

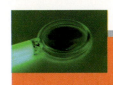

have taken them, with most being purchased through the black market.[3] Approximately 6.5 percent of male athletes and 1.9 percent of female athletes are taking anabolic steroids.[39] An estimated 2.5 percent of intercollegiate athletes take anabolic steroids.[39] The more commonly used anabolic steroids are Anavar, Dianabol, Anadrol, and Finajet.[38]

Usage of anabolic steroids is a major problem in sports that involve strength. Powerlifting, the throwing events in track and field, and American football are some sports in which the use of anabolic steroids is a serious problem.

and anabolic effects. Androgenic effects include growth development and maintenance of reproductive tissues and masculinization in males.[20] Anabolic effects promote nitrogen retention, which leads to protein synthesis in skeletal muscles and other tissues, resulting in increased muscle mass and weight, general growth, and bone maturation.[8,19]

Individuals who choose to take anabolic steroids are seeking to maximize the anabolic effects while minimizing the androgenic side effects. The problem is that no steroids exist that have only anabolic effects; they all also have androgenic effects.[41]

In 1984 the American College of Sports Medicine (ACSM) reported that anabolic steroids taken with an adequate diet could contribute to an increase in body weight and, with a heavy resistance program, to a possible significant gain in strength.[61] However, when used in mass quantities, as individual athletes typically use them, anabolic steroids can have many deleterious and irreversible side effects that constitute a major threat to the health of the user (*Focus Box 17–5*: "Examples of deleterious effects of anabolic steroids").[3]

Anabolic steroids present an ethical dilemma for the sports world.[39] It is estimated that more than a million young male and female athletes are taking or

Tetrahydrogestrinone (THG) Recently, a substance called tetrahydrogestrinone (THG) has reportedly been used by athletes to improve their performance. THG is currently thought to be undetectable on drug tests. Purveyors of THG may represent it as a dietary supplement, but it does not meet the dietary supplement definition. Rather, it is a purely synthetic "designer" steroid that is structurally related to two other synthetic anabolic steroids, gestrinone and trenbolone. It is derived by simple chemical modification from another anabolic steroid that is explicitly banned by the U.S. Anti-Doping Agency. It cannot be legally marketed without FDA approval under the agency's rigorous approval standards, and according to the FDA its use may pose considerable health risks.

Androstenedione Androstenedione is a relatively weak androgen that is produced primarily in the testes and in lower amounts by the adrenal cortex and ovaries.[47] It has been used in humans to produce transcient increases in testosterone in males and particularly in females primarily for the purpose of enhancing athletic performance. To date there is no scientific evidence or research to support the efficacy or safety of using this ergogenic aid.[26] The Anabolic Steroid Control Act of 2004 added anabolic steroids and prohormones, including androstenedione, to the list of controlled substances regulated by the Drug

Enforcement Administration. This makes possession of these substances without a prescription a crime. The use of androstenedione supplements is banned by the International Olympic Committee, the National Football League, the National Collegiate Athletic Association, and Minor League Baseball.

Human Growth Hormone Human growth hormone (HGH) is produced by the somatotropic cells of the anterior region of the pituitary gland, from which it is released into the circulatory system. The amount released varies with age and the developmental periods of a person's life. A lack of HGH can result in dwarfism. In the past, HGH was in limited supply because it was extracted from cadavers. Now, however, it can be made synthetically and is more readily available.[21]

Experiments indicate that HGH can increase muscle mass, skin thickness, connective tissues in muscle, and organ weight and can produce lax muscles and ligaments during rapid growth phases. It also increases body length and weight and decreases body fat percentage.[21]

The use of HGH by athletes throughout the world is on the increase because it is more difficult to detect in urine than are anabolic steroids.[49] There is currently a lack of concrete information about the effects of HGH on the athlete who does not have a growth problem. It is known that an overabundance of HGH in the body can lead to premature closure of long-bone growth sites or, conversely, can cause acromegaly, a condition that produces elongation and enlargement of bones of the extremities and thickening of bones and soft tissues of the face. Also associated with acromegaly is diabetes mellitus, cardiovascular disease, goiter, menstrual disorders, decreased sexual desire, and impotence. Acromegaly decreases the life span by up to 20 years. Like anabolic steroids, HGH presents a serious problem for the sports world. At this time there is no proof that an increase of HGH combined with weight training contributes to strength and muscle hypertrophy.[49]

Blood Reinjection (Blood Doping, Blood Packing, and Blood Boosting) Endurance, acclimatization, and altitude make increased metabolic demands on the body, which responds by increasing blood volume and the number of red blood cells to meet the increased aerobic demands.

Recently, researchers have replicated these physiological responses by removing 900 milliliters of blood, storing it, and reinfusing it after 6 weeks. The reason for waiting at least 6 weeks before reinfusion is that it takes that long for the athlete's body to reestablish a normal hemoglobin and red blood cell concentration. Athletes using this method have significantly improved their endurance performance. From the standpoint of scientific research, such experimentation has merit and is of interest. However, not only is the use of such methods in competition unethical, but use by nonmedical personnel could prove to be dangerous, especially when a matched donor is used.[48]

There are serious risks with transfusing blood and related blood products. The risks include allergic reactions, kidney damage (if the wrong type of blood is used), fever, jaundice, the possibility of transmitting infectious diseases (hepatitis B or HIV), and blood overload, which can result in circulatory and metabolic shock.[48]

Recreational Substance Abuse

Just as it is of the world in general, recreational substance abuse is a part of the world of sports.[17] Reasons that individuals use these substances may include the desire to experiment, to temporarily escape from problems, and to just be part of a group (peer pressure). For some people, recreational drug use leads to abuse and dependence. Drug abuse may be defined as the use of drugs for nonmedical reasons—that is, with the intent of getting high or altering mood or behavior.[17]

> **Recreational drugs include tobacco, alcohol, cocaine, and marijuana.**

Psychological versus Physical Dependence There are two general aspects of dependence: psychological and physical. Psychological dependence is the drive to repeat the ingestion of a drug to produce pleasure or to avoid discomfort. Physical dependence is the state of drug adaptation that manifests itself as the development of tolerance and, when the drug is removed, causes a withdrawal syndrome. Tolerance of a drug is the need to increase the dosage to create the effect that was obtained previously by smaller amounts. The withdrawal syndrome consists of an unpleasant physiological reaction when the drug is abruptly stopped.

Some drugs that are abused overlap with those thought to enhance performance. Examples include amphetamines and cocaine. Tobacco (nicotine), alcohol, cocaine, and marijuana are the most abused recreational drugs. The athletic trainer might also come in contact with abuse of barbiturates, nonbarbiturate sedatives, psychotomimetic drugs, or different inhalants.

Tobacco Use Although cigarettes, cigars, and pipes are becoming increasingly rare in the athletic population, the use of smokeless tobacco and the passive exposure to others who are smoking are ongoing problems.

Cigarette Smoking On the basis of various investigations into the relationship between smoking and performance, the following conclusions can be drawn:

1. There is individual sensitivity to tobacco that may seriously affect performance in instances of relatively high sensitivity. Because more than one-third of the men studied indicated tobacco sensitivity, it may be wise to prohibit smoking by athletes.

2. Tobacco smoke has been associated with as many as 4,700 different chemicals, many of which are toxic.

3. As few as 10 inhalations of cigarette smoke cause an average maximum decrease in airway conductance of 50 percent. This decrease also occurs in nonsmokers who inhale secondhand smoke.

4. Smoking reduces the oxygen-carrying capacity of the blood. A smoker's blood carries 5 to 10 times more carbon monoxide than normal. Carbon monoxide inhibits the capability of oxygen molecules to bind to the hemoglobin molecule. Thus, the red blood cells are prevented from picking up enough oxygen to meet the demands of the body's tissues. The carbon monoxide also tends to make arterial walls more permeable to fatty substances, a factor in atherosclerosis.

5. Smoking aggravates and accelerates the heart muscle cells through overstimulation of the sympathetic nervous system.

6. Total lung capacity and maximum breathing capacity are significantly decreased in heavy smokers; this fact is important to the athlete because both changes would impair the capacity to take in oxygen and make it readily available for body use.

7. Smoking decreases pulmonary diffusing capacity.

8. After smoking, an accelerated thrombolic tendency is evidenced.

9. Smoking is a carcinogenic factor in lung cancer and is a contributing factor to heart disease.

The addictive chemical of tobacco is nicotine, which is one of the most toxic drugs. When inhaled, it causes blood pressure elevation, increased bowel activity, and an antidiuretic action. Moderate tolerance and strong physical dependence occur.

Use of Smokeless Tobacco It is estimated that more than 7 million individuals use smokeless tobacco, which comes in three forms: loose-leaf, moist or dry powder (snuff), and compressed. The tobacco is placed between the cheek and the gum. Then it is sucked and chewed. Aesthetically, this habit is an unsavory one, during which an athlete is continually spitting into a container. Besides the unpleasant appearance, the use of smokeless tobacco poses an extremely serious health risk.[45] Smokeless tobacco causes bad breath, stained teeth, tooth sensitivity to heat and cold, cavities, gum recession, tooth bone loss, leukoplakia (white patches in the mouth), and oral and throat cancer. Aggressive oral and throat cancer and periodontal destruction (with tooth loss) have been associated with this habit.[10]

The major substance ingested is nitrosonornicotine, which is the drug responsible for this habit's addictiveness. It is absorbed through the mucous membranes, and within a short period of time the level of nicotine in the blood is equivalent to that of a cigarette smoker. This chemical makes smokeless tobacco a more addictive habit than smoking. The user of chewing tobacco experiences the nicotine effects without exposure to the tar and carbon monoxide associated with a burning cigarette. Smokeless tobacco increases heart rate but does not affect reaction time, movement time, or total response time among athletes and nonathletes.[10]

In sports, the biggest problem with smokeless tobacco has historically been in baseball athletes.[11] Almost one-third of rookie baseball players entering professional baseball in 1999 used smokeless tobacco. Interventions targeting young baseball players are needed to prevent and stop the use of smokeless tobacco.[15]

Passive Smoke There are dangers associated with the passive inhalation of smoke (secondhand smoke) by nonsmokers. Both smokers and nonsmokers are exposed to smoke containing carbon monoxide, nicotine, ammonia, and cyanide. Obviously, smokers inhale the greater quantity of contaminated air. However, it has been estimated that, for each pack of cigarettes smoked, the nonsmoker who shares a common air supply will inhale the equivalent of three to five cigarettes. Significant numbers of individuals exposed to passive smoke develop nasal symptoms, eye irritation, headaches, cough, and allergies to smoke. For these reasons and others, many state, local, and private sector policies have been established that restrict or ban smoking in public areas.

There is little doubt that passive smoking poses a significant health threat to the nonsmoker.

Alcohol Use Alcohol is the most widely used and abused substance.[34] Alcohol is a drug that depresses the central nervous system. It is absorbed from the digestive system into the bloodstream very rapidly. Factors that affect how rapidly absorption takes place include the number of drinks consumed, the rate of consumption, the alcohol concentration of the beverage, and the amount of food in the stomach.[54] Some alcohol is absorbed into the blood through the stomach, but the greater part is absorbed through the small intestine. Alcohol is transported through the blood to the liver, where it can be oxidized at a rate of 2/3 ounce per hour. An excess causes an increase in the level of alcohol circulating in the blood. As blood alcohol levels continue to increase, predictable signs of intoxication appear. At 0.1 percent, the person loses motor coordination; from 0.2 percent to 0.5 percent, the symptoms become progressively more profound and perhaps even life threatening.[55] Intoxication persists until the liver can metabolize the remainder of the alcohol. There is no way to accelerate the liver's metabolism of alcohol (the act of sobering up); it just takes time. Alcohol has no place in sports participation.

Approximately 20 percent of cases of alcoholism are associated with genetic reasons and 80 percent with overindulgence.[54] The individual who is suffering from alcohol abuse may display the following characteristics: mood changes, missed practices, isolation, attitude changes, fighting or inappropriate outbursts of violence, changes in appearance, hostility toward authority figures, complaints from family, and changes in peer group.[34]

Abused Illegal Drugs

Cocaine Cocaine, also known as coke, snow, toot, happy dust, and white girl, is a powerful central nervous system stimulant with effects of very short duration. Cocaine use produces immediate feelings of euphoria and excitement, decreased sense of fatigue, and heightened sexual drive. Cocaine may be snorted, taken intravenously, or smoked (freebased). The initial effects are extremely intense, and, because they are pleasurable, strong psychological dependence is developed rapidly by users who can or cannot afford to support this expensive habit.

Habitual use of cocaine will not lead to physical tolerance or dependence but will cause psychological dependence and addiction. Long-term effects include nasal congestion and damage to the membranes and cartilage of the nose if snorted, bronchitis, loss of appetite leading to nutritional deficiencies, convulsions, impotence, cocaine psychosis with paranoia, depression, hallucinations, and disorganized mental function. An overdose can lead to overstimulation of the sympathetic nervous system and can cause tachycardia, hypertension, extra heartbeats, coronary vasoconstriction, strokes, pulmonary edema, aortic rupture, and sudden death.[17]

Crack Crack is a rocklike crystalline form of cocaine that is heated in a small pipe and then inhaled, producing an immediate rush. The effects last for only a matter of minutes and are frequently followed by a state of depression. This sudden, intense stimulation of the nervous system predisposes the user to cardiac failure or respiratory failure and makes this commonly available drug extremely dangerous.

Marijuana Marijuana is one of the most abused drugs in Western society. It is more commonly called grass, weed, pot, or dope. The marijuana cigarette is called a joint, jay, number, reefer, or root.

Marijuana is not a harmless drug. The components of marijuana smoke are similar to those of tobacco smoke, and the same cellular changes are observed in the user. Continued use leads to respiratory diseases, such as asthma and bronchitis, and a decrease in vital capacity of 15 percent to 40 percent (certainly detrimental to physical performance). Among other deleterious effects are lowered sperm counts and testosterone levels. Evidence of interference with the functioning of the immune system and cellular metabolism has also been found. The most consistent sign is the increase in pulse rate, which averages close to 20 percent higher during exercise and is a definite factor in limiting performance. Some decrease in leg, hand, and finger strength has been found at higher dosages. Like tobacco, marijuana must be considered carcinogenic.[43]

Psychological effects, such as a diminution of self-awareness and judgment, a slowdown of thinking, and a shorter attention span, appear early in the use of the drug. Postmortem examinations of habitual users reveal not only cerebral atrophy but also alterations of anatomical structures, which suggest irreversible brain damage. Marijuana also contains unique substances (cannabinoids) that are stored, in much the same manner as are fat cells, throughout the body and in the brain tissues for weeks and even months. These stored quantities result in a cumulative deleterious effect on the habitual user.

A drug such as marijuana has no place in sports. Claims for its use are unsubstantiated, and the harmful effects, both immediate and long-term, are too significant to permit indulgence at any time.

Crystal Methamphetamine. This drug is used by individuals of all ages and is increasingly gaining in popularity as a club drug. It is a colorless, odorless, and highly addictive synthetic stimulant. Crystal methamphetamine resembles small fragments of glass or shiny blue-white "rocks" of various sizes. Like powdered methamphetamine, it is abused because of the long-lasting euphoric effects it produces. But it has a higher purity level and may produce even longer-lasting and more intense physiological effects than the powdered form smoked in glass pipes similar to pipes used to smoke crack cocaine; or it may be injected. A user who smokes or injects the drug immediately experiences an intense sensation followed by a high that may last 12 hours or more.

Crystal methamphetamine use is associated with numerous serious physical problems, which may include rapid heart rate, increased blood pressure, and damage to the small blood vessels in the brain that can lead to stroke. Overdoses can cause increased temperature, convulsions, and death. People who use crystal methamphetamine may have episodes of paranoia, anxiety, violent behavior, confusion, and insomnia. The drug can produce psychotic symptoms that persist for months or years after an individual has stopped using the drug.

Ecstasy. Considered the most commonly used designer drug, Ecstasy is a close derivative of methamphetamine and can be described as a hallucinogenic stimulant. Designer drugs are illicit variations of other drugs. Ecstasy is most often found in tablet, capsule, or powder form and is usually consumed orally, although it can also be injected. Ecstasy can cause euphoria and feelings of well-being, enhanced mental or emotional clarity, anxiety, and paranoia. Heavier doses can cause hallucinations, sensations of lightness and floating, depression, paranoid thinking, and violent, irrational behavior. Physical reactions can include loss of appetite, nausea, vomiting, blurred vision, increased heart rate and blood pressure, muscle tension, faintness, chills, sweating, tremors, insomnia, convulsions, and loss of control over voluntary body movements. Some reactions have been reported to persist up to 14 days after taking Ecstasy.

Abused Prescription Drugs The misuse of drugs prescribed by a physician has become a huge problem in the athletic population.[60] Two prescription medications in particular, ADHD medication and OxyContin, are being widely misused.

ADHD Medications. The abuse of medications commonly used for treating attention deficit and hyperactivity disorder (ADHD) is a relatively new phenomenon, but one that has become a major cause for concern, especially in the college population. These medications usually are amphetamines such as Ritalin, Adderall, and Dexedrine. They are stimulants, but they also decrease an individual's distractibility and facilitate concentration and focus.

Reasons for abusing or misusing stimulant medication include improving attention, partying, reducing hyperactivity, and improving grades. Some individuals are illegally or illicitly obtaining the medications for their own use or for sale. Common signs and symptoms include shakiness, rapid speech or movements, difficulty sitting still, difficulty concentrating, lack of appetite, sleep disturbance, and irritability.

OxyContin (Oxycodone) OxyContin is a prescription drug used to treat moderate to severe pain. Oxycodone is in a class of medications called opiate (narcotic) analgesics. It works by altering the way the brain and nervous system respond to pain. Although this is an extremely effective medication, it has become perhaps the most widely abused prescription drug. The drug is relatively inexpensive but may be sold on the street at 20 times the value. Tablets may be crushed, then snorted, chewed, or injected to obtain a heroin-like high. It is rare to become addicted to OxyContin when the drug is used as recommended. However, due to pharmacy break-ins, growing levels of illegal use, and increased media reports of OxyContin abuse, prescriptions are heavily regulated.

Managing a Drug Overdose Athletes, like others in society, are not immune to extreme instances of substance abuse. On occasion, an athlete can either accidentally or intentionally take too much of a particular drug or consume an excessive amount of alcohol. Sometimes the athletic trainer will get a phone call late at night from that athlete's friend or perhaps from a teammate who reports that the athlete is unconscious or not responding. They are scared that the athlete has "overdosed," and they are seeking advice as to how they should handle this emergency situation.

The athletic trainer should immediately insist that the rescue squad be called by dialing 911. In cases of suspected drug overdose, the athletic trainer should also insist that the poison control center be contacted. *Focus Box 17–6:* "Contacting the poison control center" tells how the poison control center can be contacted. It is imperative that the athletic trainer follow up to make certain that the right steps have been taken, either by telephone or by actually going to deal with the athlete in person.

DRUG TESTING IN ATHLETES

Drug testing began with the 1968 Olympic Games. In 1985, the United States Olympic Committee (USOC) began drug testing athletes involved in both national and international competitions. In 2000, the USOC was aware that its drug testing

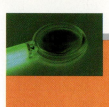

Contacting the poison control center

Each state has at least one and usually several poison control centers located in different regions of the state. The phone number of the poison control center is usually clearly accessible in the front of the phone book. The rescue squad can also contact the poison control center directly. The following information is necessary when communicating with the poison control center:

- Name and location of the person making the call
- Name and age of the person who has taken the medication
- Name and amount of the drug taken (if known)
- Time the drug was taken
- Signs and symptoms associated with the overdose, including vital signs

The experts at the poison control center will provide instructions for immediate care of the individual until the rescue squad arrives.

A Web site at Fast Health, www.fasthealth.com/poison/nc.php, provides a list of phone numbers for all the poison control centers in each state.

program lacked credibility internationally. A decision was made to turn over the drug-testing program to an independent group called the U.S. Anti-Doping Agency (USADA). Today, both the USADA and the NCAA routinely conduct drug testing.[35,52] The legality and ethics of testing only those individuals involved with sports are still open to debate.[29] The pattern of drug usage among athletes may simply reflect that of our society in general. Great care must be taken that an athlete's personal rights are not violated.[46] USADA was given full authority to execute a comprehensive national anti-doping program encompassing testing, adjudication, education, and research and to develop programs,

> **Both the NCAA and the USOC conduct drug-testing programs.**

policies, and procedures for Olympic, Pan American, and Paralympic sports in the United States. In January 1986, the member institutions of the NCAA voted overwhelmingly to expand the NCAA drug-education program to include mandatory random drug testing in specific sports throughout the year and during and after NCAA championship events.[35] The major goals of both organizations are to protect the health of athletes and to help ensure that competition is fair and equitable.[29]

Most professional teams, individual colleges and universities, and many sport clubs and individual sport governing bodies, have initiated drug-testing programs for their athletes.[29] Unfortunately, drug testing is rarely done at the high-school level because of cost constraints.

The Drug Test

There are some slight differences between NCAA and USADA drug-testing procedures and protocols. Most of these differences have to do with how the athletes are selected for random tests. The NCAA requires all athletes to sign a consent form agreeing to participate in the drug-testing program throughout the year. The USADA tests athletes on a random basis throughout the year and tests all athletes before a USOC-sanctioned competition.[29]

During the drug test, the athlete must first provide positive identification. Then, under direct observation, the athlete must urinate into two separate specimen bottles (labeled A and B), which are sealed and submitted to an official NCAA or USOC testing laboratory for analysis. In the laboratory, specimen A is used for both screening and confirmation tests. A confirmation test uses analysis techniques that are more sensitive and accurate, should a positive test result occur during the screening test. Specimen B is used only when a reconfirmation is needed for a positive test of specimen A. The athlete is then notified of a positive test result and becomes subject to sanctions from either the NCAA or the USADA.[58]

Sanctions for Positive Tests For a first-time positive test, the NCAA will declare the athlete ineligible for all regular and postseason competitions for a minimum of 1 year. During that year, the athlete may be retested at any time. The athlete must be retested with a negative result and have eligibility restored before he or she may return to competition. Additional positive tests can result in a lifetime disqualification from NCAA competition.[35]

The USADA sanctions range from 3 to 24 months of disqualification, depending on the drug, for a first-time violation, and a minimum of 2 years to a lifetime ban for subsequent positive tests.[52]

17–8 Clinical Application Exercise

A university has recently implemented a drug-testing program for athletes in all sports. The athletic director has decided that the athletic trainer is the best individual to supervise the program.

? Should the athletic trainer be willing to take on the additional responsibilities of overseeing the drug-testing program for the athletes?

Banned Substances

Both the NCAA and the United States Olympic Committee have established lists of substances that are banned from use by athletes. The lists include performance-enhancing drugs and street, or recreational, drugs, as well as many OTC and prescription drugs.

The list of drugs banned by either the NCAA or the USOC or by both is extensive and includes approximately 4,600 medications.[52] The list of drugs banned by the USOC is considerably more extensive than the NCAA list because the USOC is subject to internationally used drugs banned by the International Olympic Committee (IOC). *Focus Box 17–7: "Banned drugs—common ground"* summarizes the various categories of drugs that appear on the banned lists for the NCAA and the USOC.[29]

The athletic trainer working with athletes who may be tested for drug use by the NCAA or with world-class or Olympic athletes governed by the USOC should be thoroughly familiar with the list of banned drugs.[52] Having an athlete disqualified because of the indiscriminate use of some prescription or OTC medication would be very unfortunate. As is the case with others in the population, some athletes have conditions or illnesses that require them to take a particular medication. If that medication appears on the prohibited list, the athlete can apply for a Therapeutic Use Exemption (TUE) by completing a form that is available from the USADA, which may give that athlete permission to continue taking the needed medication.[52] Table 17–10 lists the drugs currently banned by the NCAA.

The National Federation of State High School Associations (NFHS) does not currently have a list of banned substances or specific policies on drug testing. They have left the choice of whether to drug test athletes up to individual states. To date only a few states have implemented mandatory drug-testing programs for athletes. However, they have provided guidelines for those schools wishing to institute a drug-testing program. Testing high school athletes for drugs has been occurring since the mid-1970s, when efforts to reduce drug use increased. Drug testing among high school athletes has been done infrequently and with varying degrees of success. However, court decisions in 1995 removed some hurdles for drug testing of high school athletes. Drug testing can be done for a variety of different drugs. It appears that high school drug-testing programs most commonly screen athletes for amphetamines, marijuana, cocaine, opiates, and phencyclidine (PCP). These standard drug-testing packages leave out

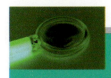

FOCUS 17–7 Focus on Organization and Administration

Banned drugs—common ground

Drugs banned by both NCAA and USOC

Alcohol*
Anti-estrogens (promote the development and maintenance of female sex characteristics)
Anabolic steroids
Diuretics
Beta blockers (used to lower blood pressure, decrease heart rate, decrease cardiac arrythmias)
Hormones (human growth hormone, corticotropin, erythropoietin, human chorionic gonadotropin, etc.)
Stimulants
Blood doping
Marijuana

Drugs banned by USADA only

Narcotics (specific drugs prohibited)
Corticosteroids** (intramuscular, intravenous, rectal, and oral use is banned; most topical and inhaled use is permitted with written permission)

Drugs banned by NCAA only

Local anesthetics

Dietary supplements

Not banned, but both groups recommend using at your own risk

*Banned only for certain sports.
**Permits with prior written Therapeutic Use Exemption (TUE).

several commonly used substances such as alcohol, tobacco, and steroids.

Dietary Supplements Many nutritional/dietary supplements contain NCAA-banned substances.[4,50] In addition, the U.S. Food and Drug Administration (FDA) does not strictly regulate the supplement industry; therefore, purity and safety of nutritional/dietary supplements cannot be guaranteed.[12] Impure supplements may lead to a positive NCAA drug test. The student-athlete is at his or her own risk when using supplements. Student-athletes should contact their institution's team physician or athletic trainer for further information.

TABLE 17–10 NCAA Banned Drug Classes

The following is a list of banned drug classes, with examples of substances under each class.

A. Stimulants

amiphenazole
amphetamine
bemigride
benzphetamine
bromantan
caffeine* (guarana)
chlorphentermine
cocaine
cropropamide
crothetamide
dextroamphetamine
diethylpropion
dimethylamphetamine
doxapram
ephedrine (ephedra, ma huang)
ethamivan
ethylamphetamine
fencamfamine
lisdexamfetamine
meclofenoxate
methamphetamine

methylenedioxymethamphetamine (MDMA) (ecstasy)
methylphenidate
nikethamide
pemoline
pentetrazol
phendimetrazine
phenmetrazine
phentermine
phenylephrine
phenylpropanolamine (ppa)
picrotoxine
pipradol
prolintane
strychnine
synephrine (citrus aurantium, zhi shi, bitter orange) and related compounds

The following stimulants are not banned:
phenylephrine
pseudoephedrine

B. Anabolic Agents

Anabolic steroids
androstenediol
androstenedione
boldenone
clostebol
dehydrochlormethyei-testosterone
dehydroepiandrosterone (DHEA)
dihydrotestosterone (DHT)
dromostanolone
epitrenbolone
fluoxymesterone
gestrinone
mesterolone
methandienone

methenolone
methyltestosterone
nandrolone
norandrostenediol
norandrostenedione
norethandrolone
oxandrolone
oxymesterone
oxymetholone
stanozolol
testosterone†
tetrahydrogestrinone (THG)
trenbolone
and related compounds
Other Anabolic Agents
clenbuterol

C. Substances Banned for Specific Sports

Rifle
  alcohol
  atenolol
  metoprolol
  nadolol
  pindolol
  propranolol
  timolol
  and related compounds

D. Diuretics

acetazolamide
bendroflumethiazide
benzthiazide
bumetanide
chlorothiazide
chlorthalidone
ethacrynic acid
flumethiazide
furosemide
hydrochlorothiazide
hydroflumethiazide
methyclothiazide
metolazone
polythiazide
quinethazone
spironolactone
triamterene
trichlormethiazide
and related compounds

E. Street Drugs

heroin
marijuana‡
THC (tetrahydrocannabinol)

F. Peptide Hormones and Analogues

corticotropin (ACTH)
growth hormone(hGH, somatotropin)
human chorionic gonadotropin (hCG)
insulin-like growth hormone (IGF-1)
leutenizing hormone (LH)
All the respective releasing factors of the above-mentioned substances also are banned.
erythropoietin (EPO)
sermorelin
darbepoetin

G. Anti-Estrogens

anastrozole
clomiphene
tamoxifen
and related compounds

Definitions of positive depend on the following:
*For caffeine—if the concentration in the urine exceeds 15 micrograms/ml.
†For testosterone—if the administration of testosterone or the use of any other manipulation has the result of increasing the ratio of the total concentration of testosterone to that of epitestosterone in the urine to greater than 6:1, unless there is evidence that this ratio is due to a physiological or pathological condition.
‡For marijuana and THC—if the concentration in the urine of THC metabolite exceeds 15 nanograms/ml.

SUMMARY

- A drug is a chemical agent used in the prevention, treatment, or diagnosis of disease; a drug may be administered either internally or externally. It is transported in an inactive substance called a vehicle.
- Pharmacokinetics is the method by which drugs are absorbed, distributed, metabolized, and eliminated or excreted by the body.
- Administering a drug is providing a single dose of medication for immediate use. Dispensing is providing the patient with a drug in a quantity sufficient to be used for multiple doses. At no time can anyone other than a person licensed by law legally prescribe or dispense drugs. In certain situations, the athletic trainer may be allowed to administer a single dose of a nonprescription medication.
- Drugs used to combat infection include local antiseptics and disinfectants, antifungal agents, and antibiotics.
- Drugs used to inhibit pain or inflammation include counterirritants and local anesthetics, narcotic analgesics, nonnarcotic analgesics and antipyretics, acetylsalicylic acid (aspirin), nonsteroidal antiinflammatory drugs, and corticosteroids.
- Drugs used to treat gastrointestinal disorders include antacids, antiemetics, carminatives, cathartics or laxatives, and antidiarrheals.
- Drugs used to treat colds and allergies include nasal decongestants, antihistamines, cough suppressants, and asthma drugs.
- Drugs used to control bleeding include vasoconstrictors, hemostatic agents, and anticoagulants.
- The athletic trainer is often responsible for the initial screening of patients who have various illnesses or injuries. Frequently, the athletic trainer must make decisions regarding the appropriate use of over-the-counter medications. Specific protocols have been established that can serve as a guide for the use of these medications by the athletic trainer.
- Substance abuse involves the use of performance-enhancing drugs and the widespread use of recreational drugs, or street drugs. The athletic trainer must be knowledgeable about substance abuse and should be able to recognize signs that an individual is engaging in substance abuse. Substance abuse has no place in the athletic population.
- The use of performance-enhancing drugs (ergogenic aids) must be discouraged because of potential health risks and to ensure equal competition. Among the more common ergogenic aids are stimulants, beta blockers, narcotic analgesics, diuretics, anabolic steroids, human growth hormone, and blood doping.
- Recreational drug abuse is of major concern. It can lead to serious psychological and physical health problems. The most prevalent substances that are abused are tobacco, alcohol, cocaine, and marijuana.
- Drug testing of athletes for the purpose of identifying individuals who may have some problems with drug abuse is done routinely by the NCAA and the USOC. The major goals of drug testing are to protect the health of athletes and to help ensure that competition is fair and equitable. Most professional teams and many individual colleges and universities have initiated drug-testing programs for their athletes. Unfortunately, drug testing is rarely done at the high-school level because of cost constraints.
- Both the NCAA and the USOC have established lists of drugs that are banned for use by athletes competing in either NCAA- or USOC-sanctioned events.

WEB SITES

NCAA Drug Testing Program:
http://www.ncaa.org/wps/wcm/connect/public/NCAA/Health+and+Safety/Drug+Testing/Drug+Testing+Landing+Page
This site provides an updated list of banned drugs and drug-testing information.

Wheeless' Textbook of Orthopaedics:
www.wheelessonline.com
Clicking on "medications" at this Web site allows the reader to search for information on dosages, indications, contraindications, and so on.

National Center for Drug Free Sport, Inc.
www.drugfreesport.com
This agency is a provider of drug-testing services, drug-screening policies, and drug-testing education programs in sport.

United States Anti-Doping Agency:
www.usantidoping.org
This organization is dedicated to eliminating the practice of doping in sport.

United States Olympic Committee:
www.olympic-usa.org
This site contains information about drug testing from the USOC.

World Anti-Doping Agency:
www.wada-ama.orgd
This site offers a comprehensive list of all medicines (over 5,000), showing which are prohibited or permitted in international sport.

SOLUTIONS TO CLINICAL APPLICATION EXERCISES

17–1 At no time can anyone other than a person licensed by law legally prescribe or dispense drugs. An athletic trainer is not permitted to administer or dispense a prescription drug. However, the athletic trainer may be allowed to administer a single dose of a nonprescription medication. The athletic trainer must be reasonable and prudent about the types of nonprescription drugs offered to the patient. If medications are administered by an athletic trainer, he or she must maintain accurate records of the types of medications administered. Each athletic trainer should be aware of state regulations and laws that pertain to the use of medications.

17–2 It is possible that this patient has exercise-induced bronchospasm (EIB). EIB may be caused by loss of heat, water, or both from the lungs during exercise or exertion, resulting from hyperventilation of air that is cooler and dryer than that in the respiratory tract. The goals of asthma therapy are to prevent chronic and troublesome symptoms, maintain normal lung function and activity levels, prevent asthma exacerbations, provide optimal pharmacotherapy with minimal adverse effects, and meet patients' expectations of and satisfaction with asthma care.

17–3 The patient should use a nonsteroidal antiinflammatory drug, such as ibuprofen or naproxen. Although acetaminophen is a drug with analgesic qualities, a nonsteroidal antiinflammatory drug (NSAID) is advantageous because of its analgesic and antiinflammatory capabilities. Aspirin is also an analgesic and antiinflammatory drug; however, aspirin is associated with more frequent side effects and adverse reactions compared with an NSAID.

17–4 Ibuprofen is an NSAID. The NSAIDs are most effective for reducing pain, stiffness, swelling, redness, and fever associated with localized inflammation. Even though NSAIDs have analgesic and antipyretic capabilities, they should not be used in cases of mild headache or increased body temperature in place of aspirin or acetaminophen. However, they can be used to relieve many other mild to moderately painful somatic conditions, such as menstrual cramps and soft-tissue injury.

17–5 The athletic trainer should let the athlete know that her drug test is designed to screen for recreational drugs rather than for performance-enhancing drugs, so this should not be a problem. Additionally, even if the test were screening for performance-enhancing drugs, it is highly unlikely that one cup of espresso would contain enough caffeine for her to test positive.

17–6 The visible signs of steroid abuse include male pattern baldness, acne, voice deepening, mood swings, aggressive behavior, gynecomastia, reduction in testicle size, and changes in libido. Because the athlete denies steroid abuse, the athletic trainer might suspect that human growth hormone has been used to achieve these results.

17–7 The athletic trainer should first point out the potential long-term effects of using smokeless tobacco, which include bad breath, stained teeth, tooth sensitivity to heat and cold, cavities (with tooth loss), gum recession, periodontal destruction, and oral and throat cancer. The trainer may also try to give the players a substitute for the tobacco, such as gum or sunflower seeds, so that their habitual need to chew on something and spit while playing baseball is satisfied.

17–8 In this case, the issue of added responsibility is irrelevant. The athletic trainer should be more concerned with how this responsibility would affect his or her ability to perform normal job functions. Athletic trainers work hard to develop a sense of trust in the athletes for whom they must provide health care. Being forced to assume a role as a police officer or enforcer can only undermine that trust. Thus, this athletic trainer should be adamant in recommending to the athletic director that some other individual assume the responsibility of overseeing the drug-testing program.

REVIEW QUESTIONS AND CLASS ACTIVITIES

1. What is the branch of science known as pharmacology, and what is the difference between a prescription and a nonprescription drug?
2. What is a drug vehicle? Give some examples of drug vehicles.
3. By what methods can drugs be administered to an individual?
4. Describe the pharmacokinetics of how a drug is handled by the body.
5. List procedures that should be followed in the selection, purchase, storage, record keeping, and safety precautions of over-the-counter drugs.
6. What are the legal implications if an athletic trainer administers prescription and nonprescription drugs?
7. List the responses that a patient may experience to a drug.
8. List examples of common drugs used to combat infection, to reduce pain and inflammation, to treat colds and allergies, to treat gastrointestinal disorders, to treat muscle dysfunctions, and to control bleeding.
9. Describe the specific protocols for administering over-the-counter medications.
10. Discuss the use of performance-enhancing drugs.
11. How do stimulants enhance performance?
12. What are the purposes of narcotic analgesic drugs? How do they affect performance?
13. What type of patient would use beta blockers? Why are they used?
14. Describe why individuals use anabolic steroids, diuretics, and growth hormone. What are their physiological effects?
15. Describe blood doping in sports. Why is it used? What are its dangers?
16. Contrast psychological and physical dependence, tolerance, and withdrawal symptoms.
17. List the dangers of smokeless tobacco. List the effects of nicotine on the body.
18. Why is cocaine use a danger to users?
19. Select a recreational drug to research. What are the physiological responses to it, and what dangers does it pose?
20. How can an individual who is abusing drugs be identified? Describe behavioral identification as well as drug testing.
21. Debate the issue of drug testing in athletics.

REFERENCES

1. Alaranta A: Use of prescription drugs in sports, *Sports Medicine* 38(6):449–63, 2008.
2. Backhouse S: Doping in sport: A review of medical practitioners' knowledge, attitudes and beliefs, *International Journal of Drug Policy* 22(11):198–202, 2011.
3. Bahrke M, Yesalis C, Kopstein A: Risk factors associated with anabolic-androgenic steroid use among adolescents, *Sports Med* 29(6):397, 2000.
4. Baume N, Mahler N, Kamber M: Research of stimulants and anabolic steroids in dietary supplements, *Scandinavian Journal of Medicine and Science in Sports* 16(1):41, 2006.
5. Beck T, Housh T, Schmidt R: The acute effects of a caffeine-containing supplement on strength, muscular endurance and

anaerobic capabilities, *J Strength Cond Res* 20(3):506, 2006.

6. Boissonnault W, Meek P: Risk factors for anti–inflammatory-drug- or aspirin-induced gastrointestinal complications in individuals receiving outpatient physical therapy services, *J Orthop Sports Phys Ther* 32(10): 510–17, 2002.

7. Bouchard M: Medications and exercise, *ACSM's Health and Fitness Journal* 16(2):34–36, 2010.

8. Brower K: Anabolic steroid abuse and dependence in clinical practice, *Physician and Sportsmedicine* 37(4):131–40, 2009.

9. Buxton I: Pharmacokinetics: The dynamics of drug absorption, distribution, metabolism, and elimination. In Brunton L: *Goodman and Gilman's the pharmacological basis of therapeutics*, New York, 2011, McGraw-Hill.

10. Cassisi NJ: Smokeless tobacco: Is it worth the risk? *NCAA Sports Sciences Education Newsletter*, Spring 2000.

11. Cooper J, Ellison J, Walsh M: Spit (smokeless)-tobacco use by baseball players entering the professional ranks, *J Athl Train* 38(2):126, 2003.

12. Earnest CP: Dietary androgen 'supplements': Separating substance from hype, *Physician Sportsmed* 29(5):63, 2001.

13. Elliott P: Nonsteroidal anti-inflammatory drugs. In Mottram D: *Drugs in sports*, New York, 2011, Taylor and Francis.

14. Feucht C: Analgesics and anti-inflammatory medications in sports: Use and abuse, *Pediatric Clinics of North America*, 57(3): 751–74, 2010.

15. Gansky S, Ellison J, Rudy D: Cluster randomized controlled trial of an athletic trainer-directed spit (smokeless) tobacco intervention for collegiate baseball athletes: Results after 1 year, *J Athl Train* 40(2):76, 2005.

16. Green G: Doping control for the team physician: A review of drug testing procedures in sport, *Am J Sports Med* 34(10):1690, 2006.

17. Green GA, Uryasz FD, Petr TA, Bray CD: NCAA study of substance use and abuse habits of college student-athletes, *Clin J Sports Med* 11(1):51, 2001.

18. Hackel J: Asthma overview, *Athletic Therapy Today* 9(2):28, 2004.

19. Hartgens F, Kuipers H: Effects of androgenicanabolic steroids in athletes, *Sports Med* 34(8):513, 2004.

20. Hartgens F, Van Marken Lichtenbelt WD, Ebbing S: Androgenic-anabolic steroid-induced body changes in strength athletes, *Physician Sportsmed* 29(1):49, 2001.

21. Holt R: Detecting growth hormone abuse in athletes, *Drug Testing and Analysis* 1(9):426–433, 2009.

22. Houglum JE: Asthma medications: Basic pharmacology, *J Athl Train* 35(2):179, 2000.

23. Houglum J: *Principles of pharmacology for athletic trainers*, Thorofare, NJ, 2010, Slack.

24. Huff P: Drug distribution in the training room, *Clin Sports Med* 17(2):214, 1998.

25. Kahanov L: Adherence to drug-dispensation and drug administration laws and guidelines in collegiate athletic training rooms: A 5-year review, *J Athl Train* 45(3):299–305, 2010.

26. Kersey RD: What athletic trainers and therapists should know about androstenedione, *Athletic Therapy Today* 6(1):59, 2001.

27. Koda-Kimble MA, Young LL: *Applied therapeutics: The clinical use of drugs*, Philadelphia, 2012, Lippincott, Williams and Wilkins.

28. Kraemer W, Gomez A, Ratamess H: Effects of vicoprofen and ibuprofen on anaerobic performance after muscle damage, *J Sport Rehabil* 11(2):104, 2002.

29. Landry G, Bernhardt D: Drug testing in the athletic setting. In Landry G, editor: *Essentials of primary care sports medicine*, Champaign, IL, 2003, Human Kinetics.

30. Loudon J: Principles of pharmacology for athletic trainers, *Physical Therapy*, 86(3):459, 2006.

31. Miller M: Questionable dispensing of medications in the athletic training room, *Athletic Therapy Today* 8(4):26, 2003.

32. Miller M, Weiler J, Baker R: National Athletic Trainers' Association position statement: Management of asthma in athletes, *J Athl Train* 40(3):224, 2005.

33. National Asthma Education and Prevention Program (NAEPP) Expert panel report 3: *Guidelines for the diagnosis and management of Asthma*. October 2007, NIH Publication 08–5846.

34. National Collegiate Athletic Association: Ergogenic drug use down: Binge-drinking on the rise according to a national study, *NCAA Sport Sciences Education Newsletter*, Winter 4:1, 1993.

35. National Collegiate Athletic Association: *NCAA drug testing program 2011–2012*, Indianapolis, 2011, NCAA.

36. Neal M: *Medical Pharmacology at a Glance*, New York, 2009, Wiley-Blackwell.

37. Nickell R: Eight principles for managing prescription medications in the athletic training room, *Athletic Therapy Today* 10(1):6, 2005.

38. Orr E: Sources of drug information for the athletic therapist, *Athletic Therapy Today* 3(2): 18, 1998.

39. Parkinson A, Evans N: Anabolic androgenic steroids: A survey of 500 users, *Med Sci Sports Exerc* 38(4):644, 2006.

40. Pearson R: Beta-blockers in sports, *Sport and Medicine Today* 4(5):15, 2001.

41. Powers M: The safety and efficacy of anabolic steroid precursors: What is the scientific evidence? *J Athl Train* 37(3):300, 2002.

42. Reents S: *Sport and exercise pharmacology*, Champaign, IL, 2000, Human Kinetics.

43. Rich B: Drugs: A common link between physicians and athletic therapists, *Athletic Therapy Today* 3(2):13, 1998.

44. Schneider AJ, Butcher RB: An ethical analysis of drug testing. In Wilson W, Derse E, editors: *Doping in elite sport: The politics of drugs in the Olympic movement*, Champaign, IL, 2001, Human Kinetics.

45. Sinusas K, Coroso J: A 10-yr study of smokeless tobacco use in a professional baseball organization, *Med Sci Sports Exerc* 38(7):1204, 2006.

46. Starkey C, Abdenour T, Finnane D: Athletic trainers' attitudes toward drug screening of intercollegiate athletes, *J Athl Train* 29(2):120, 1994.

47. Stilger V: Androstenedione and anabolicandrogenic steroids: What you need to know, *Athletic Therapy Today* 5(1):56, 2000.

48. Tokish J, Kocher M, Hawkins R: Ergogenic aids: A review of basic science, performance, side effects, and status in sports, *Am J Sports Med* 32(6):1543, 2004.

49. Trulock SC: Drug use in athletics: Abuse of the human growth hormone in amateur athletes, *Sports Med Update*, 14(4):18, 2000.

50. Tscholl P: The use of drugs and nutritional supplement in top level track and field athletes, *American Journal of Sports Medicine* 38(1):133–40, 2010.

51. U.S. Anti-doping Agency: *Athlete guide to the 2012 prohibited list*, Colorado Springs, CO, 2012, USADA.

52. U.S. Food and Drug Administration: Code of Federal Regulations Title 21 Volume 4 21CFR201.66, 2010.

53. VanHeest J, Stoppani J, Scheett T: Effects of ibuprofen and vicoprofen on physical performance after exercise-induced muscle damage, *J Sport Rehabil* 11(3):224, 2004.

54. Vella L: Alcohol, athletic performance and recovery, *Nutrients* 2(8):781–89, 2010.

55. Volpe S: Alcohol and athletic performance, *ACSM's Health and Fitness Journal* 14(3): 28–30, 2010.

56. Warrington R: Immunotherapy in asthma, *Immunotherapy*, 2(5):711–25, 2010.

57. Wennerberg D: Metered dose inhaler use and misuse by athletes, *Athletic Therapy Today* 15(5):30–33, 2010.

58. Whitehill W: The drug testing process, *Strength and Conditioning Journal* 31(6): 28–37, 2009.

59. Wilson W: Doping in elite sport: The politics of drugs in the Olympic movement, Champaign, 2001, Human Kinetics.

60. Wolf D: National Collegiate Athletic Association Division I athletes' use of nonprescription medication, *Sports Health* 3(1):25–28, 2011.

61. Yesalis CE, editor: *Anabolic steroids in sport and exercise*, ed 2, Champaign, IL, 2000, Human Kinetics.

62. Ziltener J: Non-steroidal anti-inflammatory drugs for athletes: An update, *Annals of Physical Medicine and Rehabilitation*, 53(4): 278–88, 2010.

ANNOTATED BIBLIOGRAPHY

Bahrke M, Yesalis C: *Performance enhancing substances in sport and exercise,* Champaign, IL, 2002, Human Kinetics.

A high-quality, evidence-based text on performance enhancing substances.

Beamish R: *Steroids: A New Look at Performance Enhancing Drugs,* Westport, CT, 2011, Praeger.

This book addresses a pressing issue in professional and high-performance sport—the use of steroids—by placing it within the historical context of the ongoing desire to achieve the pinnacle of human sport.

Brenner G, Stevens C: *Pharmacology,* St. Louis, 2009, Elsevier Health Sciences.

Applies the most important basic science concepts to everyday clinical problem solving and decision making in pharmacology.

Gauwitz D, Bayt P: *Administering medications,* New York, 2011, McGraw-Hill.

Provides the fundamentals of drug administration, drug laws, principles of pharmacology, drug-handling procedures, physician's orders, routes of administration, dosage calculation, and drug actions related to specific body systems and disorders.

Griffith HW: *Complete guide to prescription and nonprescription drugs,* New York, 2011, Perigee.

User-friendly reference text listing dosage and usage information, actions in the body, generic equivalents, potential adverse interactions (including those with foods and other drugs), overdose symptoms, precautions, side effects from prolonged use, and guidelines for usage.

Houglum J, Harrelson G,: *Principles of pharmacology for athletic trainers,* Thorofare, NJ, 2010, Slack.

Designed to help athletic training students understand the basic principles of pharmacology, as well as the broad classification of drugs.

Koester M: *Therapeutic Medications in Athletic Training,* Champaign, 2007, Human Kinetics.

Provides the latest information on over-the-counter and prescription medications commonly used in athletics

Magnus B, Miller M: *Pharmacology application in sports and Athletics,* Philadelphia, 2005, F.A. Davis.

Discusses pharmacological aspects of common medical conditions that certified athletic trainers may encounter in their careers. Describes the action of drugs for treating inflammation and pain, diabetes, cardiovascular arrhythmias, respiratory and gastrointestinal disorders, covers and infections. Also cover the adverse effects of performance enhancement and social drugs.

National Athletic Trainers' Association: *Consensus statement: managing prescription and nonprescription medication in the athletic training facility,* Dallas, 2009, NATA.

Discusses how athletic trainers should control the use of various medications in the clinical setting.

Reents S: *Sport and exercise pharmacology,* Champaign, IL, 2000, Human Kinetics.

Provides physicians and sports medicine specialists with information on how various commonly used drugs and supplements can affect exercise performance in their patients and athletes, and how exercise activities can drastically change the effects of drugs.

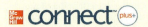

PART V

Musculoskeletal Conditions

18

The Foot

Objectives

When you finish this chapter you should be able to

- Identify the major anatomical and functional features of the foot.
- Discuss how foot injuries may be prevented.
- Explain the process for evaluating injuries to the foot.

- Identify specific injuries that occur in the foot, and discuss plans for management.
- Design rehabilitation techniques for the injured foot.

Outline

Key Terms

stance phase
swing phase
metatarsalgia
neuroma

apophysitis
apophysis
exostosis
point tenderness

Connect Highlights connect plus+

Visit connect.mcgraw-hill.com for further exercises to apply your knowledge:

- Clinical application scenarios covering evaluation of foot injuries, prevention of foot injuries, and management of foot injuries
- Click-and-drag questions covering anatomical features of the foot
- Multiple-choice questions covering injury evaluation, prevention of injury, and rehabilitation techniques for the foot
- Selection questions covering activities of the foot

Many activities involve some elements of walking, running, jumping, and changing direction. The foot is in direct contact with the ground, and the forces created by these athletic movements place a great deal of stress on the structures of the foot. Consequently, the foot has a high incidence of injury.[8,32,61]

The function of the foot is critical in walking, running, jumping, and changing direction. In one instant, the foot must act as a shock absorber to dissipate the ground reaction forces. In the next instant, it must become a rigid lever that propels the body forward, backward, or to the side.[17]

The foot forms the base for the entire kinetic chain, and different structural foot types can affect movement, stability, and the biomechanics throughout the kinetic chain.[25] Because of the stress that these movements place on the foot and because of the complex nature of the anatomical structures of this body part, recognition and management of injuries to the foot present a major challenge to the athletic trainer.

FOOT ANATOMY

Bones

The foot consists of 26 bones: 14 phalangeal, 5 metatarsal, and 7 tarsal (Figure 18–1). Additionally, there are two sesamoid bones beneath the first metatarsal.

Toes The toes are somewhat similar to the fingers in appearance but are much shorter and serve a different function. The toes are designed to give a wider base both for balance and for propelling the body forward. The first toe, or hallux, has two phalanges, and the other toes each have three phalanges.

Two sesamoid bones are located beneath the first metatarsophalangeal joint. Their functions are to assist in reducing pressure in weight bearing, increase the mechanical advantage of the flexor tendons of the great toe, and act as sliding pulleys for tendons.

Metatarsal Bones The metatarsals are the five bones that lie between and articulate with the tarsals and the phalanges, thus forming the semimovable tarsometatarsal and metatarsophalangeal joints. Although little movement is permitted, the ligamentous arrangement gives elasticity to the foot in weight bearing. The metatarsophalangeal joints permit hinge action of the phalanges, which is similar to the action between the hand and fingers. The first metatarsal is the largest and strongest and functions as the main weight-bearing support during walking and running.

The medial and lateral sesamoid bones are located on the plantar aspect of the metatarsophalangeal joint of the great toe within the flexor hallucis tendon: Their purposes are (1) to increase the mechanical efficiency of the tendon and (2) to decrease frictional stress as the tendon passes over bony prominances.

Tarsal Bones The foot has seven tarsal bones, which are located between the bones of the lower leg and the metatarsals. These bones are important for body support and locomotion. They consist of the calcaneus, talus, navicular, cuboid, and first, second, and third cuneiform bones.

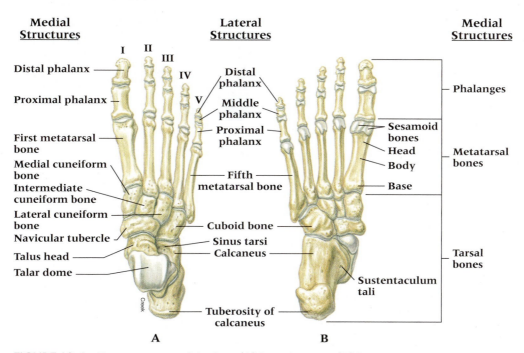

FIGURE 18–1   Bony structure of the foot. **(A)** Dorsal aspect. **(B)** Plantar aspect.

Calcaneus The calcaneus is the largest tarsal bone. It supports the talus and shapes the heel; its main functions are to convey the body weight to the ground and to serve as an attachment for both the Achilles tendon and several structures on the plantar surface of the foot.

The wider portion on the posterior calcaneus is called the tuberosity of the calcaneus. The medial and lateral tubercles are located on the inferior lateral and medial aspects and are the only parts of this bone that normally touch the ground.

Talus The irregularly shaped talus is the most superior of the tarsal bones. It is situated above the calcaneus over a bony projection called the sustentaculum tali. The talus consists of a body, neck, and head. The uppermost part of the talus is the trochlea, which articulates with the medial and lateral malleoli to form the ankle joint. The talus is broader anteriorly than posteriorly, thus preventing forward slipping of the tibia during locomotion.

Because the talus fits principally into the space formed by the malleoli, lateral movement is restricted by the stabilizing ligaments of the ankle. Because the uppermost articular surface of the talus is narrower posteriorly than anteriorly, dorsiflexion is limited. At a position of full dorsiflexion the anterior aspect of the medial collateral ligaments is taut, whereas in plantar flexion internal rotation occurs because of the shape of the talus. The average range of motion is 10 degrees in dorsiflexion and 23 degrees in plantar flexion.[68]

Navicular The navicular bone is positioned anterior to the talus on the medial aspect of the foot. Anteriorly, the navicular bone articulates with the three cuneiform bones.

Cuboid The cuboid is positioned on the lateral aspect of the foot. It articulates posteriorly with the calcaneus and anteriorly with the fourth and fifth metatarsals.

Cuneiforms The three cuneiform bones are located between the navicular and the base of the three metatarsals on the medial aspect of the foot.

Arches of the Foot

The foot is structured, by means of ligamentous and bony arrangements, to form several arches. The arches assist the foot in supporting the body weight; in absorbing the shock of weight bearing; and in providing a space on the plantar aspect of the foot for the blood vessels, nerves, and muscles.[49] There are four arches: the metatarsal, the transverse, the medial longitudinal, and the lateral longitudinal (Figure 18–2).

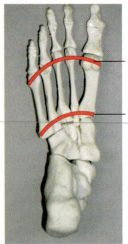

A Plantar view

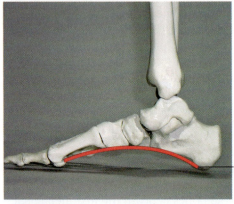

B Medial view

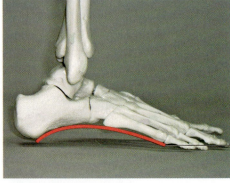

C Lateral view

FIGURE 18–2 Arches of the foot. **(A)** Metatarsal and transverse arches. **(B)** Medial longitudinal arch. **(C)** Lateral longitudinal arch.

Metatarsal Arch The metatarsal arch is shaped by the distal heads of the metatarsals. The arch has a semiovoid appearance, stretching from the first to the fifth metatarsal.

Transverse Arch The transverse arch extends across the transverse tarsal bones, primarily the cuboid and the internal cuneiform, and forms a half-dome. It gives protection to soft tissue and increases the foot's mobility.

Medial Longitudinal Arch The medial longitudinal arch originates along the medial border of the calcaneus and extends forward to the distal head of the first metatarsal. Bony support is provided by the calcaneus, talus, navicular, first cuneiform, and first metatarsal. The main supporting ligament of the longitudinal arch is the plantar calcaneonavicular ligament, which acts as a spring by returning the arch to its normal position after it has been stretched. The tendon of the posterior tibialis muscle helps reinforce the plantar calcaneonavicular ligament.

Lateral Longitudinal Arch The lateral longitudinal arch is on the outer aspect of the foot and follows the same pattern as that of the medial longitudinal arch. It is formed by the calcaneus, cuboid, and fifth metatarsal bones. It is much lower and less flexible than the inner longitudinal arch.

Plantar Fascia (Plantar Aponeurosis)

The plantar fascia is a thick, white band of fibrous tissue originating from the medial tuberosity of the calcaneus and ending at the proximal heads of the metatarsals. Along with ligaments, the plantar fascia supports the foot against downward forces (Figure 18–3). The plantar fascia is a distal continuation of fascia that runs posteriorly from the muscles of the thigh to the muscles of the calf and continues under the calcaneus, where it thickens to become the plantar fascia. It is the most superficial layer on the plantar surface of the foot, lying just between the skin and the first layer of muscles.

Articulations

The articulations (joints) of the foot are categorized into five regions: interphalangeal, metatarsophalangeal, intermetatarsal, tarsometatarsal, subtalar, and midtarsal (Figure 18–4).

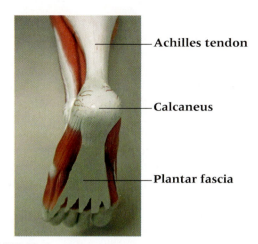

FIGURE 18–3 The Achilles tendon is continuous with the plantar fascia on the plantar surface of the foot.

Interphalangeal Joint The interphalangeal joints are located at the distal extremities of the proximal and middle phalanges at the bases of the adjacent middle and distal phalanges. These joints are designed only for flexion and extension. All interphalangeal joints have reinforcing collateral ligaments on their medial and lateral sides. Also located between the collateral ligaments on the plantar and dorsal surfaces are interphalangeal ligaments.

Metatarsophalangeal Joint The metatarsophalangeal joints are the condyloid type, which permits flexion, extension, adduction, and abduction. Each of these joints has collateral ligaments as well as plantar and dorsal metatarsophalangeal ligaments.

Intermetatarsal Joint The intermetatarsal joints are sliding joints. They include two sets of articulations. One set consists of an articulation on each side of the base of the metatarsal bones, and the second articulations are on each side of the heads of the metatarsal bone. Each of these articulations permits only slight gliding movements. Shafts of the metatarsals are

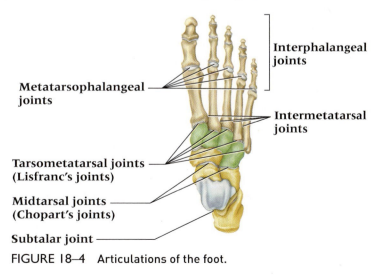

FIGURE 18–4 Articulations of the foot.

connected by interosseous ligaments. The bases are connected by plantar and dorsal ligaments, and the heads are attached by transverse metatarsal ligaments.

Tarsometatarsal Joint (Lisfranc's Joint) The tarsometatarsal joint is formed by the junction of the bases of the metatarsal bones with the cuboid and all three cuneiforms. The slight saddle shape of this joint allows for some gliding and thus for a restricted amount of flexion, extension, adduction, and abduction. Metatarsal bones are attached to the tarsal bones by the dorsal and plantar tarsometatarsal ligaments. Interosseous ligaments connect the three cuneiforms to the metatarsals. The tarsometatarsal joint is also known as Lisfranc's joint.

Subtalar Joint The subtalar joint is the articulation between the talus and the calcaneus. *Inversion, eversion, pronation,* and *supination* are normal movements that occur at the subtalar joint. Inversion is a movement of the calcaneus such that the sole of the foot turns inward, or medially. Eversion is a movement of the calcaneus such that the sole of the foot turns outward, or laterally.

In weight bearing, foot pronation is the combined movements of talar plantar flexion and adduction and calcaneal eversion. In contrast, foot supination is the combined movements of talar dorsiflexion and abduction and calcaneal inversion.[31] These movements, which occur at the subtalar joint, are triplanar movements—that is, movements that occur in all three planes simultaneously.[30] The movements of the talus during pronation and supination have profound effects on the lower extremity, both proximally and distally.

Midtarsal Joint (Chopart's Joint) The midtarsal joint, also referred to as Chopart's joint, consists of two distinct joints: the calcaneocuboid and the talonavicular joint. The midtarsal joint depends mainly on ligamentous and muscular tension to maintain position and integrity. Midtarsal joint stability is directly related to the position of the subtalar joint. If the subtalar joint is pronated, the talonavicular and calcaneocuboid joints become hypermobile. If the subtalar joint is supinated, the midtarsal joint becomes hypomobile. As the midtarsal joint becomes more or less mobile, it affects the distal portion of the foot because of the articulations at the tarsometatarsal joint.[31]

Stabilizing Ligaments

The subtalar ligaments are the interosseus talocalcaneal and the anterior, posterior, lateral, and medial talocalcaneal (Figure 18–5). A major ligament is the plantar calcaneonavicular, which passes from the medial longitudinal arch. Because of its relatively large number of elastic fibers and its primary purpose

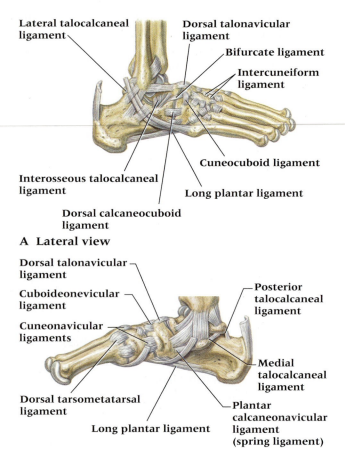

A Lateral view

B Medial view

FIGURE 18–5 Ligaments of the foot. **(A)** Lateral. **(B)** Medial.

of providing shock absorption, the plantar calcaneonavicular is commonly called the spring ligament.

The primary ligaments of the midtarsal joint are the dorsal talonavicular, bifurcate, and dorsal calcaneocuboid. The midtarsal joint is given added strength in its plantar aspect by the long plantar ligaments.

Ligaments of the anterior tarsal joints are divided into those of the cuneonavicular, cuboideonavicular, intercuneiform, and cuneocuboid joints. Each of these joints has both dorsal and plantar ligaments. The intercuneiform ligaments have three transverse bands; one band connects the first cuneiform with the second and the second with the third. A ligament also connects the third cuneiform with the cuboid bone.

Muscles and Movement

The movements of the foot are produced by numerous muscles (Figures 18–6 and 18–7). Table 18–1 summarizes the intrinsic muscles of the foot and their actions.

Dorsiflexion and Plantar Flexion Dorsiflexion and plantar flexion of the foot take place at the ankle

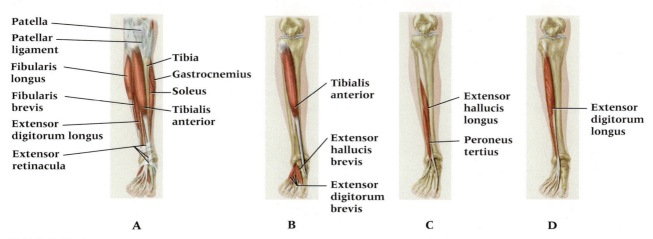

FIGURE 18–6 Muscles and tendons of the anterior aspect of the ankle and foot.

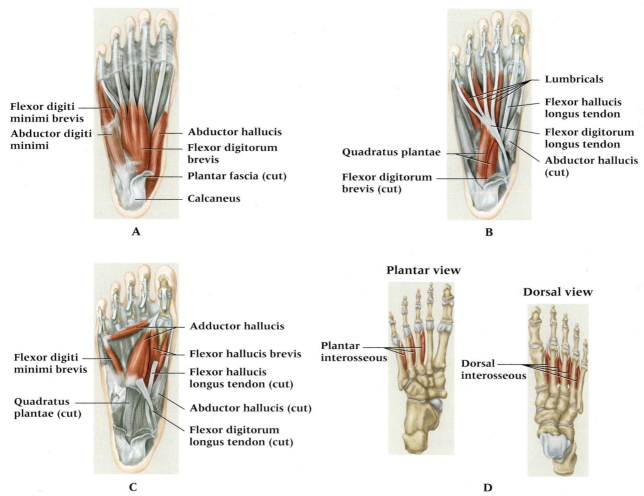

FIGURE 18–7 Intrinsic muscles of the foot. **(A)** First layer. **(B)** Second layer. **(C)** Third layer. **(D)** Fourth layer.

joint and are discussed in greater detail in Chapter 19. The gastrocnemius, soleus, plantaris, peroneus longus, peroneus brevis, tibialis posterior, flexor hallucis longus, and flexor digitorum longus muscles are the plantar flexors. Dorsiflexion is accomplished by the tibialis anterior, extensor digitorum longus, extensor hallucis longus, and peroneus tertius muscles (see Figure 18–6).

Inversion, Adduction, and Supination The medial movements of the foot are produced by the same muscles as inversion, adduction (medial movement of the forefoot), and supination (a combination of inversion and adduction). Muscles that produce these movements pass behind and in front of the medial malleolus. Muscles passing behind are the tibialis posterior (see Figure 19–5B), flexor digitorum

TABLE 18–1 Intrinsic Muscles of the Foot

Muscle	Origin	Insertion	Action	Nerve/ Nerve Root
Dorsal Muscle				
Extensor digitorum brevis	Lateral surface of the calcaneus	Tendon of the extensor digitorum longus	Extends the second through fifth toes	Deep peroneal (L5, S1)
Plantar Muscles				
First Layer				
Abductor hallucis	Calcaneus	Proximal phalanx of the great toe (with the tendon of the flexor hallucis brevis)	Abducts the great toe	Medial plantar (L4, L5, S1)
Flexor digitorum brevis	Calcaneus and plantar aponeurosis	Middle phalanx of the second through fifth toes	Flexes the second through fifth toes	Medial plantar (L4, L5, S1)
Abductor digiti minimi	Calcaneus and plantar aponeurosis	Proximal phalanx of the small toe	Abducts the small toe	Lateral plantar (S1, S2)
Second Layer				
Quadratus plantae	Calcaneus	Into tendons of the flexor digitorum longus	Aids in flexing the second through fifth toes by straightening the pull of the flexor digitorum longus	Lateral plantar (S1, S2)
Lumbricales	From tendons of the flexor digitorum longus	Into tendons of the extensor digitorum longus	Flexes the second through fifth toes	Medial and lateral plantar (L4, L5, S1, S2)
Third Layer				
Flexor hallucis brevis	Cuboid and lateral cuneiform	Proximal phalanx of the great toe	Flexes the great toe	Medial plantar (L4, L5, S1)
Adductor hallucis	*Oblique head:* second, third, and fourth metatarsals / *Transverse head:* ligaments of the metatarsophalangeal joints	Proximal phalanx of the small toe	Adducts the great toe	Lateral plantar (S1, S2)
Flexor digiti minimi brevis	Fifth metatarsal	Proximal phalanx of the small toe	Flexes the small toe	Lateral plantar (S1, S2)
Fourth Layer				
Plantar interossei	Third, fourth, and fifth metatarsals	Proximal phalanx of the same toe	Adducts the toes toward the second toe	Lateral plantar (S1, S2)
Dorsal interossei	Bases of the adjacent metatarsals	Proximal phalanges; both sides of the second toe; lateral side of the third and fourth toes	Abducts the toes from the second toe; moves the second toe medially and laterally	Lateral plantar (S1, S2)

Movements of the Foot and Toes

Toe Flexion   Toe Extension   Toe Abduction   Toe Adduction   Foot Pronation   Foot Supination

longus, and flexor hallucis longus (see Figure 19–5D). Muscles passing in front of the medial malleolus are the tibialis anterior (see Figure 19–5A) and the extensor hallucis longus (see Figure 18–6C).

Eversion, Abduction, and Pronation The lateral movements of the foot are caused by the same muscles that produce eversion, abduction (lateral movement of the forefoot), and pronation (a combination of eversion and abduction). Muscles passing behind the lateral malleolus are the fibularis longus (peroneus longus) and the fibularis brevis (peroneus brevis). Muscles passing in front of the lateral malleolus are the peroneus tertius and extensor digitorum longus (see Figure 18–6C&D).

Movement of the Phalanges The movements of the phalanges are flexion, extension, abduction, and adduction. Flexion of the second, third, fourth, and fifth distal phalanges is executed by the flexor digitorum longus and the quadratus plantar muscles. Flexion of the middle phalanges is performed by the flexor digitorum brevis, and flexion of the proximal phalanges is performed by the lumbricales and the interossei. The great toe is flexed by the flexor hallucis longus. The extension of all the middle phalanges is done by the abductor hallucis and abductor digiti quanti, the lumbricales, and the interossei. Extension of all distal phalanges is effected by the lumbricales, extensor digitorum longus, extensor hallucis longus, and extensor digitorum brevis. The adduction of the foot is performed by the interossei plantares and adductor hallucis; abduction is performed by the interossei dorsalis, abductor hallucis, and abductor digiti quanti.

Nerve Supply and Blood Supply

Nerve Supply The medial and lateral plantar nerves, which are branches of the tibial nerve, supply all of the intrinsic muscles on the plantar surface of the foot. The deep peroneal nerve supplies the extensor

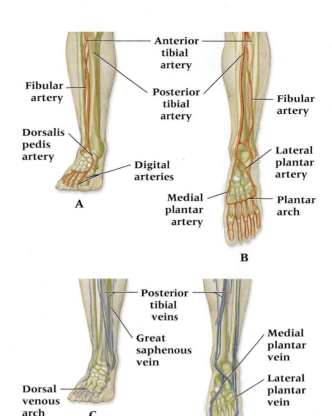

FIGURE 18–9   Blood supply of the foot. **(A)** Dorsal arteries. **(B)** Plantar arteries. **(C)** Dorsal veins. **(D)** Plantar veins.

digitorum brevis on the dorsal suface of the foot (Figure 18–8).

Blood Supply The primary blood supply for the foot comes from the anterior tibial artery and posterior tibial arteries. The dorsum of the foot is supplied by the dorsal pedal artery and the dorsal metatarsal arteries, which branch from the anterior tibial artery. The plantar aspect of the foot is supplied by the lateral plantar artery, the medial plantar artery, and the plantar arterial arch, which all branch from the posterior tibial artery (Figure 18–9A&B).

The venous drainage from the plantar surface is through the medial and lateral plantar veins into the posterior tibial vein. The venous drainage on the dorsum of the foot is through the dorsal venous arch and dorsal pedal vein into the anterior tibial vein (Figure 18–9C&D).

Surface Anatomy

Figure 18–10A shows the pertinent surface anatomy for the dorsal surface of the foot, and Figure 18–10B shows the plantar surface of the foot.

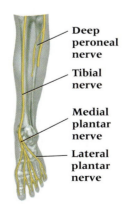

Posterior view

FIGURE 18–8   Nerves of the foot.

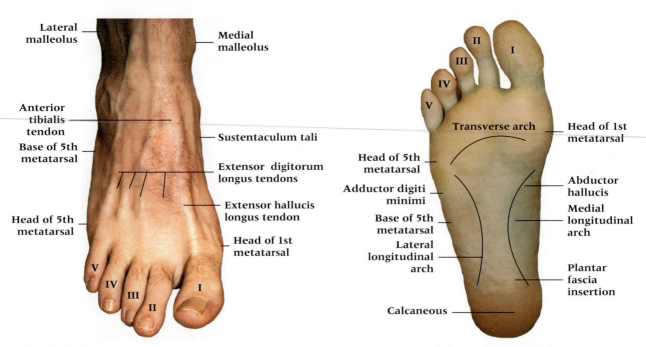

FIGURE 18–10   Surface anatomy showing pertinent landmarks of the foot from **(A)** dorsal view and **(B)** plantar view.

FUNCTIONAL ANATOMY AND FOOT BIOMECHANICS

Athletic trainers must realize, when considering foot, ankle, and leg injuries, that these segments are joined together to form a kinetic chain. Each movement of a body segment has a direct effect on proximal and distal body segments.[37] A study of lower-extremity chronic and overuse injuries related to sports participation must include some under-

> **Most people will develop foot problems at some time in their lives.**

standing of the biomechanics of the foot, especially in the act of walking and running. A number of biomechanical factors may be related to injuries of the lower-leg region.

Normal Gait

The action of the lower extremity during a complete gait cycle in walking can be divided into two primary phases (Figure 18–11). The **stance phase** starts with initial contact of the heel on the ground and ends when the toe breaks contact with the ground (toe-off). This phase accounts for about 60 percent of the total gait cycle. The stance phase involves weight bearing in a closed kinetic chain. The stance phase can be further subdivided into

> **stance phase** From initial contact to toe-off.

five periods: *initial contact, loading response, midstance, terminal stance,* and *preswing.*
At midstance and terminal stance, the body is supported by a single limb, whereas at initial contact and in the early portion of the loading response

period, there is double support with both feet on the ground.[54,70]

The time between toe-off and the subsequent initial contact is termed the **swing phase**, which is a period of non–weight bearing. The swing phase can be subdivided into three

> **swing phase** Period of non–weight bearing.

periods: *initial swing, midswing,* and *terminal swing.* In normal gait, while one leg is in the stance phase, the other is in the swing phase.

As in the walking gait, a running gait has both stance and swing phases. However, there are several differences. In running, the loading response and midstance periods occur more rapidly. There is also a period after toe-off in which neither foot is in contact with the ground and there is no time when both feet contact the ground simultaneously. In running, the stance phase accounts for only one-third of the gait cycle.

The foot's function during the stance phase of running is twofold. At heel strike, the foot acts as a shock absorber to the impact forces and then adapts to the uneven surfaces. At toe-off, the foot functions as a rigid lever to transmit the explosive force from the lower extremity to the running surface. In a heel-strike running gait, initial contact of the foot is on the lateral aspect of the calcaneus, with the subtalar joint in supination. It is estimated that 80 percent of distance runners use this heel-strike pattern, and the remainder are either midfoot or forefoot strikers.[68] Sprinters tend to be forefoot strikers, whereas a number of joggers are midfoot strikers.

At initial contact, the subtalar joint is supinated (Figure 18–12). Associated with this supination of

Stance Phase (60% of total)					Swing Phase		
Initial Contact (heel contact)	Loading Response	Midstance	Terminal Stance	Preswing (toe-off)	Initial Swing	Midswing	Terminal Swing
External Rotation of Tibia	Internal Rotation of Tibia			External Rotation of Tibia			
Supination	Pronation			Supination			

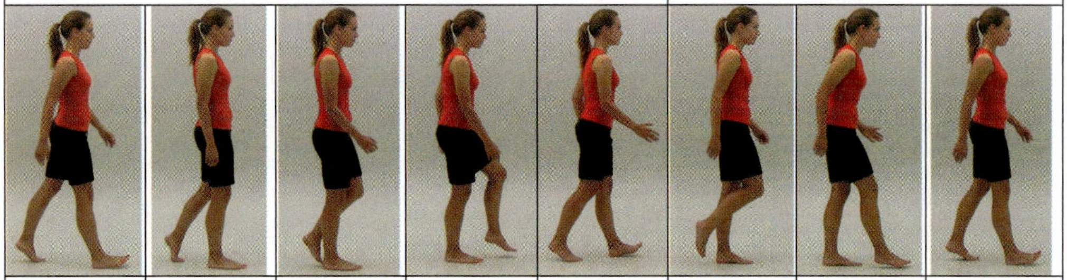

FIGURE 18–11 The stance and swing phases of a normal gait cycle.

the subtalar joint is an obligatory external rotation of the tibia.[54] As the foot is loaded, the subtalar joint moves into a pronated position until the forefoot is in contact with the running surface. The change in subtalar motion occurs between initial heel strike and 20 percent into the support phase of running.[54] As pronation occurs at the subtalar joint, there is obligatory internal rotation of the tibia. Transverse plane rotation occurs at the knee joint because of this tibial rotation. Pronation of the foot unlocks the midtarsal joint and allows the foot to assist in shock absorption and to adapt to uneven surfaces. It is important during initial impact to reduce the ground reaction forces and to distribute the load evenly on many different anatomical structures throughout the foot and leg. Pronation is normal and allows for this distribution of forces on as many structures as possible to avoid excessive loading on just a few structures. The subtalar joint remains in a pronated position through 55 to 85 percent of the stance phase, with maximum pronation being concurrent with the body's center of gravity passing over the base of support.[70]

The foot begins to resupinate and will approach the neutral subtalar position at 70 percent to 90 percent of the stance phase.[70] In supination, the midtarsal joints are locked, and the foot becomes stable and rigid to prepare for toe-off. This rigid position allows the foot to exert a great amount of force from the lower extremity to the running surface.

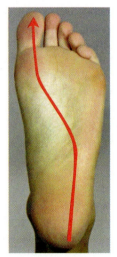

FIGURE 18–12 Foot bearing weight in walking as it moves from heel strike to toe-off.

Subtalar Joint Pronation and Supination Pronation and supination of the foot and subtalar joint are normal during the stance phase of running. However, excessive or prolonged pronation or supination often cause or contribute to overuse injuries. When structural or functional deformities exist in the foot or leg, compensation is likely to occur at the subtalar joint. The subtalar joint compensates in a manner that allows the foot to make stable contact with the ground and get into a

18-1 Clinical Application Exercise

An athletic trainer working in a sports medicine clinic observes a forefoot valgus deformity in a soccer player during a preseason screening.

? Why might this deformity be a problem? What can be done to manage this condition?

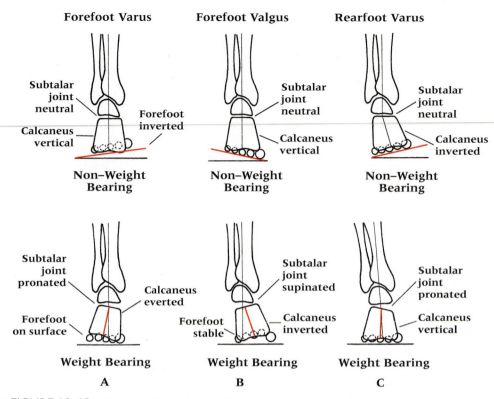

Forefoot Varus   **Forefoot Valgus**   **Rearfoot Varus**

Subtalar joint neutral — Calcaneus vertical — Forefoot inverted — **Non–Weight Bearing**

Subtalar joint neutral — Calcaneus vertical — **Non–Weight Bearing**

Subtalar joint neutral — Calcaneus inverted — **Non–Weight Bearing**

Subtalar joint pronated — Forefoot on surface — Calcaneus everted — **Weight Bearing** — **A**

Subtalar joint supinated — Forefoot stable — Calcaneus inverted — **Weight Bearing** — **B**

Subtalar joint pronated — Calcaneus vertical — **Weight Bearing** — **C**

FIGURE 18–13   Structural foot deformities in non–weight bearing and compensations in weight bearing. **(A)** Forefoot varus. **(B)** Forefoot valgus. **(C)** Rearfoot varus.

weight-bearing position (Figure 18–13). This excessive motion compensates for an existing structural deformity.[31]

Structural Deformities The most typical structural deformities of the foot that produce excessive pronation or supination include forefoot varus, forefoot valgus, and rearfoot varus (Figure 18–13).[54] These structural deformities exist in a non–weight-bearing position. Structural forefoot varus and structural rearfoot varus deformities are usually associated with excessive pronation.[51] A structural forefoot valgus causes excessive supination. The deformities usually exist in one plane, but the subtalar joint will interfere with the normal functions of the foot and make it more difficult for the joint to act as a shock absorber, to adapt to uneven surfaces, and to act as a rigid lever for toe-off. The compensation, which occurs when the foot goes into weight bearing, rather than the deformity itself, usually causes overuse injuries.[31]

Excessive Pronation Excessive or prolonged pronation during running is one of the major causes of stress injuries. Overload of specific structures results when excessive pronation is produced in the stance phase or when pronation is prolonged into the propulsive phase of running.[11] Excessive pronation during the stance phase causes compensatory subtalar joint motion such that the midtarsal joint remains

unlocked, resulting in an excessively loose foot.[23] As more motion occurs at the midtarsal joint, the first metatarsal and first cuneiform become more mobile. These bones constitute a functional unit known as the *first ray*. With pronation of the midtarsal joint, the first ray is more mobile because of its articulations with that joint. The first ray is also stabilized by the attachment of the peroneus longus tendon, which attaches to the base of the first metatarsal.[20]

The fibularis longus tendon passes posteriorly around the base of the lateral malleolus and then through a notch in the cuboid to cross the foot to the first metatarsal. The cuboid functions as a pulley to increase the mechanical advantage of the peroneal tendon. Stability of the cuboid is essential in this process. In the pronated position, the cuboid loses much of its mechanical advantage as a pulley; therefore, the peroneus longus tendon no longer stabilizes the first ray effectively. This condition creates hypermobility of the first ray and increased pressure on the other metatarsals. There is also an increase in tibial rotation, which forces the knee joint to absorb more transverse rotation motion.[31]

Prolonged pronation of the subtalar joint does not allow the foot to resupinate in time to provide a rigid lever for toe-off, resulting in a less powerful and efficient force. Thus, various foot and leg problems occur with excessive or prolonged pronation during the stance phase; these problems include stress fractures of the second metatarsal, plantar fasciitis, posterior tibial tendinitis, Achilles tendinitis, tibial stress syndrome, and medial knee pain.[30]

Excessive Supination At heel strike in prolonged or excessive supination, compensatory movement at the subtalar joint does not allow the midtarsal joint to unlock, which causes the foot to remain excessively rigid.[13] Because less movement occurs at the calcaneocuboid joint, the cuboid becomes hypomobile. The fibularis longus tendon has a greater amount of tension because the cuboid has less mobility and thus will not allow mobility of the first ray. In this case, the majority of the weight is borne by the first and fifth metatarsals. Thus, the foot cannot absorb the ground reaction forces as efficiently.[29]

Excessive supination limits tibial internal rotation. Injuries typically associated with excessive supination include inversion ankle sprains, tibial stress syndrome, peroneal tendinitis, iliotibial band friction syndrome, and trochanteric bursitis.[30]

PREVENTION OF FOOT INJURIES

Certainly, the foot is highly vulnerable to a variety of injuries. The repetitive stresses and strains incurred by the foot during athletic activities are unquestionably sufficient to cause both acute traumatic and overuse injuries. Foot injuries can best be prevented by selecting appropriate footwear, using a shoe orthotic, and paying attention to appropriate foot hygiene and care.[53,67]

Appropriate Footwear

The athletic and fitness shoe manufacturing industry has become extremely sophisticated and offers a number of options when it comes to purchasing shoes for different athletic activities. Shoe selection, parts of a shoe, and fitting were discussed in Chapter 7. Selecting an appropriate shoe is one of the most critical considerations in preventing a foot problem. Before a shoe is selected, the athletic trainer should evaluate the patient's foot to determine the existence of a structural deformity, such as a forefoot valgus or varus or a rearfoot varus. The type of shoe selected should depend on the existing structural deformity.

As noted earlier, pronation is a problem of hypermobility. Individuals who excessively pronate need stability and firmness to reduce this excess movement. Research indicates that shoe compression, compared with a barefoot condition, may actually increase pronation.[34] The ideal shoe for a pronated foot is one that is less flexible and has good rearfoot control. Conversely, supinated feet are usually very rigid. Increased cushioning and flexibility benefit this type of foot.

Several construction factors may influence the firmness and stability of a shoe. The basic form upon which a shoe is built is called the last. The upper is fitted onto a last in several ways. Each method has its own flexibility and control characteristics (Figure 18–14). A slip-lasted shoe is sewn together like a moccasin and is very flexible. A board-lasted shoe contains a piece of fiberboard to which the upper is attached, which provides a very firm, inflexible base for the shoe. A combination-lasted shoe is boarded in the back half of the shoe and slip-lasted in the front, which provides rearfoot stability with forefoot mobility.

The shape of the last may also determine shoe selection (Figure 18–15). Most individuals with excessive pronation perform better in a straight-lasted shoe—that is, a shoe in which the forefoot does not

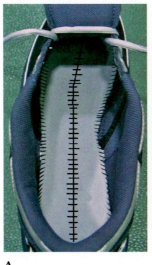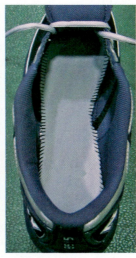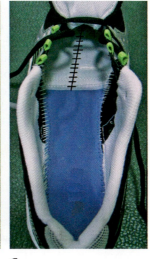

A   B   C

FIGURE 18–14   Shoe lasts. **(A)** Slip-lasted. **(B)** Board-lasted. **(C)** Combination lasted.

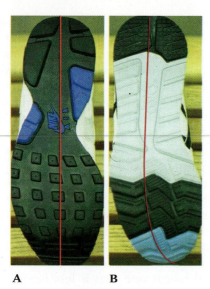

FIGURE 18–15 Shape of the last. **(A)** Straight. **(B)** Curved.

curve inward in relation to the rearfoot.[18] Midsole design also affects the stability of a shoe. The midsole separates the upper from the outsole. More dense, less yielding material is often used under the medial aspect of the foot to control pronation.

In an effort to control rearfoot movement, many shoe manufacturers have reinforced the heel counter both internally and externally, often in the form of extra plastic along the outside of the heel counter. Other factors that may affect the performance of a shoe are the outsole contour and composition, lacing systems, and forefoot wedges.[31]

Table 18–2 provides guidelines for choosing the correct shoe components based on the type of foot problem.

Shoe Orthotics

Many injuries to the foot can be prevented by using an orthotic device to correct biomechanical problems that may exist in the foot and that can cause an injury.[14] The orthotic is a plastic, rubber, or leather support that is placed in the shoe as a replacement for the existing insert. Ready-made orthotics can be purchased in sporting goods and shoe stores. Some patients need to have orthotics that are custom-fitted or made by the athletic trainer or podiatrist.[66]

The use of orthotics for correcting specific problems are discussed in the section on rehabilitation at the end of this chapter.

Foot Hygiene

Individuals who perform simple tasks—such as keeping their toenails trimmed correctly; shaving down excessive calluses; keeping their feet clean; wearing clean, correctly fitted socks; and keeping their feet as dry as possible to prevent the development of athlete's foot (see Chapter 28)—can individually and collectively reduce a number of problems that can cause them to miss days of practice or competition.

FOOT ASSESSMENT

When assessing foot injuries, athletic trainers must clearly understand that the foot is part of a kinetic chain that includes both the ankle and the lower leg.[35] Acute injuries must be differentiated from injuries with a relatively slow onset.

History

An athletic trainer making a decision about how to manage a foot injury must perform a quick assessment to determine the type of injury and its history. He or she should ask the following questions:

- Is this the first time this condition has occurred? If it has happened before, when, how often, and under what circumstances did it occur?
- How did the injury occur?
- Did it occur suddenly or come on slowly?
- Was the mechanism a sudden strain, twist, or blow to the foot?
- Where is the pain (ankle, heel, arches, toes)?
- What type of pain is the athlete experiencing?
- Is there muscle weakness?
- Is there any snapping, popping, or crepitus during movement?
- Is there any alteration in sensation?
- Can the patient point to the exact site of the pain?
- When is the pain or other symptoms more or less severe?

TABLE 18–2	Choosing the Correct Shoe Components Based on the Type of Foot Problem					
Type of Problem	**Shoe Components**					
Excessive pronation	Stiff shoe	Dense midsole, medial wedge	Good rearfoot control	Board or combination last	Straight last	Rigid or semirigid orthotic
Excessive supination	Flexible shoe	Soft midsole, lateral wedge	Rearfoot control not necessary	Slip last	Curved last	Soft or semirigid orthotic

- On what type of surface has the patient been training?
- What type of footwear is being worn during training? Is it appropriate for the type of training? Is discomfort increased when footwear is worn?

Observation

The athletic trainer should observe the patient to determine the following:

- Is the patient favoring the foot, walking with a limp, or unable to bear weight?
- Is the injured part deformed, swollen, or discolored?
- Does the foot change color when weight bearing and not weight bearing (changing rapidly from a darker to lighter pink when not weight bearing)?
- Is there pes planus (a flatfoot) or pes cavus (a high arch)?
- Is the foot well aligned? Does it maintain its shape on weight bearing?
- Do any abnormalities exist in the toes (e.g., hammertoes, mallet toes, claw toes, Morton's toe, hallux valgus, corns, bunions, plantar warts)?

Looking for Structural Deformities The first step in looking for structural deformities is to establish a position of subtalar neutral. The patient should be prone with the distal third of the leg hanging off the end of the table (Figure 18–16). A line should be drawn bisecting the leg from the start of the musculotendinous junction of the gastrocnemius to the distal portion of the calcaneus. With the patient still prone, the athletic trainer should palpate the talus while the forefoot is inverted and everted. One finger should palpate the talus at the anterior aspect of the fibula and another finger at the anterior portion of the medial malleolus. The position at which the talus is equally prominent on both sides is considered a neutral subtalar position in which the subtalar joint is neither pronated nor supinated.[31]

Once the subtalar joint is placed in a neutral position, the athletic trainer should apply mild dorsiflexion while observing the metatarsal heads in relation to the plantar surface of the calcaneus. Forefoot varus is a rigid osseous deformity in which the medial metatarsal heads are inverted in relation to the plane of the calcaneus. Forefoot varus is the most common cause of excessive pronation (see Figure 18–13A).[13] Forefoot varus can also be caused by soft-tissue tightness of the anterior tibialis muscle along with malposition of the calcaneocuboid joint. This has been referred to as forefoot supinatus and attributed to chronic subtalar joint pronation. Forefoot valgus is a rigid osseous deformity in which the lateral

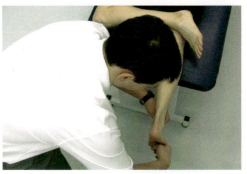

A

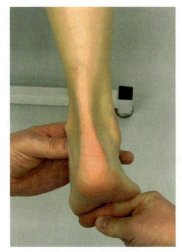

B

FIGURE 18–16 **(A)** Position for assessing existing structural deformities. **(B)** Viewing the structural deformity in subtalar neutral.

metatarsals are everted in relation to the rearfoot (see Figure 18–13B).

These rigid forefoot deformities are benign in a non–weight-bearing position; however, during weight bearing, the metatarsal heads must somehow make contact with the surface to bear weight. To accomplish this movement for a forefoot varus, the talus plantar flexes and adducts and the calcaneus everts. For the forefoot valgus, the calcaneus inverts and the talus abducts and dorsiflexes. A forefoot varus is the most common forefoot deformity.[13]

In a rearfoot varus deformity, when the foot is in a subtalar neutral position and non–weight bearing, the medial metatarsal heads are elevated, as in a forefoot varus, and the calcaneus is also in an inverted position (see Figure 18–13C).[60] For the foot to bear weight, the subtalar joint must pronate.

An equinus foot, and particularly a rigid equinus foot, is another structural deformity that is thought to be associated with poor shock absorption during running. In an equinus foot, the forefoot is plantar flexed relative to the rearfoot when the ankle is at 90 degrees of flexion. A similar condition, in which only the first metatarsal is plantar flexed relative to the rearfoot, is referred to as a plantar flexed first ray.[31]

Shoe Wear Patterns Individuals with excessive pronation often wear out the front of the running shoe under the second metatarsal. Shoe wear patterns are commonly misinterpreted by athletes who think they must be pronators because they wear out the back outside edges of their heels. However, most people wear out the back outside edges of their shoes. Just before heel strike, the anterior tibialis fires to prevent the foot from slapping forward. The anterior tibialis not only dorsiflexes the foot but also slightly inverts it, hence the wear pattern on the back edge of the shoe. An individual who excessively supinates tends to show a wear pattern on the lateral border of the shoe. The key to inspection of wear patterns on shoes is observation of the heel counter and the forefoot.[30]

Palpation

Besides determining pain sites, swelling, and deformities, palpation is used to determine and evaluate circulation.

Bony Palpation The following bony landmarks should be palpated:

Medial aspect
- Medial calcaneus
- Calcaneal dome
- Medial malleolus
- Sustentaculum tali (plantar aspect of medial calcaneus)
- Talar head
- Navicular tubercle
- First cuneiform
- First metatarsal
- First metatarsophalangeal joint
- First phalanx

Lateral aspect
- Lateral calcaneus
- Lateral malleolus
- Sinus tarsi
- Peroneal tubercle
- Cuboid bone
- Styloid process (proximal head of fifth metatarsal)
- Fifth metatarsal
- Fifth metatarsophalangeal joint
- Fifth phalanx

Dorsal aspect
- Second, third, fourth metatarsals
- Second, third, fourth metatarsophalangeal joints
- Second, third, fourth phalanges
- Third and fourth cuneiform bones

Plantar aspect
- Metatarsal heads
- Medial calcaneal tubercle
- Sesamoid bones

Soft-Tissue Palpation The following soft-tissue structures should be palpated:

Medial and plantar aspect
- Tibialis posterior tendon
- Flexor hallucis longus tendon
- Flexor digitorum longus tendon
- Deltoid ligament
- Calcaneonavicular ligament (spring ligament)
- Medial longitudinal arch
- Plantar fascia
- Transverse arch

Lateral and dorsal aspect
- Anterior talofibular ligament
- Calcaneofibular ligament
- Posterior talofibular ligament
- Peroneus longus tendon
- Peroneus brevis tendon
- Extensor hallucis longus tendon
- Extensor digitorum longus tendon
- Extensor digitorum brevis tendon
- Tibialis anterior tendon

Pulses To ensure that there is proper blood circulation to the foot, the pulse is measured at the posterior tibial and dorsalis pedis arteries (see Figure 18–9). Pulse in the dorsalis pedis artery is normally felt between the tendons of the extensor hallucis longus and extensor digitorum longus, on a line from the midpoint between the medial and lateral malleoli to the proximal end of the first intermetatarsal space.

Pulse in the posterior tibial artery is normally palpable behind the medial malleolus, 1 inch (2.5 cm) in front of the medial border of the Achilles tendon.[32]

Special Tests

Movement Assessment Both the extrinsic and the intrinsic foot muscles should be assessed for pain and range of motion during active, passive, and resistive isometric movement.

Morton's Test With the foot in a neutral position, transverse pressure is applied to the heads of the metatarsals, causing sharp pain in the forefoot. A positive test may indicate the presence of **metatarsalgia** or a **neuroma** (Figure 18–17).

> **metatarsalgia** Pain in the ball of the foot.
>
> **neuroma** A bulging that emanates from a nerve.

Neurological Assessment Reflexes and cutaneous distribution should be tested. Skin sensation should be noted for any alteration.

Tendon reflexes, such as in the Achilles tendon (S1 nerve root), should elicit a response when gently tapped. Sensation is tested by running the hands

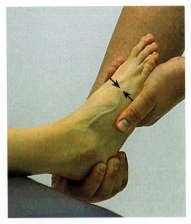

FIGURE 18–17 Morton's test to establish metatarsalgia or a neuroma.

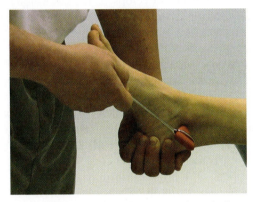

FIGURE 18–18 A positive Tinel's sign may indicate tarsal tunnel syndrome.

over the anterior, lateral, medial, and posterior surfaces of the foot and toes.

Tinel's Sign Test Tapping over the posterior tibial nerve produces tingling distal to that area. Numbness, tingling, and paresthesia may indicate the presence of tarsal tunnel syndrome (Figure 18–18).

RECOGNITION AND MANAGEMENT OF SPECIFIC INJURIES

Most people will at some time develop foot problems that can be attributed to the use of improper footwear, poor foot hygiene, or anatomical structural deviations that result from faulty postural alignments or abnormal stresses. Many activities place exceptional demands on the feet—far beyond what is considered normal. The athletic trainer should be well aware of potential foot problems and should be capable of identifying, ameliorating, and preventing them whenever possible.

Injuries to the Tarsal Region

Fractures of the Talus

Etiology Fractures of the dome of the talus usually occur either laterally from a severe inversion and dorsiflexion force, or medially from an inversion and plantar flexion force, with external rotation of the tibia on the talus.[3]

The severity of the fracture may range from a nondisplaced compression fracture to a displaced osteochondral fracture. The presence of osteochondral fragments is referred to as *osteochondritis dissecans.*

Symptoms and signs The patient often has a history of repeated trauma to the ankle. He or she feels pain on weight bearing and complains of catching and snapping along with intermittent swelling. The talar dome is tender on palpation over the anteromedial or anterolateral joint line.[3]

Management For accurate diagnosis, an X-ray is essential. Nonsurgical management is appropriate for nondisplaced subchondral compression fractures. Treatment should include protective immobilization with non–weight bearing, progressing to full weight bearing, depending on symptoms. Rehabilitation should concentrate on strengthening and regaining full range of motion in the ankle joint. If conservative treatment fails and symptoms continue or if there is a displaced osteochondral fracture, surgical removal of the loose bodies arthroscopically may be necessary. Following surgery, the patient can expect to resume activity in 6 to 8 months.[3]

Fracture of the Calcaneus

Etiology A fracture of the calcaneus most often occurs from landing after a jump or fall from a height.[41] Avulsion fractures can also occur anteriorly at the attachment of the calcaneonavicular ligament to the sustentaculum tali or posteriorly at the attachment of the talocalcaneal ligament. Anterior avulsion fractures can be misdiagnosed as tendinitis of the posterior tibialis.[27]

Symptoms and signs There is usually immediate swelling and pain and an inability to bear weight. Deformity is not normally present unless there is a displaced comminuted fracture.[43]

Management RICE must be used immediately to minimize pain and swelling before referring the athlete to X-ray for diagnosis. With nondisplaced fractures, immobilization and early range of motion exercises are recommended as soon as acute swelling and pain subside and motion is tolerated.[27]

Calcaneal Stress Fracture

Etiology Calcaneal stress fractures, along with stress fractures of the tibia and of the second metatarsal, are among the most common stress fractures in the lower extremity. A calcaneal stress fracture occurs with repetitive impact during heel strike and is most prevalent among distance runners. It is characterized by a sudden onset of constant pain in the plantar-calcaneal area.[41]

Symptoms and signs Weight bearing, particularly on heel strike in running, increases pain. Complaints of pain tend to continue after exercise stops. The fracture may fail to appear during X-ray examination; a bone scan may be a better diagnostic tool.[43]

Management Management is usually conservative for the first 2 or 3 weeks and includes rest and active range of motion exercises of the foot and ankle. Non–weight-bearing cardiovascular exercise, such as pool running, may continue during this period. After 2 weeks and when pain subsides, activity within pain limits can be resumed gradually, with the athlete wearing a cushioned shoe.

Apophysitis of the Calcaneus (Sever's Disease)

Etiology Calcaneal **apophysitis**, or Sever's disease, occurs in young, physically active patients. Sever's disease is comparable to Osgood-Schlatter disease at the tibial tubercle of the knee (see Chapter 20).[56] Sever's disease is a traction injury at the **apophysis** of the calcaneus (bone protrusion) where the Achilles tendon attaches.[57]

> **apophysitis** (a poff ah cytis) Inflammation of an apophysis.
>
> **apophysis** (a poff ah sis) Bony outgrowth, such as tubercle or tuberosity.

Symptoms and signs Pain occurs at the posterior heel below the attachment of the Achilles tendon insertion of the child or adolescent athlete. Pain occurs during vigorous activity and does not continue at rest.

Management Apophysitis, like other overuse syndromes, is best treated with rest, ice, stretching (of the Achilles tendon), and antiinflammatory medications. A heel lift can take some stress off the apophysis.

Retrocalcaneal Bursitis

Etiology Retrocalcaneal bursitis is caused by inflammation of the bursa that lies between the Achilles tendon and the calcaneus. Retrocalcaneal bursitis often occurs from the pressure and rubbing of the heel counter of a shoe. This condition is chronic, developing gradually over a long period of time, and may take many days—sometimes weeks or months—to resolve.[17]

An **exostosis** is a benign bony outgrowth or callus that protrudes from the surface of a bone and is usually capped by cartilage. An exostosis that develops on the posterior aspect of the calcaneus, called a Haglund's deformity, causes ongoing inflammation of the retrocalcaneal bursa, sometimes referred to as a "pump bump" (Figure 18–19A).[17]

> **exostosis** (ek sos toe ses) Benign bony outgrowth that protrudes from the surface of a bone and is usually capped by cartilage.

Symptoms and signs Pain may be elicited by palpating the bursa just above and anterior to the insertion of the Achilles tendon. There will likely be some swelling on both sides of the heel cord. If the source of irritation persists, a bony callus may also begin to form.

Management Initially, RICE plus NSAIDs and analgesics are used as needed. Often, the use of ultrasound can reduce the inflammation. Stretching of the Achilles tendon should be routine. A heel lift should be used to take stress off the Achilles tendon. A doughnut heel pad can be used to take pressure off the bursa and an existing exostosis (Figure 18–19B). If necessary, larger shoes with wider heel contours should be worn.[17]

Heel Contusion

Etiology Activities that demand a sudden stop-and-go response or a sudden change from a horizontal

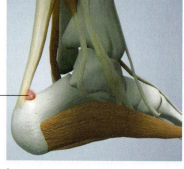
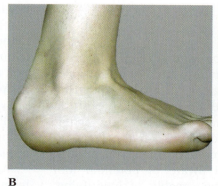
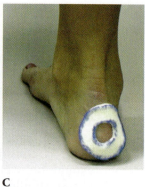

Inflammed retrocalcaneal bursa

A B C

FIGURE 18–19   **(A)** Retrocalcaneal bursitis at the attachment of the Achilles tendon to the calcaneous. **(B)** A pump bump that develops. **(C)** Can be protected using a doughnut-type pad.

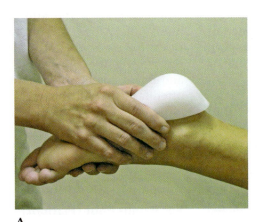
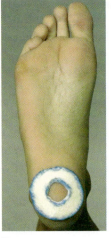

A　　　　　　　　　　　　　　**B**

FIGURE 18–20　　Heel protection. **(A)** Heel cup. **(B)** Protective heel doughnut.

to a vertical movement (e.g., basketball, jumping, or the landing in long jumping) are particularly likely to cause heel contusions.[56] The calcaneus is protected by a thick, cornified skin layer and a heavy fat pad covering, but even this thick padding cannot always protect against the impact of jumping or running.[63]

The major function of the tissue heel pad is to sustain hydraulic pressure through fat columns. Tissue compression is monitored by pressure nerve endings from the skin and plantar aponeurosis. Often, the irritation is on the lateral aspect of the heel because of the heel strike in walking or running.[39]

Symptoms and signs　When injury occurs, the patient complains of severe pain in the heel and is unable to withstand the stress of weight bearing. Often, there is warmth and redness over the tender area.[43]

Management　A contusion of the heel may develop into chronic inflammation of the periosteum. The patient should not bear weight on the heel for at least 24 hours. RICE is applied, and NSAIDs are administered. If pain when walking has subsided by the third day, the patient may resume moderate activity with the protection of a heel cup or protective doughnut (Figure 18–20). The patient should wear shock-absorbent footwear.

Cuboid Subluxation

Etiology　Pronation and trauma have been reported to be prominent causes of cuboid subluxation.[58] This condition is sometimes incorrectly confused with plantar fasciitis. However, the patient usually complains of a midfoot sprain with pain on the dorsum of the foot and/or over the anterior/lateral ankle frequently after an inversion mechanism. The primary reason for pain is the stress placed on the long peroneal muscle when the foot is in pronation. In this position, the long peroneal muscle allows the cuboid bone to move downward medially.

Symptoms and signs　This displacement of the cuboid causes pain along the fourth and fifth metatarsals as well as over the cuboid. This problem often refers pain to the heel area as well. Many times this pain is increased when the patient stands after a prolonged non–weight-bearing period.

Management　Dramatic treatment results may be obtained by manipulating to restore the cuboid to its natural position (Figure 18–21). Once the cuboid is manipulated, an orthotic often helps support it in its proper position. If manipulation is successful, quite often the patient can return to play immediately with little or no pain. The patient should wear an appropriately constructed orthotic when practicing or competing to reduce the chances of recurrence.

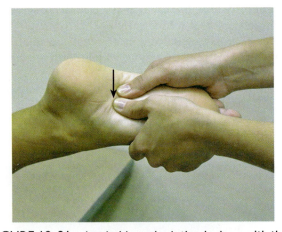

FIGURE 18–21　A cuboid manipulation is done with the patient prone. The lateral plantar aspect of the forefoot is grasped by the thumbs, with the fingers supporting the dorsum of the foot. The thumbs should be over the cuboid. The manipulation should be a thrust downward to move the cuboid into its more dorsal position. Often, a pop is felt as the cuboid moves back into place.

Tarsal Tunnel Syndrome

Etiology The tarsal tunnel is a loosely defined area behind the medial malleolus that forms a tunnel with an osseous floor and the roof composed of the flexor retinaculum. Through this tunnel pass the tibialis posterior, flexor hallucis longus, and flexor digitorum muscles with their surrounding synovial sheaths and the tibial nerve artery and vein.[52] Any condition that compromises the structures within this tunnel can cause tarsal tunnel syndrome, including tenosynovitis, previous fractures, excessive pronation, or any acute trauma.[67]

Symptoms and signs Complaints of pain and paresthesia are typical, particularly along the medial and plantar aspects of the foot. Complaints of increased pain at night are also common. Tinel's sign will be positive in cases of tarsal tunnel syndrome (see Figure 18–18). If the condition persists, motor weakness and atrophy may gradually appear, following the course of the tibial nerve.

Management Initial conservative management includes the use of antiinflammatory medication and other antiinflammatory modalities. The use of an appropriate orthotic to correct excessive pronation may effectively reduce the symptoms. Surgery may be necessary if the symptoms become recurrent.[55]

Tarsometatarsal Fracture/Dislocation (Lisfranc Injury)

Etiology Named after a French surgeon who described amputations at the tarsometatarsal joint, this is an uncommon injury that can cause long-term disability. The ankle is plantar flexed with the rearfoot locked, and there is a sudden, forceful hyper–plantar flexion of the forefoot that results in dorsal displacement of the proximal end of the metatarsals. The dorsum of the foot rolls forward, with the body weight providing the force to displace the base of the metatarsals dorsally (Figure 18–22).[65]

Symptoms and signs Symptoms may be relatively subtle. The patient complains of pain and an inability to bear weight. Swelling and tenderness are localized over the dorsum of the foot. There may be a fracture of the metatarsals. Sprain of the fourth and fifth proximal metatarsals causes ongoing pain. It is not uncommon to overlook the serious disruption of the supporting ligaments because attention is often focused on a metatarsal fracture.

Management If the athletic trainer suspects this injury, the patient should be referred to the physician for evaluation. The key to treatment is first recognizing the injury, then restoring alignment, and finally maintaining stability.[69] Closed reduction often fails, and most likely it will be necessary to do an open reduction with internal fixation to stabilize the dislocation. Potential complications include metatarsalgia, limited motion of the metatarsophalangeal joints, and long-term disability.[65]

Injuries to the Metatarsal Region

Pes Planus Foot (Flatfoot)

Etiology The term *pes planus* refers to a type of foot in which the medial longitudinal arch appears to be flat and is sometimes said to be fallen (Figure 18–23A). In general, pes planus is associated with excessive foot pronation and may be caused by a number of factors, including a structural forefoot varus deformity, shoes that are too tight, trauma that weakens supportive structures (such as muscles and ligaments), overweight, and excessive exercise that repeatedly subjects the arch to severe pounding on an unyielding surface.

Symptoms and signs The patient may complain of pain and a feeling of weakness or fatigue in the medial longitudinal

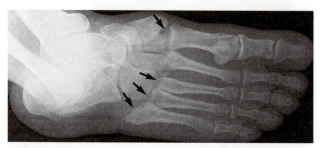

FIGURE 18–22   A Lisfranc injury is the dorsal displacement of the proximal end of the metatarsals.

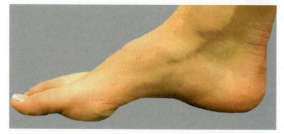

FIGURE 18–23   **(A)** Pes planus foot. **(B)** Pes cavus foot.

arch. There may be calcaneal eversion, a bulging of the navicular bone, a flattening of the medial longitudinal arch, and dorsiflexing with lateral splaying of the first metatarsal.

Management Regardless of how flattened the medial longitudinal arch appears to be, if it is not causing the individual any pain or related symptoms, then absolutely nothing should be done to try to correct the apparent problem. Attempts to do so may, in fact, create an unnecessary problem. However, if the patient is experiencing pain, an appropriately constructed orthotic designed to correct excessive pronation by using a medial wedge will most likely alleviate symptoms. In certain cases, incorporating an arch support into the orthotic or taping the arch for support may be helpful.

Pes Cavus Foot (High Arch Foot)

Etiology The term *pes cavus* refers to a type of foot that has an arch that is higher than normal (Figure 18–23B). Sometimes called *clawfoot or hollow foot*, pes cavus is not as common as pes planus. A pes cavus is generally associated with excessive supination. The accentuated high medial longitudinal arch may be congenital or may indicate a neurological disorder.[11]

Symptoms and signs In cases of pes cavus, shock absorption is poor, and thus problems such as general foot pain, metatarsalgia, and clawed or hammertoes are seen. Commonly associated with this condition are a structural forefoot valgus deformity and an abnormal shortening of the Achilles tendon. The Achilles tendon is directly linked with the plantar fascia (see Figure 18–3). Also, because of the abnormal distribution of body weight, heavy calluses develop on the ball and heel of the foot.[63]

Management As is the case with pes planus, pes cavus may be asymptomatic, in which case no attempt should be made to correct the problem. If there are associated problems, then an orthotic should be constructed using a lateral wedge to correct a structural forefoot valgus deformity. Stretching of the Achilles tendon and the plantar fascia may also be helpful.

Second Metatarsal Stress Fracture (Morton's Toe)

Etiology Normally, the first metatarsal is longer than the second. Morton's toe is a condition in which there is an abnormally short first metatarsal, and thus the second toe appears to be longer than the great toe (Figure 18–24). Much of the weight bearing is ordinarily on the first metatarsal. Because the first metatarsal is short, however, more weight must be borne by the second metatarsal instead. This uneven weight distribution becomes even more of a problem in a running gait, during which weight bearing tends to shift more to the second metatarsal.

A Morton's toe is not an injury and can be a benign condition that causes no problems. However, if the second metatarsal is subjected to more stress, particularly during running, a stress fracture could develop.[64]

Symptoms and signs Symptoms are those of stress fractures in general. The patient complains of pain both during and after activity, and there may be an area of point tenderness. A bone scan would be positive for a stress fracture. A callus is likely to form under the second metatarsal head.

Management If a Morton's toe is not causing any symptoms, nothing should be done to try to correct the problem. If a Morton's toe is associated with a structural forefoot varus deformity, an orthotic with a medial wedge would likely be helpful.

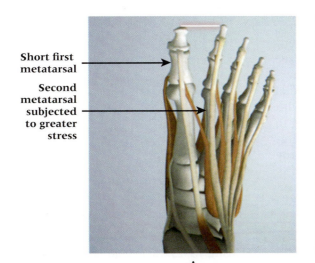
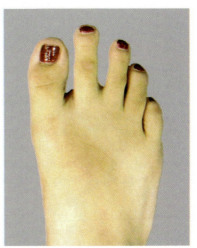

Short first metatarsal

Second metatarsal subjected to greater stress

A   **B**

FIGURE 18–24 In a Morton's toe, the first metatarsal is abnormally short.

Longitudinal Arch Strain

Etiology Longitudinal arch strain is usually caused by subjecting the musculature of the foot to increased stress produced by repetitive contact with hard surfaces. In this condition, there is a flattening or depression of the longitudinal arch while the foot is in the midsupport phase, resulting in a strain to the arch.[33] Such a strain may appear suddenly, or it may develop slowly over a considerable length of time.

Symptoms and signs As a rule, pain is experienced only during running or jumping. The pain usually appears just below the posterior tibialis tendon and is accompanied by swelling and tenderness along the medial aspects of the foot. This injury may also be associated with a sprain of the calcaneonavicular ligament as well as a strain of the flexor hallucis longus tendon.

Management The management of a longitudinal arch strain involves immediate care, consisting of RICE, followed by appropriate therapy and reduction of weight bearing. Weight bearing must be performed pain free. Arch taping technique no. 1 or 2 might be used to allow earlier pain-free weight bearing (see Figure 8–20 through 8–23).

Plantar Fasciitis Heel pain is a very common problem in the athletic and nonathletic population. This phenomenon has been attributed to several etiologies, including heel spurs, plantar fascia irritation, and bursitis.[17] *Plantar fasciitis* is a catchall term that is commonly used to describe pain in the proximal arch and heel. The plantar fascia (plantar aponeurosis) runs the length of the sole of the foot (see Figure 18–3). It is a broad band of dense connective tissue that is attached proximally to the medial surface of the calcaneus. It fans out distally, with fibers and their various small branches attaching to the metatarsophalangeal articulations and merging into the capsular ligaments. The function of the plantar fascia is to assist in maintaining the stability of the foot and in securing or bracing the longitudinal arch.[36]

Etiology Tension develops in the plantar fascia both during extension of the toes and during depression of the longitudinal arch as a result of weight bearing.[1] When the weight is principally on the heel, as in ordinary standing, the tension exerted on

the fascia is negligible. However, when the weight is shifted to the ball of the foot (on the heads of the metatarsals), fascial tension is increased. In running, because the toe-off phase involves both a forceful extension of the toes and a powerful thrust by the ball of the foot (on the heads of the metatarsals), fascial tension is increased to approximately twice the body weight.[12] Tightening of the plantar fascia during dorsiflexion, thus shortening the longitudinal arch, has been described as the "windlass" mechanism.[7]

Plantar fasciitis can occur in individuals with pes cavus, in which case the foot has too little motion, or in those with a pes planus, in which case there is too much motion.[7]

Street shoes, by nature of their design, take on the characteristics of splints and tend to restrict foot action to such an extent that the arch may become somewhat rigid. This rigidity occurs because of shortening of the ligaments and other mild abnormalities. The athlete, changing from such footwear into a flexible gymnastic slipper or soft track shoe, often experiences trauma when the foot is subjected to stress. Trauma may also result from poor running technique.

A number of anatomical and biomechanical conditions have been studied as possible causes of plantar fasciitis. Those conditions include leg length discrepancy, excessive pronation of the subtalar joint, inflexibility of the longitudinal arch, and tightness of the gastrocnemius-soleus unit.[52] Wearing shoes without sufficient arch support, running with a lengthened stride, and running on soft surfaces are also potential causes of plantar fasciitis.[48]

Symptoms and signs The patient complains of pain in the anterior medial heel, usually at the attachment of the plantar fascia to the calcaneus (Figure 18–25). The pain eventually moves into the central portion

18–4 Clinical Application Exercise

A distance runner is experiencing pain in the left arch. There is palpable tenderness in the left foot's aponeurosis, primarily in the epicondyle region of the calcaneus.

? What condition does this scenario describe, and how should it be managed?

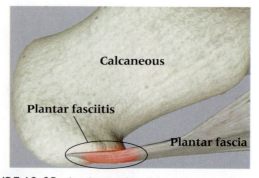

Calcaneous

Plantar fasciitis

Plantar fascia

FIGURE 18–25 In plantar fasciitis, pain usually develops at the attachment to the medial portion of the calcaneous.

Plantar Fasciitis

Injury Situation A marathon runner injured the proximal arch and heel when he stepped into a hole during a meet. The patient continued to run and work out for a week before reporting his injury to the athletic trainer.

Symptoms and Signs The patient complained of early pain in the medial arch and medial distal heel that tended to move centrally as the week progressed. He complained of severe pain when rising in the morning and after sitting for a long period. The area appeared slightly swollen with a severe, sharp pain on palpation at the plantar fascia insertion and medial aspect of the calcaneus. Pain increased with passive dorsiflexion of the great toe. An X-ray showed the beginning of a heel spur. The patient was found to have a cavus foot.

Management Plan The patient was diagnosed as having plantar fasciitis (heel spur syndrome), and a conservative plan was chosen.

Phase 1 *Acute Injury*　**GOALS:** Minimize inflammation and pain.
ESTIMATED LENGTH OF TIME (ELT): 1 week.

- **Therapy** RICE plus NSAID as needed to reduce pain and inflammation. Injection therapy consisting of a steroid and anesthetic for trigger points.
- **Exercise rehabilitation** Toe touch crutch walking. Begin heel cord stretching and rolling pin exercise to increase fascia flexibility.

Phase 2 *Repair*　**GOALS:** Gain full weight bearing and walking pattern.
ELT: 1 to 3 weeks.

- **Therapy** Ultrasound to increase blood flow. Cross-friction massage over injury site. Apply shock absorption shoe insert with cutout 1 to 2 inches (3 to 5 cm) in the tender area. Apply arch taping.
- **Exercise rehabilitation** Continue heel cord stretching and rolling pin exercise to stretch the plantar fascia. Begin a program of gradual pain-free weight bearing. Begin a program of foot flexor strengthening.

Phase 3 *Remodeling*　**GOALS:** Focus on full pain-free weight bearing while engaged in running.
ELT: 2 weeks.

- **Therapy** Ultrasound as warranted. Continue cross-friction massage. Use a heel cup and arch taping when athlete is supporting weight.
- **Exercise rehabilitation** Continue heel cord and plantar fascia stretching. Use shoes with a reinforced heel counter for heel control. Initiate foot flexor strengthening against tubular resistance. Perform general exercise to the lower leg. Begin a running program that is pain free.

Criteria for Return to Competitive Cross-Country Running

1. Proximal arch and heel are pain free.
2. Heel cord and plantar fascia are stretched.
3. Lower leg has maximum strength.
4. Patient is able to run competitively without pain.
5. Patient is psychologically ready for competition.

---

of the plantar fascia. This pain is increased when the patient rises in the morning or bears weight after sitting for a long period. However, the pain lessens after a few steps. Pain also will be intensified when the toes and forefoot are forcibly dorsiflexed. If irritation persists, a painful heel spur will probably develop at the attachment of the plantar fascia to the medial aspect of the calcaneus; the heel spur will be visible on an X-ray (Figure 18–26).

Management Management of plantar fasciitis generally requires an extended period of treatment.[61] It is not uncommon for symptoms to persist for as long as 8 to 12 weeks. Orthotic therapy is very useful in the treatment of this problem. A soft orthotic works better than a hard orthotic. An extra-deep heel cup should be built into the orthotic. The orthotic should be worn at all times, especially when the athlete rises from bed in the morning.[31] Use of a heel cup

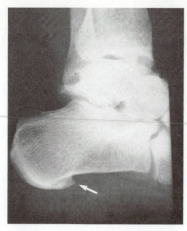

FIGURE 18–26   X-ray of a large plantar calcaneal exostotic spur.

compresses the fat pad under the calcaneus, providing a cushion under the area of irritation. When soft orthotics are not feasible, taping may reduce the symptoms. A simple arch taping or alternative taping often allows pain-free ambulation.[31] The use of a night splint to maintain a position of static stretch has also been recommended (Figure 18–27). In some cases, the athlete may need to use a short leg walking cast for 4 to 6 weeks.

The patient should engage in vigorous Achilles tendon stretching and in exercises that stretch the plantar fascia in the arch, such as rolling the plantar surface of the foot back and forth over a tennis ball, a baseball, or some other rigid, round surface.[62] Exercises that increase dorsiflexion of the great toe

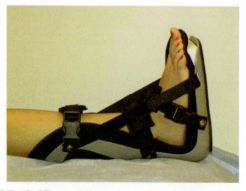

FIGURE 18–27   A night splint can be used to stretch the plantar fascia.

also may be of benefit for this problem. Stretching should be done at least three times a day. Antiinflammatory medications are recommended. Steroidal injection may be warranted at some point if symptoms fail to resolve.

Jones Fracture

Etiology   Fractures may occur to any of the metatarsals and can be caused by inversion and plantar flexion of the foot; by direct force, such as being stepped on; or by repetitive stress. By far the most common acute fracture is to the diaphysis at the base of the fifth metatarsal, which is referred to specifically as a Jones fracture (Figure 18–28).[46]

Symptoms and signs   A Jones fracture is characterized by immediate swelling and pain over the fifth metatarsal. Healing of a Jones fracture is slow and frustrating for the patient. This injury has a high nonunion rate, and the course of healing is unpredictable.[28] Nonunion fractures can occur as a result of several factors, including insufficient fracture immobilization (fixation), inadequate blood supply, chronic disease states (diabetes, renal failure, metabolic bone disease), fractures associated with tumors (pathological fractures), or infection. In a nonunion fracture, osteocytes and osteoblasts are replaced by chondroblasts. Thus, the fracture repairs itself by replacing what would normally be bone tissue with cartilage between the fractured bone ends.

Management   Treatment for a Jones fracture is controversial, but it appears that the use of crutches with no immobilization, gradually progressing to full weight bearing as pain subsides, may allow the patient to return to activity in about 6 weeks. However, nonunion may cause a refracture to occur. It has been recommended that patients be treated more aggressively using early internal fixation.[45] It has also been suggested that an electric or ultrasonic bone-growth stimulator will promote healing in a Jones fracture.[10]

Metatarsal Stress Fractures

Etiology   The most common metatarsal stress fracture in the foot involves the shaft of the second metatarsal and is often referred to as a *march fracture*. It occurs in the runner who has suddenly changed patterns of training, such as increasing mileage, running hills, or running on a harder surface. An individual who has an atypical condition,

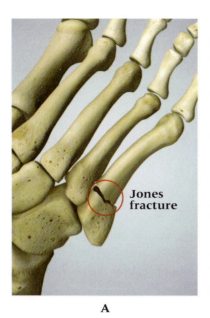 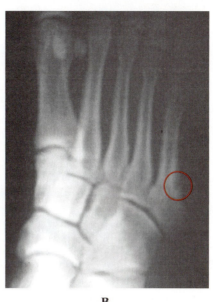

A

B

FIGURE 18–28 **(A)** A Jones fracture occurs at the neck of the fifth metatarsal. **(B)** Jones fracture X-ray.

such as a structural forefoot varus, hallux valgus, flat-foot, or short first metatarsal, is more predisposed to a second metatarsal stress fracture.[19,57]

A patient can also experience a stress fracture of the fifth metatarsal at the insertion of the peroneus brevis tendon, but this injury should not be confused with a Jones fracture.[4]

Symptoms and signs Over a 2 to 3-week period, dull pain begins to occur during exercise, then progresses to pain at rest. Pain is initially diffuse, then localizes to the site of the fracture. Patients usually report having increased the intensity or duration of their exercise program.

Management A bone scan is the best way to detect the presence of a stress fracture. Management of a metatarsal stress fracture usually consists of 2 to 4 days of partial weight bearing followed by 2 weeks of rest. Return to running should be very gradual. An orthotic that corrects excessive pronation can help take stress off the second metatarsal.[9]

Bunions (Hallux Valgus Deformities) and Bunionettes (Tailor's Bunions)?

Etiology A bunion, one of the most frequent painful deformities, occurs at the head of the first metatarsal (Figure 18–29). The term *bunion* is often used to refer to an exostosis. Commonly, a bunion is associated with a structural forefoot varus in which the first ray tends to splay outward, putting pressure on the first metatarsal head.[40] Bunions are often caused by shoes that are pointed, too narrow, or too short. It is generally believed that women's shoes play a predominant role in the development of a hallux valgus deformity.[16]

The bursa over the first metatarsophalangeal joint becomes inflamed and eventually thickens. Tendinitis may develop in the flexor tendons of the great toe.[47] The joint becomes enlarged and the great toe becomes malaligned, moving laterally toward the second toe, sometimes to such an extent that it eventually overlaps the second toe. This type of bunion is also associated with a depressed or flattened transverse arch and a pronated foot.

The bunionette, or tailor's bunion, is much less common than hallux valgus deformity, affecting the fifth metatarsophalangeal joint. In this case, the little toe angulates toward the fourth toe, causing an enlarged metatarsal head.[8]

In all bunions, both the flexor and extensor tendons are malaligned, creating more angular stress on the joint. NOTE: Sesamoid fractures and sesamoiditis can be secondary to hallux valgus.

Symptoms and signs In the beginning of bunion formation, there is tenderness, swelling, and enlargement of the joint. Poorly fitting shoes increase the irritation and pain. As the inflammation continues, angulation of the toe progresses, eventually leading to painful ambulation.

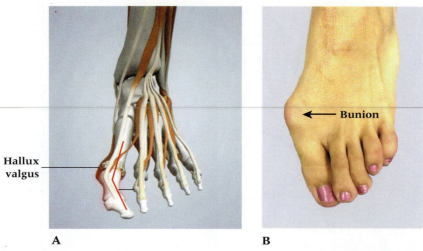

Hallux valgus

Bunion

A   B

FIGURE 18–29   (A) A Hallux valgus deformity often causes the development of a (B) bunion.

Management   Each bunion has unique characteristics. Early recognition and care can often prevent increased irritation and deformity. Following are some management procedures:

1. Wear correctly fitting shoes with a wide toe box.
2. Wear an appropriate orthotic to correct a structural forefoot varus deformity.
3. Place a felt or sponge rubber doughnut pad over the first and/or fifth metatarsophalangeal joint.
4. Wear a tape splint along with a resilient wedge placed between the great toe and the second toe (see Figure 18–28).
5. Engage in daily foot exercises to strengthen the extensor and flexor muscles. Ultimately, a surgical procedure called a bunionectomy may be necessary to correct the problem.

Sesamoiditis

Etiology   Two sesamoid bones lie within the flexors and adductor tendons of the great toe. These sesamoids transmit forces from the ground to the head of the first metatarsal. Sesamoiditis is caused by repetitive hyperextension of the great toe, which eventually results in inflammation. Sesamoiditis is most common in dancing and basketball. It is estimated that 30 percent of sesamoid injuries are sesamoiditis.[55] Fractures of the sesamoids are also common.

Symptoms and signs   The patient complains of pain under the great toe, especially during a push-off. There is palpable tenderness under the first metatarsal head.

Management   Sesamoiditis is treated with a variety of orthotic devices, including metatarsal pads, arch supports, and, most often, a metatarsal bar (Figure 18–30). Activity should be decreased to allow inflammation to subside.

Metatarsalgia

Etiology   Although *metatarsalgia* is a general term used to describe pain in the ball of the foot, it is more

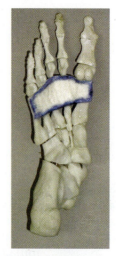

FIGURE 18–30   Metatarsal bar to treat both sesamoiditis and metatarsalgia.

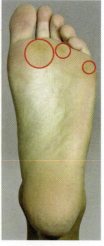

FIGURE 18–31   A heavy callus often forms under the metatarsal heads in metatarsalgia.

commonly associated with pain under the second and sometimes the third metatarsal head. A heavy callus often forms in the area of pain (Figure 18–31).[15]

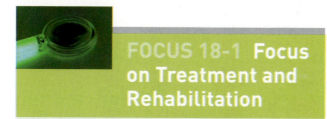

FOCUS 18-1 Focus on Treatment and Rehabilitation

Metatarsal pad support

The purpose of the metatarsal pad is to reestablish the normal relationships of the metatarsal bones. It can be purchased commercially or constructed out of felt or sponge rubber (Figure 18–34).

Materials needed

One roll of 1-inch (2.5 cm) tape, a ⅛-inch (0.3 cm) adhesive felt oval cut to a 2-inch (5 cm) circumference, and tape adherent.

Position of the patient

The patient sits on a table or chair with the plantar surface of the affected foot turned upward.

Position of the athletic trainer

The athletic trainer stands facing the plantar aspect of the patient's foot.

Procedure

1. The circular pad is placed just behind the metatarsal heads.
2. Approximately two or three circular strips of tape are placed loosely around the pad and foot.

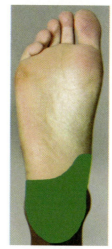

FIGURE 18–32 The Thomas heel extends anteriorly and elevates the medial aspect of the calcaneus ⅛ to ³⁄₁₆ inch (0.3 to 0.47 cm), which can help provide support to the medial longitudinal arch and relieve pronation and metatarsalgia.

gastrocnemius-soleus contracture should perform a regimen of static stretching several times per day. A patient whose metatarsal arch is depressed as a result of weakness should practice a daily regimen of exercise, concentrating on strengthening flexor and intrinsic muscles and stretching the Achilles tendon. A Thomas heel (Figure 18–32), which elevates the medial aspect of the heel from ⅛ to ³⁄₁₆ inch (0.3 to 0.47 cm) also could prove beneficial.

Metatarsal Arch Strain

Etiology The patient who has a fallen metatarsal arch or who has a pes cavus is susceptible to strain.[17] Normally, the heads of the first and fifth metatarsal bones bear slightly more weight than the heads of the second, third, and fourth metatarsal bones. The first metatarsal head bears one-third of the body weight, the fifth bears slightly more than one-sixth, and the second, third, and fourth each bear approximately one-sixth. If the foot tends to pronate excessively or if the intermetatarsal ligaments are weak, allowing the foot to spread abnormally (splayed foot), a fallen metatarsal arch may result (Figure 18–33).

Symptoms and signs The patient has pain or cramping in the metatarsal region. There is **point tenderness** and weakness in the area. Morton's test may produce pain in the metatarsals (see Figure 18–17).

> **point tenderness** Pain produced when an injury site is palpated.

Management Treatment of a metatarsal arch strain usually consists of applying a pad to elevate the depressed metatarsal heads. The pad is placed in the center and just behind the ball of the foot (metatarsal heads) (Figure 18–34).

One of the causes of metatarsalgia is restricted extensibility of the gastrocnemius-soleus complex. Because of this restriction, the patient shortens the midstance phase of the gait and emphasizes the toe-off phase, causing excessive pressure under the forefoot. This excess pressure over time causes a heavy callus to form in this region. As the forefoot bears weight, normal skin becomes pinched against the inelastic callus and produces pain.[15]

Another cause of metatarsalgia is a fallen metatarsal arch.

Symptoms and signs As the transverse arch becomes flattened and the heads of the second, third, and fourth metatarsal bones become depressed, pain can result. A cavus deformity can also cause metatarsalgia.

Management Management of metatarsalgia usually consists of applying a pad to elevate the depressed metatarsal heads. See *Focus Box 18–1: "Metatarsal Pad Support."* NOTE: The bar is placed behind and not under the metatarsal heads (Figure 18–30). Abnormal callus buildup should be removed by paring or filing. A patient for whom the etiology of metatarsalgia is primarily a

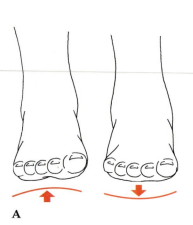 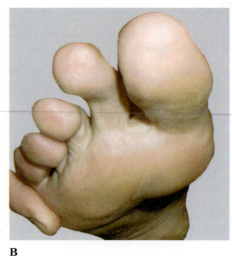

A B

FIGURE 18–33   **(A)** Normal and fallen metatarsal arch.
(B) Fallen metatarsal arch.

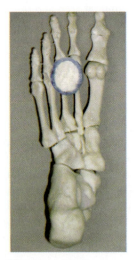

FIGURE 18–34   Metatarsal pad.

Morton's Neuroma

Etiology   Recall that a neuroma is a mass that occurs about the nerve sheath of the common plantar nerve at the point at which it divides into the two digital branches to adjacent toes. A neuroma usually occurs between the metatarsal heads and is the most common nerve problem of the lower extremity.[50] A Morton's neuroma is located between the third and fourth metatarsal heads where the nerve is the thickest because it receives branches from both the medial and the lateral plantar nerves (Figure 18–35A).[22]

Irritation increases with the collapse of the transverse arch of the foot, which puts the transverse metatarsal ligaments under stretch and thus compresses the common digital nerve and vessels. Excessive foot pronation can also be a predisposing factor, because more metatarsal shearing forces occur with the prolonged forefoot abduction.

Symptoms and signs   The patient complains of a burning paresthesia and severe intermittent pain in the forefoot that is often localized to the third web

space and radiating to the toes. The pain is often relieved with non–weight bearing.[31] Hyperextension of the toes on weight bearing, as in squatting, stair climbing, or running, can increase the symptoms. Wearing shoes with a narrow toe box or high heels can increase the symptoms. If there is prolonged nerve irritation, the pain can become constant.[22]

Management   A bone scan is often necessary to rule out a metatarsal stress fracture. A teardrop-shaped pad is placed between the heads of the third and fourth metatarsals in an attempt to splay the metatarsals apart during weight bearing, which decreases pressure on the neuroma (Figure 18–35B). Often, this teardrop pad markedly reduces pain, and the patient can continue to play despite this condition. Shoe selection also plays an important role in the treatment of neuromas. Narrow shoes, particularly women's shoes that are pointed in the toe area and certain men's boots, may squeeze the metatarsal heads together and exacerbate the problem. A shoe that is wide in the toe box area should be selected. A straight-laced shoe often provides increased space in the toe box.[66] On rare occasions, surgical excision may be required.

Injuries to the Toes

Sprained Toes

Etiology   Sprains of the phalangeal joints of the toes are caused most often by kicking some nonyielding object. Sprains result from a considerable force applied in such a manner as to extend the joint beyond its

A football player who commonly plays on artificial turf complains of pain in his right great toe.

? What type of injury frequently occurs to the great toe of an athlete who plays on artificial turf?

18–8 Clinical Application Exercise

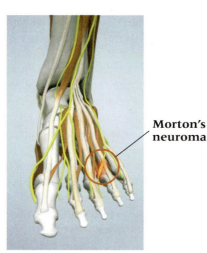

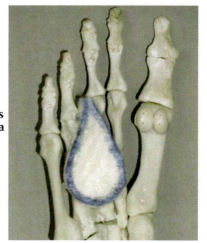

Morton's neuroma

A　　　　　**B**

FIGURE 18–35　**(A)** A Morton's neuroma between the third and fourth metatarsal heads can be treated using **(B)** a teardrop placed on the plantar surface of the foot as shown.

normal range of motion (jamming it) or to impart a twisting motion to the toe, thereby twisting and tearing the ligaments and joint capsule.

Symptoms and signs Pain is immediate and intense but is generally short lived. There is immediate swelling with discoloration appearing during the first or second day. Stiffness and residual pain may last for several weeks.

Management RICE must be applied immediately to minimize swelling. Casting or splinting of the small toes is difficult. Thus, buddy taping the injured toe to the adjacent toes is an effective technique of immobilization. The patient may begin weight bearing as soon as tolerated and may not need to be on crutches at all.

> Fractures and dislocations of the foot phalanges can be caused by kicking an object, stubbing a toe, or being stepped on.

Great Toe Hyperextension (Turf Toe)

Etiology A hyperextension of the great toe results in a sprain of the metatarsophalangeal joint, either from a single trauma or from repetitive overuse (Figure 18–36).[5] Typically, this injury occurs on unyielding synthetic turf, although it can occur on grass also. Many of these injuries occur because sports shoes made for use on artificial turf often are more flexible and allow more dorsiflexion of the great toe.

Symptoms and signs There is significant pain and swelling in and around the metatarsophalangeal joint of the great toe. Pain is exacerbated when the patient tries to push off the foot in walking and certainly in running and jumping.[16]

Management Some shoe companies have addressed this problem by adding steel or other materials to the forefoot of their turf shoes to stiffen them.[40] Flat insoles that have thin sheets of steel under the forefoot

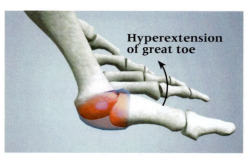

Hyperextension of great toe

FIGURE 18–36　A turf toe is a sprain of the metatarsophalangeal joint resulting from hyperextension of the great toe.

are also available. When commercially made products are not available, a thin, flat piece of thermoplastic (e.g., Orthoplast) may be placed under the shoe insole or may be molded to the foot. Taping the toe to prevent dorsiflexion may be done separately or with one of the shoe-stiffening suggestions (see Figure 8–27). Modalities of choice include ice and ultrasound. One of the major ingredients in any treatment for this injury is rest. The patient should be discouraged from returning to activity until the toe is pain free.

Fractures and Dislocations of the Phalanges

Etiology Fractures of the phalanges (Figure 18–37) usually occur by kicking an object, stubbing a toe, or being stepped on. Dislocations of the phalanges are less common than fractures. If one occurs, it is most likely to be a dorsal dislocation of the middle phalanx proximal joint. The mechanism of injury is the same as for fractures. Frequently, fractures and dislocations accompany one another.[2]

Symptoms and signs There is immediate, intense pain, which is increased when the toes are moved. In the case of a dislocation, deformity will be obvious. Swelling of the joint occurs rapidly, and there is subsequent discoloration in the area of injury.

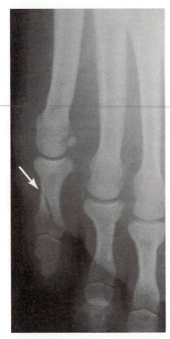

FIGURE 18–37 Fracture of the fifth phalanx.

Management Toe dislocations should be reduced by a physician. Casting of toe fractures and dislocations is unnecessary unless multiple toes are involved or unless the injury is a great toe fracture, in which case a cast may be applied for as long as 3 weeks. Otherwise, buddy taping of the injured toe to adjacent toes usually provides sufficient support.

Hallux Rigidus

Etiology Hallux rigidus is a painful condition caused by the proliferation of bony spurs on the dorsal aspect of the first metatarsophalangeal joint, resulting in impingement and a loss of both active and passive dorsiflexion.[40] Hallux rigidus is a degenerative arthritic process, resulting in changes to the articular cartilage of the metatarsal head and in synovitis. In running and jumping activities, dorsiflexion of the metatarsophalangeal joint in the great toe is essential and, if restricted, causes the foot to roll onto the lateral border to compensate.

Symptoms and signs The great toe is unable to dorsiflex, causing the patient to toe-off on the second, third, fourth, and fifth toes. Forced dorsiflexion increases pain. Walking becomes awkward because weight bearing is on the lateral aspect of the foot.

Management Management usually includes a stiffer shoe with a larger toe box. An orthosis similar to that worn for a turf toe may also be helpful. Antiinflammatory medication may help reduce the inflammatory response. An osteotomy (surgically removing a piece of bone) to remove the mechanical obstruction to dorsiflexion may allow the patient to return to a normal level of function.[40]

Hammertoe, Mallet Toe, and Claw Toe

Etiology Deformities of the smaller toes can be either fixed or flexible. A hammertoe is a flexible deformity that becomes fixed. It is caused by a flexion contracture at the proximal interphylangeal (PIP) joint (Figure 18–38A). A mallet toe is caused by a flexion contracture at the distal interphylangeal (DIP) joint involving the flexor digitorum longus tendon (Figure 18–38B). It also eventually becomes a fixed deformity in which a callus develops dorsally over the DIP joint or on the tip of the toe. In a claw toe, a flexion contracture develops at the DIP joint, but there is also a hyperextension at the metatarsophylangeal (MP) joint (Figure 18–38C). A callus develops over the PIP joint and under the metatarsal head. Deformities of the lesser toes may be congenital, but more often the conditions are caused by wearing shoes that are too short over a long period of time, thus cramping the toes.[47]

Symptoms and signs In all three conditions the MP, PIP, and/or DIP joints can become fixed. There may be blistering, swelling, pain, callus formation, and occasionally infection.

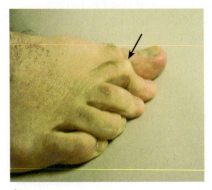
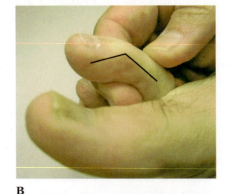
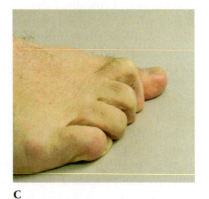

A   B   C

FIGURE 18–38 **(A)** Hammertoe. **(B)** Mallet toe. **(C)** Claw toes (all four toes).

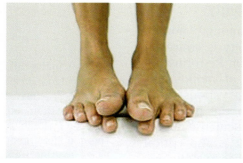

FIGURE 18–39   Overlapping toes.

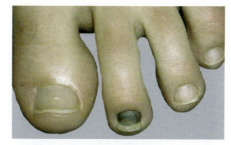

FIGURE 18–40   A subungual hematoma is blood accumulating under the nail.

Management   Conservative treatment involves relieving pressure over the toes by wearing footwear with more room for the toes. The use of padding and protective taping (see Figure 8–28) can help prevent irritation. Shaving the calluses may also help reduce skin irritation. Once the deformities become fixed, it is likely that surgical procedures that involve straightening the toes and then maintaining positioning by using K-wire (Kirshner wire) inserted longitudinally through the phalanges into the metatarsals will be necessary.[47]

Overlapping Toes
Etiology   Overlapping of the toes (Figure 18–39) may be congenital or may be brought about by improperly fitting footwear, particularly shoes that are too narrow.

Symptoms and signs   At times, the condition indicates an outward projection of the great toe articulation or a drop in the longitudinal or metatarsal arch.

Management   As in the case of hammertoes, surgery is the only cure, but some therapeutic modalities, such as a whirlpool bath, can assist in alleviating inflammation. Taping may prevent some of the contractural tension within the sport shoe.

Blood under the Toenail (Subungual Hematoma)
Etiology   Blood can accumulate under a toenail as a result of the toe being stepped on, dropping an object on the toe, or kicking another object. Repetitive shearing forces on toenails, as may occur in the shoe of a long-distance runner, may also cause bleeding into the nail bed. In any case, blood that accumulates in a confined space underneath the nail is likely to produce extreme pain and can ultimately cause loss of the nail (Figure 18–40).

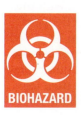

BIOHAZARD

Symptoms and signs   Bleeding into the nail bed may be either immediate or slow, producing considerable pain. The area under the toenail assumes a bluish-purple color and gentle pressure on the nail greatly exacerbates pain.

Management   An ice pack should be applied immediately, and the foot should be elevated to decrease bleeding. Within the next 12 to 24 hours, the pressure of the blood under the nail should be released by drilling a small hole through the nail into the nail bed. This drilling must be done under sterile conditions and is best done by either a physician or an athletic trainer. It is not uncommon to have to drill the nail a second time because more blood is likely to accumulate.

18–10 Clinical Application Exercise

A professional male soccer player is complaining about pain in the toes. Upon inspection, the athletic trainer observes that the second and third toes are heavily callused on the dorsal surface and on palpation realizes that the toes are stuck in a flexed, or clawlike, position.

? What is this condition, and what steps can be taken to correct this problem?

FOOT REHABILITATION

It is critical that the athletic trainer incorporate appropriate rehabilitation techniques in to the management of foot injuries. The foot is the base of support for the entire kinetic chain. Thus, injuries to the foot can affect the biomechanics of not only the foot but also the ankle, knee, hip, and spine.

General Body Conditioning

Rehabilitation techniques for managing injuries to the lower extremity in general and to the foot in particular often require that the patient be non–weight bearing for some period of time. Even if weight bearing is allowed, the injured athlete will not be able to maintain his or her level of fitness by engaging in running activities. Thus, it becomes necessary to substitute alternative conditioning activities, such as running in a pool or working on an upper-extremity ergometer (Figure 18–41).[31] The patient should certainly continue to engage in strengthening and flexibility exercises as allowed by the constraints of the injury.

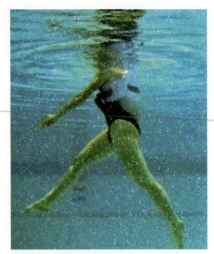

FIGURE 18–41   Pool exercises are useful in maintaining fitness while non–weight bearing.

Weight Bearing

If the patient is unable to walk without a limp, non–weight-bearing or limited weight-bearing crutch walking might be employed. Using incorrect gait mechanics certainly affects other joints within the kinetic chain, causing unnecessary pain, and tends to do more harm than good. Progressing to full weight bearing as soon as it is tolerated is generally recommended.

Joint Mobilization

Manual joint mobilization techniques are useful in maintaining or normalizing joint motions (Figure 18–42). The following joint mobilization techniques can be used in the foot:

- Anterior/posterior calcaneocuboid glides are used for increasing adduction and abduction. The calcaneus should be stabilized while the cuboid is mobilized.
- Anterior/posterior cuboidmetatarsal glides are done with one hand stabilizing the cuboid and the other gliding the base of the fifth metatarsal. These glides are used for increasing mobility of the fifth metatarsal.
- Anterior/posterior tarsometatarsal glides decrease hypomobility of the metatarsals.
- Anterior/posterior talonavicular glides also increase adduction and abduction. One hand stabilizes the talus while the other mobilizes the navicular bone.
- With anterior/posterior metatarsophalangeal glides, the anterior glides increase extension and the posterior glides increase flexion. Mobilizations are accomplished by isolating individual segments.

Flexibility

Maintaining normal flexibility is critical in the foot. Restoring full range of motion following various injuries to the phalanges is particularly important. It is also critical to engage in stretching activities in the case of plantar fasciitis (Figure 18–43). Stretching the gastrocnemius-soleus complex is also important for a number of injuries (see Figure 19–39).

Muscular Strength

Strength exercises for the foot can be done using a variety of resistance methods, including rubber tubing, towel exercises, and manual resistance.

The following are exercises commonly used in strengthening the muscles involved in foot motion:

- Writing the alphabet. With the toes pointed, the athlete writes the complete alphabet in the air three times.
- Picking up objects. The patient picks up small objects, such as marbles, with the toes and places them in a container.
- Ankle circumduction. The ankle is circumducted in as extreme a range of motion as possible (10 circles in one direction and 10 circles in the other).
- Gripping and spreading the toes. Gripping and spreading is repeated for up to 10 repetitions (Figure 18–44).
- Towel gathering. A towel is extended in front of the feet. The heels are firmly planted on the floor, with the forefoot on the end of the towel. The patient then attempts to pull the towel, with the feet, without lifting the heels from the floor. As execution becomes easier, a weight can be placed at the other end of the towel for added resistance. Each exercise should be performed 10 times (Figure 18–45A). This exercise can also be used for exercising the foot in abduction and adduction.

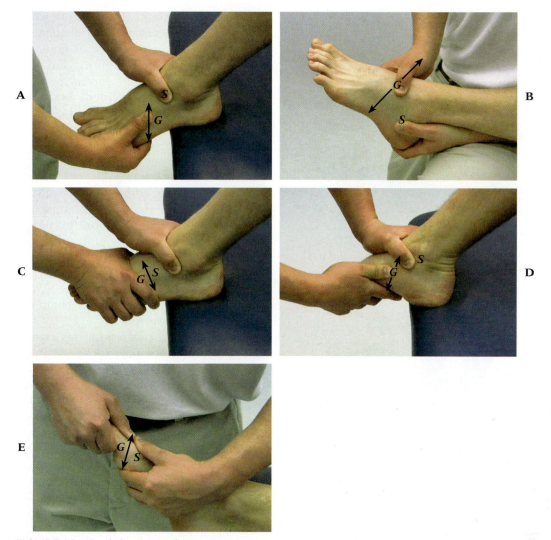

FIGURE 18–42 **(A)** Anterior/posterior calcaneocuboid glides. **(B)** Anterior/posterior cuboid-metatarsal glides. **(C)** Anterior/posterior tarsometatarsal glides. **(D)** Anterior/posterior talonavicular glides. **(E)** Anterior/posterior metatarsophalangeal glides. (S = stabilize, G = glide).

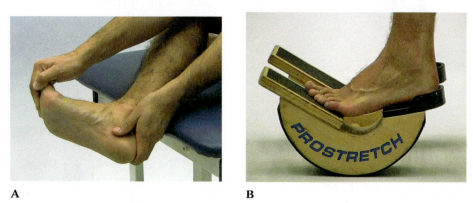

FIGURE 18–43 Plantar fascia stretches. **(A)** Manual. **(B)** Prostretch.

- Towel scoop. A towel is folded in half and placed sideways on the floor. The patient places the heel firmly on the floor and the forefoot on the end of the towel. To ensure the greatest stability of the exercising foot, it is backed up with the other foot. Without lifting the heel from the floor, the athlete scoops the towel forward with the forefoot. Again, a weight resistance can be added to the end of the towel. The exercise should be repeated up to 10 times (Figure 18–45B).

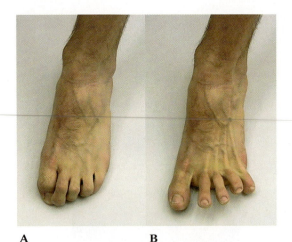

FIGURE 18–44 **(A)** Gripping and **(B)** spreading of the toes can be an excellent rehabilitation exercise for the injured foot.

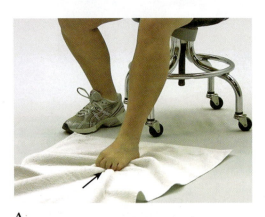

A

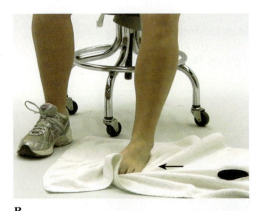

B

FIGURE 18–45 **(A)** Towel gathering exercise. **(B)** Towel scoop exercise.

Neuromuscular Control

Reestablishing neuromuscular control following foot injury is a critical component of the rehabilitative process and should not be overlooked. Although maintaining neuromuscular control while weight bearing may appear to be a rather simple motor skill for uninjured patients, neuromuscular control is compromised when injuries occur.

Muscular weakness, proprioceptive deficits, and range of motion deficits may challenge a patient's ability to maintain a center of gravity within the body's base of support, causing the patient to lose balance. Neuromuscular control in the foot is the single most important element dictating movement strategies within the closed kinetic chain. The capability of adjusting and adapting to changing surfaces while creating a stable base of support is perhaps the most important function of the foot in weight bearing.[31]

Neuromuscular control is a highly integrative, dynamic process involving multiple neurological pathways. Neuromuscular control relative to joint position sense, proprioception, and kinesthesia is essential to all performance but is particularly important to those activities that require weight bearing. Current rehabilitation protocols are therefore focusing more on closed kinetic chain exercises and neuromuscular control.

Exercises for reestablishing neuromuscular control in the foot should expose the injured patient to a variety of walking, running, and hopping exercises involving directional changes performed on varying surfaces. Balance board or wobble exercises can be useful to establish a dynamic base of support (Figure 18–46).

Exercise sandals can be incorporated into rehabilitation as a closed kinetic chain functional exercise that places increased proprioceptive demands on the patient.[6] The exercise sandals are wooden sandals with a rubber hemisphere located centrally on the plantar surface (Figure 18–47A). The patient can progress into the exercise sandals once he or she demonstrates proficiency in a barefoot single-leg stance. Prior to using the exercise sandals, the patient is instructed in the "short-foot concept"—a shortening of the foot in an anterior/posterior direction while the long toe flexors are relaxed, thus activating the short toe flexors and foot intrinsics (Figure 18–48). Clinically, the short foot appears to

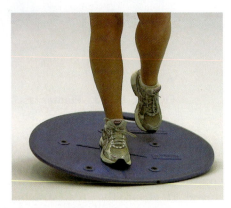

FIGURE 18–46 BAPS board exercises.

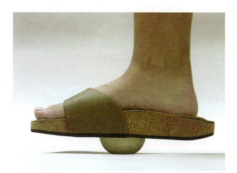

A

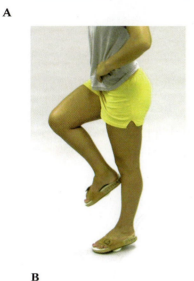

B

FIGURE 18–47 Exercise sandals are used to increase muscle activation and neuromuscular control in the foot. (OPTP Minneapolis)

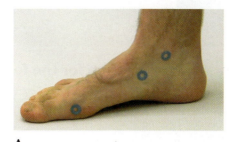

A

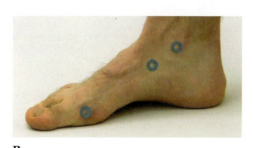

B

FIGURE 18–48 Short-foot concept. **(A)** Foot relaxed. **(B)** Intrinsic muscles contracted, shortening and elevating the arch.

enhance the longitudinal and transverse arches of the foot. Once the patient can perform the short-foot concept in the sandals, he or she progresses to walking in place and forward walking with short steps (see Figure 18–47B). The exercise sandals are excellent for increasing muscle activation in the foot and lower leg.[6]

Foot Orthotics and Taping

Throughout this chapter, references have been made to taping techniques and to the use of orthotics as means of providing additional support or correcting biomechanical abnormalities. Taping techniques are thoroughly discussed in Chapter 8, and the use of orthotics was discussed briefly earlier in this chapter. This section expands on the discussion of orthotic use relative to the various injuries described in this chapter.

The use of orthotics to correct foot deformities is a common practice by athletic trainers.[38] The normal foot functions most efficiently when no deformities are present that predispose it to injury or exacerbate existing injuries. Orthotics are used to control abnormal compensatory movements of the foot by "bringing the floor up to meet the foot."[30]

The foot functions most efficiently in a neutral position. By providing support so that the foot does not have to move abnormally, an orthotic should help prevent compensatory problems.[18] For problems that have already occurred, the orthotic provides a platform of support so that soft tissues can heal properly without undue stress (see Figure 7–26).[59]

Basically, there are three types of orthotics:[31]

1. Pads and flexible felt supports, referred to as *soft orthotics*. These soft inserts are readily fabricated and are advocated for mild overuse syndromes. Pads are particularly useful in shoes, such as spikes and ski boots, that are too narrow to hold orthotics.

2. *Semirigid orthotics* made of flexible thermoplastics, rubber, or leather.[44] These orthotics are prescribed for athletes who have increased symptoms. These orthotics are molded from a neutral cast. They are well tolerated by patients whose sports require speed or jumping.[21]

3. Functional, or *rigid, orthotics* are made from hard plastic and require neutral casting.[24] These orthotics allow control for most overuse symptoms.

Many athletic trainers make a neutral mold, put it in a box, mail it to an orthotic laboratory, and several weeks later receive an orthotic in the mail. Others like to construct the entire orthotic from start to finish, which requires a more skilled technician than does the mail-in method.[24]

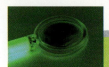
Functional progression for the foot

- Non–weight bearing
- Partial weight bearing
- Full weight bearing
- Walking
  Normal
  Heel
  Toe
  Side step/shuffle slides
- Jogging
  Straightaways on track
  Walk turns
  Jog complete oval of track
- Short sprints
- Acceleration/deceleration sprints
- Carioca
- Hopping
  Two feet
  One foot
  Alternate
- Cutting, jumping, hopping on command

A. Forefoot Varus   **B. Forefoot Valgus**   **C. Rearfoot Varus**

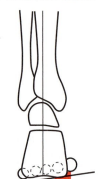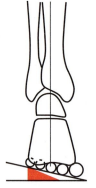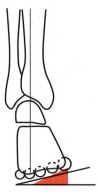

FIGURE 18–49   **(A)** Medial wedge for forefoot varus. **(B)** Lateral wedge for forefoot valgus. **(C)** Medial wedge for rearfoot varus.

Orthotics for Correcting Excessive Pronation and Supination To correct a structural forefoot varus deformity in which the foot excessively pronates, the orthotic should be the rigid type and should have a medial wedge under the head of the first metatarsal (Figure 18–49A).[26] It is also advisable to add a small wedge under the medial calcaneus to make the orthotic more comfortable.

Conversely, to correct a structural forefoot valgus deformity in which the foot excessively supinates, the orthotic should be semirigid and have a lateral wedge under the head of the fifth metatarsal (Figure 18–49B). Again, adding a small wedge under the lateral calcaneus will make the orthotic more comfortable.

To correct a structural rearfoot varus deformity, the orthotic should be semirigid and have a wedge under the medial calcaneus and a small wedge under the head of the first metatarsal (Figure 18–49C).[57]

Functional Progressions

Patients engage in functional progressions following injury to the foot in order to gradually regain the ability to walk, jog, run, change directions, and hop.[42] *Focus Box 18–2:* "Functional progression for the foot" details an appropriate functional progression for an injury to the foot.

SUMMARY

- The function of the foot is critical in running, jumping, and changing direction, and the complex nature of the anatomical structures of this body part makes recognition and management of foot injuries a major challenge to the athletic trainer.

- Many chronic and overuse injuries to the lower extremity can be related to faulty biomechanics of the foot because the foot is the part of the kinetic chain that is in direct contact with the ground.

- Essential movements that occur in the foot include pronation and supination, dorsiflexion and plantar flexion, adduction and abduction, and inversion and eversion.
- Foot injuries can best be prevented by selecting appropriate footwear, by correcting biomechanical structural deformities through the use of appropriate orthotics, and by paying attention to appropriate foot hygiene and care.
- Assessment of an injury to the foot includes a history and a palpation of soft-tissue and bony structures. In addition, observation should include a check for existing structural deformities, including forefoot varus, which might cause excessive pronation; forefoot valgus, which causes excessive supination; and rearfoot varus, which contributes to excessive pronation.
- Injuries to the foot can be classified into three categories: injuries to the tarsal region; injuries to the metatarsal region, including the arches; and injuries to the toes.
- A patient engaging in rehabilitation of an injury to the foot should maintain general body conditioning and should engage in exercises designed to regain essential joint mobility, strength, flexibility, and neuromuscular control through a series of functional progressions that gradually increase stress to the injured structures.
- The use of orthotics and taping techniques can be essential in treating many foot injuries.

WEB SITES

American College of Foot and Ankle Surgeons: www.acfas.org
Podiatric physicians and surgeons provide information on topics related to foot health.

Dr. Pribut's Running Injuries Page: www.drpribut.com/sports/spsport.html
This page lists common running injuries of the foot, ankle, knee, and hip.

Medline Plus: Foot & Ankle Disorders: www.nlm.nih.gov/medlineplus/footinjuriesanddisorders.html
This site can be a resource for many athletes related to foot injuries.

Premiere Medical Search Engine: http://www.medscape.com/
This site allows the reader to enter any medical condition and will search the Internet to find relevant articles.

Wheeless' Textbook of Orthopaedics: www.wheelessonline.com
This Web page is great for injuries, anatomy, and X-rays.

SOLUTIONS TO CLINICAL APPLICATION EXERCISES

18–1 A forefoot valgus deformity can cause excessive or prolonged supination. This condition may limit the ability of the foot and lower extremity to absorb ground reaction forces, resulting in injury. These injuries include inversion ankle sprains, tibial stress syndrome, peroneal tendinitis, iliotibial band friction syndrome, and trochanteric bursitis. The athlete can use an orthotic to correct this biomechanical problem or wear proper footwear with extra cushioning and flexibility.

18–2 Sever's disease is a traction injury to the apophysis of the calcaneal tubercle where the Achilles tendon attaches. The circulation becomes disrupted, resulting in a degeneration of the epiphyseal region.

18–3 It is likely that this athlete has a forefoot varus. To correct a structural forefoot varus deformity where the foot excessively pronates, the orthotic should be the rigid type and should have a medial wedge under the head of the first metatarsal. It is also advisable to add a small wedge under the medial calcaneus to make the orthotic more comfortable. The athletic trainer should also recommend that this patient purchase a board-lasted shoe with a medial heel wedge and a firm heel counter.

18–4 This condition is characteristic of a plantar fascial strain. It should be managed symptomatically. A doughnut placed over the epicondyle region, a heel lift, and a shoe with a stiff shank may relieve some pain. The patient should stretch the plantar muscles and gastrocnemius and perform arch exercises. Application of LowDye taping for pronation can also relieve pain.

18–5 A lateral sprain can produce an avulsion fracture of the proximal head of the fifth metatarsal bone.

18–6 Management of this stress fracture usually consists of 3 or 4 days' partial weight bearing followed by 2 weeks of rest. Return to running should be very gradual. An orthotic that corrects excessive pronation can help take stress off the second metatarsal.

18–7 This condition is a bunion, or hallux valgus deformity. It is associated with wearing dance shoes that are too pointed, narrow, or short. It may begin with an inflamed bursa over the metatarsophalangeal joint. It can be associated with a depressed transverse arch or a pronated foot.

18–8 A sprain of the first metatarsophalangeal joint (turf toe) stems from hyperextension, usually because of the unyielding surface of artificial turf. This injury is a tear of the joint capsule from the metatarsal head.

18–9 Kicking the locker with the great toe could cause a fracture of the proximal or distal phalanx. This injury may develop swelling, discoloration, and point tenderness.

18–10 This condition could be either hammertoes, mallet toes, or claw toes. It is likely that this condition developed from years of wearing shoes that were too tight or small. The athletic trainer could try padding the toes and recommend that the player wear a pair of shoes that has a larger toe box for the rest of the season. It is likely that, to permanently correct this problem, the soccer player will have to have surgery after the season.

18–11 Metatarsalgia can be caused by a restricted gastrocnemius-soleus complex that produces a pes cavus. It can also be caused by a fallen metatarsal arch that abnormally depresses the second or third metatarsal head and causes a heavy callus to develop.

18–12 The police officer has a Morton's neuroma. Conservatively, it is treated by having the patient wear a broad-toed shoe, a transverse arch support, and a metatarsal bar or teardrop pad.

REVIEW QUESTIONS AND CLASS ACTIVITIES

1. Describe the anatomy of the foot.
2. How does the foot function during the gait cycle?
3. How can an injury on the plantar surface of the foot cause soreness and pain in the knee?
4. Demonstrate an appropriate procedure for assessing injuries of the foot.
5. How does a structural forefoot varus deformity cause an individual to pronate excessively?
6. Identify the types of acute strains that occur in the region of the foot. How can they be prevented? How can they be managed?
7. What are the common fractures that occur in the foot, and how can they be managed?
8. How does plantar fasciitis occur, and what measures should be taken to treat it?
9. Where are the two most likely places for an exostosis to occur in the foot?
10. What is the difference between a pes cavus and a pes planus foot?
11. What is the difference between a Morton's toe and a Morton's neuroma?
12. How is a hallux valgus deformity related to excessive pronation?
13. Why does a Jones fracture often take such a long time to heal?
14. How would you construct the most appropriate orthotic for a patient who supinates excessively? Why?

REFERENCES

1. Allen R, Gross M: Toe flexors strength and passive extension range of motion of the first metatarsophalangeal joint in individuals with plantar fasciitis, *J Orthop Sports Phys Ther* 33(8):468, 2003.
2. Anderson R: 2010. Management of common sports-related injuries about foot and ankle, *Journal of the American Academy of Orthopedic Surgeons* 18(10):546–56.
3. Baker C, Deese M: Diagnostic and operative ankle arthroscopy. In Porter DM, editor: *Baxter's the foot and ankle in sports*, St. Louis, 2007, Mosby.
4. Bender J: Fifth metatarsal fractures: diagnosis and management, *Sports Medicine Alert* 6(3):18, 2000.
5. Bender J: Turf toe injuries: Correctly diagnosing an uncommon injury, *Sports Medicine Alert* 6(4):28, 2000.
6. Blackburn T, Hirth C, Guskiewicz K: Exercise sandals increase lower extremity electromyographic activity during functional activities, *J Athl Train* 38(3):198, 2003.
7. Bolgla L, Malone T: Plantar fasciitis and the windlass mechanism: A biomechanical link to clinical practice, *J Athl Train* 39(1):77, 2004.
8. Bruckner P: Foot pain. In Bruckner P, editor: *Clinical sports medicine*, Sydney, 2010, McGraw-Hill.
9. Cobb S: Custom-molded foot orthosis intervention and multisegment medial foot kinematics during walking, *J Athl Train* 46(4):358–65, 2011.
10. Conner C: Use of an ultrasonic bone growth stimulator to promote healing of a Jones fracture, *Athletic Therapy Today* 8(1):37, 2003.
11. Cornwall M: Common pathomechanics of the foot, *Athletic Therapy Today* 5(1):10, 2000.
12. Cornwall MW, McPoil TG: Plantar fasciitis: Etiology and treatment, *J Orthop Sports Phys Ther 2* 9(12):756, 2000.

13. Cote K, Brunet M, Gansneder B: Effects of pronated and supinated foot postures on static and dynamic postural stability, *J Athl Train* 40(1):41, 2005.
14. Dolan MG: Preventing lower extremity injury with foot orthoses, *Athletic Therapy and Training* 17(1):17–19, 2012.
15. Espinosa N: Metatarsalgia, *Journal of the American Academy of Orthopedic Surgeons* 18(8):474–85, 2010.
16. Fair J: Turf toe injuries: Continuing to increase despite decline in artificial surfaces, *Sports Med Update* 15(1):8, 2000.
17. Ferber R: Suspected mechanisms in the cause of overuse running injuries: A clinical review, *Sports Health* 1(3):242-46, 2009.
18. Genova JM, Gross MT: Effect of foot orthotics on calcaneal eversion during standing and treadmill walking for subjects with abnormal pronation, *J Orthop Sports Phys Ther* 30(11):664, 2000.
19. Glasoe W, Allen M, Kepros T: Dorsal first ray mobility in women athletes with a history of stress fracture of the second or third metatarsal, *J Orthop Sports Phys Ther* 32(11):560, 2002.
20. Glasoe WM, Allen MK, Ludewig PM: Comparison of first ray dorsal mobility among different forefoot alignments, *J Orthop Sports Phys Ther* 30(10):612, 2000.
21. Gross M, Byers J, Krafft J: The impact of custom semirigid foot orthotics on pain and disability for individuals with plantar fasciitis, *J Orthop Sports Phys Ther* 32(4):149, 2002.
22. Gulick DT: Differential diagnosis of Morton's neuroma, *Athletic Therapy Today* 7(1):38, 2002.
23. Hargrave M, Carcia C, Gansneder B: Subtalar pronation does not influence impact forces or rate of loading during a single-leg landing, *J Athl Train* 38(1):18, 2003.
24. Henry T, Cohen L: Fabricating foot orthotics, *Athletic Therapy Today* 5(1):22, 2000.

25. Hertel J, Gay J, Denegar C: Differences in postural control during single-leg stance among healthy individuals with different foot types, *J Athl Train* 37(2):129, 2002.
26. Houghlum PA, Carcia CR: Prefabricated foot orthotics decrease internal tibial rotation during hopping in females (abstract), *J Athl Train* 39(2 Suppl):S-29, 2004.
27. Hopton B: Fractures of the foot and ankle, *Surgery (Oxford)* 28(10):502–507, 2010.
28. Hunt K: Treatment of Jones fracture nonunions and refractures in the elite athlete, *American Journal of Sports Medicine* 39(9):1948–54, 2011.
29. Hunter S, Burnett G: Subtalar joint neutral and orthotic fitting, *Athletic Therapy Today* 5(1):6, 2000.
30. Hunter S, Dolan M, Davis M: *Foot orthotics in therapy and sport*, Champaign, IL, 1996, Human Kinetics.
31. Hunter S, Prentice W, Zinder S: Rehabilitation of foot injuries. In Prentice WE, editor: *Rehabilitation techniques in sports medicine and athletic training*, ed 5, New York, 2010, McGraw-Hill.
32. Hurwitz S: *Musculoskeletal examination of the foot and ankle: Making the complex simple*, Thorofare, NJ, 2011, Slack
33. Jones M, Amendola A: Navicular stress fractures, *Clin Sports Med* 25(1):151, 2006.
34. Jungers W: Biomechanics: Barefoot running strikes back, *Nature* 463:433–34, 2010.
35. Kangas J: New approach to the diagnosis and classification of chronic foot and ankle disorders: Identifying motor control and movement impairments, *Manual Therapy* 6(6):522–30, 2011.
36. Karagounis P: Treatment of plantar fasciitis in recreational athletes: Two different therapeutic protocols, *Foot and Ankle Specialists* 4(4):226–34, 2011.
37. Kindred J: Foot injuries in runners, *Current Sports Medicine Reports,* 10(5):249–54, 2011.

38. MacLean C: Short and long-term effects of a custom foot orthotic intervention on lower extremity dynamics, *Clinical Journal of Sport Medicine* 18(4):338–43, 2008.

39. Mancuso J, Cuskiewicz K, Petschauer M: Posterior foot pain in a collegiate field-hockey player, *J Sport Rehabil* 11(1):67, 2002.

40. Mann RA: Great toe disorders. In Porter DM, editor: *Baxter's the foot and ankle in sports*, St. Louis, 2007, Mosby.

41. McCarvey W, Burns M, Clanton T: Calcaneal fractures: Indirect reduction and external fixation, *Foot and Ankle International* 27(7):494, 2006.

42. McGee M: Functional progressions and functional testing in rehabilitation. In Prentice WE, editor: *Rehabilitation techniques in sports medicine and athletic training*, ed 5, St. Louis, 2010, McGraw-Hill.

43. Meyer J, Kulig K, Landel R: Differential diagnosis and treatment of subcalcaneal heel pain: A case report, *J Orthop Sports Phys Ther* 32(3):114, 2002.

44. Minert D: Foot orthoses: Materials and manufacturers, *Athletic Therapy Today* 5(1):27, 2000.

45. Mologne T: Acute Jones fractures: Operative versus non-operative treatment, *Orthopedic Trauma Directions* 7(2):1–8, 2009.

46. Mologne T, Lundeen J, Clapper M: Early screw fixation versus casting in treatment of acute Jones fractures, *Am J Sports Med* 33(7):970, 2005.

47. Nachazel KMJ: Mechanism and treatment of tendinitis of the flexor hallucis longus in classical ballet dancers, *Athletic Therapy Today* 7(2):13, 2002.

48. Neufield S: Plantar fasciitis: Evaluation and treatment, *Journal of the American Academy of Orthopedic Surgeons*, 16(6):338–46, 2008.

49. Newsham K: Strengthening the intrinsic foot muscles, *Athletic Therapy and Training* 15(1): 2010.

50. Norris R: Common foot and ankle injuries in dancers. In Solomon R, editor: *Preventing dance injuries*, ed 2, Champaign, IL, 2005, Human Kinetics.

51. Olmsted L, Hertel J: Influence of foot type and orthotics on static and dynamic postural control, *J Sport Rehabil* 13(1):54, 2004.

52. Patla CE, Abbott JH: Tibialis posterior myofascial tightness as a source of heel pain: Diagnosis and treatment, *J Orthop Sports Phys Ther* 30(10):624, 2000.

53. Peterson J: 10 steps for preventing and treating foot problems, *ACSM's Health and Fitness Journal* 6(2):44, 2002.

54. Perry J: *Gait analysis: Normal and pathological function*, Thorofare, NJ, 2010, Slack.

55. Petrizzi MJ, Richardson DG: Foot Injuries. In Birrer RB, O'Connor FG, editor: *Sports medicine for the primary care physician*, ed 3, Boca Raton, FL, 2004, CRC Press.

56. Pfeffer GB: Plantar heel pain. In Porter DM, editor: *Baxter's the foot and ankle in sports*, St. Louis, 2007, Mosby.

57. Pommering T: Ankle and foot injuries in pediatric and adult athletes, *Primary Care* 32(1):133–61, 2005.

58. Roney J: Management strategies for cuboid syndrome, *Athletic Therapy and Training* 15(5):10–13, 2010.

59. Rose J, Shultz S, Arnold B: Acute orthotic intervention does not affect muscular response times and activation patterns at the knee, *J Athl Train* 37(2):133, 2002.

60. Sandrey J, Zebas C, Bast J: Rear-foot motion in soccer players with excessive pronation under 4 experimental conditions, *J Sport Rehabil* 10(2):143, 2001.

61. Schnirring L, Mees PD: New treatment for plantar fasciitis, *Physician Sportsmed* 29(3):16, 2001.

62. Shea M: Plantar fasciitis: describing effective treatments, *Physician Sportsmed* 30(7):21, 2002.

63. Sherman KP: The foot in sport, *British Journal of Sports Medicine* 33(1):6, 1999.

64. Shindle M: Stress fractures about the tibia, foot, and ankle, *Journal of the American Academy of Orthopedic Surgeons* 20(3):167–76, 2012.

65. Simpson M: Tendonopathies of the foot and ankle, *American Family Physician*, 80(10): 1107–14, 2009.

66. Swanik C: Orthotics in sports medicine, *Athletic Therapy Today* 5(1):5, 2000.

67. Tiller R: Prevention of common pes problems, *Athletic Therapy Today* 7(6):52, 2002.

68. Valmassy R: *Clinical biomechanics of the lower extremities*, St. Louis, 1996, Mosby.

69. Wadsworth D, Eadie N: Conservative management of subtle Lisfranc joint injury: A case report, *J Orthop Sports Phys Ther* 35(3):54, 2005.

70. Whittle M: An *introduction to gait analysis*, Waltham, MA, 2007, Butterworth and Heinemann.

ANNOTATED BIBLIOGRAPHY

Alexander I: *The foot: examination and diagnosis*, New York, 1997, Churchill-Livingston.

A practical guide to clinical care of the foot and ankle; presents anatomy, biomechanics, and a systematic approach to evaluation and discusses common complaints.

Baxter DE: *The foot and ankle in sport*, St. Louis, 1995, Mosby.

A complete medical text addressing all aspects of the foot and ankle. Covers common sports syndromes, anatomical disorders in sports, unique problems, athletic shoes, orthoses, and rehabilitation.

Donatelli R: *The biomechanics of the foot and ankle*, Philadelphia, 1995, F.A. Davis.

A practical book for the therapist working directly with the patient.

Tremaine MD, Elias M: *The foot and ankle source book: everything you need to know*, New York, 1998, Contemporary Books.

Discusses common problems affecting feet and ankles, from bunions and corns to flat feet and sports injuries. Surveys the range of problems, preventive treatments, orthopedic inserts, and other health solutions to foot ailments, providing an uncommon range of disorders and treatments from self-help to surgery.

Weatherford ML: *Podiatry sourcebook*, Detroit, 2001, Omnigraphics.

Basic consumer health information about foot conditions, disease, and injuries, including bunions, corns, calluses, athlete's foot, plantar warts, hammertoes and claw toes, clubfoot, heel pain, gout, and more, along with facts about foot care, disease prevention, foot safety, choosing a foot care specialist, a glossary of terms, and resource listings for additional information.

Wolman R, Saifuddin A, Betts A: *Sports injuries: the foot, ankle and lower leg*, CD-ROM, 2003, Primal Picture Ltd.

Provides a 3-D study of the anatomy of the foot and ankle and discusses a variety of injuries related to the anatomy.

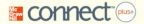

19

The Ankle and Lower Leg

■ Connect Highlights   **Mc Graw Hill** **connect**™ plus+

Visit connect.mcgraw-hill.com for further exercises to apply your knowledge:

- Clinical application scenarios covering assessment of the ankle and lower leg, etiology, symptoms and signs, and management of ankle and lower leg injuries, and rehabilitation for the ankle and lower leg
- Click-and-drag questions covering structural anatomy of the ankle and lower leg, assessment of ankle and lower leg injuries, and rehabilitation plan for the ankle and lower leg
- Multiple-choice questions covering anatomy, assessment, etiology, management, and rehabilitation of ankle and lower leg injuries
- Selection questions covering rehabilitation plan for various injuries to the ankle and lower leg
- Video identification of special tests for ankle and lower leg injuries, rehabilitation techniques for the ankle and lower leg, taping and wrapping for ankle and lower leg injuries
- Picture identification of major anatomical components of the ankle and lower leg, rehabilitation techniques of the ankle and lower leg, and therapeutic modalities for management

Like the foot, the ankle and lower leg are common sites of injury in the physically active population.[62] Ankle injuries, especially to the stabilizing ligaments, are the most frequent injuries in physical activity. This chapter focuses on traumatic and overuse injuries in the ankle and lower leg.

ANATOMY OF THE ANKLE AND LOWER LEG

Bones

The portion of the lower extremity that lies between the knee and the ankle is defined as the lower leg and contains two bones, the tibia and the fibula. The bones that form the ankle joint are the distal portion of the tibia, the distal portion of the fibula, and the talus. The calcaneus also plays a critical role in the function of the ankle joint.

Tibia With the exception of the femur, the tibia is the longest bone in the body. It serves as the principal weight-bearing bone of the leg. It is located on the medial side of the lower leg. The tibia is triangular in its upper two-thirds but is rounded and more constricted in the lower third. The most pronounced change occurs in the lower third of the shaft and produces an anatomical weakness that establishes this area as the site of most fractures occurring to the leg. The shaft of the tibia has three surfaces: posterior, medial, and lateral. The posterior and lateral surfaces are covered by muscle; the medial surface is subcutaneous and, as a result, is vulnerable to outside trauma (Figure 19–1).

Fibula The fibula is long and slender and is located along the lateral aspect of the tibia, joining it in an arthrodial articulation at the upper end, just below the knee joint, and as a **syndesmotic joint** at the lower end. Both the upper and the lower tibiofibular joints are held in position by strong anterior and posterior ligaments. The main function of the fibula is to provide for the attachment of muscles.

syndesmotic joint An articulation in which the bones are united by a ligament.

Tibial and Fibular Malleoli The thickened distal ends of both the tibia and the fibula are referred to as the medial malleolus and lateral malleolus, respectively. The lateral malleolus of the fibula extends farther distally, so that the stability created by the bony arrangement at the ankle joint is greater on the lateral aspect of the ankle than on the medial aspect (Figure 19–1).

Talus The talus, the second largest tarsal and the main weight-bearing bone of the articulation, rests on the calcaneus and receives the articulating surfaces of the lateral and medial malleoli. The talus forms a link between the lower leg and the foot, or tarsus (Figure 19–2).

Calcaneus The calcaneus is one of the tarsal bones and was discussed in Chapter 18. The calcaneus is the bone that forms the heel and to which many of the supporting ligaments of the ankle joint, as well as the Achilles tendon, attach (Figure 19–2).

Articulations

Superior and Inferior Tibiofibular Joints The tibia and fibula articulate with one another superiorly and inferiorly (tibiofibular joints). The superior tibiofibular joint is diarthrotic, allowing some gliding movements. The articulation is formed by the tibia's lateral condyle and the head of the fibula. It is surrounded by a fibrous capsule reinforced with anterior and posterior ligaments. The superior tibiofibular joint is stronger in front than in back (see Figure 19–1).

The inferior tibiofibular joint is a fibrous articulation. The articulation is between the lateral

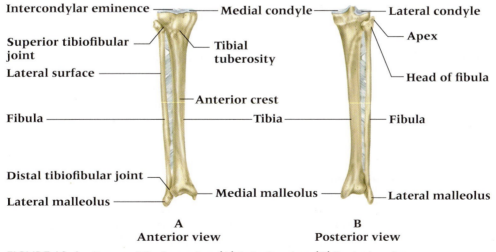

Intercondylar eminence — Medial condyle — Lateral condyle
Superior tibiofibular joint — Apex
Lateral surface — Tibial tuberosity — Head of fibula
— Anterior crest
Fibula — Tibia — Fibula
Distal tibiofibular joint
Lateral malleolus — Medial malleolus — Lateral malleolus

A
Anterior view

B
Posterior view

FIGURE 19–1 Bones of the lower leg. **(A)** Anterior view. **(B)** Posterior view.

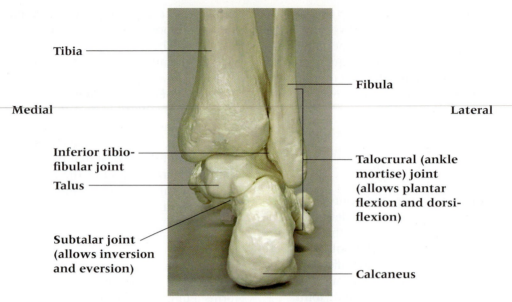

FIGURE 19–2 The ankle joint is formed by the tibia, fibula, and talus. The subtalar joint is formed by the talus and calcaneus.

malleolus and the distal end of the tibia. The joint is reinforced by the ankle ligaments (Figure 19–2).

Talocrural Joint The ankle joint, or talocrural joint, is a hinge joint (ginglymus) that is formed by the articular facet on the distal portion of the tibia, which articulates with the superior articular surface (trochlea) of the talus; the medial malleolus, which articulates with the medial surface of the trochlea of the talus; and the lateral malleolus, which articulates with the lateral surface of the trochlea (Figure 19–2). This bony arrangement is typically referred to as the

| **ankle mortise** |
| Talocrural joint formed by the tibia, fibula, and talus. |

ankle mortise. The ankle movements that occur at the talocrural joint are plantar flexion and dorsiflexion.

Subtalar Joint The anatomy and function of the subtalar joint were discussed in Chapter 18. The subtalar joint consists of the articulation between the talus and the calcaneus. The ankle movements that occur at the subtalar joint are inversion, eversion, pronation, and supination (Figure 19–2).

Stabilizing Ligaments

Tibiofibular Ligaments Joining the tibia and fibula is a strong interosseous membrane. The fibers display an oblique downward and outward pattern. The oblique arrangement aids in diffusing the forces placed on the leg. The membrane completely fills the tibiofibular space except for a small area at the superior aspect that is provided for the passage of the anterior tibial vessels. The anterior and posterior tibiofibular ligaments, which hold the tibia and fibula together and form the distal portion of the

interosseous membrane, are sometimes referred to as the syndesmotic ligaments.

Ankle Ligaments In addition to the tibiofibular ligaments, the ligamentous support of the ankle consists of three lateral ligaments and the medial, or deltoid, ligament (Figures 19–3 and 19–4).

Lateral Ligaments The three lateral ligaments are the anterior talofibular, the posterior talofibular, and the calcaneofibular (Table 19–1).

Medial Ligaments The deltoid ligament is triangular. It attaches superiorly to the borders of the medial malleolus; it attaches inferiorly to the medial surface of the talus, to the sustentaculum tali of the calcaneus, and to the posterior margin of the navicular bone. The deltoid ligament is the primary resistance to foot eversion. It, along with the plantar calcaneonavicular (spring) ligament, also helps maintain the inner longitudinal arch. Although it should be considered one ligament, the deltoid ligament includes both superficial and deep fibers (Figure 19–4). Anteriorly are the anterior tibiotalar part and the tibionavicular part. Medially is the tibiocalcaneal part, and posteriorly is the posterior tibiotalar part.

Joint Capsule

A thin articular capsule encases the ankle joint and attaches to the borders of the bone involved. It is somewhat different from most other capsules in that it is thick on the medial aspects of the joint but becomes a thin, gauzelike membrane at the back.

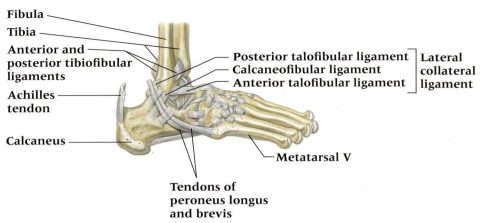

FIGURE 19–3   Lateral ligaments of the ankle.

Labels: Fibula, Tibia, Anterior and posterior tibiofibular ligaments, Achilles tendon, Calcaneus, Posterior talofibular ligament, Calcaneofibular ligament, Anterior talofibular ligament, Lateral collateral ligament, Metatarsal V, Tendons of peroneus longus and brevis

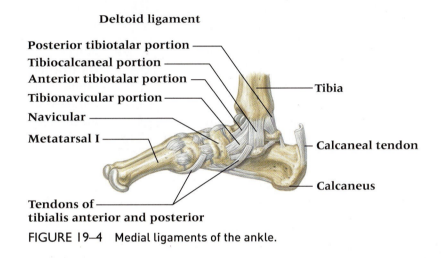

Deltoid ligament

FIGURE 19–4   Medial ligaments of the ankle.

Labels: Posterior tibiotalar portion, Tibiocalcaneal portion, Anterior tibiotalar portion, Tibionavicular portion, Navicular, Metatarsal I, Tendons of tibialis anterior and posterior, Tibia, Calcaneal tendon, Calcaneus

TABLE 19–1	Function of Key Ankle Ligaments
Ligament	**Primary Function**
Anterior talofibular	Restrains anterior displacement of talus
Calcaneofibular	Restrains inversion of calcaneus
Posterior talofibular	Restrains posterior displacement of talus
Deltoid	Prevents abduction and eversion of ankle and subtalar joint
	Prevents eversion, pronation, and anterior displacement of talus

Ankle Musculature

The movements of the talocrural joint are dorsiflexion (flexion) and plantar flexion (extension). Inversion and eversion occur at the subtalar joint. Tendons of muscles passing posterior to the malleoli produce ankle plantar flexion along with toe flexion in the foot. Muscles and their tendons passing anteriorly to the talocrural joint dorsiflex the foot and produce toe extension. The muscles that cross the ankle joint laterally cause eversion, whereas the muscles that cross the ankle joint medially cause inversion (Figure 19–5).

Muscle Compartments The musculature of the lower leg is contained within four distinct compartments, which are bounded by heavy fascia (Figure 19–6). Traumatic or overuse injury to any of these compartments can lead to swelling and neurological motor and sensory deficits.

The *anterior compartment* contains those muscles that dorsiflex the ankle and extend the toes—the tibialis anterior, extensor hallucis longus, and extensor digitorum longus muscles—and contains the anterior tibial nerve and the tibial artery.

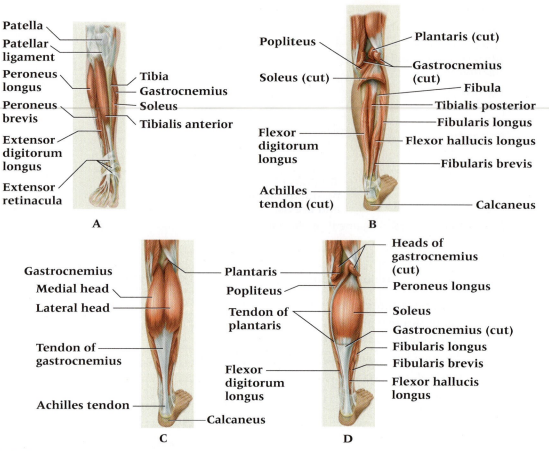

FIGURE 19–5   Muscles of the ankle and lower leg. **(A)** Anterior. **(B)** Lateral. **(C)** Superficial posterior. **(D)** Deep posterior.

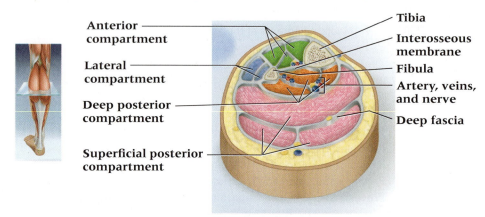

FIGURE 19–6   The four compartments of the lower leg.

The *lateral compartment* contains the fibularis longus and brevis, which evert the ankle; the peroneus tertius muscle, which assists in dorsiflexion; and the superficial branch of the peroneal nerve.

The *superficial posterior compartment* contains the gastrocnemius muscle and the soleus muscle. These muscles plantar flex the ankle.

The *deep posterior compartment* contains the tibialis posterior, flexor digitorum longus, and flexor hallucis longus muscles, which invert the ankle, and the posterior tibial artery.

Table 19–2 summarizes the muscles in the ankle and lower leg and their actions.

Nerve Supply

The lower leg is supplied by the common peroneal nerve anteriorly. The common peroneal branches into the superficial peroneal nerve and the deep peroneal nerve. The tibial nerve runs posteriorly and supplies the ankle and the foot (Figure 19–7).

Blood Supply

The ankle and lower leg are supplied by the anterior tibial artery and posterior tibial arteries. Blood drains via the peroneal vein, posterior tibial vein, and anterior tibial vein (Figure 19–8).

TABLE 19–2   Muscles of the Ankle and Lower Leg

Muscle	Origin	Insertion	Muscle Action	Nerve/Nerve Root
Anterior compartment				
Tibialis anterior	Lateral condyle and proximal two-thirds of the shaft of the tibia and the interosseous membrane	Medial surface of the first cuneiform and first metatarsal	Dorsiflexes and inverts the foot	Deep peroneal (L5, S1)
Extensor hallucis longus	Anterior surface of the middle of the fibula and the interosseous membrane	Dorsal surface of the distal phalanx of the great toe	Dorsiflexes and inverts the foot; extends the great toe	Deep peroneal (L5, S1)
Extensor digitorum longus	Lateral condyle of the tibia, proximal three-fourths of the anterior surface of the fibula, and the interosseous membrane	Dorsal surface of the phalanges of the second through fifth toes	Dorsiflexes and everts the foot; extends the toes	Deep peroneal (L5, S1)
Fibularis tertius	Distal third of the anterior surface of the fibula and the interosseous membrane	Dorsal surface of the fifth metatarsal	Dorsiflexes and everts the foot	Deep peroneal (L5, S1)
Lateral compartment				
Fibularis longus	Proximal two-thirds of the lateral surface of the fibula	Ventral surface of the first metatarsal and the medial cuneiform	Plantar flexes and everts the foot	Superficial peroneal (L4, L5, S1)
Fibularis brevis	Distal two-thirds of the fibula	Lateral side of the fifth metatarsal	Plantar flexes and everts the foot	Superficial peroneal (L4, L5, S1)
Superficial posterior compartment				
Gastrocnemius	Medial and lateral condyles of the femur	Calcaneus, via the Achilles tendon	Flexes the leg; plantar flexes the foot	Tibial (L5, S1)
Soleus	Posterior surface of the proximal third of the fibula and the middle third of the tibia	Calcaneus, via the Achilles tendon	Plantar flexes the foot	Tibial (L5, S1)
Plantaris	Posterior surface of the femur above the lateral condyle	Calcaneus, via the Achilles tendon	Flexes the leg; plantar flexes the foot	Tibial (L5, S1)
Deep posterior compartment				
Popliteus	Lateral condyle of the femur	Proximal portion of the tibia	Flexes and rotates the leg medially	Tibial (L5, S1)
Flexor hallucis longus	Lower two-thirds of the fibula	Distal phalanx of the great toe	Plantar flexes and inverts the foot; flexes the great toe	Tibial (L5, S1)
Flexor digitorum longus	Posterior surface of the tibia	Distal phalanx of the second through fifth toes	Plantar flexes and inverts the foot; flexes the toes	Tibial (L5, S1)
Tibialis posterior	Posterior surface of the interosseous membrane, the tibia, and the fibula	Navicular, cuneiforms, cuboid; second through fourth metatarsals	Plantar flexes and inverts the foot	Tibial (L5, S1)

Movements of the ankle joint.

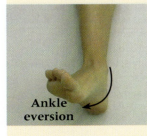
Ankle eversion

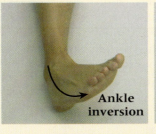
Ankle inversion

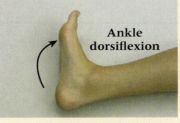
Ankle dorsiflexion

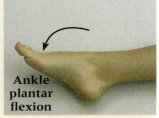
Ankle plantar flexion

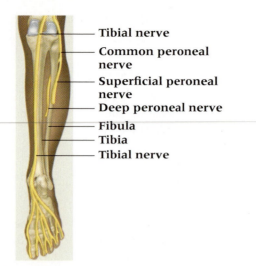

Tibial nerve
Common peroneal nerve
Superficial peroneal nerve
Deep peroneal nerve
Fibula
Tibia
Tibial nerve

FIGURE 19–7   Nerve supply of the lower leg (posterior view).

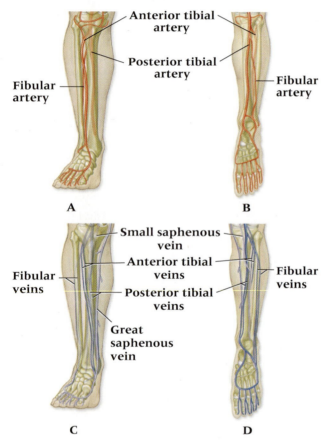

Anterior tibial artery
Posterior tibial artery
Fibular artery
Fibular artery

A   **B**

Small saphenous vein
Anterior tibial veins
Fibular veins
Posterior tibial veins
Fibular veins
Great saphenous vein

C   **D**

FIGURE 19–8   Blood supply of the lower limb.
(A) Arteries (anterior view). **(B)** Arteries (posterior view).
(C) Veins (anterior view). **(D)** Veins (posterior view).

FUNCTIONAL ANATOMY

The biomechanical motions occurring at the ankle and rear foot are complex. Anatomically, the ankle is a stable hinge joint in which the dome of the talus articulates with the distal ends of the tibia and fibula. Medial or lateral displacement of the talus is prevented by the malleoli. The arrangement of the ankle ligaments permits flexion and extension at the talocrural joint and limits inversion and eversion at the subtalar joint (see Chapter 18).[26]

> **Because the talus is wider anteriorly than posteriorly, the most stable position of the ankle is with the foot in dorsiflexion.**

The square shape of the talus contributes to ankle stability. Because the talus is wider anteriorly than posteriorly, the most stable position of the ankle is with the foot in dorsiflexion. In this position, the wider anterior aspect of the talus comes in contact with the narrower portion lying between the malleoli, gripping it tightly. By contrast, as the ankle moves into plantar flexion, the wider portion of the tibia is brought in contact with the narrower posterior aspect of the talus, which makes plantar flexion a much less stable position than dorsiflexion.

The degree of motion for the ankle joint ranges from 10 degrees of dorsiflexion to 50 degrees of plantar flexion. Normal gait mechanics require at least 20 degrees of plantar flexion and 10 degrees of dorsiflexion with the knee extended.[38]

Normal ankle function depends on the joints of the rearfoot, the most important of which is the subtalar joint. The movements of the talus during pronation and supination have profound effects on the lower extremity, both proximally and distally, as discussed in Chapter 18. The ankle joint is a critical link in the kinetic chain. Dysfunction in the ankle can lead to associated dysfunction in the knee and hip joints.

Surface Anatomy

Figure 19–9A and Figure 19–9B show the surface anatomy with pertinent landmarks for the ankle. Figure 19–10 shows the surface anatomy for the lower leg.

PREVENTING INJURY TO THE ANKLE AND LOWER LEG

Many ankle and lower leg conditions, especially sprains, can be reduced if an individual engages in the following: Achilles tendon stretching, strength training, neuromuscular control training, proper footwear, and preventive ankle taping and orthoses.[78]

Achilles Tendon Stretching

It is critical for normal gait that the ankle dorsiflex at least 10 degrees or more. A tight Achilles tendon may limit dorsiflexion and may predispose the individual to ankle injury. Anyone who engages in physical

> **Preventing ankle sprains:**
> • Achilles tendon stretching
> • Strength training
> • Neuromuscular control training
> • Footwear
> • Taping and orthoses

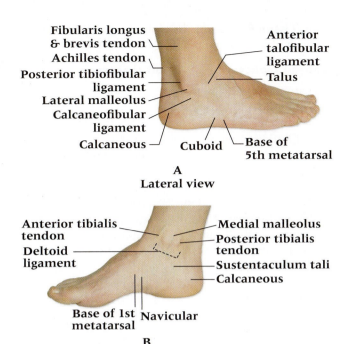

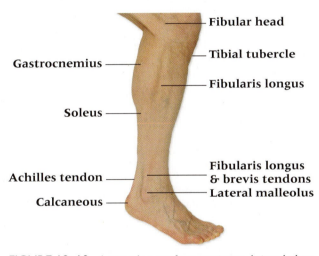

FIGURE 19–9   The foot **(A)** Lateral view. **(B)** Medial view.

FIGURE 19–10   Lower leg surface anatomy, lateral view.

activity, especially with tight Achilles tendons, should routinely stretch before and after activity.[54] To adequately stretch the Achilles tendon complex, stretching should be performed both with the knee extended and then with it flexed 15 to 30 degrees.

Strength Training

To prevent ankle injury, it is important to achieve both static and dynamic joint stability. A normal range of motion must be maintained, and the muscles and tendons that surround the talocrural joint must be kept strong.

Neuromuscular Control Training

Individuals with chronic ankle instability must develop neuromuscular control at the ankle joint.[41] Neuromuscular control involves adapting to uneven surfaces by controlling motion at the ankle joint. Ankle neuromuscular control can be enhanced by training in controlled activities on uneven surfaces or by spending time each day on a BAPS (Biomechanical Ankle Platform System) board, Bosu Balance Trainer, rocker board, or Dynadisc.

Footwear

As discussed in Chapter 7, proper footwear can be an important factor in reducing injuries to both the foot and the ankle. Shoes should not be used in activities for which they were not intended— for example, running shoes designed for straight-ahead activity should not be used to play tennis, a sport that demands a great deal of lateral movement. Cleats on a shoe should not be centered in the middle of the sole, but should be placed far enough on the border to avoid ankle sprains. High-top shoes, when worn by athletes with a history of ankle sprain, can offer greater support than low-top shoes do.[66]

Preventive Ankle Taping and Orthoses

Chapter 8 discusses the controversy surrounding the benefits of routinely taping ankles that have no history of sprain. There is some indication that tape, properly applied, can provide some prophylactic protection.[25,67] However, tape that constricts soft tissue or disrupts normal biomechanical function can create unnecessary injuries. Lace-up supports and semirigid ankle braces are increasingly being used in place of tape.[8] The sport-stirrup orthosis has been found to be superior to taping in preventing recurrent ankle sprains (see Figure 7–27). It must be emphasized that wearing a semirigid ankle brace not only alters the biomechanics at the ankle joint but also at the knee joint.[74]

ASSESSING THE ANKLE AND LOWER LEG

History

The patient's history may vary depending on whether the problem is the result of sudden trauma or is chronic. The athletic trainer should ask the patient with an acute injury to the ankle or lower leg the following questions:[7,48]

- Have you ever hurt your ankle before?
- How did you hurt your ankle?
- What did you hear when the injury occurred—a crack, snap, or pop?
- How bad was the pain, and how long did it last?
- Is there any sense of muscle weakness or difficulty in walking?

- How disabling was the injury? Could you walk right away, or were you not able to bear weight for a period of time?
- Has a similar injury occurred before?
- Was there immediate swelling, or did the swelling occur later (or at all)?
- Where did the swelling occur?

The patient with a chronic painful condition might be asked the following:

- How much does it hurt?
- Where does it hurt?
- Under what circumstances does pain occur—when bearing weight, after activity, or when arising after a night's sleep?
- What past ankle injuries have occurred?
- What first aid and therapy, if any, were given for these previous injuries?

Observation

In looking initially at the ankle, the athletic trainer should determine the following:[7,48]

- Are there any postural deviations? (Toeing in may indicate tibial torsion or genu valgum or varum; foot pronation should also be noted.)
- Is there any difficulty in walking?
- Is there an obvious deformity or swelling?
- Are the bony contours of the ankle normal and symmetrical, or is there a deviation, such as a bony deformity?
- Are the color and texture of the skin normal?
- Is there crepitus or abnormal sound in the ankle joint?
- Is heat, swelling, or redness present?
- Is the patient in obvious pain?
- Does the patient have a normal ankle range of motion?
- If the patient is able to walk, is there a normal walking pattern?

Palpation

The area of injury should be palpated to determine obvious structural deformities, areas of swelling, and points of tenderness.

Bony Palpation The following bony landmarks should be palpated:

Anterior aspect
- Fibular head
- Fibular shaft
- Lateral malleolus
- Tibial plateau
- Tibial shaft
- Medial malleolus
- Dome of the talus
- Posterior aspect

Posterior aspect
- Medial malleolus
- Lateral malleolus
- Dome of the talus
- Calcaneus
- Sustentaculum tali

Soft-Tissue Palpation The following soft-tissue structures should be palpated:

Lateral aspect
- Lateral compartment
  —Fibularis longus muscle
  —Fibularis brevis muscle
  —Fibularis tertius muscle
- Fibularis longus tendon
- Fibularis brevis tendon
- Anterior talofibular ligament
- Calcaneofibular ligament
- Posterior talofibular ligament

Medial aspect
- Deep posterior muscles
  —Posterior tibialis muscle
  —Flexor digitorum longus muscle
  —Flexor hallucis muscle
- Flexor digitorum longus tendon
- Posterior tibialis tendon
- Flexor hallucis tendon
- Deltoid ligament

Anterior aspect
- Anterior compartment
  —Anterior tibialis muscle
  —Extensor hallucis longus muscle
  —Extensor digitorum longus muscle
- Anterior tibialis tendon
- Extensor hallucis longus tendon
- Extensor digitorum longus tendon
- Fibularis tertius tendon
- Anterior tibiofibular ligament

Posterior aspect
- Superficial posterior compartment
  —Gastrocnemius muscle
  —Soleus muscle
- Achilles tendon
- Posterior tibiofibular ligament

Special Tests

Lower Leg

Lower Leg Alignment Tests Determining malalignment of the lower leg can reveal the causes of abnormal stresses applied to the foot, ankle, and lower leg as well as the knees and hip. In normal alignment of the lower extremity, anteriorly, a straight line can be drawn from the anterior superior iliac spine of the pelvis, through the patella, and to the web between the first and second toes. Laterally, a straight line can be drawn from the greater trochanter of the femur, through the center of the patella, and to just behind the lateral malleolus. Posteriorly, a straight line can be drawn from the center of the lower leg to the midline of the Achilles tendon and calcaneus.[7] A common malalignment of the lower leg is internal or external tibial torsion (Figure 19–11). In external tibial torsion, the tibial tubercle is laterally positioned; in internal tibial torsion, the tibial tubercle is medially positioned.

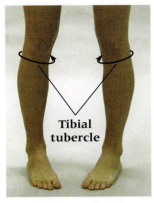
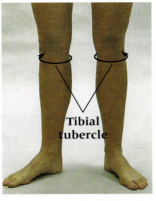

A   **B**

FIGURE 19–11   Malalignment of the lower leg. **(A)** Internal tibial torsion. **(B)** External tibial torsion.

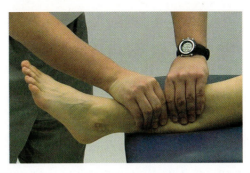

FIGURE 19–13   Compression test to check for fractures of the tibia or fibula.

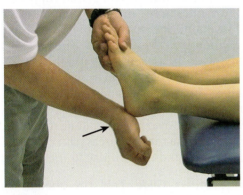

FIGURE 19–12   Percussion test to check for fractures of the ankle or lower leg.

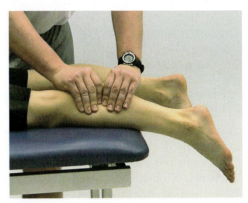

FIGURE 19–14   Thompson test to determine an Achilles tendon rupture by squeezing the calf muscle. A positive result to the test is one in which there is no plantar flexion of the foot.

Percussion and Compression Tests When fracture is suspected, a gentle percussive blow can be given to the tibia or fibula below or above the suspected site. Percussion can also be applied upward on the bottom of the heel. Such blows set up a vibratory force that resonates at the fracture, causing pain (Figure 19–12). The use of a tuning fork has also been recommended as an alternative method of providing vibration at the site of a suspected fracture.

In a compression test, the tibia and fibula are compressed either above or below the fracture site (Figure 19–13). Increased pain over the area of point tenderness may indicate a fracture, and referral should be made for X-rays.

Thompson Test The Thompson test is used to determine whether there is a rupture of the Achilles tendon. The Thompson test (Figure 19–14) is performed by squeezing the calf muscle while the leg is extended and the foot is hanging over the edge of the table. A positive Thompson sign is one in which squeezing the calf muscle does not cause the heel to move or pull upward or causes the heel to move less when compared with the uninjured leg.

Homan's Sign The test for Homan's sign gives some indication of the presence of a deep vein

thrombophlebitis. With the patient in a supine position with the knee fully extended, the ankle is passively dorsiflexed so that the calf muscles are stretched. Pain in the calf is a positive sign (Figure 19–15). The patient should be referred immediately to a physician for further diagnosis.

Ankle Stability Tests

Anterior Drawer Test The anterior drawer test is used to determine the extent of injury to the anterior talofibular ligament primarily and to the other lateral ligaments secondarily (Figure 19–16). The

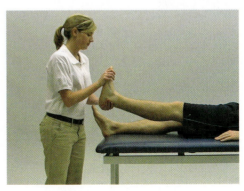

FIGURE 19–15   Homan's sign may indicate a deep vein thrombophlebitis.

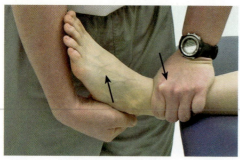

FIGURE 19–16   Anterior drawer test for ankle ligament instability.

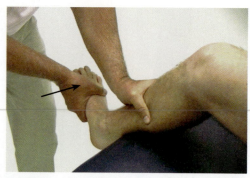

FIGURE 19–18   Kleiger's Test for injury to the deltoid ligament.

> A positive anterior drawer sign of ankle stability is when the foot slides forward, sometimes making a clunking sound as it reaches its end point.

patient sits on the edge of a treatment table with the ankle at a 90-degree angle. The athletic trainer grasps the lower tibia in one hand and the calcaneus in the palm of the other hand. The tibia is then pushed backward as the calcaneus is pulled forward. A positive anterior drawer sign occurs when the foot slides forward, sometimes making a clunking sound as it reaches its end point, and generally indicates a tear in the anterior talofibular ligament. An ankle arthrometer has been used to determine subtalar joint ligament complex laxity.[34,45]

Talar Tilt Test   Talar tilt tests are used to determine the extent of inversion or eversion injuries. With the foot positioned at 90 degrees to the lower leg and stabilized, the calcaneus is inverted. Excessive motion of the talus indicates injury to the calcaneofibular and possibly the anterior and posterior talofibular ligaments (Figure 19–17).

> A positive talar tilt occurs when the calcaneofibular ligament is sprained.

The deltoid ligament can be tested in the same manner except that the calcaneus is everted.

Kleiger's Test   Kleiger's test is used primarily to determine injury to the deltoid ligament. It can also indicate injury to the structures that support the distal ankle syndesmosis, including the anterior tibiofibular ligament, the posterior tibiofibular ligament, and the interosseous membrane. The patient should be seated with the knee flexed and the legs over the end of the table. The athletic trainer uses one hand to stabilize the lower leg and the other to hold the medial aspect of the foot and rotate it laterally (Figure 19–18). Pain over the deltoid ligament indicates injury to that structure, whereas pain over the lateral malleolus likely indicates injury to the syndesmosis.

Medial Subtalar Glide Test   The medial subtalar glide test is done to determine the presence of excessive medial translation of the calcaneus on the talus in the transverse plane.[28] The athletic trainer uses one hand to hold the talus in subtalar neutral, then glides the calcaneus in a medial direction on the fixed talus (Figure 19–19). In a positive test, there is excessive movement, indicating injury to the lateral ligaments.

Functional Tests   Muscle function is important in evaluating the ankle injury (Figure 19–20). Athletic trainers routinely have individuals with traumatic ankle sprains perform these tests. However, these

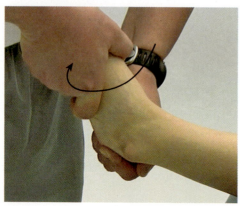

FIGURE 19–17   Talar tilt testing for lateral ankle instability.

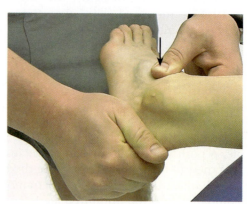

FIGURE 19–19   The medial subtalar glide test looks for excessive medial translation of the calcaneus relative to the talus, indicating injury to the lateral ligaments.

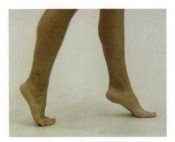
Toe walking   **Heel walking**   **Lateral walking**   **Medial walking**

FIGURE 19–20   Evaluating ankle function during walking.

tests should not be done if the patient is unable to bear weight. The following functional tests can be used:

- Walk on toes (tests plantar flexion)
- Walk on heels (tests dorsiflexion)
- Walk on lateral border of feet (tests inversion)
- Walk on medial border of feet (tests eversion)
- Hop on injured ankle

Passive, active, and resistive movements should be manually applied to determine joint integrity and muscle function.

RECOGNITION OF SPECIFIC INJURIES

Ankle Injuries

Ankle sprains are perhaps the single most common injury in a physically active population.[32] Appreciation of the anatomy and mechanics of the ankle joint and the pathomechanics and pathophysiology related to acute and chronic ankle instability is integral to the process of effectively evaluating and treating ankle injuries.[26] It is estimated that about one-third of all first-time acute ankle sprains develop into chronic ankle instability that results in recurring injury to that ankle.[32] Ankle sprains are generally caused by sudden inversion or eversion, often in combination with plantar flexion or dorsiflexion (Table 19–3). Injuries may be classified according to either location or mechanism of injury.

Inversion Ankle Sprains   Inversion ankle sprains are the most common and result in injury to the lateral ligaments. The anterior talofibular ligament is the weakest of the three lateral ligaments. Its major function is to stop forward subluxation of the talus. It is injured in an inverted, plantar flexed, and internally rotated position (Figure 19–21). A complete rupture of the talofibular ligament allows the talus to rotate about it's longitudinal axis in the transverse plane, creating what has been referred to as *rotary ankle instability*.[79] The calcaneofibular and posterior talofibular ligaments may also be injured in inversion sprains as the force of inversion is increased. Increased inversion force is needed to tear the calcaneofibular ligament (Figure 19–22).

TABLE 19–3	Mechanisms of Ankle Sprain and Ligament Injury
Mechanisms	**Area Injured**
Plantar flexion or inversion	Anterior talofibular ligament
	Calcaneofibular ligament
	Posterior talofibular ligament
	Tibiofibular ligament (severe injury)
Inversion	Calcaneofibular ligament (along with anterior or posterior talofibular ligament)
Dorsiflexion	Tibiofibular ligament
Eversion	Deltoid ligament
	Tibiofibular ligament (severe injury)
	Interosseous membrane (as external rotation increases)
	Possible fibular fracture (proximal or distal)

Occasionally, an inversion force could be of sufficient magnitude to cause a portion of the bone to be avulsed from the lateral malleolus (Figure 19–23).[62] Also, inversion can cause both an avulsion of the lateral malleolus and a fracture of the medial malleolus. This injury is known as a *bimalleolar fracture* (Pott's fracture).[62] The athletic trainer is often faced with the dilemma of deciding when a patient should be sent to the physician for X-ray to rule out a fracture. The *Ottawa ankle rules* can be used to decide whether a patient with foot or ankle pain should have a radiograph to diagnose a bone fracture in the malleoli and the midfoot.[37,59] They are most often used in an emergency room, but the guidelines can be applied by all clinicians.[47] Radiographs are only required if there is any pain in the malleolar or midfoot area and any one of the following (note that these rules do *not* apply to injuries more than 10 days old):

- Inability to bear weight for four steps (two on each foot) at the time of injury and at the time of examination
- Tenderness over the inferior or posterior pole of either malleolus, including the distal 6 cm (2.4 inches)

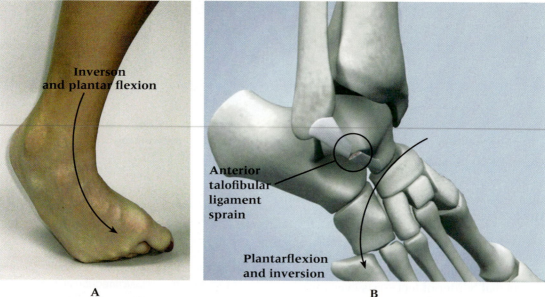

A
Anterolateral view

B
Anterolateral view

FIGURE 19–21   A mechanism of injury that involves **(A)** plantar flexion and inversion can cause **(B)** a sprain of the anterior talofibular ligament.

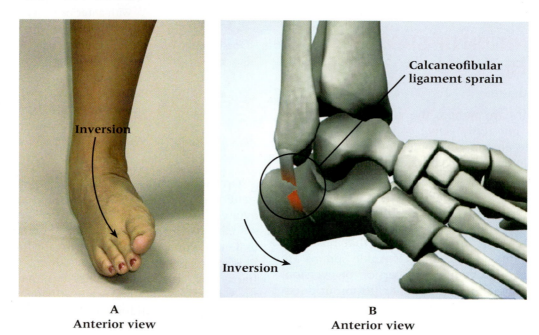

A
Anterior view

B
Anterior view

FIGURE 19–22   A mechanism of injury that involves **(A)** inversion can cause **(B)** a sprain of the calcaneofibular ligament.

- Inability to bear weight (four steps taken independently, even if limping) at the time of injury and at the time of evaluation
- Tenderness along the base of the fifth metatarsal or navicular bone

The Buffalo modification focuses on tenderness along the midline crest instead of fibular tenderness at the posterior and inferior malleolar edges.[59]

Gender does not appear to be a risk factor for suffering an ankle sprain. Patients who have suffered a previous sprain have a decreased risk of reinjury if a brace is worn, and the consensus is that generalized joint laxity and anatomical foot type are not risk factors for ankle sprains. However, the literature is divided on whether height, weight, limb dominance, ankle-joint laxity, and anatomical alignment, muscle strength, muscle-reaction time, and balance problems are risk factors for ankle sprains.[5]

Grade I Ligament Sprain   The grade 1 ligament sprain is the most common type of sprain. Lateral sprains

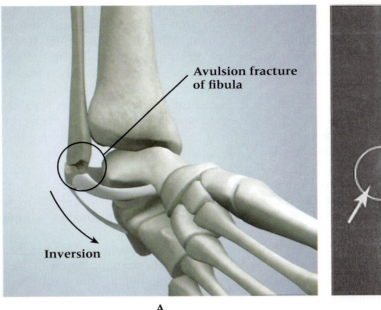
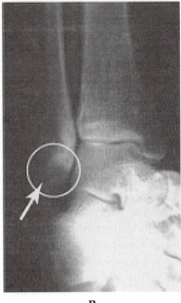

Avulsion fracture
of fibula

Inversion

A

B

FIGURE 19–23 (A) The mechanism that produces an inversion ankle sprain can also cause an avulsion fracture of the fibula. (B) X-ray showing fibular avulsion.

are probably the most frequent injury in activities in which running and jumping occur.[6]

Etiology The severity of ligament sprains is classified according to grades. In each instance, the foot is forcefully inverted, such as when a basketball player jumps and comes down on the foot of another player. Inversion sprains can also occur when an individual is walking or running on an uneven surface or suddenly steps into a hole.

Symptoms and signs Mild pain and disability occur. Weight bearing is minimally impaired. Signs are point tenderness and swelling over the ligament with no joint laxity (Figure 19–24).

Management Rest, ice, compression, and elevation (RICE) are used for 30 to 60 minutes every 2 hours for 1 to 2 days. The application of a horseshoe

pad provides focal compression and may help control edema (Figure 19–25).[36] It may be advisable for the patient to limit weight-bearing activities for 1 to 2 days, after which rehabilitation may become more aggressive. An elastic wrap might provide comfortable pressure when weight bearing begins. Early functional rehabilitation of the ankle should include range of motion exercises and isometric and isotonic strength-training exercises. In the intermediate stage of rehabilitation, a progression of proprioception-training exercises should be incorporated, followed by focusing on sport-specific activities to prepare the patient for return to competition. Anterior and posterior mobilization of the talus should begin as soon as tolerable following injury.[12] When the patient returns to weight bearing, application of tape may provide an extra measure of protection.[78] Usually, a patient can return to activity in 7 to 10 days.

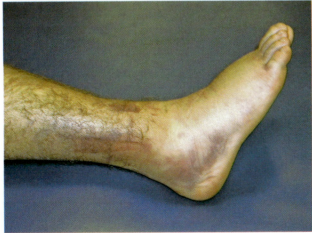

FIGURE 19–24 Typical swelling pattern for an inversion ankle sprain.

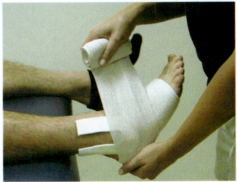

FIGURE 19–25 A horseshoe-shaped pad placed around the malleoleus provides excellent focal compression when held in place by an elastic wrap.

Grade 2 Ligament Sprain A grade 2 ligament sprain has a high incidence among active individuals and causes a great deal of disability with many days of lost time.[6]

Etiology Moderate force on the ankle while it is in a position of inversion, plantar flexion, and/or adduction can cause a grade 2 sprain.

Symptoms and signs The patient usually complains of feeling a pop or snap on the lateral side of the ankle. There is moderate pain and disability, weight bearing is difficult, and there is tenderness and edema with blood in the joint. Ecchymosis may occur, as well as a positive talar tilt test. There is also a positive anterior drawer sign between 0.16 and 0.55 inch (4 and 14 mm).[6] The anterior drawer test elicits slight to moderate abnormal motion. This injury can produce a persistently unstable ankle that is recurrently sprained and later develops traumatic arthritis.[61]

Management RICE should be used intermittently for at least 72 hours. X-ray examination should be routine for this grade of injury. Anterior and posterior mobilization of the talus should begin as soon as tolerable following injury.[12] The patient should use crutches for 5 to 10 days, gradually progressing to full weight bearing during that period. The patient will need to wear some type of protective immobilization device for 1 to 2 weeks.[6] Plantar flexion and dorsiflexion exercises in a pain-free range should begin 48 hours after the injury occurs. Early movement helps maintain range of motion and normal proprioception. Proprioceptive neuromuscular facilitation (PNF) exercise improves strength, range of motion, and proprioception. Exercise should include isometrics while the ankle is immobilized, followed by range of motion exercises, progressive resistance exercise (PRE), and balance activities lasting up to 4 weeks.[63] It has been

suggested that protection of healing structures may lead to a more optimal long-term outcome.[15]

Taping using a closed basket weave technique may protect the patient during the early stages of walking (see Figure 8–30). The patient must be instructed to avoid walking or running on uneven surfaces for 2 to 3 weeks after weight bearing has begun. NOTE: The long-term effects of a grade 2 sprain are likely to include chronic instability with a recurrence of injury.[27] Over a period of time, this instability can lead to joint degeneration and osteoarthritis. Once a grade 2 sprain has occurred, the patient must continue to engage in rehabilitative activities to minimize recurrence of injury.[46]

Grade 3 ligament sprain The grade 3 ligament sprain is relatively uncommon. When it does happen, it is extremely disabling. Often, the force causes the ankle to subluxate and then spontaneously reduce.

Etiology The grade 3 sprain is caused by a significant inversion force to the ankle, usually combined with plantar flexion, and adduction. This injury may involve tears to the anterior talofibular, calcaneofibular, or posterior talofibular ligaments as well as the joint capsule.

Symptoms and signs The patient complains of severe pain in the region of the lateral malleolus. Weight bearing is not possible because of the great amount of swelling, with or without pain. Hemarthrosis, discoloration, a positive talar tilt, and a positive anterior drawer test are present.[7] If the anterior talofibular ligament is completely disrupted, rotation of the talus about its long axis in the transverse plane results in what is referred to rotary ankle instability.

Management Normally, RICE is used intermittently for at least 3 days. It is not uncommon for the physician

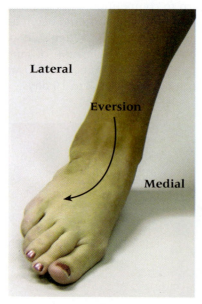

A
Anterior view

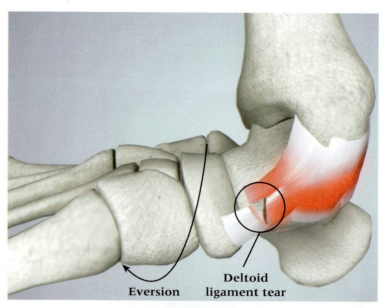

B
Medial view

FIGURE 19–26 A mechanism of injury that involves **(A)** eversion can cause **(B)** a sprain of the deltoid ligament.

to apply a dorsiflexion cast or weight-bearing brace for 3 to 6 weeks, followed by taping for 3 to 6 weeks.[38] Crutches are usually given to the athlete when the cast is removed. Isometric exercise is carried out while the cast is on, followed by range of motion exercises, PRE, and balance exercises. In some cases, surgery is warranted to stabilize the athlete's ankle. NOTE: A grade 3 ankle sprain creates significant joint laxity and instability. Because of this laxity, the ankle joint is prone to degenerative processes. However, chronic ankle instability does not necessarily have a negative effect on functional performance.[15,20]

Eversion Ankle Sprains

Etiology Eversion ankle sprains represent only about 5 percent to 10 percent of all ankle sprains. The eversion ankle sprain is less common than the inversion ankle sprain, largely because of the bony and ligamentous anatomy (Figure 19–26). As mentioned previously, the fibular malleolus extends farther inferiorly than does the tibial malleolus. This protection, combined with the strength of the thick deltoid ligament, prevents excessive eversion. More often, eversion injuries involve an avulsion fracture of the tibia before the deltoid ligament tears.[36] The deltoid ligament may also be contused in inversion sprains due to impingement between the fibular malleolus and the calcaneus. Despite the fact that eversion sprains are less common, they are more severe and may take longer to heal than inversion sprains.

A foot that excessively pronates, is hypermobile, or has a depressed medial longitudinal arch is more predisposed to eversion ankle injuries.[6]

Symptoms and signs Depending on the grade of injury, the patient complains of pain, sometimes severe, that occurs over the foot and lower leg. Usually, the patient is unable to bear weight on the foot. Both abduction and adduction cause pain, but pressing directly upward against the bottom of the foot does not produce pain.

Management X-rays are often necessary to rule out fracture. Initially, RICE and no weight bearing are recommended. NSAIDs and analgesics are given as needed. Management of eversion sprain follows the same course as for inversion sprains. The patient engages in a PRE program for the posteromedial ankle muscles, engages in balance activities, and is fitted with an inner heel wedge shoe insert. NOTE: An eversion sprain with a severity of grade 2 or more can produce significant joint instability. Because the deltoid ligament helps support the medial longitudinal arch, a sprain can cause weakness in this area, leading to excessive pronation or a fallen arch.

Syndesmotic Sprain (High Ankle Sprain)

Etiology Isolated injuries to the distal tibiofemoral joint are referred to as syndesmotic sprains,[50,64] or high ankle sprains.[72] The anterior and posterior tibiofibular ligaments are found between the distal tibia and fibula and extend up the lower leg as the interosseous ligament, or syndesmotic ligament. Sprains of the ligaments are more common than has been realized in the past.[22] These ligaments are torn with increased external rotational or forced dorsiflexion and are often injured in conjunction with a severe sprain of the medial and lateral ligament complexes (Figure 19–27).[58]

19–1 Clinical Application Exercise

A male soccer player cuts for the ball and injures his right ankle. He describes a hyperdorsiflexion mechanism of injury. X-rays were negative for this injury.

? What is this athlete's injury? What are special considerations with this injury?

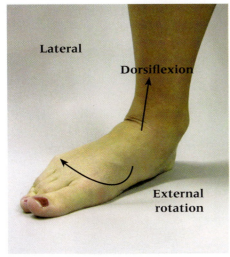

A
Anteromedial view

Lateral

Dorsiflexion

External rotation

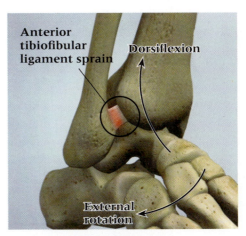

B
Anterolateral view

Anterior tibiofibular ligament sprain

Dorsiflexion

External rotation

FIGURE 19–27 A mechanism of injury that involves **(A)** hyperdorsiflexion and external rotation of the foot can cause **(B)** a sprain of the anterior tibiofibular ligament.

Initial rupture of the ligaments occurs distally at the tibiofibular ligament above the ankle mortise. As the force of disruption is increased, the interosseous ligament is torn more proximally.

Symptoms and signs The patient complains of severe pain and loss of function in the ankle region. When the ankle is passively externally rotated or dorsiflexed, there is a major pain in the lower leg, indicating a syndesmotic sprain or possibly a lateral malleolar fracture. Pain normally occurs along the anterolateral leg.[73]

Management Sprains of the syndesmotic ligaments are extremely hard to treat and often take months to heal.[50] Treatments for this problem are essentially the same as for medial or lateral sprains, with the difference being an extended period of immobilization. Functional activities may be delayed for a longer period of time than for inversion or eversion sprains.[81] It is common for this injury to require surgical intervention.

Chronic Ankle Instability Chronic ankle instability develops following about one-third of all acute ankle sprains.[3] A variety of mechanical and neuromuscular factors are thought to contribute to chronic ankle instability.[16,30] Usually, chronic ankle instability is further classified as being caused by either mechanical instability or functional instability. Mechanical instability is essentially laxity that physically allows for movement beyond the physiologic limit of the ankle's range of motion. Functional instability is a subjective feeling that the ankle is unstable as a result of recurrent ankle sprains. Functional instability has been attributed to proprioceptive and/or neuromuscular deficits that negatively impact postural control and thus stability and balance.[43]

Rehabilitation in cases of chronic ankle instability should focus on a combination of ankle strengthening and improving proprioception by challenging the neuromuscular system.[71]

Ankle Fracture/Dislocation

Etiology There are a number of mechanisms through which an ankle can be fractured or dislocated.[36,51] A foot that is forcibly abducted can produce a transverse fracture of the distal tibia and fibula. In contrast, a foot that is planted in combination with a forced internal rotation of the leg can produce a fracture to the distal and posterior tibia (Figure 19–28).

Avulsion fractures, in which a chip of bone is pulled off by the resistance of a ligament, are common in grades 2 and 3 eversion or inversion sprains.

In a *bimalleolar fracture*, both the medial malleolus of the distal tibia and the lateral malleolus of the distal fibula are fractured.

Symptoms and signs In most cases of fracture, swelling and pain are extreme. There may be some or no deformity; however, if a fracture is suspected, splinting is essential.

Management RICE is used as soon as possible to control hemorrhage and swelling. Once swelling is reduced, a walking cast or brace may be applied. Immobilization usually lasts for at least 7 to 9 weeks.[62]

Osteochondritis Dissecans

Etiology Although less common than in the knee, osteochondritis dissecans can occur in the superior medial articular surface of the talar dome. One or several fragments of articular cartilage and its underlying subchondral bone are either partially detached

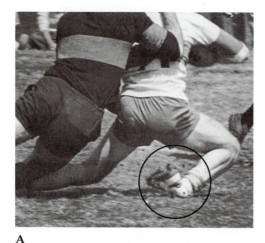

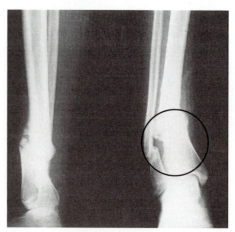

FIGURE 19–28 (A) Ankle fracture or dislocation mechanism. **(B)** X-ray of both the tibia and the fibula.

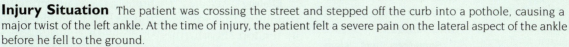

Grade 2 Inversion Ankle Sprain

Injury Situation The patient was crossing the street and stepped off the curb into a pothole, causing a major twist of the left ankle. At the time of injury, the patient felt a severe pain on the lateral aspect of the ankle before he fell to the ground.

Symptoms and Signs After the injury, the patient complained of moderate pain on the outside of his left ankle. Initially, it was painful to move the ankle. Walking on the left foot was very difficult. There was moderate tenderness over the lateral aspect of the ankle. Swelling rapidly occurred around the lateral malleoli. The ankle displayed a slight positive talar tilt and a positive anterior drawer test of 4 mm.

Phase 1 Acute Injury   **GOALS:** To control hemorrhage, swelling, pain, and spasm.
ESTIMATED LENGTH OF TIME (ELT): 2–3 days.

- **Therapy** Ice packs are applied (20 minutes) intermittently 6 to 8 times daily. X-ray examination rules out fracture. The patient should wear elastic wrap during waking hours and elevate the leg. The leg should also be elevated during sleep. Nonsteroidal antiinflammatory drugs and analgesics should be given. An air splint should be used during this period for support and compression. No weight bearing is allowed. Crutches are used to avoid weight bearing for at least 3 or 4 days or until the patient can walk without a limp with lateral support.
- **Exercise rehabilitation** The patient should begin exercise by toe gripping and spreading if there is no pain (10 to 15 times) every waking hour starting on the second day of injury. General body maintenance exercises should be conducted 3 times a week as long as they do not aggravate the injury.

Phase 2 Repair   **GOALS:** To decrease swelling, permit secondary healing to occur, restore full muscle contraction without pain, and restore 50 percent pain-free movement.
ELT: 3 weeks.

- **Therapy** All treatment should be followed immediately by exercise. Ice pack should be used (20 minutes), ice massage (7 minutes), cold whirlpool (60°F, 10 minutes), or massage above and below injury site (5 minutes). When hemorrhage is completely controlled, use whirlpool (90°F to 100°F, 10 to 15 minutes).
- **Exercise rehabilitation** The patient should crutch walk with a toe touch if he or she is unable to walk without a limp while wearing an air cast, tape, or both for 3 weeks. For the first 2 weeks, toe gripping and spreading (10 to 15 times) every waking hour. Active PNF ankle patterns 3 or 4 times daily for a pain-free range of motion. Avoid any exercise that produces pain or swelling. Ankle circumduction (10 to 15 times each direction) 2 or 3 times daily. Achilles tendon stretch from the floor (30 seconds) in each foot position (toe in, toe out, straight ahead) 3 or 4 times daily. Toe raises (10 times, 1 to 3 sets) 3 or 4 times daily. Eversion exercise using a towel or rubber tube or tire resistance 3 or 4 times daily. Shifting body weight between injured and noninjured ankle (up to 20 times 2 or 3 times daily). Wobble board exercise (1 to 3 minutes) 2 or 3 times daily. Progress to straight-ahead short-step walking if it can be done without a limp. General body maintenance exercises are conducted 3 times a week as long as they do not aggravate injury.

Phase 3 Remodeling   **GOALS:** To restore symptom-free full range of motion, power, endurance, speed, and agility.
ELT: 3–5 days.

- **Therapy** Therapeutic modalities such as whirlpool (100°F to 105°F) (20 minutes) or ultrasound (0.5 W/cm^2 at 100 percent) (5 minutes) should be used symptomatically.
- **Exercise rehabilitation** Achilles tendon stretch using slant board (30 seconds each foot position) 2 or 3 times daily. Toe raises using slant board and resistance (10 repetitions, 1 to 3 sets) 2 or 3 times daily. Resistance ankle device to strengthen anterior, lateral, and medial muscles (starting with 2 lb and progressing to 10 lb) (1 to 3 sets) 2 or 3 times daily. Wobble board for ankle proprioception (begin at 1 minute in each direction; progress to 5 minutes) 3 times daily. Walk-jog routine as long as patient is symptom free: begin with alternate walk-jog-run-walk 25 yards straight ahead, jog 25 yards straight ahead; progress to walk 25 yards in lazy S or to perform 5 figure eights, progress to figure-eight running as fast as possible; progress to run 10 figure eights or Z cuts as fast as possible and to spring up in the air on the injured leg 10 times without pain.

Criteria for Return to Normal Activity

1. The ankle is pain free during motion and no swelling is present.
2. The patient has full ankle range of motion and strength.
3. The patient is able to run, jump, and make cutting movements as well as before injury.

---

or completely detached and moving within the joint space. The mechanism of injury may be a single trauma, in which case it may be diagnosed as an osteochondral fracture, or it may be due to repeated episodes of ankle sprain.

Symptoms and signs Initially, the patient may complain of pain and effusion with signs of progressing atrophy. There may also be complaints of catching, locking, or giving way, particularly if the fragment is detached.

Management Diagnosis is usually made by X-ray, although an MRI may also show the articular cartilage overlying the osseous lesion. Incomplete and nondisplaced injuries can be immobilized with early motion and delayed weight bearing until there is evidence of healing. If the fragment is displaced, surgery is recommended to excise the fragment and minimize the risk of nonunion.

Lower Leg Injuries

Achilles Tendon Strain

Etiology Achilles tendon strains are common in sports and occur most often after ankle sprains or sudden excessive dorsiflexion of the ankle.

Symptoms and signs The resulting injury may be mild to severe. The most severe injury is a partial or complete avulsion or rupturing of the Achilles tendon. While sustaining this injury, the patient feels acute pain and extreme weakness on plantar flexion.

Management Initially, as with other acute conditions, pressure is first applied with an elastic wrap together with the application of cold. Unless the injury is minor, hemorrhage may be extensive, requiring RICE over an extended period of time. After hemorrhaging has subsided, an elastic wrap should be applied for continued pressure. Because of the tendency for acute Achilles tendon trauma to become a chronic condition, a conservative approach to therapy is required. The patient should begin stretching and strengthening the heel cord complex as soon as possible. A lift should be placed in the heel of each shoe to decrease stretching of the tendon and thus relieve some stress that contributes to chronic inflammation.

Achilles Tendinosis

Etiology Achilles *tendinitis* is an inflammatory condition that involves the Achilles tendon and/or its tendon sheath (the paratenon), in which case the condition is referred to as Achilles *tenosynovitis*. Achilles tenosynovitis causes fibrosis and scarring that can restrict the Achilles tendon's motion within the tendon sheath. Achilles tenosynovitis can occur along with, or lead to, Achilles *tendinosis*. The vast majority of people with Achilles tendon pain have Achilles tendinosis, rather than Achilles tendinitis or tenosynovitis.[2] With Achilles tendinosis, also known as Achilles tendinopathy, there is no evidence of inflammation, the injured areas of the Achilles tendon have lost their normal appearance, and the collagen fibers that make up the Achilles tendon show that the cells are disorganized, scarred, and degenerated.[2] Achilles tendinosis is a soreness and stiffness that comes on gradually and continues to worsen until treated. Often, the tendon is overloaded because of excessive tensile stress placed on it during movements of a repetitive nature, such as running or jumping. The condition worsens with repetitive weight-bearing activities, such as running or early-season conditioning in which the duration and intensity are increased too quickly with insufficient recovery time. Decreased gastrocnemius and soleus complex flexibility can also increase symptoms.

Symptoms and signs The patient often complains of generalized pain and stiffness about the Achilles tendon region that, when localized, is usually just proximal to the calcaneal insertion. Uphill running or hill workouts usually aggravate the condition. There may be reduced gastrocnemius and soleus muscle flexibility in general that may worsen as the condition progresses. Muscle testing may show a deficit when the patient performs toe raises. Initially, the patient may ignore symptoms that present at the beginning of activity and resolve as the activity progresses. Symptoms may progress to morning stiffness and discomfort with walking after periods of prolonged sitting. The tendon may be warm and painful to palpation as well as thickened, which may indicate the chronicity of the condition. Crepitus may be palpated with active plantar flexion and dorsiflexion, and pain is elicited with passive stretching. Chronic inflammation of the Achilles tendon may lead to thickening when compared with the uninvolved side (Figure 19–29).[31]

Management Achilles tendinosis may be resistant to a quick resolution because of the slower healing response of tendinous tissue. It is important to create a proper healing environment by reducing stress on the tendon. Proper shoeware and foot orthotics should be worn to address structural faults that may be causing the irritation, and flexibility exercises should be performed for the heel cord complex. Modalities such as ice can help reduce pain and inflammation early on, and ultrasound can facilitate an increased blood flow to the tendon in the later stages of rehabilitation. Cross-friction massage may be used to break down adhesions that may have formed during the healing response and to further improve the gliding ability of the paratenon. Strengthening of the gastrocnemius-soleus musculature must be progressed carefully so as not to cause a recurrence of the symptoms.[31]

Achilles Tendon Rupture A rupture of the Achilles tendon (Figure 19–30) is possible in activities that require stop-and-go action. Although most common in athletes who are 30 years of age or older, rupture of the Achilles tendon can occur in individuals of any age.[56] It usually occurs in an individual with a

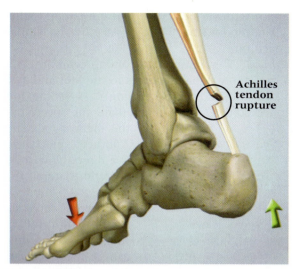

FIGURE 19–30 Achilles tendon rupture involves tearing and separation of fibers.

history of chronic inflammation and gradual degeneration caused by microtears.[2]

Etiology The initial insult normally is the result of a sudden pushing-off action of the forefoot, with the knee being forced into complete extension.[14]

> A ruptured Achilles tendon may occur because of chronic inflammation.

Symptoms and signs When the rupture occurs, the patient complains of a sudden snap that felt like something kicked him or her in the lower leg. Pain is immediate but rapidly subsides. Point tenderness, swelling, and discoloration are usually associated with the trauma. Toe raising is impossible in an Achilles tendon rupture. The major problem in Achilles tendon rupture is accurate diagnosis, especially in a partial rupture. Any acute injury to the Achilles tendon should be suspected to be a rupture. Signs indicative of a rupture are obvious indentation at the tendon site and a positive Thompson test (see Figure 19–12). An Achilles tendon rupture usually occurs 0.78 to 2.34 inches (2 to 6 cm) proximal to its insertion onto the calcaneus.

Management Usual management of a complete Achilles tendon rupture is surgical repair.[14] Nonoperative treatment consists of RICE, NSAIDs, and analgesics with a non–weight-bearing cast for 6 weeks, followed by a short-leg walking cast for 2 weeks. With this approach, there is 75 to 80 percent return of normal function.[56] Surgery is usually the choice for serious injuries, providing 75 to 90 percent return of function.[42] Exercise rehabilitation lasts for about 6 months and consists of range of motion exercises, PRE, and the wearing a heel lift in both shoes.[56]

Fibularis Tendon Subluxation/Dislocation The fibularis longus and brevis tendons pass through a

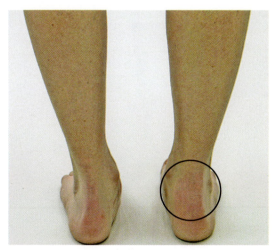

FIGURE 19–29 A thickened Achilles tendon caused by tendinosis.

common groove located behind the lateral malleolus. The tendons are held in place by the fibularis retinaculum.

Etiology   This injury most often occurs in activities that apply dynamic forces to the foot and ankle (e.g., turning and sharply cutting).[31] Wrestling, football, ice skating, skiing, basketball, and soccer have the highest incidence. Another mechanism is a direct blow to the posterior lateral malleolus. A moderate to severe inversion sprain or forceful dorsiflexion of the ankle can tear the fibularis retinaculum, allowing the fibularis tendon to dislocate out of its groove. Occasionally, the fibularis tendon ruptures instead of simply subluxing. As discussed previously, one of the major functions of the fibularis longus muscle is to pull the first metatarsal into plantar flexion.

Symptoms and signs   The patient complains that in running or jumping the tendons snap out of the groove and then back in when stress is released. Eversion against manual resistance will often replicate the subluxation. The patient experiences recurrent pain, snapping, and ankle instability. The lateral aspect of the ankle may show ecchymoses, edema, tenderness, and crepitus over the peroneal tendon.

Management   A conservative approach should be used first and should include compression with a felt pad cut in a horseshoe-shaped pattern that surrounds the lateral malleolus. This compression can be reinforced with a rigid plastic or plaster splint until acute signs have subsided, and RICE, NSAIDs, and analgesics are given as needed. The time period for this conservative care is 5 to 6 weeks, followed by a gradual exercise rehabilitation program that includes range of motion exercises, PRE, and balance training. If a conservative approach fails, surgery is required.[31]

Anterior Tibialis Tendinitis

Etiology   Anterior tibialis tendinitis is a common condition in individuals who run downhill for an extended period of time.

Symptoms and signs   There is point tenderness over the anterior tibialis tendon (Figure 19–31). The patient complains of pain when the tendon is stretched or when the muscle is contracted.

Management   The patient should be advised to rest (or at least decrease running time and distance) and to avoid hills. In more serious cases, ice packs, coupled with stretching before and after running, should help reduce the symptoms. A daily strengthening program also should be conducted. Oral anti-inflammatory medications may be required.

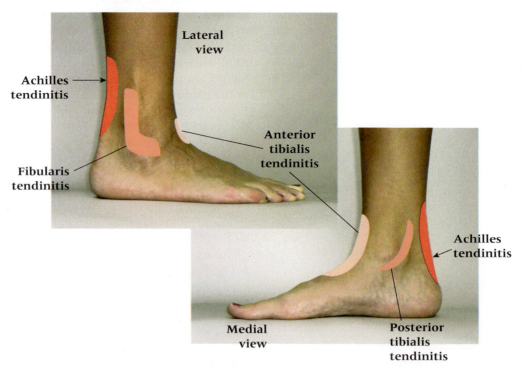

FIGURE 19–31   Common sites of tendinitis around the ankle.